CANCER EPIDEMIOLOGY

CANCER EPIDEMIOLOGY

Low- and Middle-Income Countries
and Special Populations

Edited by
Amr S. Soliman
David Schottenfeld
Paolo Boffetta

OXFORD
UNIVERSITY PRESS

OXFORD
UNIVERSITY PRESS

Oxford University Press is a department of the University of Oxford.
It furthers the University's objective of excellence in research, scholarship,
and education by publishing worldwide.

Oxford   New York
Auckland   Cape Town   Dar es Salaam   Hong Kong   Karachi
Kuala Lumpur   Madrid   Melbourne   Mexico City   Nairobi
New Delhi   Shanghai   Taipei   Toronto

With offices in
Argentina   Austria   Brazil   Chile   Czech Republic   France   Greece
Guatemala   Hungary   Italy   Japan   Poland   Portugal   Singapore
South Korea   Switzerland   Thailand   Turkey   Ukraine   Vietnam

Oxford is a registered trademark of Oxford University Press in the UK and certain other
countries.

Published in the United States of America by
Oxford University Press
198 Madison Avenue, New York, NY 10016

Library of Congress Cataloging-in-Publication Data
Cancer epidemiology : low- and middle-income countries and special populations /
edited by Amr Soliman, David Schottenfeld, Paolo Boffetta.
    p. ; cm.
Includes bibliographical references and index.
ISBN 978-0-19-973350-7 (pbk. : alk. paper)—ISBN 978-0-19-975034-4 (ebook)
I. Soliman, Amr. II. Schottenfeld, David. III. Boffetta, Paolo.
[DNLM: 1. Neoplasms—ethnology. 2. Developing Countries. 3. Socioeconomic Factors. QZ 220.1]
LC Classification not assigned
616.99′4071—dc23
2012050984

Our book is dedicated to promoting and enhancing the aspirations of health professionals who wish to pursue careers in international research in cancer epidemiology.

CONTENTS

■ SECTION 5: FUTURE DIRECTIONS AND RECOMMENDATIONS

PREFACE

Cancer Epidemiology: Low- and Middle-Income Countries and Special Populations is not intended to be a reference text in cancer epidemiology. Rather, it provides a perspective on the rationale, requisite infrastructure, and methodologic principles, and offers illustrative examples of collaborative field and laboratory-based studies that are being conducted in diverse ethnic populations, particularly those residing in low- and middle-income countries (LMICs). It should be noted that the World Health Organization predicts that there will be 16 million new cancer cases per year in 2020, and that 70% of these cases will be diagnosed in LMICs.

The book is organized into five sections. Section I—Multidisciplinary Perspectives provides an overview of conceptual orientations in planning and conducting international and crosscultural studies by an epidemiologist, pathologist, geneticist, cancer prevention specialist, and anthropologist. Each discipline interacts in identifying social, racial, cultural, lifestyle, and environmental determinants of patterns of disease risk and in addressing potential ethical issues that will require resolution before conducting studies in LMICs.

Section II—Methodological Principles in Conducting International Studies addresses core issues of quality control measures in initiating hospital-based and population-based cancer registries, certifying competencies of professional personnel, structuring, pretesting, and administering questionnaires that are culturally relevant and sensitive, collecting biological specimens, and determining the feasibility of alternative strategies in designing and conducting controlled observational and experimental studies.

Section III—Curriculum Requirements in Training Graduate Students discusses didactic and field practicum course requirements that will serve to prepare health professionals who are pursuing careers in international cancer epidemiology. This section reviews recent innovative curriculum development at schools of public health.

Section IV—Illustrative Examples of Collaborative Field Studies describes in detail research studies that have been reported or are in progress in various countries concerning the natural history of cancers of the breast, uterine cervix, lung and bronchus, upper aerodigestive tract, stomach, liver, and colon, as well as non-Hodgkin lymphoma and cancers associated with HIV infection. The chapters are organized to demonstrate the use of various methods of observation available to epidemiologists. These may include (1) descriptive and hypothesis-generating studies (e.g., migrant populations and ecological studies); (2) case-control, cohort, and "hybrid" nested and case-cohort studies that may also incorporate molecular epidemiologic methods; and (3) low-technology screening interventions and applications of primary prevention trials (e.g., chemoprevention trials and HPV vaccination).

Section V—Future Directions and Recommendations summarizes the successes and limitations of previous and on-going research in cancer epidemiology, prevention, and control in developing countries and special populations. This section outlines the essential features of infrastructure resources and priority areas of research that will be required to ensure future progress in cancer epidemiology, prevention, and control programs in these populations.

Key highlights and main points included in Section I include the unique distribution of cancer sites and risk factors in LMICs, examples of migrant studies and their usefulness in elucidating cancer etiology, and the role of biomarkers in cancer prevention. Other salient topics include challenges in implementing cancer screening and diagnostic examinations in LMICs, and the costs and benefits of incorporating genetic biomarkers in the pathologic diagnosis of neoplasms. This section also illustrates the importance of considering social norms and adaptations in diverse cultures, interpersonal relationships, and ethical and professional obligations that will serve to ensure fairness and equity when conducting cancer epidemiologic research in LMICs.

Important highlights from Section II include presentations concerning feasibility, methodologic principles, and illustrative examples of conducting case-control and cohort studies in LMICs, including incorporating molecular technology that measures individual indicators of exposure, susceptibility, and prognosis.

Section III illustrates key issues related to the growing need of cancer epidemiology research training in LMICs. Training of students in LMICs should be based on assessment of the needs of communities, as well as advancing learning and skill development of students in special population research. Institutional and community agencies in LMICs can benefit from student involvement in the testing and investigation of research hypotheses or of clinical questions that may have been revealed by student projects. The section provides details about the status of teaching cancer epidemiology in medical schools and schools of public health in the United States and internationally, offering examples of specific curricula and opportunities for field research training. The section also describes programs for educating and training clinicians and scientists in cancer epidemiology who are from LMICs through affiliations with nonuniversity institutions in the United States and other developed countries.

Section IV illustrates the experience with the hepatitis B virus and its targeted eradication by universal immunization and the challenges in treatment and management of chronic complications. Other examples are HIV and cervical cancer and the role of community motivation, health care system development, and primary and secondary prevention in combating infectious diseases in LMICs. The section thoroughly describes suggested policies and guidelines for down-staging and early detection of breast cancer.

In addition to addressing LMICs in general, the book reports on specific studies conducted in Africa, Asia, Central and South America, and the Middle East, as well as studies in Australia, Europe, North America, and in populations that migrate from LMICs to developed countries. The overall objective is to facilitate future advances by trained health professionals by reviewing the current status of cancer epidemiologic research and training opportunities in LMICs.

Amr S. Soliman
David Schottenfeld
Paolo Boffetta

ACKNOWLEDGMENTS

We wish to thank Melanie Wells at the University of Nebraska Medical Center for her exceptional skills in editorial support and coordination of all communications.

CONTRIBUTORS

HABIBUL AHSAN, M.D., M.MED.SC.
Center for Cancer Epidemiology and
    Prevention
Department of Health Studies
The University of Chicago
Chicago, Illinois USA

BENJAMIN O. ANDERSON, MD
Chair and Director, Breast Health Global
    Initiative
Joint Member, Fred Hutchinson Cancer
    Research Center
Professor of Surgery and Global
    Health-Medicine
University of Washington
Seattle, Washington USA

TIMOTHY M. BLOCK, PH.D.
President and Director, Institute for
    Hepatitis and Virus Research
President and Director, Hepatitis B
    Foundation
Director, Drexel Institute for
    Biotechnology and Virology Research
Professor, Microbiology and Immunology
Drexel University College of Medicine
Doylestown, Pennsylvania USA

PAOLO BOFFETTA, M.D.
Director, Institute for Translational
    Epidemiology
Associate Director, Tisch Cancer Institute
Mount Sinai School of Medicine
New York, New York USA
Vice-President, Research
International Prevention Research Institute
Lyon, France

ROBERT M. CHAMBERLAIN, PH.D.
Professor of Epidemiology
University of Texas
M.D. Anderson Cancer Center
Austin, Texas USA
University of Nebraska Medical Center
College of Public Health
Omaha, Nebraska USA

YU CHEN, PH.D., M.D.
Professor, Department of Environmental
    Medicine
New York University
Medical Center
New York, New York USA

STEVEN S. COUGHLIN, PH.D.
Professor, Department of Epidemiology
Rollins School of Public Health
Emory University
Atlanta, Georgia USA
Epidemiology Program
Post-Deployment Health
Office of Public Health
Department of Veterans Affairs
Washington, D.C. USA

MARIA PAULA CURADO, M.D., PH.D.
Senior Researcher
International Prevention Research Institute
Lyon, France

JEAN-MARIE DANGOU, PH.D.
Regional Adviser for Cancer Control
Disease Prevention & Control Cluster (DPC)
WHO Regional Office for Africa
CitéDjoué, Brazzaville, Congo Republic

Maria Iniesta Doñate , M.D., Ph.D.
Research Fellow
University of Michigan School of
  Medicine
Internal Medicine
Ann Arbor, Michigan USA

**Kyle Esdaille, Dr.P.H., M.P.H.,
C.P.H.**
School of Community Health and Policy
Morgan State University
Baltimore, Maryland USA

**Jessica M. Faupel-Badger, Ph.D.,
M.P.H**
Deputy Director
Cancer Prevention Fellowship Program
Division of Cancer Prevention
National Cancer Institute
Bethesda, Maryland USA

Rolando Herrero, M.D., Ph.D.
Head of Prevention and Implementation
  Group
International Agency for Research on
  Cancer
Lyon, France

Kelly Hirko, MPH
Ph.D. Candidate
University of Michigan School of Public
  Health
Department of Epidemiology
Ann Arbor, Michigan USA

Farhad Islami, M.D., Ph.D.
Instructor
Digestive Disease Research Center
Tehran University of Medical
  Sciences
Tehran, Iran
Tisch Cancer Institute and Institute of
  Transitional Epidemiology
Mount Sinai School of Medicine
New York, New York USA

Shamagonam James, Ph.D.
Specialist Scientist
Health Promotion Research and
  Development Unit
Medical Research Council
Pietermaritzburg, South Africa

**Farin Kamangar, M.D., Ph.D.,
M.H.S., M.P.H.**
Professor and Chairman
Department of Public Health Analysis
School of Community Health and Policy
Morgan State University
Baltimore, Maryland USA

Kardinah, M.D.
National Cancer Center
Dharmais Hospital
Jakarta, Indonesia

Laurence N. Kolonel, M.D., Ph.D.
Professor
Cancer Epidemiology Program
University Hawaii Cancer Center
Honolulu, Hawaii USA

W. Thomas London, M.D.
Chairman
Fox Chase Cancer Center
Institutional Review Board
Philadelphia, Pennsylvania USA

Hongxia Ma, M.D., Ph.D.
Instructor
Department of Epidemiology &
  Biostatistics
School of Public Health
Nanjing Medical University
Nanjing, Jiangsu Province
China

Anthony Mbewu, M.B.B.S., M.D., F.R.C.P
Honorary Professor of Medicine and
  Cardiology
Department of Medicine
Faculty of Health Sciences
University of Cape Town
Cape Town, South Africa

Sam M. Mbulaiteye, M.D.
Investigator
Infections and Immunoepidemiology
  Branch
Division of Cancer Epidemiology and
  Genetics
National Cancer Institute
National Institutes of Health
Department of Health and Human Services
Rockville, Maryland USA

KATHERINE A. McGLYNN, PH.D., M.P.H.
Deputy Chief
Hormonal and Reproductive
 Epidemiology Branch
Division of Cancer Epidemiology and
 Genetics
National Cancer Institute
National Institutes of Health
Department of Health and Human Services
Rockville, Maryland USA

STEPHANIE MELKONIAN, B.A.
Graduate Research Assistant
Center for Cancer Epidemiology and
 Prevention
Department of Health Studies
The University of Chicago
Chicago, Illinois USA

SOFIA D. MERAJVER, M.D., PH.D.
Professor of Internal Medicine and
 Epidemiology
University of Michigan
School of Medicine
School of Public Health
Ann Arbor, Michigan USA

RAUL MURILLO, M.P.H.
General Director
Instituto Nacional de Cancerología de
 Columbia
Bogotá, Colombia

NASHEEN NAIDOO, M.B.B.CH., M.P.H.
Senior Scientist
Health Promotion Research and
 Development Unit
Medical Research Council of South Africa
Cape Town, South Africa

TWALIB NGOMA, M.D.
Executive Director
Ocean Road Cancer Institute
Dar es Salaam, Tanzania

KOLA OKUYEMI, M.D., M.P.H.
Professor
Director, Medical School Program in
 Health Disparities Research
Family Medicine and Community Health
University of Minnesota
Minneapolis, Minnesota USA

OLUFUNMILAYO I. OLOPADE, M.D., F.A.C.P.
Professor of Medicine and Human
 Genetics
Director, Cancer Risk Clinic
The University of Chicago Medicine
Chicago, Illinois USA

OLUWAFEMI OLUWOLE, M.SC.
Global Health Initiative
University of Chicago
Chicago, Illinois USA

SONG-YI PARK, PH.D.
Assistant Specialist
Cancer Epidemiology Program
University of Hawaii Cancer Center
Honolulu, Hawaii USA

YOULIN QIAO, M.D.
Director, Department of Cancer
 Epidemiology
Cancer Institute of the Chinese Academy
 of Medical Sciences
Peking Union Medical College
Beijing, People's Republic of China

PRISCILLA REDDY, PH.D.
Deputy Executive Director
Population Health, Health Systems and
 Innovation (PHHSI)
Human Sciences Research Council Cape
 Town, South Africa

KEN RESNICOW, PH.D.
Professor
Department of Health Behavior & Health
 Education
University of Michigan School of Public
 Health
Ann Arbor, Michigan USA

KARINA BRAGA RIBEIRO, PH.D.
Adjunct Professor
Department of Social Medicine
Faculdade de CiênciasMédicas da Santa
 Casa de São Paulo
Director
Division of Epidemiology
Fundação Oncocentro de São Paulo
São Paulo, Brazil

RENGASWAMY SANKARANARAYANAN, M.D.
Head, Early Detection & Prevention
  Section
Head, Screening Group
International Agency for Research on
  Cancer
World Health Organization
Lyon, France

DAVID SCHOTTENFELD, M.D., M.S.
John G. Searle Professor Emeritus of
  Epidemiology
Professor Emeritus of Internal
  Medicine
University of Michigan School of Public
  Health and Medical School
Ann Arbor, Michigan USA

RONEL SEWPAUL, M.SC.
Scientist
Health Promotion Research and
  Development Unit
Medical Research Council of South
  Africa
Tygerberg, Cape Town
South Africa

HONGBING SHEN, M.D., PH.D.
Professor of Epidemiology
Department of Epidemiology &
  Biostatistics
School of Public Health
Nanjing Medical University
Nanjing, Jiangsu Province
China

AMR S. SOLIMAN, M.D., PH.D.
Professor and Chair of Epidemiology
Director of Cancer Epidemiology Education
  in Special Populations Program
University of Nebraska Medical Center
College of Public Health
Omaha, Nebraska USA

DOMINIQUE SIGHOKO, PH.D.
Department of Medicine
Center for Clinical Cancer Genetics and
  Global Health
University of Chicago
Chicago, Illinois USA

SOMANATHAN THARA, M.D.
Additional Professor of Pathology
Division of Cytopathology
Regional Cancer Centre
Trivandrum, India

DAVID B. THOMAS, M.D., DR.P.H.
Senior International Research Advisor,
  Breast Health Global Initiative
Member, Division of Public Health
  Sciences
Fred Hutchinson Cancer Research Center
Professor, Public Health Sciences
University of Washington
Seattle, Washington USA

YONGLAN ZHENG, PH.D.
Department of Medicine
Center for Clinical Cancer Genetics and
  Global Health
University of Chicago
Chicago, Illinois USA

CANCER EPIDEMIOLOGY

1

Multidisciplinary Perspectives

CHAPTER 1

BURDEN OF CANCER IN LOW- AND MIDDLE-INCOME COUNTRIES

MARIA PAULA CURADO, PAOLO BOFFETTA, DAVID SCHOTTENFELD, JEAN-MARIE DANGOU, KARINA BRAGA RIBEIRO

INTRODUCTION

Cancer was considered a disease of the affluent world. The burden of disease and death in low- and medium-income countries (LMICs) was traditionally dominated by infectious diseases, perinatal conditions, malnutrition, and accidents. This pattern has rapidly changed during the last 20–30 years as a result of a number of factors, all related to improved economic conditions: increasing control of infectious and perinatal diseases, aging of the population, and increasing prevalence of risk factors for chronic diseases. As a result of this trend, cancer mortality is currently the second leading cause of death in LMICs, while it remains the leading cause of death in high-income countries (HICs).[1] About 12.7 million cancer cases and 7.6 million cancer deaths are estimated to have occurred in 2008 worldwide, with 56% of the cases and 64% of the deaths in LMICs (Figure 1.1).

Cancer is the leading cause of death in economically developed countries, and it is the second main cause of death in developing countries.[1] Of the 7.5 million deaths from cancer worldwide in 2008, an estimated 1.5 million were from cancers due to infections. Cervical cancer accounted for about half of the infection-related burden of cancer in women, and in men liver and gastric cancers accounted for more than 80%.[3] In this chapter, we will review the descriptive epidemiology of cancer in LMICs and discuss cancer registration as the most important source of reliable data on the burden of cancer in LMICs.

SOURCES OF DATA

Incidence data (the number of newly diagnosed cases) are derived from population-based cancer registries, which may cover entire national populations but more often cover smaller, subnational areas. In developing countries, they usually cover only urban environments, such as major cities. Data on burden of cancer from most LMICs are of limited quality.[4] When cancer registries are not available, death certificate data have served as the basis for total and cause-specific cancer mortality for 25% to 50% of the LMICs.[5] In most African countries and in some large countries in Asia there are no vital data at hand (Figure 1.2).

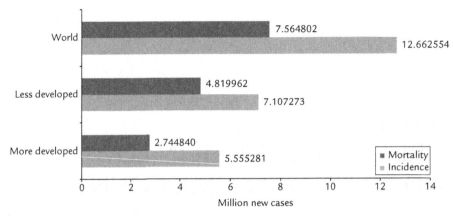

FIGURE 1.1 Estimated new cancer cases and deaths in the world in 2008.[2]

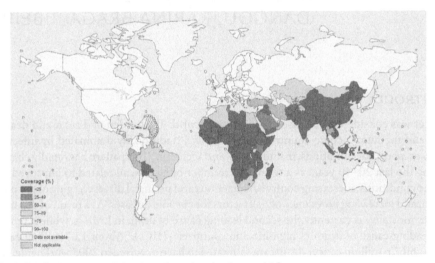

FIGURE 1.2 Coverage of death registration in the world.[5]

Underenumeration of cancer cases, particularly in elderly persons and in rural areas, is a potential limitation of many available sources of data.

Systematic data on global cancer incidence and mortality are available from the *Globocan* project:[2] the most recent data refer to 2008 and concern 20 regions of the world, including all regions of Africa, Asia (excluding Japan), Latin America, and the Caribbean, as well as Melanesia, Micronesia, and Polynesia.

■ CANCER REGISTRATION

Cancer incidence data play a major role in monitoring of cancer control activities and policies in a country.[6] Population-based cancer registries (PBCRs) are the main source of information on cancer incidence. In HICs, where health care facilities are sufficient, it is possible to produce cancer incidence data that are reliable for monitoring the burden of cancer. However, in LMICs, where health care facilities are scarce, cancer registration activities are limited due to lack of resources, and data may be of lesser quality in comparison with international standards. Therefore, limitations in the accuracy and reproducibility of cancer registration data may reflect overall weaknesses in the health care system. Geographical coverage by PBCRs in the world ranges from 80% in North America to 1% in Africa (Table 1.1).

There is lack of cancer incidence data in Africa, Asia, and Latin America, although a growing number of PBCRs are active. The resource requirements for sustaining PBCRs in these regions are a major factor impeding timely release of cancer incidence data. Without accurate and reliable information the countries' cancer control interventional policies are unlikely to be successful.

The main task of cancer registration is to identify patterns of incident cases of cancer in a defined population over a period of time. Cancer registration must be a continuous activity of collecting incident cases in a way to ensure consistent results over time and comparability with other registries. Therefore, the official demographic profile of the underlying population must be available, with information about the population distribution by age group and gender. This will make it possible to calculate the incidence rates in the area covered by the PBCR. Aside from population data, it is possible to perform cancer registration if the PBCRs have access to all sources of data where cancer diagnosis and treatment is carried out, such as hospitals, clinics, and pathology and imaging laboratories. In general, the main sources of information on cancer incidence cases in LMICs are cancer hospitals or general hospitals treating cancer patients. Usually in these hospitals there is a pathology laboratory where the morphological diagnosis is established.

A national population-based cancer registry covers the whole population of the country. To establish this kind of cancer registry in LMIC is challenging and will depend on the local resources, budget, adequate physical facilities, and informatics equipment. This type of cancer registry is rare in LMIC; however, one initiative in West Africa is the Gambia National Cancer Registry. This PBCR was created as a part of the Gambia Hepatitis Intervention Project for the purpose of evaluating the efficacy of hepatitis B vaccination in reducing the burden of liver cancer incidence in that country.[8] The most common type of PBCR in LMIC is the regional cancer registry that covers a defined population within a country; usually it is an urban registry collecting data from a metropolitan area. There are a few rural cancer registries in LMIC, such as in Barshi, India.[9] The size of the population included in regional cancer registries can range from a few thousands to millions, depending on the country's resources.

Setting and adhering to quality control standards is essential for the production of internationally comparable cancer incidence rates. Data comparability, however, goes beyond

TABLE 1.1 Population based cancer registries coverage by continent[7]

CONTINENT	COUNTRIES INCLUDED/ SUBMITTED DATA	PBCR INCLUDED/ SUBMITTED DATA	GEOGRAPHIC COVERAGE BY CONTINENT (%)	POPULATION COVERAGE IN MILLIONS (%)
Africa	5/14	5/16	31	8.8 (1%)
Asia	15/18	44/77	57	152.3 (4%)
Europe	29/30	100/120	83	238.8 (33%)
North America	2/2	54/58	93	258.5 (80%)
Oceania	4/6	11/13	85	23 (73%)
South and Central America	8/11	11/29	38	22.7 (4.3%)

definition and collection of standardized data. The diagnostic and treating capacity of the countries and the access to the health care system or the existence of screening programs have to be equally considered, as they pose an inherent problem in achieving data completeness and quality. In LMIC, and especially in some regions of Africa, Asia, and Latin America, the scarcity of health care facilities impedes the access of the patient to the health care system. Limitations in existing diagnostic and treatment facilities result in incomplete case registration and underestimation of the cancer incidence. Moreover, limited diagnostic services may result in inaccurate diagnosis. In LMICs, quality control indicators of cancer registration data point to the weaknesses of the health system that influence the quality above and beyond the cancer registrars' performance.[4] These indicators have to be interpreted with caution, taking into account the deficiencies of the health care system. For example, for some Asian and for most African registries, the low percentage of microscopically verified (MV) cases may be related to the low number of pathology laboratories for the size of the population, resulting in incomplete case ascertainment and lack of specificity in the morphologic classification of each cancer case.[10]

Death certificates are valuable tools for identifying missed cases. Although a low percentage of death-certificate-only (DCO) cases is highly desirable, it is an indicator of a problem when registries are reporting zero percent of DCO cases. It indicates that quality control for completeness has not been performed, thus making it more likely that some cases are missed. At the same time, a very high percentage of DCO cases is an indicator of suboptimal completeness and quality, because the date of diagnosis cannot be determined accurately and there is selective registration of the more lethal cancers. In African countries, in particular, there is wide range in the percentage of DCO due to (1) the lack of an official death certificate form, (2) availability of death certificates through an official national center, and (3) recording of the cause of death by a layperson. Similar limitations are found in Asia, where the death certificates are often signed by an inexperienced individual instead of a medical doctor, thereby leading to errors in identifying the cause of death.

Countries with PBCRs and reliable data on cancer incidence over long periods have valuable tools for monitoring the cancer burden and also for assessing the effectiveness of cancer control programs in the coverage area. PBCRs that adhere to quality control standards are significant contributors in evaluating cancer control interventions and fostering epidemiologic research. When the commitment to the registry is continuous, trends over time and successful policies can be supervised. From a research point of view, we can investigate or detect new risk factors by using quality PBCR data. The registry in the city of Cali, Colombia, is a good example for monitoring cancer trends in Latin America; it has been producing cancer incidence data continuously for the past 40 years. Similarly, in Asia, the cancer registry of Bombay city (Mumbai), India, has been producing cancer incidence data since 1964.

Unfortunately, few LMICs have long-term cancer incidence data available. It is therefore extremely important to expand the coverage and quality of PBCRs in all LMICs in order to promote better research and facilitate the design or monitoring of cancer control policies. Discontinuity of registration impedes the monitoring of the cancer burden or the performance of a cancer control measure adopted in the coverage area, and it precludes identifying the changes that have occurred during that period.

Cancer registration in LMICs is a challenge, and there is no magical solution when war, infectious diseases, and epidemics such as HIV/AIDS hinder health care organizations. PBCRs in LMICs will remain as individual initiatives whether connected or not to international research projects. These projects can assist local governments in recognizing the importance of cancer registration for cancer control and epidemiological and etiological research.

▪ DESCRIPTIVE EPIDEMIOLOGY OF CANCER IN LMICS

In this section we describe the patterns of cancer incidence, mortality, and trends in LMICs as defined by the United Nations.[11] The main sources of data are *Cancer Incidence in Five Continents*,[12] *Globocan*,[5] and *Cancer in Africa*.[13] Given the heterogeneity in cancer incidence, mortality and underlying risk factors, we describe the epidemiology of cancer separately for Africa and LMICs in Asia and Latin America.

Cancer in Africa

The estimated number of new cancer cases in Africa for 2008 was 325,000 in men and 390,600 in women; the corresponding estimates of cancer deaths were 267,000 and 274,800 in men and women, respectively. The case-fatality ratio (the ratio of deaths to incident cases in the time period) was approximately 82% in men and 70% in women. In both sexes, the pattern of cancer incidence in Africa is rather heterogeneous.[2]

Among African men, the overall age-adjusted cancer incidence rate was 114/100,000. However, a wide variation in incidence was present, with relatively high rates being observed in South Africa (254.8/100,000) and Uganda (156.9/100,000) and lower rates in Sudan (81.6/100,000) and Niger (68.6/100,000). In the continent as a whole, prostate and liver cancers are the most common cancers in males (Figure 1.3): the high rate of liver cancer, in particular, indicates that control of hepatitis B infection has not been achieved.

Another high-incidence cancer related to infectious agents is Kaposi sarcoma, with particularly high rates in eastern and southern Africa. Lung cancer is the most common cancer in northern African men, but it exhibits relatively low rates in the other regions of the continent. Prostate cancer is most common in southern Africa, with rates above 50 per 100,000 men, whereas in other regions rates range from 5 to 23 per 100,000. These large differences in incidence may be due to screening activities in southern Africa, but genetic factors might also play a role.[14] Non-Hodgkin lymphoma incidence rates are intermediate (under 10 per 100,000) but are relatively common in all regions. Esophageal squamous cell cancer is a highly lethal cancer with elevated rates, in particular, in eastern and southern Africa. This neoplasm needs to be further studied to improve early diagnosis and to implement preventive measures. Alcohol consumption, infections, and dietary factors, including mycotoxin contamination, are among the suspected risk factors.[15] The mortality patterns for men in Africa are dominated by lung, liver, and esophageal cancer; mortality rates for Kaposi sarcoma and prostate cancer are relatively increased in all regions.

The overall cancer incidence among African women ranges from 98/100,000 in central Africa to 180/100,000 in southern Africa (Figure 1.4).

These rates are two to three times lower in comparison with those in HIC. The most common cancers are cervical and breast cancer. Cancer of the cervix is the most common cancer in eastern, central, and western Africa, with rates as high as 30 to 35/100,000.

Breast cancer shows a relatively high incidence in all regions, but particularly in countries of northern Africa with rates above 30/100,000. In other regions rates are similar to those of cervical cancer, with the exception of eastern Africa, where they are lower. Liver cancer is the third most common female cancer in central and western Africa, with rates about 10/100,000, while its incidence is lower in the other regions. The incidence of esophageal and colon cancers is increasing among women and men in eastern and southern Africa. The incidence of other cancers is relatively low in African women.

In both men and women, the pattern of cancer in Africa is dominated by neoplasms linked to chronic infections (HPV, HBV, HIV, HHV8). This provides ample opportunities for

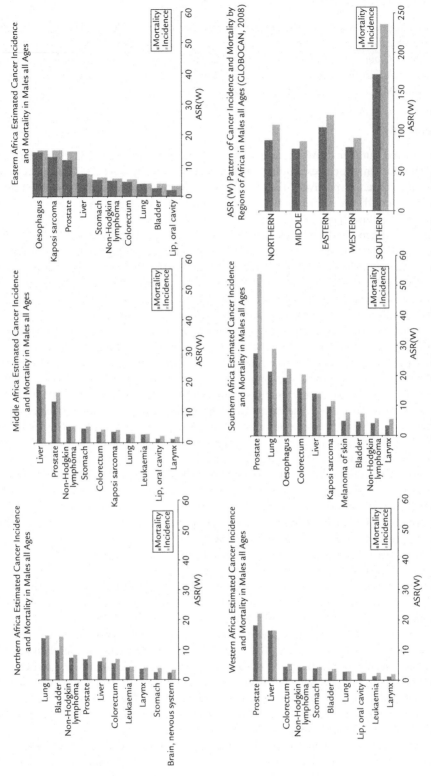

FIGURE 1.3 Age standardize rates by world population ASR(W) of cancer incidence and mortality in males by African region.[2]

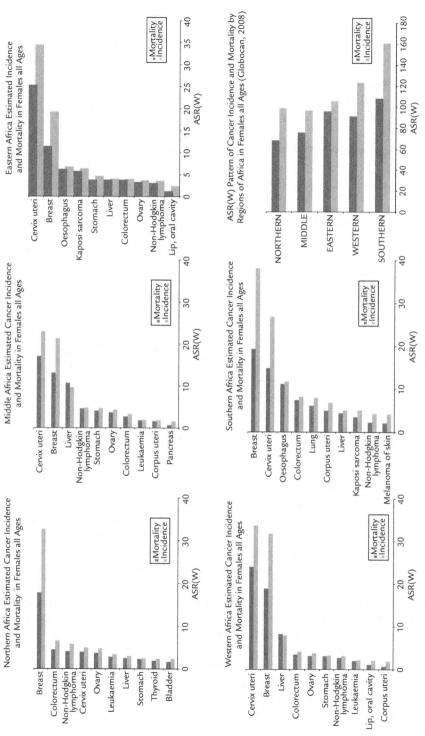

FIGURE 1.4 ASR(W) of cancer incidence and mortality in females by African regions.[2]

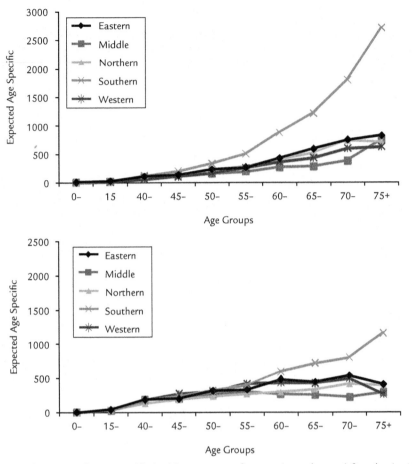

FIGURE 1.5 Expected age-specific incidence rates of cancer in males and females in Africa for all cancers excluding non–skin melanoma.[2]

primary prevention through vaccination and control of the underlying infection. In addition, cancers related to lifestyle, such as lung cancer (in northern African men), breast cancer, and colon cancer, are rapidly becoming major contributors to the overall burden of the disease.

Most African countries are undergoing a rapid demographic transition (Figure 1.5): with the aging of the population, the overall cancer burden will increase even if age-specific rates will not.

An analysis of temporal trends would be useful to better understand current patterns and predict future scenarios. However, no PBCR exists in Africa that has been operating over a sufficient period to allow for meaningful trend analyses. Short of such data, a cross-sectional analysis of age-specific incidence rates for the main cancers is informative in understanding current and future trends in incidence. In particular, breast cancer age-specific rates have steadily increased in postmenopausal women from southern Africa; however, in the other regions rates have been higher in premenopausal women (Figure 1.6). This finding illustrates a different degree of evolution of the epidemic of breast cancer in the various parts of the continent.

A similar pattern is shown for prostate cancer (Figure 1.7).

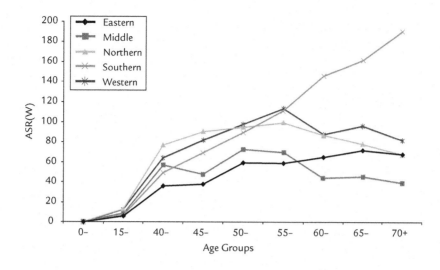

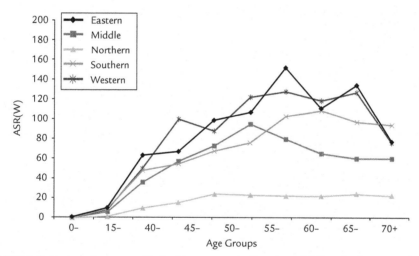

FIGURE 1.6 Expected age specific incidence rate in females of Africa for breast and cervix cancer.[2]

Cancer in Low- and Medium-Income Countries of Asia

In Asia, the highest incidence and mortality rates are registered in countries located in the eastern part of the continent, such as China, Korea, and Mongolia. Incidence rates range from above 200/100,000 in men and more than 150/100,000 in women. The lowest incidence and mortality rates are observed in south-central Asia (Figure 1.8).

In men, lung cancer is the most common cancer in all regions of Asia, with rates ranging from 13 to 45/100,000 and being the highest in eastern Asia and the lowest in south-central Asia. Infection-related cancers such as stomach and liver cancers also have high incidence in eastern and south-eastern Asia. The incidence of cancers of the lower digestive tract is increasing. South-central Asia (i.e., India and neighboring countries) shows a peculiar

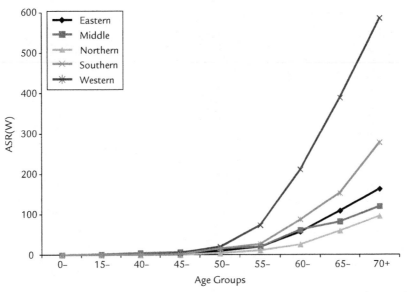

FIGURE 1.7 Expected age specific incidence of prostate cancer based on world population by African regions.[2]

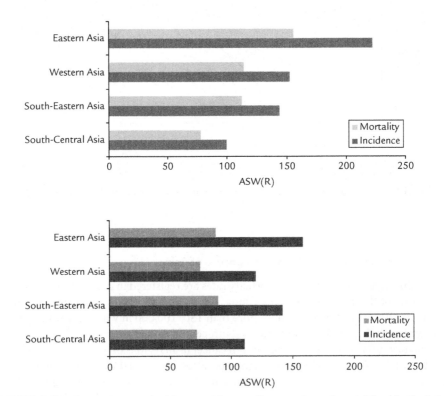

FIGURE 1.8 Estimated cancer incidence and mortality rates in males and females in Asia.[2]

pattern, as head and neck cancer is the second most common cancer in men. Patterns of cancer mortality follow closely those of incidence, since the most common cancers (lung, stomach, and liver cancers) are highly fatal (Figure 1.9).

Therefore the burden of cancer incidence and mortality in Asian men is dominated by two groups: tobacco-related cancers (lung and head and neck) and infection-related cancers (liver and stomach).

Breast cancer is the most common cancer among women in LMICs of Asia, although the rates are about half of those in HICs.[2] Cervical cancer, however, is the most common cancer in southern-central Asia, with rates similar to those of breast cancer. For the other anatomical sites, excluding genital cancer, there is no clear pattern, but gastrointestinal cancers (i.e., esophagus, stomach, and colon-rectum) are relatively frequent (Figure 1.10).

Analysis of temporal trends for overall cancer incidence in the two major Asian LMICs (China and India) shows increasing rates in Chinese women, stable rates in Chinese males, and decreasing rates in Indian men and women (Figure 1.11).

Time trend analysis of specific cancers shows a decrease in lung cancer incidence among Chinese men but not Chinese women, while liver cancer incidence is relatively stable among Indian men (Figure 1.12).

Among cancers in the genital organs, prostate cancer incidence is increasing in China and is stable in India, where the rates are about 70% lower in comparison with those of HICs (Figure 1.13).

Cervical cancer incidence rates are decreasing in India, while they are stable (and much lower) in China.

Overall, cancer represents an increasing cause of morbidity and mortality in Asian LMICs. Infection-related cancers remain a major contributor to the overall burden, but the role of lifestyle factors is rapidly growing. The increase in the incidence of breast cancer is the most striking aspect of this trend, probably due to the rapid changes in reproductive habits of Asian women (lower number of pregnancies, later age at first pregnancy).[16]

Cancer in Latin America

Latin America has a growing population, and most of the countries are under transition to middle- and upper middle-income countries. The overall age-adjusted cancer incidence is 174.5/100,000 in men and 155.7/100,000 in women. Among men, the highest rates are observed in Uruguay (354.4/100,000), Argentina (232.1/100,000), and Cuba (213.4/100,000), while in women the highest rates are registered in Uruguay (230.7/100,000), Argentina (193.0/100,000), and Honduras (181.6/100,000). In this region of South and Central America and the Caribbean, average total cancer mortality rates are estimated as 109.3/100,000 in men and 86.6/100,000 in women (Figure 1.14).

Among men in Latin America the most common cancer is prostate cancer: rates are particularly high in the Caribbean (around 60/100,000), intermediate in South America, and lower in Central America (Figure 1.15).

Lung cancer is the second most common cancer in men; the highest rates are observed in the Caribbean (up to 26/100,000), while in the other regions the rates are lower (around 10/100,000). Stomach cancer is the third most common cancer; rates are particularly high in Central and South America. Estimated mortality rates in men are high for lung cancer (27/100,000) and prostate cancer (12–25/100,000). For all other cancers, mortality rates are below 10/100,000.

Among women in Latin America, breast cancer is the most common cancer: rates are highest (45/100,000) in South America (Figure 1.16).

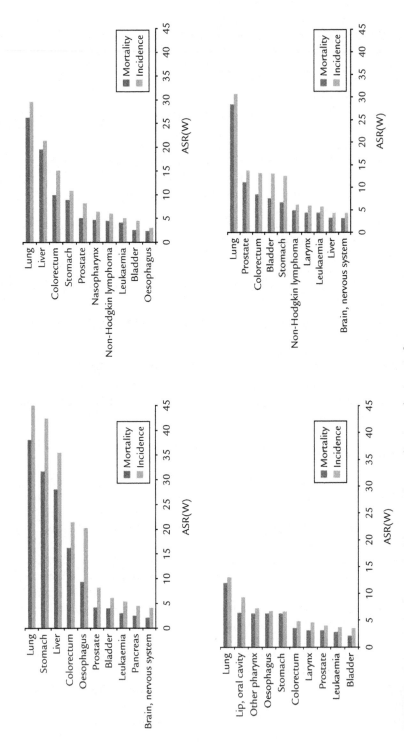

FIGURE 1.9 ASR(W) of cancer incidence and mortality in males in Asia.[2]

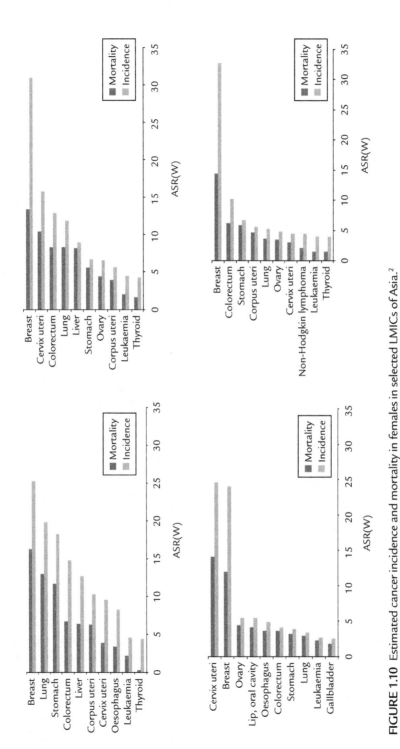

FIGURE 1.10 Estimated cancer incidence and mortality in females in selected LMICs of Asia.[2]

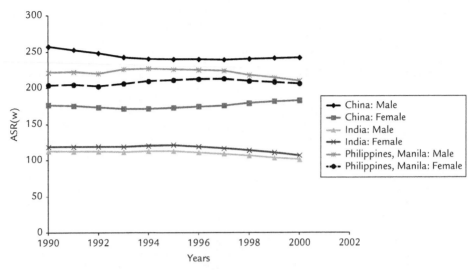

FIGURE 1.11 Incidence trends of all cancers excluding non–skin melanoma in selected countries of Asia.[2]

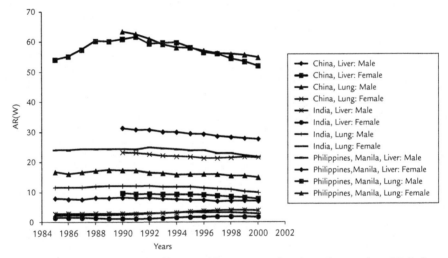

FIGURE 1.12 Incidence trends of lung and liver cancers in selected countries of Asia.[2]

The second most common malignancy is cervical cancer, whose rates are about half in comparison with breast cancer. The pattern for other cancers is rather heterogeneous within this region: lung and endometrial cancers are relatively frequent in the Caribbean, while stomach, liver, and colon cancers are more common in Central and South America.

An analysis of temporal trends in cancer incidence is feasible for several population-based cancer registries from Brazil, Colombia, Costa Rica, and Ecuador (Figure 1.17).

Stomach cancer rates are declining in both sexes in most populations, while colon cancer incidence is increasing in Brazil and Costa Rica, although rates remain rather low

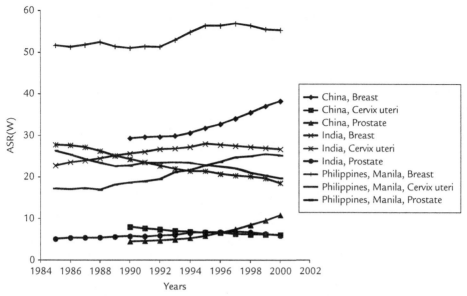

FIGURE 1.13 Trends on cancer incidence of breast, cervix and prostate cancers in females and males of selected LMICs of Asia.[2]

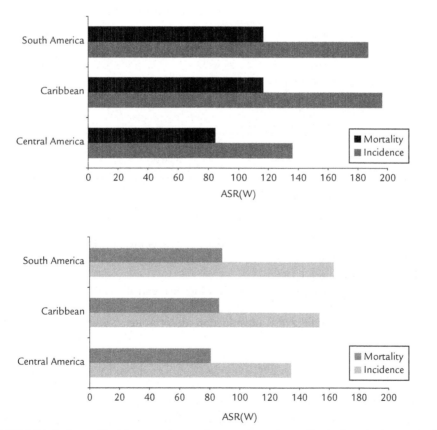

FIGURE 1.14 Estimated incidence and mortality rates by regions of Latin America by gender.[2]

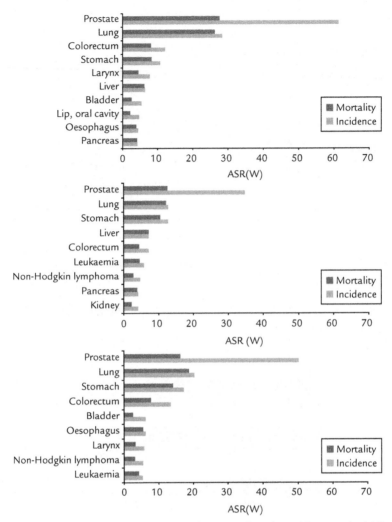

FIGURE 1.15 Estimated incidence and mortality rates for selected low- and middle-income countries of Latin America in men.[2]

(around 10/100,000). The incidence of breast cancer is increasing in all populations in Latin America, while that of cervical cancer is decreasing, although the slope is different in different countries (Figure 1.18).

The incidence of prostate cancer is rapidly increasing in all countries, notably in Brazil (Figure 1.19).

This pattern may reflect the introduction of prostate cancer screening in these populations.

▪ DISCUSSION

Cancer represents an increasing burden of disease in LMICs. Although overall age-standardized cancer incidence rates in LMICs are approximately half of those of HICs (160.3/100,000 vs. 300.1/100,000 in men and 138.0/100,000 vs. 225.5/100,000 in women), the difference is smaller for overall cancer mortality rates (119.3/100,000 vs.

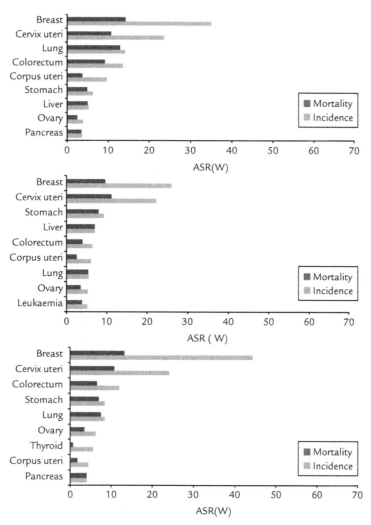

FIGURE 1.16 Estimated incidence and mortality rates for selected low and middle income countries of Latin America in women.[2]

143.9/100,000 in men and 85.4/100,000 vs. 87.3/100,000 in women).[17] This pattern is explained by the importance of cancers with high fatality in LMICs (liver, stomach, and esophageal cancer), as well as by the higher mortality from preventable or curable cancers such as cervical and breast cancer. These global figures mask a complex, heterogeneous pattern of cancer in LMIC, however, as described in the previous sections on the basis of three main regions and in recent reviews that analyzed more detailed groups of countries.[1,17,18]

The increasing availability of good-quality data on cancer incidence and mortality in LMICs leads to the identification of global patterns, as well as features specific to a given population. Two major trends in cancer occurrence can be identified in LMICs: the progressive decline in the role of infection-related cancers, and the increase in importance of cancers related to lifestyle factors.

Despite the fact that infection-related cancers still represent in LMICs an estimated 22.9% of all cancers,[3] the incidence of the most important cancers associated with biological agents is declining in most countries, and the growing availability of effective vaccines

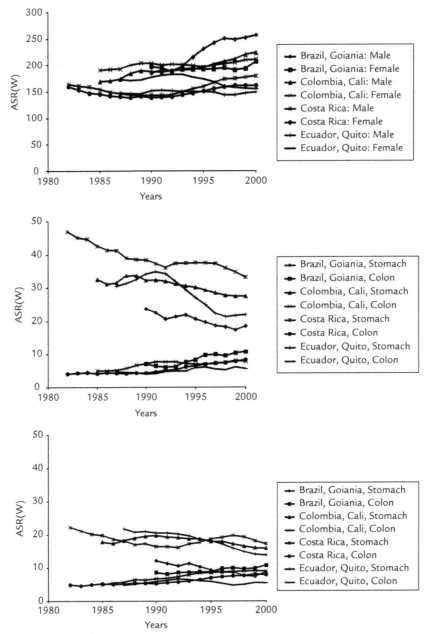

FIGURE 1.17 Estimated trends to all cancers except non melanoma skin cancer in selected countries of Latin America.[2]

against HBV and HPV will accelerate this pattern. The experience of Taiwan, a high-risk country for liver cancer in which nationwide HBV vaccination has been implemented in children since the 1980s, is exemplary (Figure 1.20).

In the case of other important cancer-causing agents such as *H. pylori* and HIV, for which vaccination will not be feasible in the foreseeable future, effective treatments are available and are likely to become more affordable in LMICs.

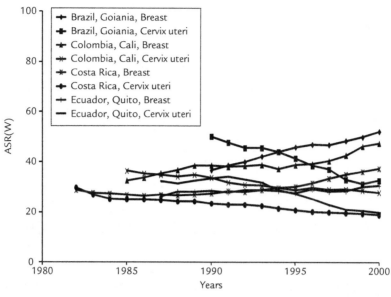

FIGURE 1.18 Trends in breast and cervix cancer incidence in selected countries of Latin America.[2]

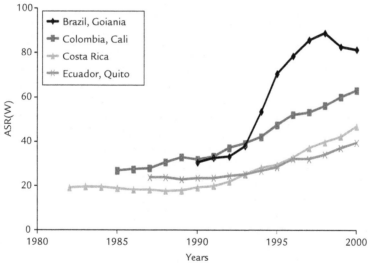

FIGURE 1.19 Trends in breast and cervix cancer incidence in selected countries of Latin America.[2]

The increase in the occurrence of lifestyle-related cancers represents a major challenge for LMICs, as it is linked to economic development, which entails major improvements in many other aspects of health, in particular infant mortality, reproductive morbidity and mortality, and infection diseases. In this respect, LMIC seem to replicate the experience of HIC, with an increase in the prevalence and severity of exposure to known risk factors such as tobacco smoking, overweight/obesity, and sedentary life. Other lifestyle changes leading

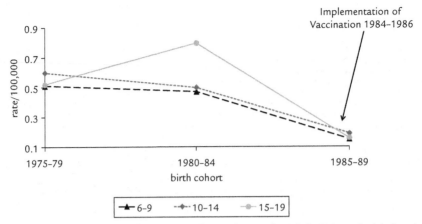

FIGURE 1.20 Temporal trends in age-specific incidence of HCCs in Taiwan by birth cohort—Effect of nationwide HBV vaccination.[19]

to an increase in cancer risk—such as reduced number of pregnancies and later age at first pregnancy, two important risk factors of breast, endometrial, and ovarian cancer—are so intimately linked to development and improved quality of life that it seems impossible to counteract them. Addressing modifiable lifestyle-related risk factors of cancer represents a key health priority of LMICs, especially because these are also the main determinant of other major chronic diseases.[20]

In addition to these global trends, the descriptive epidemiology of cancer in LMICs leads to the observation of defined patterns affecting specific populations. Burkitt lymphoma in sub-Saharan Africa is a well-known example.[21] The high incidence of gallbladder and extra-hepatic biliary tract cancer in several areas of the world, such as northern India and the Andean region,[22] is another example. Studies in such high-risk populations might lead to discoveries with implications that extend beyond the local region.

Cancer epidemiology in LMICs is a growing discipline: following the recent economic development in many LMICs, an increasing number of PBCRs have been established, often as part of national cancer control plans. In parallel, more opportunities for etiological and prevention research have been recognized.[23] Taken together, these efforts are likely to help mitigate the impact of cancer on the health of these populations. Supporting data collection in PBCRs and hospital cancer registries would be very important. These instruments have been neglected in LMICs due to a lack of knowledge about their role as a source of information to monitor cancer. The maintenance of information systems with timely data will make it possible to plan effective cancer control strategies in LMICs.

■ SUMMARY

Cancer mortality was viewed in prior decades as a public health burden impacting selectively the affluent world. The cumulative burden of diseases in low- and medium-income countries (LMICs) was traditionally dominated by epidemic infectious diseases, maternal and perinatal conditions, malnutrition, and accidents. This pattern has undergone demographic transition during relatively recent decades, as a result of multiple factors including improving economic conditions, increasing urbanization, aging of the population implementation of programs of prevention and control of infectious and perinatal diseases, and increasing prevalence of potentially avoidable lifestyle and environmental risk factors that are considered causal for various chronic degenerative diseases. Of current significance, cancers of various organ sites and morphology represent an increasing proportionate burden of diseases in LMICs. The maintenance of quality controlled cancer registration systems with timely data will enable the planning and implementation of effective cancer control interventions in LMICs.

ACKNOWLEDGMENT

The authors acknowledge Kim Coppens for helping in the final version of the manuscript with the figures and references.

REFERENCES

1. Mathers C, Fat DM, Boerma JT, World Health Organization. *The global burden of disease: 2004 update.* Geneva, Switzerland: World Health Organization; 2008.

2. Ferlay J, Shin HR, Bray F, Forman D, Mathers C, Parkin DM. GLOBOCAN 2008 v1.2, cancer incidence and mortality worldwide: IARC Cancer Base no. 10 [internet]. 2010. Available from: http://globocan.iarc.fr, accessed 07/02/2012.

3. de Martel C, Ferlay J, Franceschi S, et al. Global burden of cancers attributable to infections in 2008: A review and synthetic analysis. *Lancet Oncol.* 2012;13(6):607–615.

4. Curado MP, Voti L, Sortino-Rachou AM. Cancer registration data and quality indicators in low and middle income countries: Their interpretation and potential use for the improvement of cancer care. *Cancer Causes Control.* 2009;20(5):751–756.

5. World Health Organization. Coverage of vital registration of deaths, 2000–2008. Available from: http://www.who.int/healthinfo/statistics/, accessed 11/03/2010.

6. Parkin DM. The evolution of the population-based cancer registry. *Nat Rev Cancer.* 2006;6(8):603–612.

7. Curado MP, International Agency for Research on Cancer, International Association of Cancer Registries. *Cancer incidence in five continents, volume IX.* Lyon : Geneva: International Agency for Research on Cancer; Distributed by WHO Press, World Health Organization; 2008.

8. Bah E, Hall AJ, Inskip HM. The first 2 years of the Gambian national cancer registry. *Br J Cancer.* 1990;62(4):647–650.

9. Parkin DM, Whelan SL, Ferlay J, Raymond L, Young J. Cancer incidence in five continents, volume VII. Lyon, France: International Agency for Research on Cancer; 1997.

10. Ogwang MD, Zhao W, Ayers LW, Mbulaiteye SM. Accuracy of Burkitt lymphoma diagnosis in constrained pathology settings: Importance to epidemiology. *Arch Pathol Lab Med.* 2011;135(4):445–450.

11. United Nations Population Division. International human development indicators. Available from: http://hdr.undp.org/en/statistics/, accessed 02/02/2011.

12. Ferlay J, Parkin DM, Curado MP, et al. Cancer incidence in five continents, volumes I to IX: IARC CancerBase no.9. Lyon, France: International Agency for Research on Cancer; 2010.

13. Parkin DM, International Agency for Research on Cancer. *Cancer in Africa: Epidemiology and prevention.* Lyon, France: IARC Press; 2003.

14. Chu LW, Ritchey J, Devesa SS, Quraishi SM, Zhang H, Hsing AW. Prostate cancer incidence rates in Africa. *Prostate Cancer.* 2011;2011:947870.

15. Naidoo R, Ramburan A, Reddi A, Chetty R. Aberrations in the mismatch repair genes and the clinical impact on oesophageal squamous carcinomas from a high incidence area in South Africa. *J Clin Pathol.* 2005;58(3):281–284.

16. Breast cancer in developing countries. *Lancet.* 2009;374(9701):1567.

17. Jemal A, Bray F, Center MM, Ferlay J, Ward E, Forman D. Global cancer statistics. *CA Cancer J Clin.* 2011;61(2):69–90.

18. Bray F, Jemal A, Grey N, Ferlay J, Forman D. Global cancer transitions according to the human development index (2008–2030): A population-based study. *Lancet Oncol.* 2012;13(8):790–801.

19. Chang MH, You SL, Chen CJ, et al. Decreased incidence of hepatocellular carcinoma in hepatitis B vaccinees: A 20-year follow-up study. *J Natl Cancer Inst.* 2009;101(19):1348–1355.

20. Probst-Hensch N, Tanner M, Kessler C, Burri C, Kunzli N. Prevention—a cost-effective way to fight the non-communicable disease epidemic: An academic perspective of the united nations high-level NCD meeting. *Swiss Med Wkly.* 2011;141:w13266.

21. Parkin DM, Sohier R, O'Conor GT. Geographic distribution of Burkitt's lymphoma. *IARC Sci Publ.* 1985;(60)(60):155–164.

22. Randi G, Franceschi S, La Vecchia C. Gallbladder cancer worldwide: Geographical distribution and risk factors. *Int J Cancer.* 2006;118(7):1591–1602.

23. Sankaranarayanan R, Boffetta P. Research on cancer prevention, detection and management in low- and medium-income countries. *Ann Oncol.* 2010;21(10):1935–1943.

CHAPTER 2

MIGRANT STUDIES

SONG-YI PARK AND LAURENCE N. KOLONEL

INTRODUCTION

Migrants are individuals who move from one geographic area to another, sometimes over long distances or in large groups. Human migration usually means movement from one country (home country or country of origin) to another (host country or adopted country), which is known as "international migration," although sometimes it refers to movement from one region to another within a country ("internal migration").[1-8] Because studies of disease in migrant populations provide unique research opportunities that would not have been created intentionally, epidemiologic studies of migrants are often referred to as *natural experiments*. Migrants often undergo extreme changes in exposures to risk factors for disease and may have substantially different disease rates in the host country from those in the home country. The corresponding changes in risk for different cancers have been widely used for inferences on the relative importance of environmental factors versus inherited predisposition in cancer etiology.[9]

OPPORTUNITIES FOR EPIDEMIOLOGIC RESEARCH ON MIGRANTS

International Migration

In 2010, 214 million people, representing 3.1% of the world population, are estimated to be international migrants, and 60% of the world's migrants currently reside in more developed regions.[10,11] A major proportion of international migration takes place from low- and middle-income countries to high-income countries, since the main reason for translocation to another country is to seek better living environments, including jobs, education, and safety.[12]

Migration to developed countries causes dramatic changes in exposures and subsequently in disease patterns. Such rapid and extreme changes in exposure and disease rates can help identify meaningful risk factors for cancer, especially those related to lifestyle.[13] Migrant studies permit comparisons between genetically similar groups with widely different rates of cancer incidence. This type of study may identify populations particularly susceptible to certain types of cancer. For instance, colorectal cancer rates for Japanese migrants to the United States increased rapidly to surpass the level of the host population.[14] Migrant studies can also offer insights into the relative contributions of genetics and environment to the risk of specific cancers. A particular potential of migrant studies is to suggest critical periods of life when relevant exposures have their greatest impact on cancer risk. In some instances, cancer rates in first generation migrants may be used to infer rates in the home country when such data are not available;[15] however, because even first generation migrants may experience dramatic changes in cancer rates,[16] caution must be exercised when using migrant data for this purpose. The magnitude of change in cancer rates among migrants can suggest the extent of risk reduction achievable through successful public health interventions.[17]

Internal Migration

Today, internal migration is important in most countries, and in some it is far greater than international migration.[18] For example, 140 million people were estimated to migrate internally in China in 2003 compared with a mere 450,000 people who migrated internationally for work.[19] In Indonesia, it is estimated that more than 23 million citizens migrate each year, but only 10% of these migrants move internationally.[20] In many poor countries, rural-rural migration still dominates, with laborers from poorer regions traveling to more agriculturally prosperous, often irrigated, areas that provide more work. In India, for instance, rural-rural migration accounted for roughly 62% of all movement in 1999–2000 according to National Sample Survey data.[18] Although still not the main form of migration in many developing countries, rural-urban migration is rapidly gaining in importance, especially in the urbanizing economies of Asia as rural-urban wage differentials grow and the economic gains from migration increase.

It appears that even internal migration within a country can generate sufficient lifestyle change to influence cancer rates. Research on internal migrants can be used to determine whether place of birth or place of adult residence is the stronger predictor of disease.[8] Such research can also determine the effects on disease risk of movement from a high-risk to low-risk area or vice versa or of movement from a rural to an urban area. In particular, countries with rapid social and economic changes provide special research opportunities, since differences in environment between rural and urban area tend to be extreme, mostly due to urban-centered development, while genetic and cultural inheritance is similar between the two areas. Unfortunately, few studies have been published on internal migration and cancer particularly in a country under cultural and economic transition, probably because nationwide cancer registries have not been established or are relatively new.

■ TYPES OF MIGRANT STUDIES

Comparison of Groups with Same Origin and Different Living Environments

Comparison of cancer incidence and mortality rates between the home country and the migrant group in the host country has been the basis of most migrant studies.[17] The two groups are genetically similar but are exposed to different environments. Examples include comparisons of cancer incidence rates among Japanese migrants to the United States with corresponding rates in Japan,[16] and comparisons of cancer incidence rates among Indians living in Singapore, the United Kingdom, and the United States with corresponding rates in the home country, India (Figure 2.1).[21] Studies of internal migration are generally of this type. For example, breast cancer incidence rates of migrants from the south (low-risk area) to the north (high-risk area) in Italy were compared with the stable population of the south.[2]

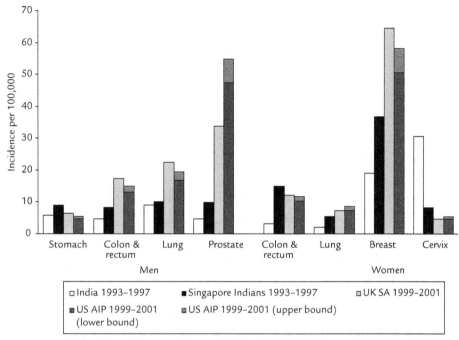

FIGURE 2.1 Cancer incidence in India, Singapore Indians, UK South Asians (SA) and US Asian Indians and Pakistanis (AIP): rates were age-adjusted to the 1960 Segi world population. *(Source: Adapted[21])*

Comparison of Groups with Different Origin and Same Living Environment

Comparisons have also been made between the migrants and the indigenous population or other migrant groups in the host country. In this instance, the groups compared are genetically different but share the same environment. For example, cancer incidence and mortality among Asian Americans of Chinese, Filipino, Vietnamese, and Korean have been compared with US whites (Figure 2.2).[22]

Comparison within the Migrant Group

Comparisons have been made within the migrant group, for example by duration of residence in the host country,[23–29] age at migration,[28,30–33] and between first generation migrants and their descendants in the host country.[16,34–37] For certain cancer sites, analyses by anatomic region within the organ[34,36,38] or by histologic subtype[39–42] may be possible.

Population versus Individual-Level Studies

Most migrant studies are descriptive in nature. Studies with information on exposures have usually only had population-level data and typically were ecologic in design.[17] For example, cancer rates in the home and host countries have been examined in relation to per capita intakes based on national food disappearance data.[43] Case-control and cohort studies have the advantages of information obtained at the individual levels and the ability to control for confounders. Unfortunately, it is very rarely feasible to carry out a true cohort study on migrants, which would involve enrolling individuals at the time of their migration, and

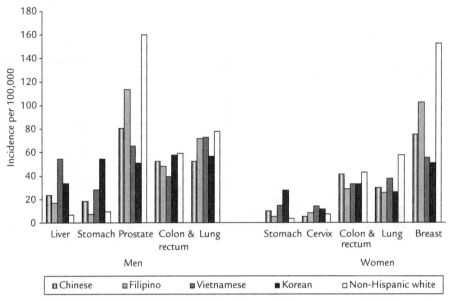

FIGURE 2.2 Cancer incidence among Asian American ethnic groups and non-Hispanic whites, California: rates for the period 2000–2002 were age-adjusted to the standard US year 2000 population. The majority of these ethnic groups (68–78%) are first generation migrants based on the 2000 US Census. *(Source: Adapted[22])*

following the cohort to obtain disease incidence, deaths, and losses to follow-up.[9] Therefore, only a limited number of case-control studies[28,31,32,44–48] and cohort studies[33,49–55] have been conducted among migrants. In recent years, migrant studies have progressed from relatively simple comparisons of incidence and mortality rates to studies that utilize a wider range of appropriate epidemiologic methods.[9]

▦ ISSUES IN MIGRANT STUDIES

International Migration

Bias in Incidence Comparisons
Caution is needed in comparisons of cancer incidence across countries. The completeness of case ascertainment, definition used to establish cases, diagnostic coding schemes applied, and rates of histologic confirmation of diagnoses may all differ between the home and host countries. Also, screening practices may differ, which can have a substantial effect not only on observed incidence rates but on the stage distribution of the tumors.[52,56] Exposures of migrants to more intensive screening in the host country would lead initially to a higher incidence of disease because of the identification of previously undetected, more advanced cancers (detection bias); subsequent screening would detect proportionally more cancers at earlier stages. Utilization of screening by migrants may also differ from that of the native-born population in the host country[22,57–59] and quality of denominator data for incidence computations vary across countries. An important consideration is whether the sources of the numerator data (usually cancer registries) and the denominator data (usually national censuses) use consistent definitions for the migrant population of interest.[17]

Bias in Mortality Comparisons

Because mortality reflects not only incidence but also treatment, survival, and competing causes of death, it is a poor measure of disease risks, except for highly fatal cancers. Considerations for mortality comparisons between countries include possible differences in accuracy of cause-of-death assignment, screening programs, access to medical care, quality of cancer treatment, available treatment modalities, and consequently survival rates.[17] Although health care in general might be better in the host country than the home county, migrants may experience cultural barriers or other obstacles that limit their access, leading to higher disease-specific mortality rates compared with those for their descendants[60] or the indigenous population.[61]

Selection Bias

Migrant populations are a nonrandom (self-selected) sample of the population of their country of origin. Selective migration is an important factor which may influence mortality or morbidity rates because migrants may be either more or less healthy than, or differ on other characteristics from, their non-migrant counterparts. They may derive disproportionately from a particular socioeconomic stratum: most often, migrants reflect a lower tier group seeking economic opportunity in the host country,[62,63] although sometimes they constitute a more educated group seeking better professional opportunities in the host country.[63] They may also reflect a religious or other persecuted group[24] and may come from a particular region of a country that has different cancer rates than the country as a whole. There may be undefined selection factors that influence the willingness to migrate as well as the levels of exposure to risk factors for cancer.

Confounding Factors

Several demographic variables recorded by cancer registries or on death certificates can be considered as confounders if they are related to both cancer risk and migrant status. This includes date of diagnosis/death, marital status, place of residence, and possibly ethnic group, occupation, or socioeconomic status (such as employment status, income, educational level, etc).[9] Migrants are rarely distributed homogeneously in their host county: they tend to settle in certain area, generally in urban areas, and the establishment of a migrant society in a place tends to draw later migrants to settle there. Social class and occupation are also known to be strong factors related to cancer risk, and it is often clear from census data that migrants are over-represented in specific occupational categories, and are atypical of the general population in their socioeconomic profile.[9]

Internal Migration

Selection Bias

Similar to international migrants, internal migrants are likely to be a selective group. For instance, the migrant population in China tends to be younger and is more likely to be male and single than the general population, although more women and families have also started to migrate in recent years and more people are settling in cities. Indicators of socioeconomic status place these migrants below the socioeconomic status of the urban population but above their rural counterparts.[64]

Bias in Incidence or Mortality Comparisons

Comparison of cancer rates within a country can utilize consistent sources for the numerator data and the denominator data. However, certain factors that affect cancer rates may vary between regions. There may be substantial difference in accessibility to medical care between rural and urban areas, and even among residents of the same urban area due to socioeconomic or other differences. Although they move to urban areas where more health care facilities are available, migrants often become the urban poor and they are largely excluded from urban public health services.[65] For instance, in China, the outsider status of migrants in the health care system of the cities and lack of medical insurance are widespread problems in migrant workers.[64]

▨ KNOWLEDGE GAINED FROM MIGRANT STUDIES

General Principles

The effect of internal and international migration on migrants' health is complex, and much variation exists among migrant groups. Many factors can influence the disease patterns of a particular migrant group, including the environments of the original and new countries, selection bias in those who choose to migrate, when the migration takes place (both age and calendar time), where the migrants originate, where they resettle, and even the process of migration itself.[8]

Findings from migration studies of cancer are site-specific. In general, incidence rates among migrants for any particular cancer shift toward the prevailing rates in the host country. Thus, migrants may benefit from a lower risk in the host region or country or, conversely, may suffer from a higher risk in the host locale.[17] An increased incidence of cancer in the host country implies that exposure to risk factors is higher in the host country than in the home country or, conversely, that exposure to protective factors is lower. Because generally the host country is more prosperous and has a higher standard of living than the home country (the most common reason for migration), changes in socioeconomic status should also be considered. An obvious area of dramatic changes in the lives of migrants relates to diet. Although overall food availability is usually greater in the host country, certain ethnic foods or other traditional recipe ingredients may not be readily available in the new setting. On the contrary, decreased incidence of cancer among migrants in the host country implies that exposures to risk factors are lower in the host country than in the home country, although greater exposure to protective factors could also contribute to the lower rates. For example, exposure to foods that increase cancer risk may be lower in the host country, and exposure to foods that are protective may be higher. Lower cancer rates could also reflect more intensive screening in the host country if the screening program identifies precursor lesions that can be treated definitively.[17]

Insights into changes in cancer risk and particularly the relative influence of acculturation on cancer pattern can be obtained by comparing generations of migrants in the host country and examining the effects of duration of residence in the host country and age at migration.[17] For a cancer with a higher incidence in the host country, cancer rates in the second generation of migrants would be expected to be higher than in the first generation because the first generation would have experienced the exposure levels of the lower-risk home country for a portion of their early lives (illustrated by breast cancer in Figure 2.3). First generation migrants with a longer time of residence in the host country would have greater cumulative exposure to risk factors in the new country and consequently higher incidence rates than shorter-term migrants (illustrated by malignant melanoma in Figure 2.4). The effect of age at migrant on cancer risk depends on the period of life when the influence of risk factors is greatest (illustrated by breast cancer in Figure 2.5). If the influence of a particular risk factor is greater during early life, migration during adulthood (most migrants are working-age

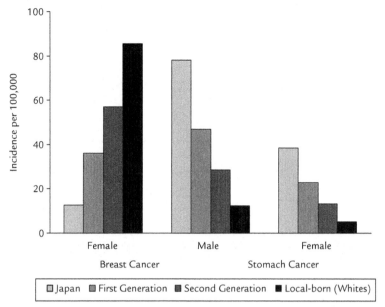

FIGURE 2.3 Typical patterns of change in cancer incidence among migrants populations: breast and stomach cancer in Japanese migrants to Hawaii. Rates for the period 1973–1977 were age-adjusted to the world standard population. Japanese rates are from the Osaka Prefecture registry. *(Source: Adapted[16,122])*

adults) would have less impact on the migrating generation and would result in a greater difference between first and second generation migrants in the host country. On the contrary, for a cancer with a lower incidence in the host country, one would expect rates to be higher in the first generation than in the second generation (illustrated by stomach cancer in Figure 2.3), to show continued declines with duration of residence among first generation migrants (illustrated by cervical cancer in Figure 2.4), and to be higher in individuals who migrated at later ages if an early period of life was critical for the effects of exposure.[17]

Cancer rates in migrants do not always fall between those in the native and the host countries. Although the change in incidence between home and host countries usually shows a gradual increase over several generations, in a few instances a more abrupt change can be seen, such that rates comparable to those prevailing in the host country are achieved in the first generation (illustrated by colon cancer in Figure 2.6). Many factors may account for these exceptions, including variations in genetic susceptibility to risk factors, and sociological variables such as educational and career opportunities.[17]

Site-Specific Observations

International Migration
The following review will focus on breast, prostate, and colorectal cancers that generally show an increased incidence among migrants in the host country, and stomach, lung, and cervical cancers for which rates generally decrease in the host country.

BREAST CANCER
Breast cancer is the most common non-skin cancer among women and displays marked variation by race and ethnicity.[66,67] While the relative importance of some of the risk factors

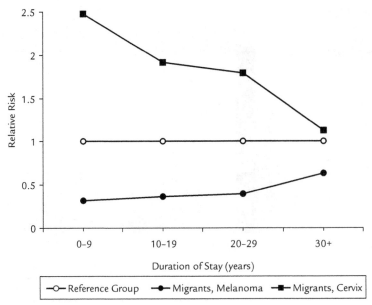

FIGURE 2.4 Effect of the duration of residence on cancer incidence in migrants: cervical cancer and cutaneous malignant melanoma in European migrants to Israel. Israeli-born residents were the reference group. *(Source: Adapted[119])*

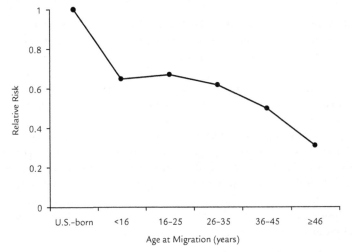

FIGURE 2.5 Effect of age at migration on cancer incidence in migrants: breast cancer risk in female migrants to the United States from Asia. US-born Asian women were the reference group. *(Source: Adapted[31])*

(e.g., family history, age at menarche) might be ethnicity-dependent,[68,69] findings from migrant studies typically relate most interethnic and international differences in rates to lifestyle or behavioral factors.[66]

Most studies of breast cancer incidence have entailed migrations from countries with lower rates to countries with higher rates.[17] The results showed that under these circumstances cancer incidence generally increased in the migrants to levels intermediate between

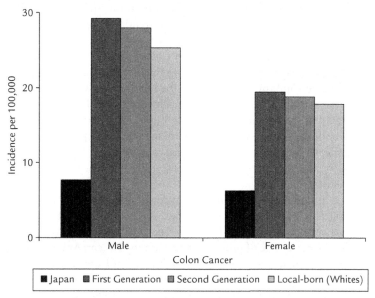

FIGURE 2.6 Unusual pattern of change in cancer incidence among migrant populations: colon cancer in Japanese migrants to Hawaii. Rates for the period 1973–1977 were age-adjusted to the world standard population. Japanese rates are from the Osaka Prefecture registry. *(Source: Adapted[16,122])*

the home and host countries. For example, Japanese migrants to Hawaii and California showed incidence rates that more than doubled in the first (migrating) generation compared with rates in Japan for the same period.[16] Rates increased further in the second generation, although they were still considerably lower (at all ages) than those for white women;[16] a similar pattern was reported for Chinese,[70] Korea,[71] and Asian Indian migrants[21] to the United States.

There are few examples for breast cancer of migrations from higher-risk to lower-risk countries. One study reported on migrants from the United Kingdom and Ireland, with higher incidence rates, to Australia, with lower incidence rates. The incidence of breast cancer among these migrants in Australia was 20% higher than that of native-born women.[23] A few exceptions, in which breast cancer incidence rates did not increase in migrants to higher-risk host countries, have been reported,[70,72,73] possibly reflecting slower acculturation to the new environment. Overall, these findings confirm the important influence of environmental, or exogenous, factors on breast cancer risk.

Age at migration showed an effect on breast cancer risk among Japanese,[30] Asian (Japanese, Chinese, Filipino),[31] and Hispanic migrants[28] to the United States; women who migrated at younger ages had a higher incidence rate than did those who migrated at later ages. Longer duration of residence in the host country was associated with an increased risk among Jewish migrants from Europe and North Africa to Israel[24] and Hispanic women in the United States.[28]

Mortality data have been examined often because incidence data were not available for the group of interest. However, because of the impact of mammography screening, treatment, and competing causes of death, the mortality data entail problems of interpretation. In a study of migrants to Australia and Canada from countries with higher breast cancer mortality rates than these two host countries, the investigators tended to find lower mortality rates than in the home country, whereas migrants from countries with lower mortality rates than Australia and Canada tended to show an opposite trend.[74] Japanese immigrants to Brazil showed breast cancer mortality intermediate between the home and host country.[75] Breast cancer mortality rates in Polish migrants to the United States,[76] England and Wales,[77] and Australia[75] were higher than those in Poland and similar to those of the native-born populations, whereas they were intermediate between the home and host countries in France.[78] In the latter study, the authors found that after adjusting for place of residence, age, and social status, the mortality rate was similar to that in the home, rather than the host, country.

Overall, the findings from previous studies confirm that both premigration and postmigration environmental exposures influence breast cancer risk.

PROSTATE CANCER

Migrations have primarily occurred to host countries with higher prostate cancer incidence rates than the migrants' home countries. Thus the rates among migrants were nearly always increased and generally were intermediate between the home and host countries.[21,73,79–84] For example, the incidence rate of prostate cancer among Korean Americans was four-fold higher than among their native counterparts in Korea, and was a quarter of that in US whites.[71] Chinese immigrants to Canada also showed an intermediate incidence rate between Canadian-born residents and Chinese living in Shanghai.[85]

Some exceptions to this pattern have been reported. In California, the incidence among Japanese and Spanish surnamed migrants was much higher than in the home countries, and was similar to that of US-born residents, suggesting the importance of environmental factors acting relatively later in life.[30] Similarly, in Canada, Asian Indian surnamed men showed a much higher incidence rate than did their counterparts in the home country, with the incidence similar to that of the general population in Canada.[86]

In Australia, the incidence of prostate cancer among migrants from certain Asian countries (Philippines, Indonesia, Hong Kong, Malaysia/Singapore) was already similar to that of native-born Australians within a couple of decades; however, this was not seen for migrants from other Asian countries (Vietnam, India/Sri Lanka, China/Taiwan).[63] In California, Filipino and Japanese men had a substantially higher incidence rate than did Vietnamese and Korean men[22]. This difference by country of origin could not be readily explained, although the migrants groups with the higher rates tended to be of higher socioeconomic standing, not generally a risk factor for prostate cancer, however. The risk of prostate cancer among migrants to Brazil from Italy, Spain, and Portugal was similar to that of the native-born white population of Brazil after adjusting for several variables (age, calendar period, social class, civil status, extent of histologic verification, proportion of death certificate-only cases).[87] First generation immigrants from Cuba and Puerto Rica living in Florida had prostate cancer incidence rates similar to whites, whereas Mexican immigrants showed a lower rate.[88] Both selection and detection bias may play an important role in these exceptions.

Prostate cancer incidence was 10-times higher in the first generation of Japanese migrants in Hawaii compared with the population in Japan, but was not further increased in the second generation; in both generations, the rates were much lower than among whites in Hawaii[16] The high rates in the first relative to the second generation may indicate detection bias, reflecting more intense screening in Hawaii than in Japan and the identification of previously undiagnosed cases. Longer duration of residence in the host country was associated with an increased risk of prostate cancer in Asian migrants to the United States,[25] in Jewish migrants from Europe to Israel[23], and in Latino immigrants to Sweden.[53] Unlike breast cancer, prostate cancer showed little effect of age at migrant in a study of Japanese and Hispanic migrants to California.[30]

Mortality data on prostate cancer present the same problems as breast cancer data, as this also is an organ site subject to screening. Although screening was primarily by digital rectal examination prior to the era of prostate-specific antigen (PSA) testing, the frequency and regularity of physician visits could have contributed to significant intercountry differences in state at diagnosis and thus to mortality from the disease.[17] Most migrants studied were from countries with lower prostate cancer mortality rates than the host countries, and for the most part their rates in the host countries were intermediate.[75,76,89–91]

COLON AND RECTAL CANCER

For colorectal cancer, although general trend has been for the rates of migrants to move to an intermediate level between the risks of the home and host countries, several groups exhibited a complete transition in risk to that of the host country. For example, first generation migrants to the United States and Australia from the low-risk countries of Japan, Poland, Scandinavia, Cuba, and Puerto Rica all showed colorectal cancer rates similar to those of the native-born population.[16,36,88,92,93] Because migration usually occurs during adulthood, this implies that an exposure later in life critically affects the risk of this cancer; it also implies that in migrant groups whose rates undergo a complete transition to the host country rates, acculturation occurs rather rapidly and/or the migrant population has a greater genetic susceptibility to the effects of the pertinent exposure.[17]

Among migrant groups displaying their complete transition, Japanese Americans have been studied most extensively. In a study of Japanese migrants to Hawaii, the incidence of colon cancer in the home country, Japan, was 25% that of whites in Hawaii, whereas the incidence for first generation migrants and their descendents was the same as, or slightly higher than, that of whites (Figure 2.6).[16] The increased rate in migrants was unlikely to be explained by a greater use of screening in the United States, as an autopsy study found that Japanese in Hawaii had a much higher prevalence of (asymptomatic) adenomatous polyps than Japanese in Japan.[94] More recent data also showed that Japanese living in Hawaii had a higher incidence of colon cancer than did the local whites.[95] Confirming the importance of the host country rates on the experience of migrants, the incidence of colon cancer among Japanese migrants to Brazil, a low-risk country, remained low.[80] Migrants to Israel from the Middle East/Asia showed a slight increase in colon cancer incidence with duration of residence, although their risk remained lower than that of the Israeli-born; in contrast, immigrants from Africa showed no convergence toward the host country rates.[24]

European and American migrants to Israel who lived on a kibbutz provide an example of a migrant population that experienced a decrease in the incidence of large bowel cancer; the colorectal cancer incidence among these migrants was much lower than that in either their home country or in the general Israeli population.[96]

The findings from mortality studies of colon and rectal cancers were largely consistent with those from the incidence studies. There was a shift in rates toward those prevailing in the host country, whether the migrants came from higher-risk or lower-risk countries. Similarly, duration of residence in the host country correlated with the extent of the changes.[26,27,43,97] Interestingly, studies of Polish migrants to several countries were relatively uniform in showing complete transition in their colon or colorectal cancer mortality rates to those of the host countries.[43,76,98,99] The consistent convergence in rates among Polish migrants suggests that they, along with the Japanese, may be particularly susceptible to the major risk factors for cancers of the large bowel. It seems unlikely that the mortality increase could be explained entirely by detection bias in the host countries or more accurate assignment of cause of deaths, as no increases were seen for rectal cancer. Furthermore, in one instance, the mortality results were confirmed with incidence data.[92]

STOMACH CANCER

Most investigations of stomach cancer in migrants have involved populations moving from high-risk areas to low-risk areas. The general pattern was for the risk among migrants to decrease toward that of the host country but to remain elevated.[17] For instance, the incidence rate among Korean Americans was around half that of the native population in Korea, but was still more than four-fold higher than among the US whites.[71] Complete transition to the rates of the host country often took two or more generations. The continued elevation in risk among first generation migrants could be accounted for by the lasting effect of an exposure early in life or by incomplete acculturation in the host country, although the former explanation has been favored. In a study of Japanese migrants to Hawaii, the investigators found that, compared to local whites, the risk of stomach cancer in the home country, Japan, was sevenfold higher, whereas the risk was fourfold higher in Japanese migrants and twofold higher in their descendants.[16] In a later calendar period, the elevation in rates among the descendants of high-risk migrant groups persisted for Japanese but not for Chinese in the United States.[38] Migration from Japan to Brazil, a medium risk country, also resulted in a decline in stomach cancer incidence to a level intermediate between the home and host countries, although the rates for Japanese migrants to Brazil were more than twofold higher than those for Japanese migrants to the United States, a low-risk country.[80] This example underscores the importance of the prevailing level of risk in the host country to the experience of the migrants. An exception to this pattern of convergence of risk was seen in migrants from Puerto Rico to New York City, among whom rates remained at the relatively high levels of the home country.[100-102] Because Puerto Rico is a US commonwealth, there is free movement between the two, which was suggested as a reason for the lack of convergence in this instance.

The effect of duration of residence was examined in migrants to Israel. Migrants from Europe and the former USSR showed a modest decrease in stomach cancer risk with longer duration in Israel, but those who migrated from the Middle East/Asia and Africa did not.[15,24]

As noted, several observations suggest that an exposure early in life has a lasting effect on the risk of stomach cancer. This is consistent with an etiologic role of Helicobactor pylori, because infection with this bacterium is usually acquired during childhood[102]; moreover, *H. pylori* prevalence varies geographically[80,104,105] and by ethnicity.[106]

Most mortality studies have also investigated migrants from high to low-risk areas, and generally found that the mortality rates of migrants moved toward that of the host country, in agreement with the studies of incidence. Because treatment of stomach cancer is not particularly effective, mortality rates are more useful indicators of risk for this cancer than for most others. Evidence of continued excess mortality was found among descendants of Japanese immigrants to the United States[89,107] and to Brazil,[75] of Italian immigrants to Canada,[108] and among the former Soviet Union migrants to Israel and Germany[54] but not of Chinese immigrants to the United States.[91] The complete transition to the prevailing host country rates in US-born Chinese may reflect a larger number of generations in the United States and a greater degree of acculturation compared with the other migrant group studies. The rates among migrants to Australia from higher-risk European countries decreased with longer residence but remained higher than the native-born rates.[26,43]

Mortality studies also showed that stomach cancer rates among low-risk migrants can increase upon migration to a high-risk area. The rates of immigrants to Argentina from Paraguay increased to an intermediate level.[5]

LUNG CANCER

Lung cancer rates have generally been higher in the host than the home country, and the incidence in the migrants most frequently was intermediate.[81-84,102] Lung cancer rates among migrant Indian women in four countries (India, Singapore, United Kingdom, and United States) were very different: compared to native Indians, lung cancer rates were 3 times higher among those in Singapore, 4 times higher among those in the United Kingdom and United States, and 16 times higher among US whites.[21] Several exceptions, in which higher incidence rates were seen in the migrants than in the native population of the host country, were reported from Australia. For example, the incidence of lung cancer among both male and female migrants from the United Kingdom was higher than among native-born Australians, which was not surprising, as lung cancer incidence in the United Kingdom exceeded that of the white population of Australia at the time.[23,62,109,110] Similarly, lung cancer incidence rates among females Chinese migrants from Asia to Australia were much higher than among the native-born Australia women,[62,63] which was also not unexpected, as Chinese women in Asia have particularly high rates of lung cancer (largely due to a disproportionately higher frequency of adenocarcinomas).[111]

In Hawaii, the incidence of lung cancer was compared between two generations of Japanese migrants. The rate in the first generation, for both males and females, was approximately double the rate in Japan, but the rate in the second generation was lower than in the first generation and not much higher than in Japan.[16]

Because tobacco smoking is a strong risk factor for lung cancer in most parts of the world, incidence rates in migrants can be assumed to reflect smoking behavior. The latency period between first exposure to tobacco smoke and the appearance of clinical disease is relatively long, so smoking habits prior to migration would be expected to have a major influence on the observed incidence of lung cancer among first generation migrants in the host country.[17] Thus, observations of higher incidence rates of lung cancer among migrants to Australia from the United Kingdom[23,62,109,110] and to England/Wales from Scotland and Ireland[112] could be accounted for by the higher prevalence of smoking in the migrants compared with the native-born populations.[23,112] In some instance, however, the observed difference in lung cancer rates between migrants and local-born populations could not be explained by smoking differences, but data on smoking prior to migration were not available.[46,62,63,113,114] Differences in patterns of smoking or in susceptibility to the carcinogens in tobacco smoke between migrants and native population might also contribute to such discrepancies.[115,116]

Because routine screening for lung cancer is uncommon and the disease is highly fatal, mortality data on lung cancer show relations similar to those for incidence. For example, Chinese female migrants in Australia had higher lung cancer mortality than local-born Australia women,[117] thus paralleling the incidence findings noted above.[62,63] Similarly, Italian migrants to Canada had lower mortality from lung cancer than other Canadian-born residents,[108] as was found in another study based on incidence.[46] Finally, the observation of higher lung cancer incidence in first than in second generation Japanese migrants to Hawaii[16] was reflected in mortality data for first and second generation Japanese and Chinese migrants in the United States.[118]

CERVICAL CANCER

Migration has generally occurred from countries at high risk for cervical cancer to those at lower risk. Almost universally, the risk among migrants declined to levels intermediate between the home and host countries.[17] In Korean Americans, cervical cancer incidence decreased to less than 50% of that in the native population in Korea but was still slightly higher than that of US whites.[71] Among migrants living in the low-risk host country of Israel, longer duration of residence was associated with a lower incidence of cervical cancer.[15,24]

The incidence of cervical cancer in US-born Japanese women was similar to that in US whites and was less than half that of Japanese migrants.[16] The general decrease in risk among migrants has been attributed to increased cytologic screening,[119] leading to definitive treatment of precancerous lesions and possibly to reduced prevalence of human papilomavirus infection as a result of changes in sexual practices in the host country. Among Asian ethnic groups in the United States, large variation existed in cervical cancer incidence: Vietnamese women had the highest and Asian Indian/Pakistani women had the lowest rate, compared to Chinese, Filipino, Japanese, and Korean women.[120] This was attributed partly to the fact that immigration histories and screening behaviors vary across these ethnic groups.[22]

An exception to the usual trend was seen in migrants from the Indian subcontinent to England,[81,121] Australia,[63] and the Unites States,[21] who had lower incidence rate for cervical cancer than the host populations, as well as their home populations. Selection bias may have accounted for this finding.

Internal Migration

Since studies on internal migration and cancer rates have been performed in only a small number of countries, the following summaries are organized by country, instead of by cancer site.

Several interesting studies on internal migrants have been conducted in Italy. Women who migrated from the low-risk south to the higher-risk north showed increased incidence rates for intestinal, breast, and tobacco-related tumors, although migration in the reverse direction did not reduce cancer incidence.[2] Based on mortality data, it appeared that various environmental factors and/or genetic elements must influence the risk of different cancers after migration, not only between the north and the south, but also among provinces.[8] For lung and stomach cancer, place of birth in Italy rather than place of residence was a major risk indicator.[4] The authors reported that dietary habits in the first years of life may have induced an increased risk that could not be reversed by subsequent dietary changes. However, for colorectal cancer mortality, place of residence was found to be a stronger predictor than was place of birth in Italy.[5]

Stomach cancer mortality varied from place to place within England and Wales, and the proportional mortality was more closely related to county of birth.[1] This association was found in migrants both out of, and into, high-risk areas.

In the United States, striking differences in cancer mortality were found between southern-born blacks who moved to New Jersey and those born in New Jersey.[6] Southern-born black male and female migrants had an all-cancer mortality rate 31% and 10% higher, respectively, than their New Jersey counterparts. In particular, the Southern-born blacks showed significantly higher rates for cancers of the cervix, esophagus, male lung, prostate, and stomach than did the New Jersey-born blacks.

In Finland, a clear dose-response relation was found between occupational exposures and lung cancer among migrant workers but not among the native urban dwellers. The lung cancer risk of migrant men who worked in heavily exposed industries was more than twice that of native urban men in similar jobs.[3] The authors speculated that although the joint effect of smoking and occupational exposure was the main explanatory factor for high risk of lung cancer in migrant males, environmental and psychosocial factors also might have a contributory effect.

A study in Spain showed that internal migrants had less access to preventive services, such as cervical cancer screening, which was almost completely accounted for by their lower socioeconomic status. Thus, migration can be seen as a social factor that puts people at risk of falling into lower socioeconomic status leading to poor access to screening.[7]

CONCLUSIONS

Past studies of migrants have contributed essential information to research on the etiology of cancer. Foremost, they have shown the dominant role of environmental factors in determining cancer risk. New opportunities for research have resulted from recent internal migrations in many countries, particularly low- and middle-income countries in Asia. Studies in these migrant groups can be strengthened if comprehensive lifestyle information, such as dietary and physical activity practices, can be collected at the group or individual level, as well as data on other variables necessary to control for confounding in the analyses.

SUMMARY

Migration between countries or other geographically separated areas often leads to extreme changes in exposures to risk factors for disease, and, consequently, to different disease rates in the migrants and their descendants from the prevailing rates in the home country. The substantial changes in rates of different cancers among migrants over relatively short time intervals have been widely used to assess the relative importance of environmental factors versus inherited predisposition in cancer etiology. Various types of migration studies have been conducted, including comparisons of groups with the same origin but different living environments; comparison of groups with different origins but the same living environment; and comparisons within migrant groups by migration-related factors. Several methodological issues arise in migrant studies, including bias in incidence or mortality comparisons across countries, selection bias, and confounding factors that are related to both cancer risk and migrant status. Although findings from migration studies of cancer vary by site, in general, the incidence rates among migrants shift toward the prevailing rates in the host country. For example, breast cancer incidence rates in female migrants to the United States (most of whom arrived from countries with relatively low rates) increased to levels intermediate between the risks of the home and host countries, whereas cervical cancer rates (which were usually high in their native countries) declined in the US to levels intermediate between the home and host countries. Past studies of migrants have contributed essential information to research on the etiology of cancer, particularly showing the dominant role of environmental factors in determining cancer risk. New opportunities for research have resulted from recent internal migrations in many countries, especially low- and middle-income countries in Asia. Studies in these migrant groups can be strengthened if comprehensive information on lifestyle factors and potential confounders could be available at the group or individual level.

REFERENCES

1. Coggon D, Osmond C, Barker DJ. Stomach cancer and migration within England and Wales. *Br J Cancer.* 1990;61(4):573–574.
2. Rosso S, Patriarca S, Vicari P, Zanetti R. Cancer incidence in Turin: The effect of migration. *Tumori.* 1993;79(5):304–310.
3. Tenkanen L. Migration to towns, occupation, smoking, and lung cancer: Experience from the Finnish-Norwegian lung cancer study. *Cancer Causes Control.* 1993;4(2):133–141.
4. Ceppi M, Vercelli M, Decarli A, Puntoni R. The mortality rate of the province of birth as a risk indicator for lung and stomach cancer mortality among Genoa residents born in other Italian provinces. *Eur J Cancer.* 1995;31A(2):193–197.
5. Fascioli S, Capocaccia R, Mariotti S. Cancer mortality in migrant populations within Italy. *Int J Epidemiol.* 1995;24(1):8–18.
6. Greenberg M, Schneider D. Migration and the cancer burden of New Jersey blacks. *N J Med.* 1995;92(8):509–511.

7. Sanchez V, Rohlfs I, Borras JM, Borrell C. Migration within Spain, level of education, and cervical cancer screening. *Eur J Cancer Prev.* 1997;6(1):31–37.

8. McKay L, Macintyre S, Ellaway A. Migration and health: A review of the international literature. Glasgow: Medical Research Council; 2003;MRC Social & Public Health Science Unit, Occasional Paper No.12.

9. Parkin DM, Khlat M. Studies of cancer in migrants: Rationale and methodology. *Eur J Cancer.* 1996;32A(5):761–771.

10. United Nations, Department of Economic and Social Affairs, Population Division. International migration report 2006: A global assessment. New York: United Nations; 2009.

11. International Organization for Migration. Facts & figures. http://www.iom.int/jahia.Jahia/about-migration/facts-and-figures/lang/en. Updated 2010. Accessed 05/03, 2010.

12. Hammar T. *International migration, immobility and development: Multidisciplinary perspectives.* Oxford; New York: Berg; 1997:x, 316 p.

13. Prentice RL, Sheppard L. Validity of international, time trend, and migrant studies of dietary factors and disease risk. *Prev Med.* 1989;18(2):167–179.

14. Marchand LL. Combined influence of genetic and dietary factors on colorectal cancer incidence in Japanese Americans. *J Natl Cancer Inst Monogr.* 1999;(26)(26):101–105.

15. Iscovich J, Howe GR. Cancer incidence patterns (1972–91) among migrants from the Soviet Union to Israel. *Cancer Causes Control.* 1998;9(1):29–36.

16. Kolonel LN, Hinds MW, Hankin JH. Cancer patterns among migrants and native-born Japanese in Hawaii in relation to smoking, drinking, and dietary habits. In: Gelboin HV, MacMahon B, Matsuchima T, Sugimura T, Takayama S, Takebe H, eds. *Genetic and environmental factors in experimental and human cancer.* Tokyo: Japan Scientific Societies Press; 1980:327–340.

17. Kolonel LN, Wilkens LR. Migrant studies. In: Schottenfeld D, Fraumeni JF, eds. *Cancer epidemiology and prevention.* 3rd ed. New York: Oxford University Press; 2006:xviii, 1392 p.

18. Deshingkar P, Grimm S. Internal migration and development: A global perspective. Geneva: International Organization for Migration; 2005;19.

19. Ping H, Shaohua Z. Internal migration in China: Linking it with development. Paper for Regional Conference on Migration and Development in Asia; Lanzhou, China. 2005.

20. Lu Y. Test of the 'healthy migrant hypothesis': A longitudinal analysis of health selectivity of internal migration in Indonesia. *Soc Sci Med.* 2008;67(8):1331–1339.

21. Rastogi T, Devesa S, Mangtani P, et al. Cancer incidence rates among south Asians in four geographic regions: India, Singapore, UK and US. *Int J Epidemiol.* 2008;37(1):147–160.

22. McCracken M, Olsen M, Chen MS, Jr, et al. Cancer incidence, mortality, and associated risk factors among Asian Americans of Chinese, Filipino, Vietnamese, Korean, and Japanese ethnicities. *CA Cancer J Clin.* 2007;57(4):190–205.

23. McMichael AJ, Giles GG. Cancer in migrants to Australia: Extending the descriptive epidemiological data. *Cancer Res.* 1988;48(3):751–756.

24. Parkin DM, Steinitz R, Khlat M, Kaldor J, Katz L, Young J. Cancer in Jewish migrants to Israel. *Int J Cancer.* 1990;45(4):614–621.

25. Whittemore AS, Kolonel LN, Wu AH, et al. Prostate cancer in relation to diet, physical activity, and body size in blacks, whites, and Asians in the United States and Canada. *J Natl Cancer Inst.* 1995;87(9):652–661.

26. McCredie M, Williams S, Coates M. Cancer mortality in migrants from the British isles and continental Europe to New South Wales, Australia, 1975–1995. *Int J Cancer.* 1999;83(2):179–185.

27. McCredie M, Williams S, Coates M. Cancer mortality in east and southeast Asian migrants to New South Wales, Australia, 1975–1995. *Br J Cancer.* 1999;79(7–8):1277–1282.

28. John EM, Phipps AI, Davis A, Koo J. Migration history, acculturation, and breast cancer risk in Hispanic women. *Cancer Epidemiol Biomarkers Prev.* 2005;14(12):2905–2913.

29. Norredam M, Krasnik A, Pipper C, Keiding N. Cancer incidence among 1st generation migrants compared to native Danes—a retrospective cohort study. *Eur J Cancer.* 2007;43(18):2717–2721.

30. Shimizu H, Ross RK, Bernstein L, Yatani R, Henderson BE, Mack TM. Cancers of the prostate and breast among Japanese and white immigrants in Los Angeles county. *Br J Cancer.* 1991;63(6): 963–966.

31. Ziegler RG, Hoover RN, Pike MC, et al. Migration patterns and breast cancer risk in Asian-American women. *J Natl Cancer Inst.* 1993;85(22):1819–1827.

32. McCormack VA, Mangtani P, Bhakta D, McMichael AJ, dos Santos Silva I. Heterogeneity of breast cancer risk within the south Asian female population in England: A population-based case-control study of first-generation migrants. *Br J Cancer.* 2004;90(1):160–166.

33. Azerkan F, Zendehdel K, Tillgren P, Faxelid E, Sparen P. Risk of cervical cancer among immigrants by age at immigration and follow-up time in Sweden, from 1968 to 2004. *Int J Cancer.* 2008;123(11):2664–2670.

34. Shimizu H, Mack TM, Ross RK, Henderson BE. Cancer of the gastrointestinal tract among Japanese and white immigrants in Los Angeles county. *J Natl Cancer Inst.* 1987;78(2):223–228.

35. Herrinton LJ, Stanford JL, Schwartz SM, Weiss NS. Ovarian cancer incidence among Asian migrants to the United States and their descendants. *J Natl Cancer Inst.* 1994;86(17):1336–1339.

36. Flood DM, Weiss NS, Cook LS, Emerson JC, Schwartz SM, Potter JD. Colorectal cancer incidence in Asian migrants to the United States and their descendants. *Cancer Causes Control.* 2000;11(5):403–411.

37. Stirbu I, Kunst AE, Vlems FA, et al. Cancer mortality rates among first and second generation migrants in the Netherlands: Convergence toward the rates of the native Dutch population. *Int J Cancer.* 2006;119(11):2665–2672.

38. Kamineni A, Williams MA, Schwartz SM, Cook LS, Weiss NS. The incidence of gastric carcinoma in Asian migrants to the United States and their descendants. *Cancer Causes Control.* 1999;10(1):77–83.

39. Akazaki K, Stemmerman GN. Comparative study of latent carcinoma of the prostate among Japanese in Japan and Hawaii. *J Natl Cancer Inst.* 1973;50(5):1137–1144.

40. Correa P, Sasano N, Stemmermann GN, Haenszel W. Pathology of gastric carcinoma in Japanese populations: Comparisons between Miyagi prefecture, Japan, and Hawaii. *J Natl Cancer Inst.* 1973;51(5):1449–1459.

41. Yanagihara ET, Blaisdell RK, Hayashi T, Lukes RJ. Malignant lymphoma in Hawaii-Japanese: A retrospective morphologic survey. *Hematol Oncol.* 1989;7(3):219–232.

42. Herrinton LJ, Goldoft M, Schwartz SM, Weiss NS. The incidence of non-Hodgkin's lymphoma and its histologic subtypes in Asian migrants to the united states and their descendants. *Cancer Causes Control.* 1996;7(2):224–230.

43. McMichael AJ, McCall MG, Hartshorne JM, Woodings TL. Patterns of gastro-intestinal cancer in European migrants to Australia: The role of dietary change. *Int J Cancer.* 1980;25(4):431–437.

44. Haenszel W, Berg JW, Segi M, Kurihara M, Locke FB. Large-bowel cancer in Hawaiian Japanese. *J Natl Cancer Inst.* 1973;51(6):1765–1779.

45. Holman CD, Armstrong BK. Cutaneous malignant melanoma and indicators of total accumulated exposure to the sun: An analysis separating histogenetic types. *J Natl Cancer Inst.* 1984;73(1):75–82.

46. Terracini B, Siemiatycki J, Richardson L. Cancer incidence and risk factors among Montréal residents of Italian origin. *Int J Epidemiol.* 1990;19(3):491–497.

47. Whittemore AS, Wu-Williams AH, Lee M, et al. Diet, physical activity, and colorectal cancer among Chinese in North America and China. *J Natl Cancer Inst.* 1990;82(11):915–926.

48. Brown LM, Gridley G, Wu AH, et al. Low level alcohol intake, cigarette smoking and risk of breast cancer in Asian-American women. *Breast Cancer Res Treat.* 2010;120(1):203–210.

49. Stemmermann GN. The pathology of breast cancer in Japanese women compared to other ethnic groups: A review. *Breast Cancer Res Treat.* 1991;18 Suppl 1:S67–S72.

50. Swerdlow A. Mortality and cancer incidence in Vietnamese refugees in England and Wales: A follow-up study. *Int J Epidemiol.* 1991;20(1):13–19.

51. Monroe KR, Hankin JH, Pike MC, et al. Correlation of dietary intake and colorectal cancer incidence among Mexican-American migrants: The multiethnic cohort study. *Nutr Cancer.* 2003;45(2):133–147.

52. Norredam M, Krasnik A, Pipper C, Keiding N. Differences in stage of disease between migrant women and native Danish women diagnosed with cancer: Results from a population-based cohort study. *Eur J Cancer Prev.* 2008;17(3):185–190.

53. Beiki O, Ekbom A, Allebeck P, Moradi T. Risk of prostate cancer among Swedish-born and foreign-born men in Sweden, 1961–2004. *Int J Cancer.* 2009;124(8):1941–1953.
54. Ronellenfitsch U, Kyobutungi C, Ott JJ, et al. Stomach cancer mortality in two large cohorts of migrants from the former Soviet Union to Israel and Germany: Are there implications for prevention? *Eur J Gastroenterol Hepatol.* 2009;21(4):409–416.
55. Winkler V, Ott JJ, Holleczek B, Stegmaier C, Becher H. Cancer profile of migrants from the former Soviet Union in Germany: Incidence and mortality. *Cancer Causes Control.* 2009;20(10):1873–1879.
56. Weber MF, Banks E, Smith DP, O'Connell D, Sitas F. Cancer screening among migrants in an Australian cohort; cross-sectional analyses from the 45 and up study. *BMC Public Health.* 2009;9:144.
57. Kagawa-Singer M, Pourat N. Asian American and Pacific Islander breast and cervical carcinoma screening rates and healthy people 2000 objectives. *Cancer.* 2000;89(3):696–705.
58. Maxwell AE, Crespi CM. Trends in colorectal cancer screening utilization among ethnic groups in California: Are we closing the gap? *Cancer Epidemiol Biomarkers Prev.* 2009;18(3):752–759.
59. Vermeer B, Van den Muijsenbergh ME. The attendance of migrant women at the national breast cancer screening in the Netherlands 1997–2008. *Eur J Cancer Prev.* 2010;19(3):195–198.
60. Chuang SC, Chen W, Hashibe M, Li G, Zhang ZF. Survival rates of invasive breast cancer among ethnic Chinese women born in East Asia and the United States. *Asian Pac J Cancer Prev.* 2006;7(2):221–226.
61. Uiters E, Deville W, Foets M, Spreeuwenberg P, Groenewegen PP. Differences between immigrant and non-immigrant groups in the use of primary medical care; a systematic review. *BMC Health Serv Res.* 2009;9:76.
62. McCredie M, Coates MS, Ford JM. Cancer incidence in migrants to New South Wales. *Int J Cancer.* 1990;46(2):228–232.
63. Grulich AE, McCredie M, Coates M. Cancer incidence in Asian migrants to New South Wales, Australia. *Br J Cancer.* 1995;71(2):400–408.
64. Hu X, Cook S, Salazar MA. Internal migration and health in China. *Lancet.* 2008;372(9651):1717–1719.
65. Song S, Zhu E. Urban poor in China. *The Chinese Economy.* 2009;42:44–62.
66. Andreeva VA, Unger JB, Pentz MA. Breast cancer among immigrants: A systematic review and new research directions. *J Immigr Minor Health.* 2007;9(4):307–322.
67. American Cancer Society. Cancer facts & figures 2009. Atlanta: American Cancer Society, Inc.; 2009.
68. Nomura AM, Lee J, Kolonel LN, Hirohata T. Breast cancer in two populations with different levels of risk for the disease. *Am J Epidemiol.* 1984;119(4):496–502.
69. Pike MC, Kolonel LN, Henderson BE, et al. Breast cancer in a multiethnic cohort in Hawaii and Los Angeles: Risk factor-adjusted incidence in Japanese equals and in Hawaiians exceeds that in whites. *Cancer Epidemiol Biomarkers Prev.* 2002;11(9):795–800.
70. Stanford JL, Herrinton LJ, Schwartz SM, Weiss NS. Breast cancer incidence in Asian migrants to the United States and their descendants. *Epidemiology.* 1995;6(2):181–183.
71. Lee J, Demissie K, Lu SE, Rhoads GG. Cancer incidence among Korean-American immigrants in the United States and native Koreans in South Korea. *Cancer Control.* 2007;14(1):78–85.
72. Kolonel LN. Cancer incidence among Filipinos in Hawaii and the Philippines. *Natl Cancer Inst Monogr.* 1985;69:93–98.
73. Minami Y, Staples MP, Giles GG. The incidence of colon, breast and prostate cancer in Italian migrants to Victoria, Australia. *Eur J Cancer.* 1993;29A(12):1735–1740.
74. Kliewer EV, Smith KR. Breast cancer mortality among immigrants in Australia and Canada. *J Natl Cancer Inst.* 1995;87(15):1154–1161.
75. Iwasaki M, Mameri CP, Hamada GS, Tsugane S. Cancer mortality among Japanese immigrants and their descendants in the state of Sao Paulo, Brazil, 1999–2001. *Jpn J Clin Oncol.* 2004;34(11):673–680.
76. Staszewski J, Haenszel W. Cancer mortality among the Polish-born in the United States. *J Natl Cancer Inst.* 1965;35(2):291–297.
77. Adelstein AM, Staszewski J, Muir CS. Cancer mortality in 1970–1972 among Polish-born migrants to England and Wales. *Br J Cancer.* 1979;40(3):464–475.

78. Tyczynski J, Parkin D, Zatonski W, Tarkowski W. Cancer mortality among Polish migrants to France. *Bull Cancer*. 1992;79(8):789–800.

79. Dunn JE. Cancer epidemiology in populations of the United States—with emphasis on Hawaii and California—and Japan. *Cancer Res*. 1975;35(11 Pt. 2):3240–3245.

80. Tsugane S, de Souza JM, Costa ML, Jr, et al. Cancer incidence rates among Japanese immigrants in the city of Sao Paulo, Brazil, 1969–78. *Cancer Causes Control*. 1990;1(2):189–193.

81. Winter H, Cheng KK, Cummins C, Maric R, Silcocks P, Varghese C. Cancer incidence in the south Asian population of England (1990–92). *Br J Cancer*. 1999;79(3–4):645–654.

82. Le GM, Gomez SL, Clarke CA, Glaser SL, West DW. Cancer incidence patterns among Vietnamese in the United States and Ha Noi, Vietnam. *Int J Cancer*. 2002;102(4):412–417.

83. Gomez SL, Le GM, Clarke CA, Glaser SL, France AM, West DW. Cancer incidence patterns in Koreans in the US and in Kangwha, South Korea. *Cancer Causes Control*. 2003;14(2):167–174.

84. Mousavi SM, Brandt A, Weires M, Ji J, Sundquist J, Hemminki K. Cancer incidence among Iranian immigrants in Sweden and Iranian residents compared to the native Swedish population. *Eur J Cancer*. 2010;46(3):599–605.

85. Luo W, Birkett NJ, Ugnat AM, Mao Y. Cancer incidence patterns among Chinese immigrant populations in Alberta. *J Immigr Health*. 2004;6(1):41–48.

86. Hislop TG, Bajdik CD, Saroa SR, Yeole BB, Barroetavena MC. Cancer incidence in Indians from three areas: Delhi and Mumbai, India, and British Columbia, Canada. *J Immigr Minor Health*. 2007;9(3):221–227.

87. Bouchardy C, Khlat M, Mirra AP, Parkin DM. Cancer risks among European migrants in Sao Paulo, Brazil. *Eur J Cancer*. 1993;29A(10):1418–1423.

88. Pinheiro PS, Sherman RL, Trapido EJ, et al. Cancer incidence in first generation U.S. Hispanics: Cubans, Mexicans, Puerto Ricans, and new Latinos. *Cancer Epidemiol Biomarkers Prev*. 2009;18(8):2162–2169.

89. Haenszel W, Kurihara M. Studies of Japanese migrants. I. mortality from cancer and other diseases among Japanese in the United States. *J Natl Cancer Inst*. 1968;40(1):43–68.

90. De Stefani E, Parkin DM, Khlat M, Vassallo A, Abella M. Cancer in migrants to Uruguay. *Int J Cancer*. 1990;46(2):233–237.

91. Hanley AJ, Choi BC, Holowaty EJ. Cancer mortality among Chinese migrants: A review. *Int J Epidemiol*. 1995;24(2):255–265.

92. Kune S, Kune GA, Watson L. The Melbourne colorectal cancer study: Incidence findings by age, sex, site, migrants and religion. *Int J Epidemiol*. 1986;15(4):483–493.

93. Moradi T, Delfino RJ, Bergstrom SR, Yu ES, Adami HO, Yuen J. Cancer risk among Scandinavian immigrants in the US and Scandinavian residents compared with US whites, 1973–89. *Eur J Cancer Prev*. 1998;7(2):117–125.

94. Stemmermann GN, Yatani R. Diverticulosis and polyps of the large intestine. A necropsy study of Hawaii Japanese. *Cancer*. 1973;31(5):1260–1270.

95. Curado MP, International Agency for Research on Cancer., International Association of Cancer Registries. *Cancer incidence in five continents, volume IX*. Lyon :Geneva: International Agency for Research on Cancer ;Distributed by WHO Press, World Health Organization; 2008.

96. Rozen P, Hellerstein SM, Horwitz C. The low incidence of colorectal cancer in a "high-risk" population: Its correlation with dietary habits. *Cancer*. 1981;48(12):2692–2695.

97. Geddes M, Balzi D, Buiatti E, Khlat M, Parkin D. Cancer in Italian migrants. *Cancer Causes Control*. 1991;2(2):133–140.

98. Newman AM, Spengler RF. Cancer mortality among immigrant populations in Ontario, 1969 through 1973. *Can Med Assoc J*. 1984;130(4):399–405.

99. Matos EL, Khlat M, Loria DI, Vilensky M, Parkin DM. Cancer in migrants to Argentina. *Int J Cancer*. 1991;49(6):805–811.

100. Warshauer ME, Silverman DT, Schottenfeld D, Pollack ES. Stomach and colorectal cancers in Puerto Rican-born residents of New York City. *J Natl Cancer Inst*. 1986;76(4):591–595.

101. Menendez-Bergad B, Blum S. Stomach cancer in a native and migrant population in Puerto Rico and New York City, 1975 to 1979. *Bol Asoc Med P R*. 1989;81(3):95–98.

102. Polednak AP. Cancer incidence in the Puerto Rican-born population of Long Island, New York. *Am J Public Health.* 1991;81(11):1405–1407.

103. Malaty HM, El-Kasabany A, Graham DY, et al. Age at acquisition of helicobacter pylori infection: A follow-up study from infancy to adulthood. *Lancet.* 2002;359(9310):931–935.

104. Graham DY, Malaty HM, Evans DG, Evans DJ, Jr, Klein PD, Adam E. Epidemiology of helicobacter pylori in an asymptomatic population in the united states. Effect of age, race, and socioeconomic status. *Gastroenterology.* 1991;100(6):1495–1501.

105. Zhang L, Blot WJ, You WC, et al. Helicobacter pylori antibodies in relation to precancerous gastric lesions in a high-risk Chinese population. *Cancer Epidemiol Biomarkers Prev.* 1996;5(8):627–630.

106. Graham DY, Klein PD, Opekun AR, et al. Epidemiology of campylobacter pylori infection: Ethnic considerations. *Scand J Gastroenterol Suppl.* 1988;142:9–13.

107. Buell P, Dunn JE, Jr. Cancer mortality among Japanese Issei and Nisei of California. *Cancer.* 1965;18:656–664.

108. Balzi D, Geddes M, Brancker A, Parkin DM. Cancer mortality in Italian migrants and their offspring in Canada. *Cancer Causes Control.* 1995;6(1):68–74.

109. McMichael AJ, Bonett A, Roder D. Cancer incidence among migrant populations in South Australia. *Med J Aust.* 1989;150(8):417–420.

110. McCredie M, Coates MS, Ford JM. Cancer incidence in migrants to New South Wales from England, Wales, Scotland and Ireland. *Br J Cancer.* 1990;62(6):992–995.

111. Gao YT, Blot WJ, Zheng W, et al. Lung cancer among Chinese women. *Int J Cancer.* 1987;40(5):604–609.

112. Harding S, Rosato M. Cancer incidence among first generation Scottish, Irish, West Indian and South Asian migrants living in England and Wales. *Ethn Health.* 1999;4(1–2):83–92.

113. McCredie M, Coates M, Grulich A. Cancer incidence in migrants to New South Wales (Australia) from the Middle East, 1972–91. *Cancer Causes Control.* 1994;5(5):414–421.

114. Raz DJ, Gomez SL, Chang ET, et al. Epidemiology of non-small cell lung cancer in Asian Americans: Incidence patterns among six subgroups by nativity. *J Thorac Oncol.* 2008;3(12):1391–1397.

115. Stephens EA, Taylor JA, Kaplan N, et al. Ethnic variation in the CYP2E1 gene: Polymorphism analysis of 695 African-Americans, European-Americans and Taiwanese. *Pharmacogenetics.* 1994;4(4):185–192.

116. Le Marchand L, Donlon T, Lum-Jones A, Seifried A, Wilkens LR. Association of the hOGG1 Ser326Cys polymorphism with lung cancer risk. *Cancer Epidemiol Biomarkers Prev.* 2002;11(4):409–412.

117. Zhang YQ, MacLennan R, Berry G. Mortality of Chinese in New South Wales, 1969–1978. *Int J Epidemiol.* 1984;13(2):188–192.

118. Thomas DB, Karagas MR. Cancer in first and second generation Americans. *Cancer Res.* 1987;47(21):5771–5776.

119. Steinitz R, Parkin DM, Young JL, Bieber CA, Katz L. Cancer incidence in Jewish migrants to Israel, 1961–1981. *IARC Sci Publ.* 1989;(98)(98):1–311.

120. Wang SS, Carreon JD, Gomez SL, Devesa SS. Cervical cancer incidence among 6 Asian ethnic groups in the United States, 1996 through 2004. *Cancer.* 2010;116(4):949–956.

121. Barker RM, Baker MR. Incidence of cancer in Bradford Asians. *J Epidemiol Community Health.* 1990;44(2):125–129.

122. Waterhouse J, Muir CS, Shanmugaratnam K, Powell J. Cancer incidence in five continents, IV. Lyon, France: International Agency for Research on Cancer; 1982;*IARC Scientific Publications* No. 42.

CHAPTER 3

OPPORTUNITIES FOR MOLECULAR PATHOLOGY RESEARCH

KELLY HIRKO, MARIA INIESTA DOÑATE,
SOFIA D. MERAJVER

INTRODUCTION

An individual's whole-genome code is known to confer susceptibility or resistance to multiple diseases, cancer among them. In the course of the lifespan, starting in utero, environmental factors influence cancer risk through interactions with human tissues and with the genomic material. Furthermore, the timing diversity, and complexity of multiple exposures would influence cancer risk, with some periods being especially critical for increased susceptibility. Understanding the cellular and molecular pathways involved from exposure to carcinogens to cancer is a major challenge in cancer research.

Epidemiologic research has historically focused primarily on the association between exposure and disease risk. Increasingly, however, the focus has enlarged recently to include research on the etiologic mechanisms linking exposure to disease and that branch of the discipline is currently referred to as "molecular epidemiology." Molecular epidemiology has opened up the "black box" that comprises the integrated genotypic and phenotypic events and pathways from exposure to disease, by carefully examining the broad array of intermediate events between exposure and disease occurrence or progression.[1] To this end, the focus of the work of modern molecular epidemiology involves the integration and interrelationships of biologic measures of exposures, genetic susceptibility, and outcomes[1]. The identification of specific factors on the disease pathway influencing risk and susceptibility to disease furthers our understanding of the overall disease process and operationally suggests potential targets for prevention research.

Molecular epidemiology in cancer research accomplishes the merging of molecular biology and epidemiology in the study of the causation of cancer and of tissue conditions that are antecedents to cancer to positively impact cancer prevention.[2] This field was introduced in the early 1980s by Perera and Weinstein, who described it as "an approach in which advanced laboratory methods are used in combination with analytical epidemiology to identify at the biochemical or molecular level specific exogenous agents and/or host factors that play a role in human cancer causation."[2] This work provided an initial robust framework for the application of novel molecular techniques to aid in the detection of carcinogens and host factors that may modify susceptibility to them. By combining

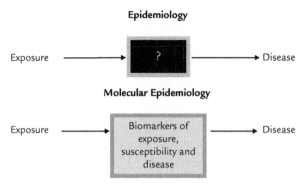

FIGURE 3.1 From "black box" to the "modern" molecular epidemiology.

epidemiological methods with laboratory procedures that assay for cellular and biochemical markers of host susceptibility, carcinogens and their metabolites, as well as for early human responses to carcinogens, researchers are now able to predict cancer risks more precisely than ever.

The main goal of this discipline is to contribute to the prevention of cancer by multiple avenues, notably by the following main goals: (1) providing evidence that specific environmental agents pose human carcinogenic hazards, (2) establishing their mechanisms, of causation of cancer, (3) identifying specific subpopulations who are at special risk and stratifying the risk levels of the whole population, and (4) using this information to suggest or to develop new and more effective strategies to reduce risk.[3] All of these goals provide evidence for the enormous potential of molecular epidemiology in cancer prevention through the early identification of "at risk" populations and the rapid assessment of intervention efficacy.[4] Molecular epidemiologic research has flourished during the last decade and is now widely recognized as an independent and rich discipline.

▪ BIOMARKERS

In the context of epidemiological studies, a biomarker is defined as a substance, structure, or process that (1) can be measured in the human body or its products and (2) may influence the incidence or outcome of disease in human populations.[5] Biomarkers can be effectively used in multiple roles: before cancer diagnosis in risk assessment and screening, at diagnosis, and after diagnosis for monitoring therapy, selecting additional therapy and detecting recurrence.[6] Biomarkers can be utilized in cancer research to discover fundamental mechanisms in the induction of cancer, to increase the accuracy of exposure assessment to potential carcinogens, to identify genetic and/or acquired susceptibility factors that contribute to the risk for cancer, and to predict cancer outcomes in exposed populations.[7] Biomarkers can elucidate the multistage mechanisms involved in carcinogenesis and can be used to measure the exposures that induce the DNA damage, the quantity and quality of the damage itself, or individual susceptibility to damage that underlies many cancers.[8] Further, biomarkers can be utilized to assess interventions and response to treatment. The study of biomarkers offers opportunities to explore biological markers at critical stages in the carcinogenesis pathway from acquired genetic susceptibilities, to exposure assessment to the many gene-environment interactions that influence the development and detection of cancer.

Classification of Biomarkers

Biomarkers are generally classified into those of exposure, intermediate (markers of early response), disease, and susceptibility.[9] Biomarkers in cancer can be further categorized into markers of altered structure/function, markers of cancer subtypes, and markers of prognosis. These classifications are however, evolving as whole genome and broad expression data have become available. For instance, chromosomal aberrations that were once considered biomarkers of exposure are now classified as markers of disease. Further, DNA adducts can be used to identify both biomarkers of exposure and biomarkers of susceptibility to disease. For example, assays with antibodies to polycyclic aromatic hydrocarbons (PAH)—DNA adducts have been utilized to identify high-risk segments of the population that have been exposed to PAH and may be at increased risk for lung cancer.[10]

Biomarkers of Exposure

Exposure assessment in epidemiologic research is challenging and often relies on medical records or questionnaire data, which may not have been collected explicitly for an epidemiologic study. In the latter instance, misclassification of exposure information can potentially lead to substantial bias in epidemiologic studies. Biomarkers offer an attractive alternative for assessing, corroborating, and/or quantifying exposure, as they can quantify the biologically relevant exposure without relying on data based on an individual's recall. Exposures to a potential carcinogen can be measured as a specific chemical or metabolite or as a genotoxic material in blood, urine, feces or tissues.[8] Biomarkers of exposure include chemicals and their metabolites, as well as DNA adducts, which occur when carcinogenic chemicals bond with a segment of DNA. Biomarkers of exposure have been utilized in studies of infectious agents, such as HPV infection and oral cancer risk,[11] nutrients, such as folate and cancer risk;[12] DNA adducts have proven useful in studies of the molecular etiology of liver cancer[13,14] and endogenous compounds, such as sex hormones which are implicated in breast cancer risk.[9,15] Complex patterns of exposures in the environment and through consumption of certain types of foods characterize the environmental determinants of risk in high-resource settings, as well as in low-resource and mid-resource regions that are undergoing rapid growth and development. Modern integrated assessment models are required to fully define the attributable risk of the single and combined exposures.

Biomarkers of Intermediates (Early Response or Early Biologic Effects)

Biomarkers of early biological effects measure events in the pathway from exposure to disease. Carcinogenic agents may cause cellular damage triggering cellular response and repair mechanisms. Biomarkers can be utilized to identify these cellular responses on multiple pathways involved in cancer development. Aflatoxins, fungal toxins produced mainly by *Aspergillus flavi*, commonly contaminate legumes, maize, groundnuts, and other crop seeds, play an important role in modifying risk of liver cancer associated with hepatitis B by inducing mutations and exacerbating a state of chronic inflammation. After being metabolized in the liver, the toxin binds to the guanine moiety in DNA, resulting in carcinogenic mutations—for example in codon 249 of the TP53 tumor suppressor gene.[16] This mutation is common in primary liver cancers from areas of high exposure to aflatoxin and serves as a robust indicator of possible exposure.[17] When quantifying this mutation, DNA adducts serve as a biomarker of early response to exposure to aflatoxins. Another example of a biomarker of early response involves the CA assay, which is widely used as a validated method for detecting exposure to ionizing radiation as radiation induces chromosomal aberrations, which can be easily detected in this assay.[18,19]

Biomarkers of Susceptibility, Disease and Prognosis

Biomarkers can also be used to identify groups at high risk for developing disease, as well as for the purpose of conveying prognosis. For example, the BRCA1 or BRCA2 (breast cancer 1 or 2) genes are commonly used for risk assessment in individuals exhibiting a personal history of early onset or bilateral breast cancer or ovarian cancer or a family history of these cancers. Deleterious mutations in these genes confer a moderately to highly increased risk of breast and ovarian cancer.[20] Single nucleotide polymorphism (SNP), which are common DNA sequence variations between individuals have also been utilized to understand modifiers of susceptibility among carriers; an example of this includes associations between SNPs in repair genes and lung cancer risk.[21]

Prostate specific antigen (PSA), is normally produced in small quantities by prostate cells but when this antigen level is elevated, it may be indicative of potentially underlying prostate cancer. This biomarker is commonly used for prostate cancer screening purposes, although its usefulness at the population level is highly controversial and its use is being much more narrowly defined. In order to be effective for screening purposes, a biomarker must be cost effective and highly specific in order to minimize the unwarranted psychological burden, cost and invasiveness of follow-up procedures that accompany false positive results; determining the appropriate balance between the sensitivity/specificity ratio and the cost/benefit analyses is the purview of comparative effectiveness research, an important multi disciplinary activity that spans the scholarly gap between medicine and public health.

Biomarker Validation

The analytic validity of a biomarker refers to the accuracy with which it measures its target[22]. Thus, the validity of a biomarker is often dependent on the assay employed. Assays must be highly sensitive (detecting the biomarker if it is present, even in minute amounts) and specific (not detecting the marker if it is absent). There is potential variability within the biomarker itself that should also be considered when assessing validity. For example, biologic markers may have half lives or their concentrations may vary according to the time of day the sample is acquired, due to circadian or other rhythms. Therefore, it is critical to standardize laboratory methods used to derive marker samples. These issues are especially imperative when validating biomarkers from multiple studies.

There has been dramatic progress in the application of biomarkers to human studies of cancer causation, yet there remains limited availability of validated biomarkers in clinical use or in population assessment to allocate resources or to implement prevention strategies. Validation of biomarkers involves addressing the reliability (reproducibility) of a newly developed marker, by blindly measuring replicate samples.[9] Biomarker validation is a lengthy process involving human field studies, which is one of several major reasons why so few markers have been integrated in clinical practice.

▪ STUDY DESIGNS: ADVANTAGES AND LIMITATIONS

Cohort, case-control, and cross-sectional study designs are useful for conducting molecular epidemiology research. Cross-sectional studies evaluate exposure and disease at a single time point. A general limitation with the cross-sectional approach is the temporal ambiguity, the inability to demonstrate that the exposure preceded disease. However, this approach is still useful for understanding population-level data to generate hypotheses and guide future research. An example of this design in molecular epidemiology involves measuring the prevalence of gene variants in a given population and correlating them with disease occurrence and other disease phenotypic characteristics, termed expressivity.

Case-control studies involve comparing exposure information between individuals with and without the disease of interest. For example, researchers could employ this design to compare levels of blood markers for suspected carcinogens between cases and controls to determine if the levels differ between groups. However, because of changes in environmental exposures over time, cohort studies with repeated measures of biomarkers of exposure and intermediate outcomes may be preferable to case-control studies, unless case-control studies are nested in an underlying cohort of a well-defined population for which biologic samples stored at the beginning of the study are later analyzed for exposures.[22]

Cohort studies involve classifying participants according to exposure status and following them longitudinally for disease occurrence and expressivity of disease. These studies allow for repeated measures of exposure and therefore may be better suited for certain markers of exposure. This design also allows for assessment of an exposure's effect on a multitude of outcomes. Prospective cohort studies are the gold standard in validating biomarkers. Although these studies can be costly and time consuming, they also provide a unique design for nesting comparative studies of implementation of strategies that either ameliorate exposure or actively interrupt the carcinogenesis pathway. If used in this context, longitudinal cohort studies offer the most powerful substrate for definitive efficacy studies, which may justify and indeed mitigate the initial costs.

REVIEW OF IMPORTANT KEY FINDINGS IN MOLECULAR EPIDEMIOLOGY

In recent years, molecular epidemiology has made critical contributions to our understanding of cancer etiology and prevention. These include the evidence of aflatoxin's hepatocellular carcinogenicity (HCC) in humans as mentioned already, the elucidation of the mechanisms of tobacco-related carcinogenesis, and the relation between human papillomavirus (HPV) and different human cancers, among others. In this section we will discuss some of the most relevant findings due to their great importance in cancer prevention and public health and because they illustrate how different types of challenges in the field were overcome.

Hepatitis B virus infection and aflatoxins were known risk factors for hepatocellular carcinoma (HCC), but their molecular pathogenic mechanisms were unknown until Bressac et al[23] and Hsu et al[24] found p53 mutations in hepatocellular carcinomas from Africa and China, respectively. Both groups found a single point mutation at codon 249, position 3 and both studies suggested that G-T transversions could be induced by exposure to an environmental factor prevalent both in Africa and Asia, a major candidate being aflatoxin B1 (AFB1). Since those two reports appeared, a very large amount of data has been published in support of the occurrence of such TP53 mutations in HCC in many regions of the world. *In vitro* studies have supported this finding, showing that AFB1 can induce this mutation.[25] The molecular marker of aflatoxin-induced mutagenesis (the specific G to T transversion within codon 249 of the TP53 gene) helped to establish that aflatoxin is a human liver carcinogen, responsible for a high proportion of HCC in geographic areas with high dietary exposure to aflatoxin, including regions of southeast Asia and sub-Saharan

Africa.[26] This example of such a specific association between a particular class of mutagen and a well defined, single TP53 mutation is especially notable. Two main factors may contribute to this unique situation: site-specific mutagenesis by aflatoxin, and the selection of p.R249S, as a protein which contributes to hepatocarcinogenesis in a unique way.[27] These findings were crucial in establishing a molecular marker of exposure that in time led to the implementation of robust measures for primary prevention. At the present time, it is possible to detect this mutant protein at an early stage of HCC development, through a simple blood test based on plasma DNA; however, more work is required to assess how, and in which context, such a biomarker may be applicable, either for monitor ongoing exposure to aflatoxin or to detect early liver cancer.[27]

Tobacco adducts and cancer. Most of the molecular epidemiologic research on lung cancer has targeted tobacco smoke and polycyclic aromatic hydrocarbons (PAHs) as model carcinogens. PAHs are found in tobacco smoke, in outdoor air from fossil fuel combustion, in indoor air from cooking, heating, and smoking, and in the diet. PAHs, such as benzo(a) pyrene, form adducts with DNA, a mechanism considered to be a critical early event in PAH-induced tumorigenesis.

Since 1982, several molecular epidemiologic case-control studies have found associations between PAH-DNA or related aromatic-DNA adducts measured in white blood cells (WBCs) and lung cancer.[28,29] Whereas the earlier studies were subject to the limitations of retrospective studies, two later investigations nested within prospective cohort studies, found adducts to be predictive of lung cancer within specific exposure groups.[30,31] A meta-analysis of aromatic/PAH-DNA adducts and lung cancer concluded that current smokers with high levels of adducts have an increased risk of lung cancer.[32]

HPV and cancer. HPV is considered essentially a necessary causative agent of cervical cancer (with HPV DNA detectable in 99.7% of cervical cancer specimens), although it is not a sufficient cause. HPV has also been implicated in the pathogenesis of other anogenital cancers, oropharynx cancers and nonmelanoma skin cancers. Studies have demonstrated that between 46–94% of anal cancers[33] and 60–65% of vaginal cancers[34] harbor HPV DNA. The overall prevalence of HPV in penile cancers is estimated to range from 15% to 71%,[35] although, more work is needed on the reliability of viral DNA assessment in penile cancer, given that HPV can infect the penile shaft, scrotum, and other anogenital skin.[33] A population-based case-control study of HPV and squamous cell carcinomas (SCC) of the skin detected HPV antibodies more frequently in SCC patients than in controls, supporting a role for HPV types in the pathogenesis of SCC.[36] In a systematic review of worldwide head and neck SCC, HPV prevalence was estimated at 25.9%.[37]

Molecular epidemiologic studies of HPV have also been utilized to predict patient outcomes in cancers. One such study found that HPV16 copy number was positively associated with response to therapy and with overall and disease specific survival in head and neck squamous cell carcinoma of the larynx and oropharynx.[38] A randomized study in India demonstrated that DNA testing of HPV was associated with a significant reduction in the numbers of advanced cervical cancers and deaths from cervical cancer as compared to cytologic testing or visual inspection of the cervix with acetic acid (VIA).[39]

The identification of HPV as a major etiologic agent for cervical cancer has increased its medical importance and stimulated research into developing primary and secondary prevention strategies such as vaccines and cervical cancer screening campaigns. The examples described above are amongst many others in which molecular epidemiology has not only contributed to the understanding of human cancer, but also has implemented measures for primary and secondary prevention.

■ CURRENT PERSPECTIVES AND CHALLENGES

During the last decade, molecular epidemiology has greatly evolved due to the rapid developments in human genomics/genetics like the completion of the Human Genome Project, the Haplotype Map (HapMap) project and the first phase of the Encyclopedia of DNA Elements (ENCODE) project. The Human Genome Project, completed the first-pass sequencing in 2002 and created a database of information on the sequences of the chemical base pairs and genes in human DNA.[40] The International HapMap project developed a map of the common patterns of DNA sequence variation in the human genome by determining the genotypes of one million or more sequence variants, their frequencies, and the degree of association between them, in DNA samples from populations with ancestry from parts of Africa, Asia and Europe.[41] The HapMap findings are critical for the implementation of genome-wide association studies (GWAS) to facilitate research on genetic factors contributing to disease susceptibility. The National Genome Research Institute (NHGRI) embarked on the ambitious ENCODE project in 2003 to delineate all the functional elements encoded in the human genome sequence.[42] Taken together, these public research consortium projects extend our understanding of genetic regulation and expression associated with disease susceptibility. Detailed understanding of the human genome as a whole, of both the coding and non coding regions, is enabling already many opportunities for research to address disease susceptibility and etiology, as well as to develop targeted therapeutic strategies.

Epigenetic Modulation of Cancer Biomarkers

Epigenetics refers to heritable changes in gene expression that are not due to any alteration of the DNA sequence.[43] Thus, genes can be modulated, activated, or suppressed in response to environmental stimuli through specific protein complexes that respond to the stimuli by binding to specific DNA regulatory sequences. Significant progress has been made in the basic understanding of how various epigenetic changes, such as DNA methylation, histone modification, miRNA expression, and higher order chromatin structure changes affect gene expression.[44] DNA hypomethylation in tumors as compared with the normal-tissue counterparts was one of the first epigenetic alterations to be described in human cancer.[45] Understanding these epigenetic alterations can lead to the identification of novel biomarkers for cancer detection and targeted therapeutic approaches in clinical cancer care.

Metabolomic Signatures and Biomarkers

Metabolomics is the study of the metabolic response to stimuli, involving the systematic investigation of the abundance of metabolites and metabolic pathway intermediates in biological fluids, tissues, and cells.[46] The field holds promise of being quite useful for the detection of biomarkers in cancer development and progression and of providing tools and targets in the field of drug discovery and tailored therapeutic approaches for the treatment of cancer. One recent study used metabonomic methods to detect a novel biomarker pattern of two urinary metabolites which demonstrated better overall diagnostic performance than a single metabolite in discriminating bladder cancer patients from healthy controls.[47] Further studies have used metabonomics to delineate subpopulations susceptible to adverse events from chemotherapy, thus demonstrating an important potential therapeutic role in the assessment of treatment viability for cancer patients prior to commencing chemotherapy.[48]

Proteomics

Proteomics is the study of proteins in a cell or in body fluids, involving the use of technologies to identify and quantify broadly the patterns of protein expression, which may reveal special patterns of biomarkers of disease and progression.[49] Proteomic research has been utilized to describe proteins that are overexpressed in certain aggressive prostate cancer cells, and may promote cell growth, migration and invasion,[50] providing important clues about the process of carcinogenesis at the molecular level. This discipline has also led to the identification of novel biomarkers for the diagnosis of gastric adenocarcinoma,[51] colorectal cancer,[52] as well as the early detection of squamous cell cancer of the lung.[53] Many studies are in progress and the technical detection sensitivity and specificity continues to improve in this promising new field.

Bioinformatics

The field of bioinformatics emerged from the extensive advances in genomics and the need for standardized data management capabilities to facilitate the analysis of these increasingly complex datasets. Bioinformatics merges science, biology, computer science, and information technology to enable the discovery of new biological insights, as well as to create a global perspective from which unifying principles in biology can be discerned.[54] With the vast genomic data now publicly available, the application of metabonomics and proteomics to discover biomarkers of early diagnosis of cancer relies on bioinformatics tools to effectively extract complex and vast data for analysis. Bioinformatics can be utilized to bridge the gap between biological knowledge and clinical therapy by facilitating the rapid identification of new targets for further experimental validation.[55]

GWAS Studies

Genome-wide association studies (GWA study or GWAS) have become very common in the recent years. GWAS are an examination of genetic variation across a given genome, designed to identify genetic associations with observable traits. These studies normally require two groups of participants: people with the disease (cases) and similar people without (controls). After genotyping each participant, the set of markers, such as single nucleotide polymorphism (SNPs) are compared between groups. SNP is a DNA sequence variation occurring when a single nucleotide differs between members of a species with minor allele frequency of more than 1%. If genetic variations are more frequent in people with the disease, the variations are said to be "associated" with the disease. The associated genetic variations are then considered as pointers to the region of the human genome where the disease-causing problem is likely to reside.

GWAS have recently assayed hundreds of thousands of SNPs in thousands of individuals identifying hundreds of associations of common genetic variants with more than 80 diseases and traits. These studies have progressed from assaying fewer than 100,000 SNPs to more than one million and sample sizes have also increased. An online catalog has been developed where SNP-trait associations from published GWAS are reported (www.genome.gov/gwastudies).

One of the challenges for a successful GWAS in the future will be to apply the findings in a way that accelerates drug and diagnostics development, including better integration of genetic studies into the drug-development process and a focus on the role of genetic variation in maintaining health as a blueprint for designing new drugs and diagnostics.

CHALLENGES

Selection bias, information bias, and confounding are all potential sources of error in epidemiologic research. Selection bias occurs when participation in the study is affected by exposure status. Ensuring high response rates and selection into the study independent of exposure status can limit the potential for selection bias in molecular epidemiologic studies. Information bias refers to misclassification of exposure or disease status. The varying stability of biomarkers may be a source of misclassification and bias in molecular epidemiologic studies, especially for chronic exposures. Ensuring proper selection into studies and objective measurements of exposure and disease are imperative in any epidemiologic study. Confounding occurs when there is a mixing of effects of exposure with other factors that influence disease. It is critical to have information on potential confounding factors so that these can be adjusted for in the analysis of the study to ensure that we are properly accounting for the effect of a given exposure on the disease. Unpublished data in molecular epidemiology are very frequent, due to the relative novelty of this discipline, the quick decrease in interest for markers that are less fashionable, the lack of funding or difficulty in recruiting subjects, and the use of data for survey purposes.[56] This publication bias could be deterring progress in biomarker validation and incorporation into clinical practice. Further, molecular studies are often based on a single sample and this makes it difficult to acquire information on cumulative exposures or time-related exposures. Methods to overcome limitations in molecular studies, including small sample size and limited power of studies to show effects must also be addressed. There is a need to conduct large epidemiological studies including biological markers, to answer questions that have been raised by preliminary studies, such as the possible association between cancer and metabolic polymorphisms, or the presence of intermediate end points as predictors of future cancer development.[57]

Finally, molecular epidemiology needs to evolve to address limitations of the field, such as the need for technology to quantify biomarkers in blood at low concentrations. Advances of this caliber will lead to more breakthroughs in our understanding of cancer etiology.

FUTURE APPLICATIONS

The opportunity to apply molecular methods for continued development in the field of cancer epidemiology is great. Molecular epidemiologic studies have created vast opportunities to further explore the susceptibility genes and their interactions with carcinogens. Future research should focus on biomarkers that indirectly affect disease risk through epigenetic mechanisms. Further, the role of specific nutritional factors and the modulating effect of genetic polymorphisms in cancer need to be explored through the development and validation of new biomarkers. By building reliable biomarker databases, a promising future is the integration of information from the genome programs to expand the scientific frontiers on etiology, health risk prediction and prevention of environmental disease.[18]

Our knowledge of individual susceptibility to disease remains limited and biomarkers in this area need to be further explored in order to effectively alter the disease process. Accounting for interindividual differences in research may lead to tailored approaches to treatment.

Many biomarkers can be useful in assessing exposure, early deleterious molecular and biologic effects, and potential risk for a group or population; most are not, however, sufficiently characterized or validated for routine use in screening, diagnosis or quantitative estimation of individual risk of developing cancer.[4] The development and validation of biomarkers relevant to the carcinogenic process must continue to be an area of focus among epidemiologists. New molecular technologies need to be incorporated into epidemiologic studies going forward.

An imperative focus for future molecular epidemiology research is on the neglected populations in low and middle-income countries where the technology and personnel needed for molecular epidemiologic research remains to be cultivated. We stand to gain potentially valuable new information from molecular research conducted in low and middle-income countries where substantial differences in exposure and disease patterns exist.

■ SUMMARY

Despite the limitations of molecular epidemiology, there remains great potential for altering carcinogenesis by focusing research on biomarkers in the pathways from exposure to disease, in an integrated multidisciplinary manner. Understanding this complex process holds the hope to allow us to interrupt the natural history of the disease, either by altering its course or, since it could enable us to detect exposures to small amounts of a harmful compound, including those found in mixtures, by removing its cause altogether. Biomarkers offer a promising approach to this challenge and the tools of integrated assessments in environmental science offer the novel methodologies needed to attack this important problem.[57]

■ ACKNOWLEDGMENT

Work supported in part by the Breast Cancer Research Foundation (SDM), the Avon Foundation (SDM), and the Center for Global Health (SDM, KH).

■ REFERENCES

1. Schulte PA, Perera FP. *Molecular epidemiology: Principles and practices.* San Diego: Academic Press; 1993:xx, 588 p.
2. Perera FP, Weinstein IB. Molecular epidemiology and carcinogen-DNA adduct detection: New approaches to studies of human cancer causation. *J Chronic Dis.* 1982;35(7):581–600.
3. Perera FP. Molecular epidemiology: On the path to prevention? *J Natl Cancer Inst.* 2000;92(8):602–612.
4. Perera FP, Weinstein IB. Molecular epidemiology: Recent advances and future directions. *Carcinogenesis.* 2000;21(3):517–524.
5. Application of biomarkers in cancer epidemiology. Workshop report. *IARC Sci Publ.* 1997;(142)(142):1–18.
6. Ludwig JA, Weinstein JN. Biomarkers in cancer staging, prognosis and treatment selection. *Nat Rev Cancer.* 2005;5(11):845–856.
7. Albertini RJ. Mechanistic insights from biomarker studies: Somatic mutations and rodent/human comparisons following exposure to a potential carcinogen. *IARC Sci Publ.* 2004;(157)(157):153–177.
8. Albertini RJ. Biomarker responses in human populations: Towards a worldwide map. *Mutat Res.* 1999;428(1–2):217–226.
9. Adami H, Hunter DJ, Trichopoulos D. *Textbook of cancer epidemiology.* Oxford ;New York: Oxford University Press; 2008:xxxiii, 748 p.
10. Perera FP, Santella RM, Brenner D, Young TL, Weinstein IB. Application of biological markers to the study of lung cancer causation and prevention. *IARC Sci Publ.* 1988;(89)(89):451–459.
11. Mork J, Lie AK, Glattre E, et al. Human papillomavirus infection as a risk factor for squamous-cell carcinoma of the head and neck. *N Engl J Med.* 2001;344(15):1125–1131.
12. Rossi E, Hung J, Beilby JP, Knuiman MW, Divitini ML, Bartholomew H. Folate levels and cancer morbidity and mortality: Prospective cohort study from Busselton, Western Australia. *Ann Epidemiol.* 2006;16(3):206–212.

13. Yu MW, Lien JP, Chiu YH, Santella RM, Liaw YF, Chen CJ. Effect of aflatoxin metabolism and DNA adduct formation on hepatocellular carcinoma among chronic hepatitis B carriers in Taiwan. *J Hepatol.* 1997;27(2):320–330.

14. Ross RK, Yuan JM, Yu MC, et al. Urinary aflatoxin biomarkers and risk of hepatocellular carcinoma. *Lancet.* 1992;339(8799):943–946.

15. Kaaks R, Berrino F, Key T, et al. Serum sex steroids in premenopausal women and breast cancer risk within the European prospective investigation into cancer and nutrition (EPIC). *J Natl Cancer Inst.* 2005;97(10):755–765.

16. Hall AJ, Wild CP. Liver cancer in low and middle income countries. *BMJ.* 2003;326(7397):994–995.

17. IARC Working Group on the Evaluation of Carcinogenic Risks to Humans. Some traditional herbal medicines, some mycotoxins, naphthalene and styrene. *IARC Monogr Eval Carcinog Risks Hum.* 2002;82: 1–556.

18. Bonassi S, Au WW. Biomarkers in molecular epidemiology studies for health risk prediction. *Mutat Res.* 2002;511(1):73–86.

19. Bender MA, Griggs HG, Bedford JS. Mechanisms of chromosomal aberration production. 3. chemicals and ionizing radiation. *Mutat Res.* 1974;23(2):197–212.

20. Robson ME, Chappuis PO, Satagopan J, et al. A combined analysis of outcome following breast cancer: Differences in survival based on BRCA1/BRCA2 mutation status and administration of adjuvant treatment. *Breast Cancer Res.* 2004;6(1):R8–R17.

21. Hung RJ, Brennan P, Canzian F, et al. Large-scale investigation of base excision repair genetic polymorphisms and lung cancer risk in a multicenter study. *J Natl Cancer Inst.* 2005;97(8):567–576.

22. Rothman KJ, Greenland S, Lash TL. *Modern epidemiology.* Philadelphia: Wolters Kluwer Health/ Lippincott Williams & Wilkins; 2008:x, 758 p.

23. Bressac B, Kew M, Wands J, Ozturk M. Selective G to T mutations of p53 gene in hepatocellular carcinoma from southern Africa. *Nature.* 1991;350(6317):429–431.

24. Hsu IC, Metcalf RA, Sun T, Welsh JA, Wang NJ, Harris CC. Mutational hotspot in the p53 gene in human hepatocellular carcinomas. *Nature.* 1991;350(6317):427–428.

25. Aguilar F, Hussain SP, Cerutti P. Aflatoxin B1 induces the transversion of G→T in codon 249 of the p53 tumor suppressor gene in human hepatocytes. *Proc Natl Acad Sci U S A.* 1993;90(18):8586–8590.

26. Parkin DM, Bray F, Ferlay J, Pisani P. Global cancer statistics, 2002. *CA Cancer J Clin.* 2005;55(2): 74–108.

27. Gouas D, Shi H, Hainaut P. The aflatoxin-induced TP53 mutation at codon 249 (R249S): Biomarker of exposure, early detection and target for therapy. *Cancer Lett.* 2009;286(1):29–37.

28. Tang D, Santella RM, Blackwood AM, et al. A molecular epidemiological case-control study of lung cancer. *Cancer Epidemiol Biomarkers Prev.* 1995;4(4):341–346.

29. Wiencke JK, Thurston SW, Kelsey KT, et al. Early age at smoking initiation and tobacco carcinogen DNA damage in the lung. *J Natl Cancer Inst.* 1999;91(7):614–619.

30. Tang D, Phillips DH, Stampfer M, et al. Association between carcinogen-DNA adducts in white blood cells and lung cancer risk in the physicians health study. *Cancer Res.* 2001;61(18):6708–6712.

31. Perera FP, Mooney LA, Stampfer M, et al. Associations between carcinogen-DNA damage, glutathione S-transferase genotypes, and risk of lung cancer in the prospective physicians' health cohort study. *Carcinogenesis.* 2002;23(10):1641–1646.

32. Veglia F, Loft S, Matullo G, et al. DNA adducts and cancer risk in prospective studies: A pooled analysis and a meta-analysis. *Carcinogenesis.* 2008;29(5):932–936.

33. Schiffman M, Kjaer SK. Chapter 2: Natural history of anogenital human papillomavirus infection and neoplasia. *J Natl Cancer Inst Monogr.* 2003;(31)(31):14–19.

34. IARC Working Group on the Evaluation of Carcinogenic Risks to Humans. Human papillomaviruses. *IARC Monogr Eval Carcinog Risks Hum.* 1995;64:1–378.

35. Rubin MA, Kleter B, Zhou M, et al. Detection and typing of human papillomavirus DNA in penile carcinoma: Evidence for multiple independent pathways of penile carcinogenesis. *Am J Pathol.* 2001;159(4):1211–1218.

36. Karagas MR, Nelson HH, Sehr P, et al. Human papillomavirus infection and incidence of squamous cell and basal cell carcinomas of the skin. *J Natl Cancer Inst.* 2006;98(6):389–395.

37. Kreimer AR, Clifford GM, Boyle P, Franceschi S. Human papillomavirus types in head and neck squamous cell carcinomas worldwide: A systematic review. *Cancer Epidemiol Biomarkers Prev.* 2005;14(2):467–475.

38. Kumar B, Cordell KG, Lee JS, et al. Response to therapy and outcomes in oropharyngeal cancer are associated with biomarkers including human papillomavirus, epidermal growth factor receptor, gender, and smoking. *Int J Radiat Oncol Biol Phys.* 2007;69(2 Suppl):S109–S111.

39. Sankaranarayanan R, Nene BM, Shastri SS, et al. HPV screening for cervical cancer in rural India. *N Engl J Med.* 2009;360(14):1385–1394.

40. Lander ES, Linton LM, Birren B, et al. Initial sequencing and analysis of the human genome. *Nature.* 2001;409(6822):860–921.

41. International HapMap Consortium. The international HapMap project. *Nature.* 2003;426(6968): 789–796.

42. ENCODE Project Consortium. The ENCODE (ENCyclopedia of DNA elements) project. *Science.* 2004;306(5696):636–640.

43. Holliday R. The inheritance of epigenetic defects. *Science.* 1987;238(4824):163–170.

44. Huang Y, Nayak S, Jankowitz R, Davidson NE, Oesterreich S. Epigenetics in breast cancer: What's new? *Breast Cancer Res.* 2011;13(6):225.

45. Feinberg AP, Vogelstein B. Hypomethylation distinguishes genes of some human cancers from their normal counterparts. *Nature.* 1983;301(5895):89–92.

46. Beckonert O, Keun HC, Ebbels TM, et al. Metabolic profiling, metabolomic and metabonomic procedures for NMR spectroscopy of urine, plasma, serum and tissue extracts. *Nat Protoc.* 2007;2(11):2692–2703.

47. Huang Z, Lin L, Gao Y, et al. Bladder cancer determination via two urinary metabolites: A biomarker pattern approach. *Mol Cell Proteomics.* 2011;10(10):M111.007922.

48. Backshall A, Sharma R, Clarke SJ, Keun HC. Pharmacometabonomic profiling as a predictor of toxicity in patients with inoperable colorectal cancer treated with capecitabine. *Clin Cancer Res.* 2011;17(9):3019–3028.

49. Sellers TA, Yates JR. Review of proteomics with applications to genetic epidemiology. *Genet Epidemiol.* 2003;24(2):83–98.

50. Kong L, Schafer G, Bu H, Zhang Y, Zhang Y, Klocker H. Lamin A/C protein is overexpressed in tissue-invading prostate cancer and promotes prostate cancer cell growth, migration and invasion through the PI3K/AKT/PTEN pathway. *Carcinogenesis.* 2012;33(4):751–759.

51. Ahn HS, Shin YS, Park PJ, et al. Serum biomarker panels for the diagnosis of gastric adenocarcinoma. *Br J Cancer.* 2012;106(4):733–739.

52. Fan NJ, Gao CF, Wang CS, et al. Discovery and verification of gelsolin as a potential biomarker of colorectal adenocarcinoma in the Chinese population: Examining differential protein expression using an iTRAQ labelling-based proteomics approach. *Can J Gastroenterol.* 2012;26(1):41–47.

53. Zeng GQ, Zhang PF, Deng XM, et al. Identification of novel biomarkers for early detection of human lung squamous cell cancer by quantitative proteomics. *Mol Cell Proteomics.* 2012;11(6): M111.013946-1-M111.013946-16.

54. National Center for Biotechnology Information. NCBI bioinformatics factsheet. http://www.ncbi.nlm.nih.gov/About/primer/bioinformatics.html. Updated 2004.

55. Desany B, Zhang Z. Bioinformatics and cancer target discovery. *Drug Discov Today.* 2004;9(18): 795–802.

56. Taioli E, Bonassi S. Methodological issues in pooled analysis of biomarker studies. *Mutat Res.* 2002; 512(1):85–92.

57. Bonassi S, Neri M, Puntoni R. Validation of biomarkers as early predictors of disease. *Mutat Res.* 2001; 480-481:349–358.

CHAPTER 4

OPPORTUNITIES IN GENETIC EPIDEMIOLOGY IN DEVELOPING COUNTRIES

DOMINIQUE SIGHOKO, OLUWAFEMI OLUWOLE, YONGLAN ZHENG, OLUFUNMILAYO I. OLOPADE

INTRODUCTION

Cancer imposes a major disease burden worldwide, with considerable variation among countries and regions. According to the International Agency for Research on Cancer (IARC), the global cancer burden doubled in the last 30 years with an estimated 12 million of new cancer cases diagnosed in 2008[1] and an estimated 22 million of new cancer cases projected by the year 2030.[2,3] In developing countries, the burden of cancer has long been overshadowed by the focus on infectious and other diseases. Lack of reliable data on cancer incidence has also hindered progress on effective cancer control policies. Although cancers caused by infectious agents remain high in less developed countries; 22.9% compared to 7.4% in more developed countries,[4] the progressive control of infectious diseases and the increase in life expectancy in low and middle income countries (LMICs) has considerably changed the distribution of the global burden of cancer.[3,5] Nowadays, more than half of the global cancer burden (56% in 2008)[1] is borne by low- and middle-income countries.[6,7]

Currently, it is estimated that more than 72% of all cancer deaths occur in LMICs and this is expected to increase considerably across Asia, Africa, and Latin America.[8,9] In 2008, lung (12.7%), breast (10.9%), and colorectal (9.7%) cancers were the top three leading cancers worldwide[1] but, in sub-Saharan Africa specifically, the main cancer sites are cervical, breast, liver, and prostate cancer.[10] Cervix and liver cancers have become highly preventable while breast and prostate cancers are highly treatable, yet they remain leading causes of mortality in LMICs partly due to lack of awareness, lack of structured programs for cancer prevention, delay in diagnosis and treatment and poor infrastructure for effective management of cancer. Breast (female) and cervical cancers are the top two leading causes of cancer deaths for women in most developing countries, whereas lung, stomach, and liver cancers are leading causes of death in males.[11] It is projected that aging of the population, as well as adoption of other behavioral risk factors such as smoking, sedentary lifestyle, and westernized diets, which reflect improvements in socioeconomic status, will in turn increase cancer burden in LMICs.[11,12]

While much of what is known about cancer prevention and treatment comes from studies conducted in developed countries,[13] cancer control activities in LMICs are in infancy, making it difficult to estimate the costs and effectiveness of various prevention and treatment strategies. This creates an unprecedented opportunity for LMICs to leverage emerging technologies to gain a better understanding of the variety of lifestyle and environmental exposures, as well as genetic factors that can inform cancer prevention and management strategies in these regions. With the number of new cases projected to increase substantially, LMICs simply cannot afford to set up the large hospital based systems to treat cancer without impacting development in other areas of the economy. As such researchers in LMICs must lead the creation of innovative approaches to stem the looming cancer epidemic in LMICs by "leap frogging" to take advantage of some of the scientific discoveries that are transforming cancer treatment and prevention in developed countries. Without innovative research and improved access to appropriate diagnostic and treatment centers, the increasing burden of cancer poses a serious threat to already overwhelmed health care systems. In this review, we discuss emerging opportunities to translate genomics to meaningful cancer control activities in LMICs and identify knowledge gaps to spur research in the field.

■ CANCER INCIDENCE AND MORTALITY IN DEVELOPING COUNTRIES

Incidence and mortality of cancer in males and females vary dramatically between geographic regions. In 2008, the number of new cancer cases was estimated at 12.7 million and the number of cancer deaths at 7.6 million in the world.[1,2] While the overall age-adjusted rate incidence (age standardized rate (ASR) per 100,000) for all cancers combined in economically developed countries are nearly twice as high as in LMICs in both male and females (300 vs. 160), mortality rates for all cancers combined in developed countries are only 21% higher in males and 2% higher in females.[11] The reason for the differences in the incidence and mortality of cancers in different geographical regions are multifactorial. Factors such as family structure, genetics, environment, lifestyle, sociocultural practices, behavioral pattern, and economics may all play a role and interact to contribute to higher or lower risks for specific cancers.[14] While the incidence of cancers related to infection such as cervical, liver, or stomach cancers remain high in less developed countries,[15] the incidence of prostate, colorectal, female breast, and lung cancers are 2–5 times higher in developed countries partly as a result of cancer screening programs that are virtually nonexistent in LMICs.[11] Lack of awareness and screening when coupled to poor access to diagnosis lead to late stage diagnosis in many LMICs compared to developed countries. This makes death rates from most cancers significantly higher in LMICs.[16,17] A study of cancer survival rates around the world indicates substantially lower survival rates in Africa, Brazil and eastern Europe compared to those in North America, Australia, and Japan.[18,19] Brazil and many countries in eastern Europe including Russia are undergoing rapid transformation of their economies and with economic progress, rapid expansion of their health investments. Africa remains underdeveloped with very limited resources. Thus, our focus will be restricted to African countries in an attempt to encourage broader thinking on making investments in genomics and biotechnology to foster innovations that will accelerate progress in cancer control in Africa and throughout the African Diaspora.

▨ GENETIC DIVERSITY OF AFRICAN POPULATION

According to the UN population prospect, after Asia, the African continent is the world's second largest and second most populous continent.[20] With over one billion people in more than 50 countries, the African continent has an extensive cultural and genetic diversity.[21,22] Africa is recognized as the birthplace and the oldest settlements of modern humans and as such the continent holds a unique significance for human population genetics, which may improve our understanding of overall genetic diversity across populations.[23] For example, African Americans in the United States are believed to be predominantly from Niger-Kordofanian (~71%) and other African (~8%) populations; with the remaining (~13%) from European populations, although admixture levels vary considerable among individuals.[24] Africa shows the highest levels of within-population and between-population genetic diversity; and that genetic diversity declines with distance away from Africa.[25] Thus, understanding the diverse genetic complexity of African populations is important for future understanding of the history of human evolution and more importantly, for the design and interpretation of studies designed to explore genetic and environmental risk factors for common diseases such as cancers among populations of African ancestry. Therefore, considering the increasing prevalence of cancer in African populations, it is necessary to explore the influence of both environmental and genetic factors because neither can be considered in isolation.[26] Recently, the Human Heredity and Health in Africa (H3Africa) Initiative has started to investigate the genetic and environmental diversity in Africa as well as their interactions in order to improve the health of African populations (http://h3africa.org/). This creates new opportunities to integrate genomics in cancer control activities in Africa.

▨ CANCER PREDISPOSITION: THE ROLE OF GENETICS

Mutations (changes of genetic materials, DNA) caused by carcinogens, lead to cell abnormalities and may bring errors in DNA replication and subsequent accumulation of these harmful damages evolves to more malignant events as cancer progresses. Nearly two decades ago, linkage analysis in families of European ancestry segregating common cancers, successfully led to the cloning of many cancer susceptibility genes. Examples include BRCA1 and BRCA2 (BRCA1/2) for breast and ovarian cancers, as well as APC and the mismatch repair (MMR) genes MLH1, MSH2, MSH6 and PMS2 for colorectal cancer (CRC). Mutations of these genes are highly penetrant, and contribute to high rates of age-dependent relative risk (RR ≥ 10.0) in mutation cancers. Later, candidate gene sequencing identified many rare moderate-penetrance mutations in genes such as CHEK2 and PALB2 for breast cancer and MUTYH for CRC. Individuals carrying mutations in these genes have higher cancer risks than nonmutation carriers in control populations (odds ratio (OR) ≥ 2.0).

In addition to the highly penetrant genetic mutations, recent advances in human genome and DNA microarray techniques have made large-scale genotyping more affordable. Consequentially, numerous common and low-penetrance susceptibility alleles have been discovered to confer a typically per-allele OR of 1.1–1.6 to common cancers including breast, lung, prostate cancers, among others. Given that genetic factors have been identified to play important roles in cancer development, we believe that LMICs could develop policies that take advantage of the cancer family history to gain a better understanding of how testing for mutations in cancer predisposing genes or cancer susceptibility alleles in numerous genes could be used to develop polygenic risk models and integrated into cancer control interventions at the personal and population level, especially for the leading causes of cancer deaths in Africa.

■ **GENETIC EPIDEMIOLOGY OF COMMON CANCERS IN AFRICA**

Breast Cancer

Breast cancer is the first or second most frequently diagnosed cancer and cause of cancer death for women in most sub-Saharan Africa countries.[10] While there is paucity of reliable cancer statistics, recent studies in Africa showed that breast cancer rates are increasing in most African countries. In 2008, 68,000 women were reportedly diagnosed with breast cancer in Africa with a corresponding 37,000 deaths.[2] In sub-Saharan Africa, 75% of the cases of BC occur in women under 50 years of age, and most of them occur before or around menopause. For unknown reasons, the highest incidence is observed in multiparous women (average number of children 5 and aged between 40 to 44 years.[27-31] The etiology of breast cancer in Africa remains largely understudied. Despite the well-established role of reproductive factors on breast cancer risk among women of western countries, few studies have assessed the role of reproductive factors on the Africa continent. Available studies, although mostly hospital-based have confirmed the role of reproductive factors on breast cancer risk in African women. The Nigerian Breast Cancer Study remains the largest study among African women to date. In a report involving 1388 Nigerian women (819 breast cancer cases and 569 controls), parity ($\geq$7 children, Odds Ratio (OR) = 0.52, 95% Confidence Interval (CI): 0.30–0.89), extended breastfeeding period (>96 months, OR = 0.54, 95% CI: 0.34–0.85) and later onset of menstruation ($\geq$19 years, OR = 0.56, 95% CI: 0.35–0.91) were all shown to be protective against breast cancer in Nigerian women by our group.[32] We have also shown that the highest tertile of waist-hip ratio was associated with breast cancer risk; especially among postmenopausal women (OR = 2.67, 95% CI: 1.05–6.80),[33] a finding consistent with what is established in the literature. However, it should be noted that, the protective effects of reproductive life seems to be restricted to hormone-dependent estrogen/progesterone receptor-positive (ER+/PR+) breast cancer.[34-38] Breast cancer among African women is more frequently negative for ER and/or PR[39-43] as well as negative for human epidermal growth factor receptor (HER2) (termed triple-negative breast cancer) compared to that of Caucasian women.[39-42] Apart from reproductive life factors, genetic mutations are believed to play important role in the development of breast cancer, especially early onset disease as manifested in African women.

About 5%–10% of breast cancer cases are thought to be hereditary in nature, resulting directly from gene mutations which are inherited from a parent.[44] The most common cause of hereditary breast cancer is inherited mutations in the *BRCA1/2* genes, which account for about 10–20% of inherited susceptibility to breast cancer.[44,45] Indeed, women with these inherited mutations also have an increased risk for developing other cancers, particularly ovarian cancer.[46,47] BRCA 1 and BRCA2 genes (*BRCA1/2*) are tumor suppressor genes that are involved in many crucial cellular pathways.[48] In normal cells, they help prevent cancer by repairing damaged DNA and therefore maintain genome stability. However, if an individual inherits a mutated copy of either gene from a parent, there is a high risk of developing breast cancer during one's lifetime.[49] In other words, high risk of breast cancer occurs in individuals from families that segregate *BRCA1/2* mutation with risk as high as 40–87% for members of families with *BRCA1*.[50] Women with these mutations have higher risk of developing breast cancer at a younger age and in both breasts compared to women who are *BRCA1/2* mutation negative.[44] Family history of breast cancer has been identified as a risk factor for these mutations in Africa and other countries.[51] Currently, very little is known about the prevalence of these mutations in African populations especially populations from sub-Saharan Africa.

A few studies from Nigeria, Sudan, and South Africa[52] have assessed the role of these mutations on breast and ovary cancer risk. In the first ever report from Africa, among Nigerian breast cancer patients, mostly diagnosed under the age of 40 years, 4% had BRCA1/2 mutations with two protein-truncating mutations (Q1090X and 17422insG) in BRCA1 and 3034del4 or 3036del4 in BRCA2.[53] In another recent study from Nigeria, sixteen different BRCA1 mutations (seven of which had never been reported previously) and thirteen different BRCA2 mutations (six of which had never been reported previously) were detected in women with breast cancer with the frequency of BRCA1 and BRCA2 mutations being 7.1% and 3.9%, respectively among the women.[54] Report from Central Sudan has also documented deleterious BRCA1/2 mutations among a small consecutive series of patients with breast cancer (34 females, 1 male) selected by age at onset less than 40 years. Five truncating mutations, one of which (in BRCA2) was in the male patient were identified. A large number of nontruncating variants including 3 unclassified variants predicted to affect protein product and not co-occurring with a truncating mutation in the same gene were also identified. These data suggest that BRCA1/2 deleterious mutations represent an important etiological factor for breast cancer in Central Sudan.[27] Furthermore, it has been reported that BRCA1 mutation was mostly associated with basal-like phenotype, a phenotype[55-57] that occurs at a higher prevalence among premenopausal African Americans[58] who share common ancestry with African women and West African women in particular. Until now, few studies have assessed similarities in BRCA mutations among West African women and African American.

In view of the significant genetic diversity in the African Diaspora, we were interested in determining whether 11 recurrent mutations identified in our Nigerian breast cancer study, along with a previously identified BRCA1 mutation, 943ins10, contribute significantly to breast cancer risk in the African Diaspora. After screening 260 African American and 118 Barbadian breast cancer patients, six of the 11 recurrent mutations identified in our previous study were also identified in a second cohort of Nigerian breast cancers but none of the recurrent mutations in the Nigerian study were identified in breast cancer cases from Barbados or the United States. We concluded that Nigerian breast cancer patients from Ibadan carry a unique spectrum of BRCA1/2 mutations, many of which are recurrent among presumably unrelated probands and may represent complex population substructures. These data suggest that an approach particularly based on recurrent mutations is not sufficient to understand the BRCA1/2 associated breast cancer risk in African populations. We have also conducted replication studies of 22 SNPS previously identified as breast cancer susceptibility loci in populations of European or Asian ancestry and could not replicate any of the index SNPs in women of European ancestry.[59] As cost of sequencing is considerably reduced, high throughput DNA sequencing of BRCA1/2 and genotyping of population specific genomic markers will be essential for identifying at-risk individuals in African populations and should be incorporated into cancer control strategies in low-resource settings.

Cervical Cancer

Worldwide, cervical cancer is the third most common cancer among female, with 529,000 cases diagnosed in 2008.[1] High-risk regions include eastern, western, and southern Africa, south-central Asia, middle Africa, and South America where more than 85% of these cases occur. In sub-Saharan Africa, cervical cancer is the most frequent cancer and the leading cancer-related cause of death among women; 75,100 of new cases and 53,000 cases of death in 2008.[1] It represents about one-quarter of all female cancers in sub-Saharan Africa.[60]

Cervical cancer ASRs ranged from 15.42 in The Gambia,[31] 36 in Nigeria,[29] and 52.4 in Uganda.[61] Women affected by this disease are mostly young and multiparous, with an average age at diagnosis of 44 years and 6 children on average.[31]

The natural history of cervical cancer is well known and makes it one of the most preventable chronic noncommunicable diseases. Infection by Human Papillomavirus (HPV), the necessary and central cause of cervical cancer,[62] is highly prevalent among African women.[63–65] Genomic analysis has allowed better classification of the virus. The high-risk HPV genotypes 16 and 18 infections accounting for nearly 70% of total new cases worldwide.[66] The eight most common genotypes (HPV 16, 18, 45, 31, 33, 52, 58, and 35) account for nearly 90% of cervical cancer cases.[67,68] In sub-Saharan Africa, HPV-31, 35, 51, 52, 53, and 58 have also been identified,[63–65,69,70] and more work should be done to genotype all cervical cancer cases in Africa. Infection with high-risk human papillomavirus (HPV) has been identified to be the major risk factor among vulnerable women.[71] Indeed, it has been reported that human deficiency virus (HIV)-positive women have higher rates of cervical intraepithelial neoplasia (CIN) than do HIV-negative women.[72,73] HIV infection is a risk factor for cervical cancer and both viruses (HIV and HPV) are prevalent in sub-Saharan Africa. In several countries of Africa such as Benin, Cameroon, Nigeria, Tanzania, Kenya, and South Africa, women affected by HIV have been shown to be at greater risk of cervical squamous intraepithelial lesions than HIV negative women.[63,74–78] The high burden of cervical cancer in many African countries and elsewhere in medically underserved populations may be largely due to lack of screening that detects precancerous and early stage cervical cancer.[79] Indeed, stage of disease at the moment of diagnosis is in general the most determinant factor to predict survival. Therefore continued population-based screening of at-risk populations is vital.

In addition to pap smear screening, visual screening tests, such as visual inspection with acetic acid (VIA) and Lugol's iodine (VILI) have been shown to be among the most efficient method for cervical cancer diagnosis and treatment. A study performed in India where the incidence of cervical cancer is among the highest have reported that VIA, VILI, and cytology to detect high-grade CIN were 64.5%, 64.5%, and 67.7%, respectively, for the sensitivity and 84.2%, 85.5% and 95.4% for the specificities.[80] However the lower cost, the immediate availability of results and therefore a possibility of a rapid treatment management make the visual inspection screening the efficient method of screening and treatment for LMICs.[81,82] In Africa, visual inspection screening has been shown to be an efficient screening test in several countries of Africa.[83–85] Furthermore, a study performed in Mali has shown that visual inspection screening can be easily integrated into the health services as a routine screening test for cervical cancer diagnosis.[86] However, progress in this area is recent and sub-Saharan Africa still faces the highest mortality rate. Most women affected by cervical cancer are diagnosed at an advanced stage due to lack of awareness.[87–89] Population-based studies on cervical cancer survival in different geographic regions have also identified that African American women were at 55% increased risk of dying from cervical cancer (hazard ratio (HR) = 1.55, 95% CI: 1.40–1.72) whereas Hispanic women were at 11% decreased risk of death (HR = 0.89, 95% CI: 0.81–0.99).[90] In this study, the major differential survival advantage among the Hispanic women was attributed to the fact that Hispanic women were diagnosed with cervical cancer at early stage compared to African American women.

In 2006, the U.S. Food and Drug Administration approved the vaccine Gardasil, the first HPV vaccine for the prevention of cervical cancer and associated precancerous lesions due to HPV types 6, 11, 16, and 18 in person aged from 9 to 26 years. A study by Sue J. Goldie on health and economic outcomes of HPV 16, 18 vaccination in 72 GAVI

(Global Alliance for Vaccines and Immunization) eligible countries showed that although the costs of HPV vaccination was somewhat higher than traditional vaccines, HPV 16, 18 vaccination would be cost-effective even in the poorest countries and that, making an HPV 16, 18 vaccine accessible and affordable to these countries could prevent the deaths of close to 5 million women vaccinated as young adolescent girls in the next two decades.[91] However, to make progress in eradicating cervical cancer, clinical researchers in LMICs must continue to characterize other genotypes and monitor determinants of success of vaccination programs.

Prostate Cancer

Worldwide, prostate cancer is the second most common cancer among men with an estimated 914,000 new cases diagnosed in 2008 and the sixth leading cause of death from cancer among men. There were 258,000 deaths in 2008 attributed to prostate cancer.[1] In sub-Saharan Africa, prostate cancer is the most frequently diagnosed cancer in men in 46 countries of sub-Saharan Africa[3,92] and the first leading cause of cancer death for males.[92] The age standardized rates (ASRs) ranged from 3.4 in The Gambia[38] to 25.9 in Abuja[29] to 39.6 in Uganda-Kampala,[61] where it represents the second and most common cancers among men, respectively. With the growth and aging of the global population, the burden of prostate cancer is expected to grow to 1.7 million new cases and 499,000 new deaths by 2030.[1]

Geographic variation has been reported in the incidence rate of prostate cancer in Africa. The incidence of prostate cancer in southern Africa has been reported to be twice as high as the highest rate in western Africa and nearly seven-fold higher than the lowest regional rate in Northern Africa.[92] Data suggest that the high incidence rate in southern Africa might reflect population-based screening leading to increased diagnosis, rather than true disease occurrence. Indeed, the lower life expectancy and the lack of cancer screening programs and therefore cancer detection in most countries in sub-Saharan Africa can explain the lower rate of the burden in West Africa countries such as The Gambia. However, high prostate cancer rates have been reported among western and southern African descendants in Jamaica and Trinidad and Tobago,[92] suggesting the role of genetic susceptibility.[93,94]

The only well-established risk factors for prostate cancer are older age, black men of African origin, and a family history of the disease.[95] A positive family history of prostate cancer has been suggested to play a major role, especially among men of African ancestry. For example, it has been suggested that approximately 10–15% of men with prostate cancer have at least one relative who is also affected.[96,97] A meta-analysis of 11 case-control studies and 2 cohort studies identified a higher risk of developing prostate cancer among first degree relatives (OR=2.5, 95% CI: 2.2–2.8).[98] In all but one of these studies, the OR was observed to be greater if a brother was affected than if a father was affected (OR=3.4, 95% CI: 2.9–4.1 vs. OR=2.5, 95% CI: 2.1–3.1). In addition, relatives of individuals with early onset prostate cancer were also observed to have higher risk of developing prostate cancer over that of late onset cancer cases. The OR associated with a positive family history was greater if a man was diagnosed at age <65 years than at age >64 (OR=4.3 vs. OR=2.4). Also, studies have reported that relatives with a stronger family history would be at a higher risk of prostate cancer compared to relatives of a single case, suggesting that the more affected first-degree relatives in a family, the higher the risk to other male relatives. For example, a report showed that the estimated OR of developing prostate cancer increased from 2.2 to 4.9 to 10.9 if there were one, two, or three or more affected first-degree relatives, respectively.[99] The main finding from these studies suggested that there is shared familial risk factor for prostate cancer within families and relatives, possibly genetic, at least for men with positive family history. According to these findings, the important modifiers of risk related to familial history of prostate cancer can be summarized in three ways: (1) the status of the affected relative, (2) the age of the affected relative, and (3) the number of relatives with prostate cancer.

Another commonly argued risk factor for prostate cancer among African populations is environmental exposure. However, in the search for susceptibility alleles for prostate cancer, the risk variant rs6983267 at 8q24, has been reported to be significantly associated with prostate cancer in African American populations (OR = 1.43, 95% CI: 1.17–1.75, P = 0.035). It provides further support for the hypothesis of a genetic contribution underlying prostate cancer risk.[100] 8q24 region has been confirmed by a recently conducted genome-wide association study (GWAS) which also identified a new risk variant on chromosome 17q21 (rs7210100, per allele OR = 1.5, $P = 3.4 \times 10^{-13}$). The study found the risk allele occurring in approximately 4–7% of men of African descent, including Ghanaian men (7%), but <1% in other non-African populations.[101] Considering the low rate of westernization in Africa, the observation that total incidence rates of prostate cancer in Africa, even in the earlier period, were slightly higher than those among African Americans is consistent with the GWAS findings suggesting some risk loci may be specific to African populations. Whether 8q24 and 17q21 in combination with other potential risk variants play an important role in prostate cancer in African men remains unclear. Their underlying biological mechanisms need to be further investigated.

Thus, there is tremendous opportunity for identifying inherited susceptibility to prostate cancer pending the adoption of genetic testing in Africa. It may be necessary to focus on (1) identifying clusters of three or more first-degree relatives with prostate cancer, (2) prostate cancer in each of three generations in paternal or maternal lineage and, (3) identifying two or more first- or second-degree relatives with a prostate cancer under the age of 65 and (4) identifying at risk relative of cases diagnosed under 55 years. Such individuals should be enrolled in longitudinal studies which will enable observation of repeated prostate cancer outcomes across and within paternal or maternal lineage over time.

Liver Cancer

Worldwide, liver cancer is the fifth most common cancer in men (522,000 cases, 7.9% of the total) and the seventh in women (226,000 cases, 6.5% of the total), with almost 85% of the cases occurring in developing countries, especially eastern and south-eastern Asia and middle and western Africa.[1] With an estimated number of 696,000 deaths in 2008, liver cancer is the third cause of death by cancer in the world.[1] The geographical distribution of mortality is similar to the incidence rate; 5 years survival below 10%.[1] In sub-Saharan Africa, liver cancer is the second most common cancer among men and the third among female. There were an estimated total of 29,172 new cases in males and 15,072 cases in females in 2008 with corresponding mortality of 28,532 and 14,756, respectively.[10] Recent data showed that ASRs ranged from 14.4 in Harare-Zimbabwe to 32.84 per 100,000 person-years in The Gambia for men and around 14 for women.[38] Areas of high incidence of liver cancer mainly include countries of West Africa, where cases comprise a quarter or more of all cancer cases.[102]

Hepatocellular carcinoma (HCC) develops from parenchyma cells (hepatocytes) and represents 75–90% of primary liver cancer.[103] As cervical cancer, liver cancer is related to infection mainly caused by the chronic infection with Hepatitis B virus (HBV) and C (HCV) which are responsible for 70–85% of liver cancer burden in the world.[104] HCC is also caused by alcohol consumption and exposure to aflatoxin B1 a mycotoxin produce by *fungus aspergillus* specially *aspergillus flavus* and *aspergillus parasiticus*. Human exposure to aflatoxins is mainly through consumption of contaminated staples, such as maize and peanuts. Contaminations are often the result of inappropriate storage, which leads to the infestation by aflatoxin-producing fungi.[105] While in western countries liver cancer is mainly due to HCV chronic infection and alcohol consumption, in LMICs and sub-Saharan Africa in particular HCC is mainly due to HBV chronic infection and the exposition to aflatoxin B1, which together have a multiplicative effect on the risk to develop HCC.[105,106] The prevalence of HBV is over 10% in central, western, and eastern Africa and between 5–10% in southern Africa.[107] A study by Gouas et al. showed that regions of the world with high incidence of HCC correspond to regions of the world where the chronic carriage of HBV is high as well as higher prevalence of somatic mutation of *TP53* at codon 249.[108] Indeed, aflatoxin B1 induces G>T transversions and is associated with a substitution at *TP53* codon 249 (AGG to AGT, R240S) which is the most common *TP53* mutation in hepatocellular carcinoma.[109–111]

Recent trends in liver cancer showed that, while rates were stable or decreasing among men, they were increasing among women. Indeed two population-based studies in East Africa (Uganda) and West Africa (The Gambia) showed that liver cancer rate has increased by more than 50% among females in Uganda, and 27% in The Gambia.[38,112] Several hypotheses such as increased exposure to HCV observed among women as well as the increased prevalence of obesity have been given as explanations for these changes. Available studies assessing the role of HCV in HCC risk suggested a RR of 1.1 to 62[107] and indicated that the risk of chronic infection by HCV and HBV may be additive[113,114] and may act synergistically in increasing HCC risk.[115] A study performed in The Gambia between 1997 and 2001 showed that among liver cancer patients, 32% of women were Hepatitis C virus positive, as compared to 16% of men $(P = 0.03)$.[114] Furthermore, recent meta-analyses have found that in West Africa, the prevalence of obesity has doubled (114%) over the 15 past years. In this study, women were more likely to be obese than men (OR = 3.16, 95% CI: 2.51–3.98 vs. OR = 4.79, 95% CI: 3.30–6.95 in urban and rural areas, respectively).[116] A meta-analysis of 11 cohort studies has shown a substantial association between excess bodyweight and increased risk of liver cancer. This study also reported that, compared with persons of normal weight, the relative risk of liver cancer among the obese was 1.89 (95% CI: 1.51–2.36).[117] Currently very few data on liver cancer trends and obesity as a risk factor for liver cancer in Africa are available. Nevertheless the role of obesity and HCV exposition among women deserves further attention in hepatocellular carcinoma prevention strategies.

Although there is no vaccine against HCV, hepatitis B vaccine is available. The first universal HBV vaccination program was launched in Taiwan. After 20 years, chronic HBV infection rates in the general population below 20 years of age have revealed a remarkable reduction from 10–17% before the vaccination program to 0.7–1.7% after the program.[118] In 2004, GAVI reported that 50% of low-income countries included hepatitis B vaccine in their routine immunization programs and reported that 296 million children were immunized against hepatitis B virus from 2009 to 2011.[119] Developing countries should include Hepatitis B in their immunization programs and supplemental efforts are needed to prevent and diagnose HCC early among adults in Africa.

Family history of liver cancer could be an important risk factor in the development of liver cancer in Africa. Familial clustering of HCC has been reported among eastern Asian countries where liver cancer is also common. Family history was found to be related to HCC risk, even in subjects without hepatitis B or C serum marker after adjusting for confounding variables.[120,121] Also, a recent study in southern Europe reported a significant HCC risk in subjects with a family history of liver cancer, after adjusting for several risk factors, including HbsAg and/or anti-HVC positivity (OR = 2.38, 95% CI: 1.01–5.53).[122] In the United States, history of liver cancer in a first-degree relative was also found to be significantly associated with HCC development independent of HBV and HCV (AOR = 5.7, 95% CI: 1.2–27.3). Therefore, there could be much to discover about a link between family history of liver cancer and development of HCC in sub-Sahara Africa.

Colorectal Cancer

Colorectal cancer (CRC) is the fifth and the fourth most commonly diagnosed cancer and the sixth and fifth most common cause of death by cancer in males and females respectively in sub-Saharan Africa.[92] In 2008, 26,816 cases and 20,889 deaths were estimated in sub-Saharan Africa.[10] This is far lower than the over 1.2 million new cases and 608,700 deaths world estimates in 2008.[2] Previous studies have shown CRC to be a rare disease in Africans: ASR ≥ 0,93 in The Gambia and ≥ 7.5 in Uganda-Kampala,[38,61] where it represents 2–6% of all malignant tumors.[38,123,124] However, CRC incidence rates are rapidly increasing in several African countries historically known to be at low risk, including Nigeria,[125,126] Ghana,[127] Tunisia,[128] and Egypt.[129,130] In these areas, CRC now accounts for about 10–50% of all malignant tumors. Such unfavorable trends are thought to reflect a combination of risk factors, such as changes in dietary pattern, obesity, and smoking.[131,132]

Predisposing factors in the development of CRC include the presence of premalignant conditions such as familial Lynch syndrome (LS),[125,133] which results from the accumulation of MMR gene mutations.[134] LS is characterized by an early age of colorectal onset (mean, 44 years) and can occur in multiple individuals within a family with an advanced transformation rate which is due to mutation and subsequent inactivation of MMR genes, especially *MLH1* and *MSH2*[135] African populations frequently show loss of expression of *MLH1* and *MSH2* genes which are mutated to a variable extent in the germline of patients with LS.[136] This has been confirmed by two studies in South Africa which identified and linked mutations in *MLH1* and *MSH2* with CRC. The studies found that 36%[137] and 40%[138] of young black patients had abnormal expression of both genes and thus may predispose relatives of carriers to LS.[139] Similarly, mutations of *MLH1* and *MSH2* were also identified in CRC in African Americans who shared genetic resemblance with the African (blacks).[140]

The International Collaborative Group on LS has established some phenotypic criteria (commonly referred to as the Amsterdam and Bethesda criteria) for diagnosing LS disorder in a family.[141] In their recommendations, the criteria for diagnosing LS risks should pertain primarily to a family history of colorectal cancer, such as (1) the existence of three or more relatives with histologically verified colorectal cancer, one of whom is a first-degree relative of the two; (2) colorectal cancer involving at least two generations; and (3) one or more cases of colorectal cancer diagnosed before the age of 50 in the family.[142] However, in many developing regions such as Africa, it is difficult to obtain a family history from affected individuals due to language barriers, fears of isolation and overall patient reluctance to follow up after initial diagnosis. Therefore, in addition to obtaining comprehensive family history, morphological and molecular tests for LS through by universal screening of tumors by immunohistochemistry could identify loss of MLH1, MSH2, MSH6 and PMS2 and indicate possible carriers of germline mutations in the *MLH1, MSH2, MSH6 and PMS2* genes may be an important step in ascertaining risk of developing CRC within a family.

▦ CANCER PREVENTION: WHAT WE COULD BE DOING

Effective cancer prevention can only be accomplished if there is clear knowledge of the causal factors or predisposing causes for different types of cancers. As earlier pointed out, the prevalence of cancers and cancer mortality are on the rise in Africa. This is a major concern, especially in areas with limited resources, where over a quarter of disease-related deaths are linked to cancer. Several factors have been implicated to be responsible for the rapid increase in prevalence and incidence of cancer in Africa, including changes in lifestyle and the emergence of westernization.[107] Unless prevention can reduce the incidence of cancer, the number of new cases has been projected to increase to about 9 million in developing countries in 2020.[143] Yet there are many feasible ways to fight the rise of cancer in Africa, such as increasing the population's awareness of the increasing burden of cancer, making genetic testing and counseling more common, and encouraging collaborative research on the application of low-technology tools to obtain evidence on the most cost-effective approaches to prevention of cancer in low-resource settings.

Increase Public Awareness

One of the major reasons that the fatality of cancer is on the rise in developing countries is that majority of the population lack awareness of the early stage signs and symptoms of cancer. Nearly one-third of cancer cases are treatable if detected early.[144] However, many patients with cancers, especially breast cancer, are diagnosed too late for curative interventions to be effective. For example, in Kenya 73%[145] of breast cancer patients reported for treatment more than three months after noticing symptoms due to lack of knowledge of the serious nature of the symptoms.[146] Studies In Mali, Cameroon, and Nigeria revealed that patients affected by breast cancer initially consult lower tier health professional and that, access to knowledgeable health professionals remains mainly motivated by the appearance of symptoms of the disease and by the pressure of their inner circle, with a long delay between the initial consultation by a lower tier health professional and the consultation with a specialized doctor.[147] Poverty, local belief and lack of acceptance of orthodox treatment were among the reasons for the delay.[148,149] This delay of the disease presentation is also due to lack of communication between patients and health professionals. In Nigeria a study found that 73.4% of women affected by breast cancer had a delay of more than 3 months after the initial hospital contact. This delay was partly due to Institutional or physician barriers and partly due to patients.[150] In addition, the poor organization of the health care system also has a role in patients' delay.[151]

More can be done to save lives in Africa if cancer can be detected early and if cancer health education, information, and communication are increased. Cancer awareness education is needed to educate communities that (1) cancer is not necessarily a death sentence, (2) risks can be reduced through healthy lifestyle, and (3) early detection can increase chances of successful treatment. Public health agencies, government, nongovernmental organizations, and private donors can play significant roles in strengthening existing cancer control programs by establishing national or district cancer control programs that provide educational services about prevention, including cancer risk assessment and genetic testing and early detection of cancer. This would be particularly valuable in areas and regions where adequate facilities for treatment of cancer are not available. Through methods such as educational posters and onsite knowledge-sharing centers, the emphasis should be to create awareness regarding early symptoms of cancer, teaching the importance of personal hygiene and a healthy lifestyle, and educating the people to realize that many of the cancer cases, if detected and reported at an early stage, can be fully cured. The result of the general public knowing that more effective treatment may result from early detection and early presentation for treatment may lead to a macrolevel reduction in pain and significant decrease in the loss of life.

Family-Based Risk Assessment and Counseling for High-Risk Patients

The initial management of any patient with a suspected inherited cancer syndrome is genetic counseling and genetic testing if available. Genetic counseling is a multistep process, which includes education regarding the genetics of cancer, the likelihood of developing cancer, the likelihood of carrying a genetic susceptibility mutation, and the implications of a hereditary disease for the patient's family.[152]

Since inherited genetic mutations have a 50% chance of being passed on, individuals with family members known to have cancer need to be referred for risk assessment and genetic testing to confirm the presence of mutations. Early testing for genetic predisposition has recently received more recognition for being part of an effective comprehensive cancer control strategy.[153,154] Because healthy lifestyle and education on the avoidance of cancer risk factors may prevent the occurrence of cancer in predisposed persons, it is encouraged that individuals get tested if they have a known history of cancer in the family; especially if they have immediate relatives affected by cancer. In the case of breast cancer, the overall goal of genetic counseling is to ensure that women have been sufficiently educated regarding inherited breast/ovarian cancer in order to make informed decisions concerning genetic testing and available preventive options.[155] This is necessary for the affected patients to make informed decisions on the appropriate choice of surgery or treatment needed. Previous studies have indicated that the majority of newly diagnosed breast cancer patients at high risk of being *BRCA1/2* mutation carriers will accept rapid genetic counseling and testing, and that the DNA test results can have a substantial impact on the choice of surgery.[156,157] In resource poor settings, this may not be attainable but the newly diagnosed cancer patient can now provide a mechanism to reach at risk relatives.

While genetic counseling and testing may be beneficial at reducing cancer risk, patients may also be more psychologically vulnerable since they may exhibit more cancer-related anxiety due to their recent diagnosis and treatment. By providing counseling that fits the specific socio cultural need of patients, baseline higher anxieties have been found to decrease after genetic counseling. Studies indicated that although disclosure of test results following genetic counseling and testing may increase short-term distress, there is no evidence to suggest that there is a sustained increased in levels of distress as a result of counseling or testing.[158–161] Results from these studies are consistent with a recent meta-analysis of 12 published studies on genetic counseling for breast cancer. Results indicated that genetic counseling led to significant decreases in generalized anxiety (average weighted effect $r = -0.17$, $P < 0.01$).[162] Studies are needed from resource poor settings to guide implementation of genetic counseling programs.

Determining a patient's specific genetic abnormality can provide helpful prognostic information. However, while genetic counseling and testing are provided routinely to high-risk individuals in developed countries and have demonstrated benefits in cancer prevention and treatment,[163] such practices are very much unavailable in developing countries. Recent data suggest that cancer screening especially mammographic screening is not sustainable in developing countries due to limited resources and low breast cancer incidence and prevalence rates;[16] however, recent advances in genetic counseling and testing can open new possibilities of offering cancer patients with suspected hereditary form of the disease the opportunity for better treatment options to lower risks both to themselves and family members. Testing for predisposing genes will allow the identification of individuals at increased risk and the reassurance for those who are not. This may form a cost-effective clinical standard practice for dealing with high-penetrance familial cancer syndromes.

Genes, Physical and Social Environment

Although cancer risk factors may be multifactorial, the interaction between genes and the physical and social environment in the development of cancer is increasingly recognized. As mentioned earlier, some of the risk factors involved in the development of cancer include changes in lifestyle, occupation, and environmental exposures. While most of the current research in LMICs has focused on the influence of these factors in the origin and progression of cancer,[164–167] interactions between genes and the various nongenetics factors may be driving the rapid increase in cancer prevalence and incidence. Therefore, researchers should begin to collect clinical, sociodemographic, and genomic data of large cohorts in population-based genetic epidemiological studies to learn as much as possible about the multifactorial genetic and nongenetic causes of cancer. Given LMICs' restricted resources, lack of human capacity, and large sample sizes needed to generate reliable data, it would be prudent to foster collaborative research between investigators from developed countries and LMICs on the relative roles of genetic and nongenetics factors in the causation of cancer. Generating this kind of data would be useful in prioritizing cancer prevention and management programs based on varied cancer incidence and prevalence rates in different regions.

The Age of Personalized Risk Assessment and Prevention

Literature on cancer control in resource poor settings is dominated by descriptive epidemiology, on the basis of registries and case-control studies assessing cancer risk factors. There is increasing evidence of genetic linkage to cancer onset and development which represents important aspects of cancer research that can no longer be overlooked in developing countries. By coupling the awareness of genetic predisposition—through genetic testing and counseling—with healthy lifestyle choices, individuals can gain control over their own health and reduce the cost of care. There are substantial gains to be made in LMICs by applying genetic information to achieve more effective cancer control activities.

■ SUMMARY

Cancer imposes a major disease burden worldwide, with considerable variation among countries and regions. While much of what is known about cancer prevention and treatment comes from studies conducted in developed countries, cancer control activities in LMICs are in infancy, making it difficult to estimate the costs and effectiveness of various prevention and treatment strategies. This creates an unprecedented opportunity for LMICs to leverage emerging technologies to gain a better understanding of the variety of lifestyle and environmental exposures, as well as genetic factors that can inform cancer prevention and management strategies in these regions. Researchers and health professionals in LMICs must lead the creation of innovative approaches to stem the looming cancer epidemic in LMICs by "leap frogging" to take advantage of some of the scientific discoveries that are transforming cancer treatment and prevention in developed countries.

▦ REFERENCES

1. Ferlay J, Shin H, Bray F, Forman D, Mathers C, Parkin DM. Estimates of worldwide burden of cancer in 2008: GLOBOCAN 2008. *International Journal of Cancer*. 2010;127(12):2893–2917.
2. International Agency for Research on Cancer. GLOBOCAN 2008: Cancer incidence, mortality and prevalence worldwide. 2008.
3. Bray F, Jemal A, Grey N, Ferlay J, Forman D. Global cancer transitions according to the human development index (2008–2030): A population-based study. *Lancet Oncol*. 2012;13(8):790–801.
4. de Martel C, Ferlay J, Franceschi S, et al. Global burden of cancers attributable to infections in 2008: A review and synthetic analysis. *Lancet Oncol*. 2012;13(6):607–615.
5. Levitt NS, Steyn K, Dave J, Bradshaw D. Chronic noncommunicable diseases and HIV-AIDS on a collision course: Relevance for health care delivery, particularly in low-resource settings—insights from South Africa. *Am J Clin Nutr*. 2011;94(6):1690S–1696S.
6. Boyle P. The globalisation of cancer. *Lancet*. 2006;368(9536):629–630.
7. Fontham ET. Infectious diseases and global cancer control. *CA Cancer J Clin*. 2009;59(1):5–7.
8. Braithwaite D, Wernli KJ, Anton-Culver H, Engstrom P, Greenberg ER, Meyskens F. Opportunities for cancer epidemiology and control in low- and middle-income countries: A report from the American society for preventive oncology international cancer prevention interest group. *Cancer Epidemiol Biomarkers Prev*. 2010;19(7):1665–1667.
9. Brown BJ, Ajayi SO, Ogun OA, Oladokun RE. Factors influencing time to diagnosis of childhood cancer in Ibadan, Nigeria. *Afr Health Sci*. 2009;9(4):247–253.
10. International Agency for Research on Cancer (IARC). The GLOBOCAN project. GLOBOCAN 2008. Web site: http://globocan.iarc.fr/. Updated 2010.
11. Jemal A, Bray F, Center MM, Ferlay J, Ward E, Forman D. Global cancer statistics. *CA Cancer J Clin*. 2011;61(2):69–90.
12. Thun MJ, DeLancey JO, Center MM, Jemal A, Ward EM. The global burden of cancer: Priorities for prevention. *Carcinogenesis*. 2010;31(1):100–110.
13. Rastogi T, Hildesheim A, Sinha R. Opportunities for cancer epidemiology in developing countries. *Nat Rev Cancer*. 2004;4(11):909–917.
14. Plesnicar S, Plesnicar A. Cancer: A reality in the emerging world. *Semin Oncol*. 2001;28(2):210–216.
15. Jemal A, Center MM, DeSantis C, Ward EM. Global patterns of cancer incidence and mortality rates and trends. *Cancer Epidemiol Biomarkers Prev*. 2010;19(8):1893–1907.
16. Harford JB. Breast-cancer early detection in low-income and middle-income countries: Do what you can versus one size fits all. *Lancet Oncol*. 2011;12(3):306–312.
17. Kanavos P. The rising burden of cancer in the developing world. *Ann Oncol*. 2006;17 Suppl 8:viii15–viii23.
18. Coleman MP, Quaresma M, Berrino F, et al. Cancer survival in five continents: A worldwide population-based study (CONCORD). *Lancet Oncol*. 2008;9(8):730–756.
19. Sankaranarayanan R. Cancer survival in Africa, Asia, the Caribbean and Central America. Introduction. *IARC Sci Publ*. 2011;(162)(162):1–5.
20. United Nations, Department of Economic and Social Affairs, Population Division. World population prospects: The 2010 revision, CD-ROM edition. 2011.
21. Sellier J, Le Fur A, Brun Bd. *Atlas des peuples d'Afrique*. Paris: La Découverte; 2005.
22. Lewis MP, ed. *Ethnologue: Languages of the world, sixteenth edition*. Dallas, TX: SIL International; 2009. Online version: http://www.ethnologue.com/.
23. Campbell MC, Tishkoff SA. African genetic diversity: Implications for human demographic history, modern human origins, and complex disease mapping. *Annu Rev Genomics Hum Genet*. 2008;9:403–433.
24. Tishkoff SA, Reed FA, Friedlaender FR, et al. The genetic structure and history of Africans and African Americans. *Science*. 2009;324(5930):1035–1044.
25. Patterson N, Price AL, Reich D. Population structure and eigenanalysis. *PLoS Genet*. 2006;2(12):e190.
26. Piniewski-Bond J, Celestino PB, Mahoney MC, et al. A cancer genetics education campaign: Delivering parallel messages to clinicians and the public. *J Cancer Educ*. 2003;18(2):96–99.

27. Awadelkarim KD, Aceto G, Veschi S, et al. BRCA1 and BRCA2 status in a central Sudanese series of breast cancer patients: Interactions with genetic, ethnic and reproductive factors. *Breast Cancer Res Treat*. 2007;102(2):189–199.

28. Ekanem VJ, Aligbe JU. Histopathological types of breast cancer in Nigerian women: A 12-year review (1993–2004). *Afr J Reprod Health*. 2006;10(1):71–75.

29. Jedy-Agba E, Curado MP, Ogunbiyi O, et al. Cancer incidence in Nigeria: A report from population-based cancer registries. *Cancer Epidemiol*. 2012;36(5):e271–e278.

30. Mbonde MP, Amir H, Schwartz-Albiez R, Akslen LA, Kitinya JN. Expression of estrogen and progesterone receptors in carcinomas of the female breast in Tanzania. *Oncol Rep*. 2000;7(2):277–283.

31. Sighoko D, Bah E, Haukka J, et al. Population-based breast (female) and cervix cancer rates in the Gambia: Evidence of ethnicity-related variations. *Int J Cancer*. 2010;127(10):2248–2256.

32. Huo D, Adebamowo CA, Ogundiran TO, et al. Parity and breastfeeding are protective against breast cancer in Nigerian women. *Br J Cancer*. 2008;98(5):992–996.

33. Adebamowo CA, Ogundiran TO, Adenipekun AA, et al. Waist-hip ratio and breast cancer risk in urbanized Nigerian women. *Breast Cancer Res*. 2003;5(2):R18–R24.

34. Bah E, Parkin DM, Hall AJ, Jack AD, Whittle H. Cancer in the Gambia: 1988–97. *Br J Cancer*. 2001;84(9):1207–1214.

35. Clavel-Chapelon F, E3N-EPIC Group. Differential effects of reproductive factors on the risk of pre- and postmenopausal breast cancer. results from a large cohort of French women. *Br J Cancer*. 2002;86(5): 723–727.

36. Elsie KM, Gonzaga MA, Francis B, et al. Current knowledge, attitudes and practices of women on breast cancer and mammography at Mulago Hospital. *Pan Afr Med J*. 2010;5:9.

37. Nggada HA, Yawe KD, Abdulazeez J, Khalil MA. Breast cancer burden in Maiduguri, north eastern Nigeria. *Breast J*. 2008;14(3):284–286.

38. Sighoko D, Curado MP, Bourgeois D, Mendy M, Hainaut P, Bah E. Increase in female liver cancer in the Gambia, West Africa: Evidence from 19 years of population-based cancer registration (1988–2006). *PLoS One*. 2011;6(4):e18415.

39. Adesunkanmi AR, Lawal OO, Adelusola KA, Durosimi MA. The severity, outcome and challenges of breast cancer in Nigeria. *Breast*. 2006;15(3):399–409.

40. Bhikoo R, Srinivasa S, Yu T, Moss D, Hill AG. Systematic review of breast cancer biology in developing countries (part 1): Africa, the Middle East, Eastern Europe, Mexico, the Caribbean and South America. *Cancers*. 2011;3(2):2358.

41. Fregene A, Newman LA. Breast cancer in sub-Saharan Africa: How does it relate to breast cancer in African-American women? *Cancer*. 2005;103(8):1540–1550.

42. Gukas ID, Jennings BA, Mandong BM, et al. Clinicopathological features and molecular markers of breast cancer in Jos, Nigeria. *West Afr J Med*. 2005;24(3):209–213.

43. Huo D, Ikpatt F, Khramtsov A, et al. Population differences in breast cancer: Survey in indigenous African women reveals over-representation of triple-negative breast cancer. *J Clin Oncol*. 2009;27(27): 4515–4521.

44. Fackenthal JD, Olopade OI. Breast cancer risk associated with BRCA1 and BRCA2 in diverse populations. *Nat Rev Cancer*. 2007;7(12):937–948.

45. Ponder BA, Antoniou A, Dunning A, Easton DF, Pharoah PD. Polygenic inherited predisposition to breast cancer. *Cold Spring Harb Symp Quant Biol*. 2005;70:35–41.

46. Antoniou A, Pharoah PD, Narod S, et al. Average risks of breast and ovarian cancer associated with BRCA1 or BRCA2 mutations detected in case series unselected for family history: A combined analysis of 22 studies. *Am J Hum Genet*. 2003;72(5):1117–1130.

47. Sowter HM, Ashworth A. BRCA1 and BRCA2 as ovarian cancer susceptibility genes. *Carcinogenesis*. 2005;26(10):1651–1656.

48. Welcsh PL, King MC. BRCA1 and BRCA2 and the genetics of breast and ovarian cancer. *Hum Mol Genet*. 2001;10(7):705–713.

49. Balmain A, Gray J, Ponder B. The genetics and genomics of cancer. *Nat Genet*. 2003;33 Suppl:238–244.

50. Chen S, Parmigiani G. Meta-analysis of BRCA1 and BRCA2 penetrance. *J Clin Oncol.* 2007;25(11):1329–1333.

51. Rosenberg L, Kelly JP, Shapiro S, Hoffman M, Cooper D. Risk factors for breast cancer in South African women. *S Afr Med J.* 2002;92(6):447–448.

52. Pegoraro RJ, Moodley M, Rom L, Chetty R, Moodley J. P53 codon 72 polymorphism and BRCA 1 and 2 mutations in ovarian epithelial malignancies in black South Africans. *Int J Gynecol Cancer.* 2003;13(4):444–449.

53. Gao Q, Adebamowo CA, Fackenthal J, et al. Protein truncating BRCA1 and BRCA2 mutations in African women with pre-menopausal breast cancer. *Hum Genet.* 2000;107(2):192–194.

54. Fackenthal JD, Zhang J, Zhang B, et al. High prevalence of BRCA1 and BRCA2 mutations in unselected Nigerian breast cancer patients. *Int J Cancer.* 2012;131(5):1114–1123.

55. Foulkes WD, Stefansson IM, Chappuis PO, et al. Germline BRCA1 mutations and a basal epithelial phenotype in breast cancer. *J Natl Cancer Inst.* 2003;95(19):1482–1485.

56. Olopade OI, Grushko T. Gene-expression profiles in hereditary breast cancer. *N Engl J Med.* 2001;344(26):2028–2029.

57. Atchley DP, Albarracin CT, Lopez A, et al. Clinical and pathologic characteristics of patients with BRCA-positive and BRCA-negative breast cancer. *J Clin Oncol.* 2008;26(26):4282–4288.

58. Carey LA, Perou CM, Livasy CA, et al. Race, breast cancer subtypes, and survival in the Carolina breast cancer study. *JAMA.* 2006;295(21):2492–2502.

59. Huo D, Zheng Y, Ogundiran TO, et al. Evaluation of 19 susceptibility loci of breast cancer in women of African ancestry. *Carcinogenesis.* 2012;33(4):835–840.

60. Parkin DM, Sitas F, Chirenje M, Stein L, Abratt R, Wabinga H. Part I: Cancer in indigenous Africans—burden, distribution, and trends. *The Lancet Oncology.* 2008;9(7):683.

61. Parkin DM, Nambooze S, Wabwire-Mangen F, Wabinga HR. Changing cancer incidence in Kampala, Uganda, 1991–2006. *Int J Cancer.* 2010;126(5):1187–1195.

62. Walboomers JM, Jacobs MV, Manos MM, et al. Human papillomavirus is a necessary cause of invasive cervical cancer worldwide. *J Pathol.* 1999;189(1):12–19.

63. Dartell M, Rasch V, Kahesa C, et al. Human papillomavirus prevalence and type distribution in 3603 HIV-positive and HIV-negative women in the general population of Tanzania: The PROTECT study. *Sex Transm Dis.* 2012;39(3):201–208.

64. Piras F, Piga M, De Montis A, et al. Prevalence of human papillomavirus infection in women in Benin, West Africa. *Virol J.* 2011;8:514.

65. Wall SR, Scherf CF, Morison L, et al. Cervical human papillomavirus infection and squamous intra-epithelial lesions in rural Gambia, West Africa: Viral sequence analysis and epidemiology. *Br J Cancer.* 2005;93(9):1068–1076.

66. Munoz N, Castellsague X, de Gonzalez AB, Gissmann L. Chapter 1: HPV in the etiology of human cancer. *Vaccine.* 2006;24 Suppl 3:S3/1–10.

67. Munoz N, Bosch FX, Castellsague X, et al. Against which human papillomavirus types shall we vaccinate and screen? The international perspective. *Int J Cancer.* 2004;111(2):278–285.

68. Smith JS, Lindsay L, Hoots B, et al. Human papillomavirus type distribution in invasive cervical cancer and high-grade cervical lesions: A meta-analysis update. *Int J Cancer.* 2007;121(3):621–632.

69. Didelot-Rousseau MN, Nagot N, Costes-Martineau V, et al. Human papillomavirus genotype distribution and cervical squamous intraepithelial lesions among high-risk women with and without HIV-1 infection in Burkina Faso. *Br J Cancer.* 2006;95(3):355–362.

70. Xi LF, Toure P, Critchlow CW, et al. Prevalence of specific types of human papillomavirus and cervical squamous intraepithelial lesions in consecutive, previously unscreened, West-African women over 35 years of age. *Int J Cancer.* 2003;103(6):803–809.

71. Castellsague X, Diaz M, de Sanjose S, et al. Worldwide human papillomavirus etiology of cervical adenocarcinoma and its cofactors: Implications for screening and prevention. *J Natl Cancer Inst.* 2006;98(5):303–315.

72. Conti M, Agarossi A, Parazzini F, et al. HPV, HIV infection, and risk of cervical intraepithelial neoplasia in former intravenous drug abusers. *Gynecol Oncol.* 1993;49(3):344–348.

73. Wright TC, Jr, Ellerbrock TV, Chiasson MA, Van Devanter N, Sun XW. Cervical intraepithelial neoplasia in women infected with human immunodeficiency virus: Prevalence, risk factors, and validity of papanicolaou smears. New York cervical disease study. *Obstet Gynecol.* 1994;84(4):591–597.

74. Atashili J, Adimora AA, Ndumbe PM, et al. High prevalence of cervical squamous intraepithelial lesions in women on antiretroviral therapy in Cameroon: Is targeted screening feasible? *Cancer Epidemiol.* 2012;36(3):263–269.

75. Desruisseau AJ, Schmidt-Grimminger D, Welty E. Epidemiology of HPV in HIV-positive and HIV-negative fertile women in Cameroon, West Africa. *Infect Dis Obstet Gynecol.* 2009;2009:810596.

76. Dim CC, Ezegwui HU, Ikeme AC, Nwagha UI, Onyedum CC. Prevalence of cervical squamous intraepithelial lesions among HIV-positive women in Enugu, south-eastern Nigeria. *J Obstet Gynaecol.* 2011;31(8):759–762.

77. Horo A, Jaquet A, Ekouevi DK, et al. Cervical cancer screening by visual inspection in Côte d'Ivoire, operational and clinical aspects according to HIV status. *BMC Public Health.* 2012;12:237.

78. De Vuyst H, Ndirangu G, Moodley M, et al. Prevalence of human papillomavirus in women with invasive cervical carcinoma by HIV status in Kenya and South Africa. *Int J Cancer.* 2012;131(4):949–955.

79. Mathew A, George P. Trends in incidence and mortality rates of squamous cell carcinoma and adenocarcinoma of cervix—worldwide. *Asian Pacific Journal of Cancer Prevention.* 2009;10(4):645.

80. Deodhar K, Sankaranarayanan R, Jayant K, et al. Accuracy of concurrent visual and cytology screening in detecting cervical cancer precursors in rural India. *Int J Cancer.* 2012;131(6):E954–E962.

81. Sangwa-Lugoma G, Mahmud S, Nasr SH, et al. Visual inspection as a cervical cancer screening method in a primary health care setting in Africa. *Int J Cancer.* 2006;119(6):1389–1395.

82. Saxena U, Sauvaget C, Sankaranarayanan R. Evidence-based screening, early diagnosis and treatment strategy of cervical cancer for national policy in low- resource countries: Example of India. *Asian Pac J Cancer Prev.* 2012;13(4):1699–1703.

83. Lewis KC, Tsu VD, Dawa A, Kidula NA, Chami IN, Sellors JW. A comparison of triage methods for Kenyan women who screen positive for cervical intraepithelial neoplasia by visual inspection of the cervix with acetic acid. *Afr Health Sci.* 2011;11(3):362–369.

84. Lewis KD, Sellors JW, Dawa A, Tsu VD, Kidula NA. Report on a cryotherapy service for women with cervical intraepithelial neoplasia in a district hospital in western Kenya. *Afr Health Sci.* 2011;11(3):370–376.

85. Moon TD, Silva-Matos C, Cordoso A, Baptista AJ, Sidat M, Vermund SH. Implementation of cervical cancer screening using visual inspection with acetic acid in rural Mozambique: Successes and challenges using HIV care and treatment programme investments in Zambezia province. *J Int AIDS Soc.* 2012;15(2):17406.

86. Teguete I, Muwonge R, Traore CB, Dolo A, Bayo S, Sankaranarayanan R. Can visual cervical screening be sustained in routine health services? Experience from Mali, Africa. *BJOG.* 2012;119(2):220–226.

87. Denny L. Cervical cancer treatment in Africa. *Curr Opin Oncol.* 2011;23(5):469–474.

88. Francis SA, Battle-Fisher M, Liverpool J, et al. A qualitative analysis of South African women's knowledge, attitudes, and beliefs about HPV and cervical cancer prevention, vaccine awareness and acceptance, and maternal-child communication about sexual health. *Vaccine.* 2011;29(47):8760–8765.

89. Mbamara SU, Ikpeze OC, Okonkwo JE, Onyiaorah IV, Ukah CO. Knowledge, attitude and practice of cervical cancer screening among women attending gynecology clinics in a tertiary level medical care center in southeastern Nigeria. *J Reprod Med.* 2011;56(11–12):491–496.

90. Patel DA, Barnholtz-Sloan JS, Patel MK, Malone JM, Jr, Chuba PJ, Schwartz K. A population-based study of racial and ethnic differences in survival among women with invasive cervical cancer: Analysis of surveillance, epidemiology, and end results data. *Gynecol Oncol.* 2005;97(2):550–558.

91. Goldie SJ, O'Shea M, Campos NG, Diaz M, Sweet S, Kim SY. Health and economic outcomes of HPV 16, 18 vaccination in 72 GAVI-eligible countries. *Vaccine.* 2008;26(32):4080–4093.

92. Jemal A, Bray F, Forman D, et al. Cancer burden in Africa and opportunities for prevention. *Cancer.* 2012;118(18):4372–4384.

93. Bock CH, Schwartz AG, Ruterbusch JJ, et al. Results from a prostate cancer admixture mapping study in African-American men. *Hum Genet.* 2009;126(5):637–642.

94. Miller DC, Zheng SL, Dunn RL, et al. Germ-line mutations of the macrophage scavenger receptor 1 gene: Association with prostate cancer risk in African-American men. *Cancer Res.* 2003;63(13):3486–3489.

95. Platz EA, Giovannucci E. Prostate cancer. In: Schottenfeld D, Fraumeni JF, eds. *Cancer epidemiology and prevention.* New York: Oxford University Press; 2006:1128–1150.

96. Hayes RB, Liff JM, Pottern LM, et al. Prostate cancer risk in U.S. blacks and whites with a family history of cancer. *Int J Cancer.* 1995;60(3):361–364.

97. Whittemore AS, Wu AH, Kolonel LN, et al. Family history and prostate cancer risk in black, white, and Asian men in the United States and Canada. *Am J Epidemiol.* 1995;141(8):732–740.

98. Schaid DJ. The complex genetic epidemiology of prostate cancer. *Hum Mol Genet.* 2004;13 Spec No 1:R103–R121.

99. Steinberg GD, Carter BS, Beaty TH, Childs B, Walsh PC. Family history and the risk of prostate cancer. *Prostate.* 1990;17(4):337–347.

100. Haiman CA, Patterson N, Freedman ML, et al. Multiple regions within 8q24 independently affect risk for prostate cancer. *Nat Genet.* 2007;39(5):638–644.

101. Haiman CA, Chen GK, Blot WJ, et al. Genome-wide association study of prostate cancer in men of African ancestry identifies a susceptibility locus at 17q21. *Nat Genet.* 2011;43(6):570–573.

102. International Agency for Research on Cancer (IARC). Cancer epidemiology. http://www.iarc.fr/en/publications/pdfs-online/epi/sp153/index.php. Published 2008.

103. McGlynn KA, Tarone RE, El-Serag HB. A comparison of trends in the incidence of hepatocellular carcinoma and intrahepatic cholangiocarcinoma in the United States. *Cancer Epidemiol Biomarkers Prev.* 2006;15(6):1198–1203.

104. Perz JF, Armstrong GL, Farrington LA, Hutin YJF, Bell BP. The contributions of hepatitis B virus and hepatitis C virus infections to cirrhosis and primary liver cancer worldwide. *J Hepatol.* 2006;45(4):529.

105. Williams JH, Phillips TD, Jolly PE, Stiles JK, Jolly CM, Aggarwal D. Human aflatoxicosis in developing countries: A review of toxicology, exposure, potential health consequences, and interventions. *Am J Clin Nutr.* 2004;80(5):1106–1122.

106. Wogan GN. Aflatoxin carcinogenesis: Interspecies potency differences and relevance for human risk assessment. *Prog Clin Biol Res.* 1992;374:123–137.

107. Parkin DM, Ferlay J, Hamdi-Cherif M, et al, eds. *Cancer in Africa: Epidemiology and prevention. 4.3 Cervix cancer.* Lyon: IARC Press; 2003; No. IARC Scientific Publications No. 153.

108. Gouas D, Shi H, Hainaut P. The aflatoxin-induced TP53 mutation at codon 249 (R249S): Biomarker of exposure, early detection and target for therapy. *Cancer Lett.* 2009;286(1):29–37.

109. Bressac B, Kew M, Wands J, Ozturk M. Selective G to T mutations of p53 gene in hepatocellular carcinoma from southern Africa. *Nature.* 1991;350(6317):429–431.

110. Hsu IC, Metcalf RA, Sun T, Welsh JA, Wang NJ, Harris CC. Mutational hotspot in the p53 gene in human hepatocellular carcinomas. *Nature.* 1991;350(6317):427–428.

111. Ozturk M. P53 mutation in hepatocellular carcinoma after aflatoxin exposure. *Lancet.* 1991;338(8779):1356–1359.

112. Ocama P, Castelnuovo B, Kamya MR, et al. Low frequency of liver enzyme elevation in HIV-infected patients attending a large urban treatment centre in Uganda. *Int J STD AIDS.* 2010;21(8):553–557.

113. Kew MC, Welschinger R, Viana R. Occult hepatitis B virus infection in southern African blacks with hepatocellular carcinoma. *J Gastroenterol Hepatol.* 2008;23(9):1426–1430.

114. Kirk GD, Lesi OA, Mendy M, et al. The gambia liver cancer study: Infection with hepatitis B and C and the risk of hepatocellular carcinoma in West Africa. *Hepatology.* 2004;39(1):211–219.

115. Parkin DM, Bray FI, Devesa SS. Cancer burden in the year 2000. The global picture. *Eur J Cancer.* 2001;37 Suppl 8:S4–S66.

116. Abubakari AR, Lauder W, Agyemang C, Jones M, Kirk A, Bhopal RS. Prevalence and time trends in obesity among adult West African populations: A meta-analysis. *Obes Rev.* 2008;9(4):297–311.

117. Larsson SC, Wolk A. Overweight, obesity and risk of liver cancer: A meta-analysis of cohort studies. *Br J Cancer.* 2007;97(7):1005–1008.

118. Chang MH. Cancer prevention by vaccination against hepatitis B. *Recent Results Cancer Res.* 2009; 181:85–94.

119. GAVI Alliance. Hepatitis B vaccine support. GAVI Alliance: Types of support. Web site: http://www. gavialliance.org/support/nvs/hepb/. Updated 2012.

120. Donato F, Gelatti U, Chiesa R, et al. A case-control study on family history of liver cancer as a risk factor for hepatocellular carcinoma in North Italy. Brescia HCC study. *Cancer Causes Control.* 1999;10(5):417–421.

121. Evans AA, Chen G, Ross EA, Shen F, Lin W, London WT. Eight-year follow-up of the 90,000-person Haimen city cohort: I. hepatocellular carcinoma mortality, risk factors, and gender differences. *Cancer epidemiology, biomarkers & prevention: a publication of the American Association for Cancer Research, cosponsored by the American Society of Preventive Oncology.* 2002;11(4):369.

122. Turati F, Edefonti V, Talamini R, et al. Family history of liver cancer and hepatocellular carcinoma. *Hepatology.* 2012;55(5):1416–1425.

123. Holcombe C, Babayo U. The pattern of malignant disease in North-East Nigeria. *Trop Geogr Med.* 1991;43(1–2):189.

124. Okobia M, Aligbe J. Pattern of malignant diseases at the University of Benin teaching hospital. *Trop Doct.* 2005;35(2):91.

125. Abdulkareem FB, Abudu EK, Awolola NA, et al. Colorectal carcinoma in Lagos and Sagamu, southwest Nigeria: A histopathological review. *World J Gastroenterol.* 2008;14(42):6531–6535.

126. Irabor DO, Arowolo A, Afolabi AA. Colon and rectal cancer in Ibadan, Nigeria: An update. *Colorectal Dis.* 2010;12(7 Online):e43–e49.

127. Dakubo JC, Naaeder SB, Tettey Y, Gyasi RK. Colorectal carcinoma: An update of current trends in Accra. *West Afr J Med.* 2010 May-Jun;29(3):178–183.

128. Missaoui N, Jaidaine L, Abdelkader AB, Trabelsi A, Mokni M, Hmissa S. Colorectal cancer in central Tunisia: Increasing incidence trends over a 15-year period. *Asian Pac J Cancer Prev.* 2011;12(4):1073–1076.

129. Abou-Zeid AA, Khafagy W, Marzouk DM, Alaa A, Mostafa I, Ela MA. Colorectal cancer in Egypt. *Dis Colon Rectum.* 2002;45(9):1255–1260.

130. Soliman AS, Bondy ML, Levin B, et al. Colorectal cancer in Egyptian patients under 40 years of age. *Int J Cancer.* 1997;71(1):26–30.

131. Center MM, Jemal A, Ward E. International trends in colorectal cancer incidence rates. *Cancer Epidemiology Biomarkers & Prevention.* 2009;18(6):1688–1694.

132. de Kok IMCM, Wong CS, Chia KS, et al. Gender differences in the trend of colorectal cancer incidence in Singapore, 1968–2002. *Int J Colorectal Dis.* 2008;23(5):461.

133. Soliman AS, Bondy ML, Levin B, et al. Familial aggregation of colorectal cancer in Egypt. *Int J Cancer.* 1998;77(6):811–816.

134. Raut CP, Pawlik TM, Rodriguez-Bigas MA. Clinicopathologic features in colorectal cancer patients with microsatellite instability. *Mutat Res.* 2004;568(2):275–282.

135. Lynch HT, de la Chapelle A. Hereditary colorectal cancer. *N Engl J Med.* 2003;348(10):919–932.

136. Olopade OI, Cummings S. Genetic counselling for cancer: Part II. *Principles and Practice of Oncology.* 1996;10(2):1–11.

137. Cronje L, Paterson AC, Becker PJ. Colorectal cancer in South Africa: A heritable cause suspected in many young black patients. *S Afr Med J.* 2009;99(2):103–106.

138. Hameed F, Goldberg PA, Hall P, Algar U, van Wijk R, Ramesar R. Immunohistochemistry detects mismatch repair gene defects in colorectal cancer. *Colorectal Dis.* 2006;8(5):411–417.

139. Peltomaki P, Vasen HF. Mutations predisposing to hereditary nonpolyposis colorectal cancer: Database and results of a collaborative study. The international collaborative group on hereditary nonpolyposis colorectal cancer. *Gastroenterology.* 1997;113(4):1146–1158.

140. Weber TK, Chin HM, Rodriguez-Bigas M, et al. Novel hMLH1 and hMSH2 germline mutations in African Americans with colorectal cancer. *JAMA*. 1999;281(24):2316–2320.

141. Umar A, Boland CR, Terdiman JP, et al. Revised Bethesda guidelines for hereditary nonpolyposis colorectal cancer (lynch syndrome) and microsatellite instability. *J Natl Cancer Inst*. 2004;96(4):261–268.

142. Vasen HF, Mecklin JP, Khan PM, Lynch HT. The international collaborative group on hereditary non-polyposis colorectal cancer (ICG-HNPCC). *Dis Colon Rectum*. 1991;34(5):424–425.

143. Salminen E, Izewska J, Andreo P. IAEA's role in the global management of cancer-focus on upgrading radiotherapy services. *Acta Oncol*. 2005;44(8):816–824.

144. World Health Organization (WHO), Regional Office for Europe. Cancer. What we do: Data and evidence, health topics, events. Web site: http://www.euro.who.int/en/what-we-do/health-topics/noncommunicable-diseases/cancer. Updated 2012.

145. Otieno E, Micheni J, Kimende S, Mutai K. Delayed presentation of breast cancer patients. *The East African Medical Journal*. 2010;87(4):147–150.

146. Almuammar A, Dryden C, Burr JA. Factors associated with late presentation of cancer: A limited literature review. *Journal of Radiotherapy in Practice*. 2010;9(2):117.

147. Ly M, Diop S, Sacko M, Baby M, Diop CT, Diallo DA. Breast cancer: Factors influencing the therapeutic itinerary of patients in a medical oncology unit in Bamako (Mali). *Bull Cancer*. 2002; 89(3):323–326.

148. Ekortarl A, Ndom P, Sacks A. A study of patients who appear with far advanced cancer at Yaoundé General Hospital, Cameroon, Africa. *Psychooncology*. 2007;16(3):255–257.

149. Ukwenya AY, Yusufu LM, Nmadu PT, Garba ES, Ahmed A. Delayed treatment of symptomatic breast cancer: The experience from Kaduna, Nigeria. *S Afr J Surg*. 2008;46(4):106–110.

150. Ezeome ER. Delays in presentation and treatment of breast cancer in Enugu, Nigeria. *Niger J Clin Pract*. 2010;13(3):311–316.

151. Anorlu RI, Orakwue CO, Oyeneyin L, Abudu OO. Late presentation of patients with cervical cancer to a tertiary hospital in Lagos: What is responsible? *Eur J Gynaecol Oncol*. 2004;25(6):729–732.

152. Berlina JF, Fay AM. Familial cancer risk special interest group of the national society of genetic counselors. Risk assessment and genetic counseling for hereditary breast and ovarian cancer: Recommendations of the national society of genetic counselors. *J Genet Counsel*. 2007;16(3):397–406.

153. Anderson K, Jacobson JS, Heitjan DF, et al. Cost-effectiveness of preventive strategies for women with a BRCA1 or a BRCA2 mutation. *Ann Intern Med*. 2006;144(6):397–406.

154. Brown ML, Riley GF, Schussler N, Etzioni R. Estimating health care costs related to cancer treatment from SEER-medicare data. *Med Care*. 2002;40(8 Suppl):IV-104–117.

155. Peshkin BN, Isaacs C. Evaluation and management of women with BRCA1/2 mutations. *Oncology (Williston Park)*. 2005;19(11):1451–1459; discussion 1459–68 1474.

156. Evans DG, Lalloo F, Hopwood P, et al. Surgical decisions made by 158 women with hereditary breast cancer aged <50 years. *Eur J Surg Oncol*. 2005;31(10):1112–1118.

157. Schwartz MD, Lerman C, Brogan B, et al. Utilization of BRCA1/BRCA2 mutation testing in newly diagnosed breast cancer patients. *Cancer Epidemiol Biomarkers Prev*. 2005;14(4):1003–1007.

158. Bowen DJ, Burke W, McTiernan A, Yasui Y, Andersen MR. Breast cancer risk counseling improves women's functioning. *Patient Educ Couns*. 2004;53(1):79–86.

159. Lerman C, Hughes C, Benkendorf JL, et al. Racial differences in testing motivation and psychological distress following pretest education for BRCA1 gene testing. *Cancer Epidemiol Biomarkers Prev*. 1999;8(4 Pt 2):361–367.

160. Schlich-Bakker KJ, ten Kroode HF, Ausems MG. A literature review of the psychological impact of genetic testing on breast cancer patients. *Patient Educ Couns*. 2006;62(1):13–20.

161. Watson M, Lloyd S, Davidson J, et al. The impact of genetic counselling on risk perception and mental health in women with a family history of breast cancer. *Br J Cancer*. 1999;79(5–6):868–874.

162. Meiser B, Halliday JL. What is the impact of genetic counselling in women at increased risk of developing hereditary breast cancer? A meta-analytic review. *Soc Sci Med*. 2002;54(10):1463–1470.

163. Garber JE, Offit K. Hereditary cancer predisposition syndromes. *J Clin Oncol*. 2005;23(2):276–292.

164. Coyle YM. The effect of environment on breast cancer risk. *Breast Cancer Res Treat*. 2004;84(3):273–288.

165. Dey S, Soliman AS, Hablas A, et al. Urban-rural differences in breast cancer incidence in Egypt (1999–2006). *Breast*. 2010;19(5):417–423.

166. McCormack VA, Schuz J. Africa's growing cancer burden: Environmental and occupational contributions. *Cancer Epidemiol*. 2012;36(1):1–7.

167. Mzileni O, Sitas F, Steyn K, Carrara H, Bekker P. Lung cancer, tobacco, and environmental factors in the African population of the northern province, South Africa. *Tob Control*. 1999;8(4):398–401.

CHAPTER 5

CANCER SCREENING IN LOW- AND MEDIUM-INCOME COUNTRIES

RENGASWAMY SANKARANARAYANAN, SOMANATHAN THARA, YOULIN QIAO, TWALIB NGOMA, RAUL MURILLO

INTRODUCTION

The objective of cancer screening is to prevent death from invasive cancer and improve quality of life by early detection and treatment of persons with early preclinical, asymptomatic cancers or precancerous lesions by the application of a relatively simple, inexpensive test to a large number of apparently healthy persons in order to classify them as likely or unlikely of having the disease of interest. The usefulness of screening as a control option for a given cancer site will depend upon the suitability of the disease for early detection and treatment, the availability of suitable, affordable, easy to use, acceptable, and accurate screening tests to detect the disease in early stages and the availability of affordable and effective treatment to cure the cancer.

Large-scale population-based screening has been a major intervention for control of cancers of the uterine cervix, breast, and colon and rectum in many developed countries. Cervical cancer screening has been particularly effective in reducing mortality to the tune of 60–80% within two to three decades from the initiation of programs,[1] whereas population-based mammography screening programs have reduced breast cancer deaths by 20–25% in population based programs in developed countries.[2]

We describe and discuss the current status and performance of ongoing cervical, breast, colorectal, and oral cancer screening programs in low- and medium-income countries (LMIC) in Latin America, South and South East Asia in terms of organization, coverage, process indicators, and outcome measures, as well as their overall impact on cancer prevention and control. The estimated burden of these cancers, in terms of incident cases and deaths in LMIC around 2008, is given in Table 5.1.[3] We also describe the results of various studies undertaken in LMIC to evaluate different screening approaches and the impact of the evidence generated in catalyzing new programs and strengthening the existing ones, as well as the new research directions in the context of improving screening outcomes.

TABLE 5.1 Global burden of oral, large bowel, breast and uterine cervical cancer, 2008[3]

	MALE		FEMALE		TOTAL	
	NO. OF CASES	NO. OF DEATHS	NO. OF CASES	NO. OF DEATH	NO. OF CASES	NO. OF DEATH
ORAL CANCER						
World	170,903	83,254	92,958	44,697	263,861	127,951
Less developed regions	107,736	61,235	64,164	35,766	171,900	97,001
COLORECTAL CANCER						
World	663,612	320,595	570,099	288,049	1,233,711	608,644
Less developed regions	273,945	154,436	232,352	134,136	506,297	288,572
BREAST CANCER						
World	–	–	1,383,523	458,367	1,383,523	458,367
Less developed regions			691,281	268,879	691,281	268,879
CERVICAL CANCER						
World	–	–	529,409	274,883	529,409	274,883
Less developed regions	–	–	452,902	241,724	452,902	241,724

▦ CRITERIA FOR SUITABILITY OF CANCER SCREENING

Suitable Cancers and Suitable Tests

A cancer may be considered suitable for screening if it has a long natural history with a long detectable preclinical phase, facilitating the detection of precancerous lesions, or early preclinical invasive cancer, if suitable tests are available to detect the preclinical disease, and if effective treatment is available. Suitable tests are those which are easy to apply, noninvasive or very slightly invasive, safe, acceptable, inexpensive, affordable, and accurate in identifying those with a high probability of disease and no disease. The application of cancer screening as a cancer control option in a given country, setting or region will depend upon the public health importance of disease in terms of incidence and mortality and the ability and efficiency of the health care services to meet the demands of diagnostic, treatment, and follow-up care services arising out of a screening program.

A potential benefit from screening can be expected if the reduction of risk surpasses the potential harms of the intervention and if most clinical cases of a disease go through a detectable preclinical phase and, in the absence of intervention, most cases in the preclinical phase progress to symptomatic and clinically detectable progressive disease and death. If a significant proportion of the preclinical cases do not progress to overt clinical disease or if most of the clinical cases do not pass through a detectable preclinical phase or they pass through a very short preclinical detectable phase, screening is unlikely to be of benefit. These are important considerations in assessing any potential benefit from screening.

Evaluation of Screening Programs

Although it would seem that screening is beneficial, such an undertaking should be supported by evidence using process (operational or input) and outcome measures from appropriately designed and conducted studies and population-based screening programs. The process measures useful to evaluate screening programs include number and proportion of targeted subjects screened, number of times each subject is screened, number and proportion of people screened positive, screen-positive subjects undergoing diagnostic investigations and treatment, subjects diagnosed with disease, positive predictive value of the screening test, total costs of the program, and cost per case found. The useful outcome measures to assess the success of screening programs include stage distribution of cancer, case fatality, survival rates, incidence rate of disease (if the screening test identifies disease in the precancerous phase), cancer specific death rate in the population invited for screening, safety and acceptability of the interventions, quality of life and cost-effectiveness of the entire program.

Organized and Opportunistic (Unorganized, Spontaneous) Screening Programs

Screening programs may be organized or opportunistic. Organized programs are characterized by centralized screening invitations to a well-defined target population, systematic call and recall for screening, delivery of test results, investigations, treatment and follow-up care, centralized quality assurance and a program database with linkages with other information systems such as cancer and death registration systems for monitoring and evaluation of the program. Examples of organized programs for cervix, breast and colorectal cancer screening exist in countries such as Finland, the Netherlands, United Kingdom, and Australia.

In opportunistic programs, screening tests are provided to subjects on request or coincidentally during routine health care interactions with patients and there is no predetermined eligible population. Screening programs are unorganized in many developed countries such as the United States, France, Germany, and Japan. Organized screening programs have shown the greatest effect, while using fewer resources than opportunistic programs. The critical components of successful screening programs are high coverage of target population with accurate, quality assured screening tests and of screen-positive persons with diagnostic investigations, treatment and follow-up care. These are most cost-effectively met within organized screening programs.

Cervical Cancer Screening Programs in Low- and Medium-Resource Countries

Of the estimated 529,000 new cervical cancer cases and 275,000 cervical cancer deaths world-wide around 2008, four-fifths occurred in LMICs (Table 5.1).[3] More than a 15-fold variation in incidence rates of cervical cancer has been observed worldwide.[4] It is quite likely that the burden of disease in developing countries, such as sub-Saharan African countries is underestimated, given the grossly inadequate diagnostic and treatment services and cancer information systems. Reported age-adjusted cervical cancer mortality rates exceed 10 per 100,000 women in most developing countries.[3,5] It is estimated that 358,000 maternal deaths occurred in the world around 2008 and, given the inadequate investments in cervical cancer prevention in LMIC, cervical cancer deaths are likely to exceed maternal deaths in the near future. The high burden of cervical cancer in LMICs is due to the high prevalence of human papillomavirus (HPV) infection (>10% in women aged 30 years or more), the lack of effective early detection programs and inadequate health systems to provide diagnostic and treatment services. The five-year survival rates for cervical cancer varied from 13 to 67% in LMICs, indicating advanced stages at diagnosis and inadequate treatment[6] (Table 5.2).

TABLE 5.2 Five-year survival rates (%) from cancer in African, Asian and Latin American countries[6]

	TONGUE	MOUTH	LARGE BOWEL	BREAST	CERVIX
LOW-INCOME COUNTRIES (PER CAPITA GROSS NATIONAL INCOME (GNI) <996 USD)					
The Gambia	–	–	4	12	22
Uganda	–	–	8	46	13
Pakistan	39	41	–	–	–
LOWER MIDDLE-INCOME COUNTRIES(PER CAPITA GNI 996–3945 USD)					
China	67 (64–68)*	67 (44–71)*	44 (36–63)*	82 (58–90)*	67 (48–79)*
India	23 (12–30)	37 (26–45)	28 (6–31)	52 (31–54)	46 (10–48)
Philippines	–	–	40	47 (40–55)	37
Thailand	32 (24–33)	36 (22–42)	35 (31–44)	63 (57–66)	61 (54–63)
UPPER MIDDLE-INCOME COUNTRIES (PER CAPITA GNI 3946–12,195 USD)					
Costa Rica	–	–	–	70	53
Turkey	–	–	52	77	63
HIGH-INCOME COUNTRIES (PER CAPITA GNI >12,195 USD)					
South Korea	53 (52–60)	52 (48–54)	60 (57–64)	79 (78–81)	79 (76–79)
Saudi Arabia	–	–	–	64	–
Singapore	44	49	52	76	66

Figures in brackets indicate minimum and maximum survival within different populations in the country.

*Source of GNI: http://www.globalforumhealth.org/Glossary/Classification-of-countries-by-income-level.

Cervical cancer is very suitable for screening as it has a long natural history with slowly progressing and readily detectable and treatable precancerous lesions. It is caused by persistent infection with one of the oncogenic types HPV.[7] The peak risk of HPV infection is soon after the onset of sexual activity, usually between the ages of 14 and 20 years and a second peak around menopause has been observed for some developing countries.[8] In most infected women HPV infection usually resolves spontaneously, but it may persist in some women leading to the occurrence, persistence and progression of precancerous lesions such as cervical intraepithelial neoplasia (CIN), particularly grade 2 and 3 CIN and adenocarcinoma in situ. If undetected and untreated, the precursor lesions may progress to invasive cervical cancer over a period of 5–15 years. Early detection of precancerous lesions by screening and prevention of oncogenic HPV infection by vaccination are complimentary approaches of cervical cancer prevention. Early clinical diagnosis constitutes a third approach to disease control, where the emphasis is on prompt diagnosis of early stages (stages I and IIA) of invasive cancer among symptomatic women and offering effective treatment.

Screening tests such as conventional cytology (Pap smear), liquid-based cytology (LBC), visual inspection with acetic acid (VIA), visual inspection with Lugol's iodine (VILI) and human papillomavirus (HPV) testing can accurately identify women with CIN, as well as early, asymptomatic, preclinical invasive cancer, if these are carried out with quality assurance and by well-trained providers. Colposcopy is a useful diagnostic tool to triage women with positive tests, to assess the nature and extent of lesions and to direct biopsies and treatment. Effective treatment methods for CIN include cryotherapy, cold coagulation, laser ablation, loop electrosurgical excision procedure (LEEP), laser conization, and cold knife conization.

Cervical cancer is the most widely screened cancer and Pap smear is the most widely used cervical screening test in the world. Pap smear is still the workhorse of current screening programs in developed countries and LMIC, although new perspectives for alternative screening tests such as LBC, HPV testing and visual screening are developing rapidly in the light of new research findings.[1,9–11] It has been shown that Pap smear screening, at the population level, every three to five years can reduce cervical cancer incidence up to 80% and has been largely responsible for the substantial decline in cervical cancer incidence and mortality in developed countries of Europe, North America, Japan, Australia and New Zealand in the last 5 decades.[1] Such benefits can only be achieved if quality is optimal at every step in the screening process, from information dissemination and invitation of the eligible target population, to performance of the screening test and follow-up, and treatment of women diagnosed with cervical neoplasia.

Population-Based Cytology Screening Programs in LMICs

Population-based, large-scale cytology screening programs with colposcopy and CIN treatment services have been ongoing nationally over the last 30–40 years in LMIC such as Argentina, Cuba, Costa Rica, Chile, Mexico, Panama, Venezuela and Uruguay and regionally in Brazil, Peru, Colombia, Ecuador and Bolivia. Many of these programs suffered from a combination of suboptimal cytology testing, lack of quality assurance, poor coverage of women at risk, and inadequate follow-up of screen-positive women with diagnosis and treatment and consequently had very little impact on disease burden for several years after their introduction. While poor quality cytology reflected the several challenges in providing quality assured testing, the lack of coverage for diagnosis and treatment reflected the inadequate health care infrastructure, human resources and lack of program logistics for awareness, delivery of results, diagnosis, and treatment.

Substantial improvements in coverage in Chile, Costa Rica, Mexico, Puerto Rica, certain regions of Brazil, Colombia, and Uruguay have resulted in a reduced burden of disease in recent years. More than 70% of the women between 30 and 60 years have received at least a single round of screening and more than 50% have received a Pap smear in the preceding three years in these countries. Efforts are ongoing to reorganize programs in Argentina, Brazil, Panama, and other Latin American countries.

It is interesting to examine the progress in cervical cancer screening in the Republic of Korea, Singapore, Thailand, Hong Kong special administrative region (SAR) and Taiwan in the Asian region, which have evolved from low- to high-income economies over the last four decades. Repeated audits of the programs, improvement in health care services and increase in gross national incomes prompted reorganization of screening in the mid 1990s, which have led to more efficient programs in Singapore, Taiwan, Hong Kong SAR and the Republic of Korea. Pap smear (LBC since 2004) screening is provided once in three years to women aged 25–64 years and the incidence of cervical cancer in Singapore has declined from 18.1 in 1968 to 10.6 per 100 000 women in 2002, with the biggest decline in the Indian ethnic group[4,12,13] (Figure 5.1). There was a 60% reduction in mortality in Singapore during 1970 to 2005 (Figure 5.1). Reorganization of the cytology screening program in 1999 in the Republic Korea has improved coverage from 22.4% in 1998 to 58% in 2007

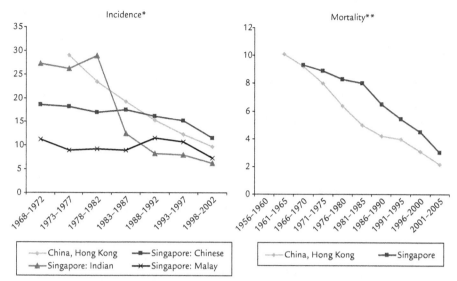

FIGURE 5.1 Trends in age standardized cervical cancer incidence and morality rates in selected Asian countries. *International Agency for Research on Cancer. Cancer Incidence in Five Continents Volumes I to IX. Available at: http://ci5.iarc.fr/CI5i-ix/ci5i-ix.htm **World Health Organization. Mortality database. Available at: http://www who int/whosis/en/

among women aged 30–60 years.[14,15] The cervical cancer incidence and mortality rates in Korea declined from 19 to 15 per 100,000 women and from 5.9 to 3.2 per 100,000 during 1992 and 2002, respectively.[16] Pap smear screening is offered to women aged 25–64 years once in three years in Hong Kong SAR where the life time coverage reached 72% in 2008 and the age-standardized incidence rates declined from 25 per 100 000 women in 1983 to 9 per 100,000 in 2007 and mortality declined from 6 to 2 per 100 000, respectively (Figure 5.1). The Taiwanese government launched a national cervical cancer screening program in 1995 with annual Pap smears offered to women aged 30 years and above and 61% of target women had at least one Pap smear by 2001. The cervical cancer incidence and mortality rates declined by 48% during 1995–2006 and the incidence of carcinoma in situ increased by 70% during 1995–2000 and decreased by 20% during 2000–2005.[17,18]

The age-standardized incidence rates ranged between 17.8 to 28.9 per 100,000 women during 2000–2003 in different provinces of Thailand.[4] A pilot Pap smear screening project in Nakhon Phanom province showed the feasibility of integrating cervical cancer screening and treatment services in routine health services.[19] A screen and treat demonstration program with VIA and cryotherapy in 4 districts of Roi-et province established the safety, acceptability and feasibility of a VIA screen and treat approach.[20] The above findings led to a government policy to provide screening with Pap smear or VIA, leading to the initiation of the first phase of an organized cytology screening project in 75 provinces in 2005 as a five-year program and the expansion of VIA screen and treat program targeting women aged 30–45 years to 29 provinces in 2006. Both programs have resulted in more than 8 of the 13 million target women aged 30–60 years being screened in the past 5 years. Bangladesh has recently launched an opportunistic nationwide VIA screening project through the routine health services; around 300,000 women are screened annually and efforts are underway to further expand the program.[21]

Cervical cancer screening programs are yet to be effectively implemented in many high risk LMICs in Asia such as India, China, Sri Lanka, Philippines, Vietnam, and Indonesia, among others. It is estimated that less than 2 million opportunistic smears are taken annually in China and India, the two large countries contributing substantially to the global burden of disease. Mass cytology screening programs do not exist anywhere in mainland Africa, except in South Africa where a national policy to provide Pap smears at 30, 40, and 50 years of age exists and coverage is less than 20% and is yet to be realized in a large scale. Even though cytology screening is wide spread in Mauritius, screen-positive women are seldom diagnosed and treated, with no appreciable impact on disease burden over the last three decades. Although there are small scale screening outlets providing VIA screening in the capitals of some sub Saharan African countries, they are far from evolving into large-scale programs. Cumulatively, less than 120,000 women are screened annually with VIA in the entire sub-Saharan Africa.

Cervical cancer is a major public health problem in Mexico where mortality rates remained stable, around 17 per 100,000 women, during the 1980s. Although Mexico has had a national cervical cancer screening program since 1974 to provide a Pap smear once in three years for women aged 25–64 years, coverage was poor for many years with no impact on cervical cancer mortality until 2000. Since 2000, the annual coverage has reached around 25% and at least 60% of the target women have received a smear in the preceding three years.[22] The steady decline in cervical cancer mortality rates from 17 per 100,000 women in 1989 to 10 in 2006 has been attributed to both increasing coverage and reduced birth rates[22,23] (Figure 5.2).

Two decades of opportunistic annual screening from the mid-sixties to the mid-eighties did not significantly reduce cervical cancer mortality in Chile. The program reorganization in 1987 targeting women aged 25–64 years every three years, optimizing existing resources, program logistics, quality assurance and timeliness of diagnosis and treatment, has led to more than 70% coverage of target women over a 3-year period with more than 80% of those with abnormal Pap smears receiving diagnosis and treatment and 100% of the

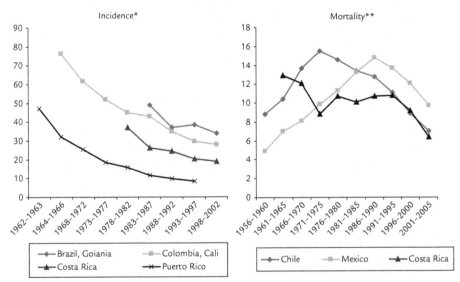

FIGURE 5.2 Trends in age standardized cervical cancer incidence and morality rate in selected Latin American countries. *International Agency for Research on Cancer. Cancer Incidence in Five Continents Volumes I to IX. Available at: http://ci5.iarc.fr/CI5i-ix/ci5i-ix.htm **World Health Organization. Mortality database. Available at: http://www who int/whosis/en/

public laboratories subjected to external quality control. As a consequence, the age-adjusted cervical cancer mortality declined from 12.8 in 1980 to 6.8 per 100,000 women in 2001[23,24] (Figure 5.2).

The screening program in Costa Rica offers a Pap smear every two years for women aged 25–69 years and coverage has improved substantially in recent years, with 78% having had a Pap smear in the preceding three years.[25] The cervical cancer incidence rates have declined from 25 per 100,000 women in 1980 to around 15 per 100,000 in 2002[4,12] and mortality rates have declined by 40% since 1995. Cervical cancer mortality rates are much lower in urban areas such as Buenos Aires in Argentina, Sao Paolo and Campinas in Brazil and Cali in Colombia than the rural and national rates, reflecting inequalities in screening and treatment coverage (Figure 5.2).[26–28]

Alternative Screening Tests and New Paradigms for cervical Screening in LMIC
The challenges and resources required to organise cytology screening and the limited impact of such programs in several Latin American countries have prompted the search for and evaluation of alternative screening tests and paradigms that require one or two visits to complete the screening and diagnosis/treatment processes, as well as the reorganization of existing programs and more effective utilization of resources in some countries.[24,29,30]

VISUAL INSPECTION WITH ACETIC ACID (VIA) AND LUGOL'S IODINE (VILI)
VIA is the most widely studied visual test that involves naked eye inspection of the cervix, using a bright torch light or a halogen focus lamp, 1 minute after the application of 3–5% acetic acid.[31] A positive test is characterized by well-defined acetowhite areas close to the squamocolumnar junction (SCJ) or to the external os, on the entire cervix or on a cervical growth. It is a simple, affordable test that can be rapidly taught to primary health workers, nurses and doctors, and gives immediate results to permit a "single visit" approach that permits screening and treatment in the same session.[32,33] The sensitivity of VIA to detect CIN 2 and 3 lesions and invasive cervical cancer varied from 37 to 95% and the specificity varied from 49 to 97% in several cross-sectional studies in developing countries.[32,34,35] When conventional cytology was concurrently evaluated, the sensitivity of VIA was found to be higher than or similar to that of cytology, but with lower specificity. However, VIA accuracy is substantially reduced in older premenopausal women, due to the movement of the SCJ and transformation zone in to the endocervical canal.

VILI involves naked eye examination of the cervix immediately after the application of Lugol's iodine and a positive result is based on the appearance of definite mustard-yellow lesions on the cervix close to the SCJ or the os, on the entire cervix or on a cervical growth.[31] VILI has been investigated in fewer studies than VIA and its sensitivity varied between 44–92% and specificity between 75–85% in cross-sectional studies in India, Africa and Latin America.[34–37] It seems that concurrent use of both VIA and VILI is advisable when individual women seek screening or early diagnosis services.

The reported sensitivities for VIA and VILI are likely to be overestimates, given the wide variation in the quality of reference diagnostic standards used in different studies; it appears that a quality assured single VIA or VILI has an average sensitivity around 50% and specificity around 85% to detect high-grade CIN in study settings. Quality assurance for visual tests is yet to be standardized and test providers require constant monitoring and frequent re-training. The useful quality assurance procedures and indices include freshly prepared 3–5% acetic acid on a daily basis, periodic re-training of providers and reproducibility studies and monitoring the following process measures regularly: test positivity rates between 7–15%, positive predictive value for any grade of CIN not less than 20%, positive predictive value for CIN 2–3 lesions not less than 10%, and interobserver agreement exceeding 70%.

In a randomized controlled trial in South Africa, a VIA-based screen-and-treat intervention reduced the cumulative prevalence of CIN 2 and 3 lesions by 37% at 6 months and by 32% at 36 months follow-up as compared to a delayed evaluation ("control") group (Table 5.3); there was a significant 38% reduction in the prevalence of CIN 3 lesions at 36 months follow-up following this intervention.[38,39] The effectiveness of a single round of VIA screening by nurses in reducing cervical cancer incidence and mortality was addressed in a randomized trial in Dindigul district, South India.[9] A 25% reduction in cervical cancer incidence and a 35% reduction in cancer mortality in the intervention group, with the greatest reduction in incidence and mortality rates in the 30–39 year age group, compared to a control group to receive routine care were observed 7 years from the beginning of screening in this study (Table 5.4).

TABLE 5.3 Magnitude of reduction in cervical intraepithelial neoplasia grade 2 or 3 (CIN 2 and 3) lesions at 36 months after human papillomavirus (HPV) DNA or visual inspection with acetic acid (VIA) based 'screen and treat' approach in South Africa[39]

CHARACTERISTIC	HPV SCREEN-AND-TREAT (N = 2163)	VIA SCREEN-AND-TREAT (N = 2227)	DELAYED EVALUATION CONTROL GROUP (N = 2165)
Cumulative frequency of CIN 2 and 3 lesions	29 (1.5%)	71 (3.8%)	105 (5.6%)
Rate ratio (95% CI)	0.27 (0.17–0.43)	0.68 (0.50–0.92)	1.0
Percentage of CIN 2 and 3 prevented (95% CI)	73 (60–85)	32 (11–53)	–

TABLE 5.4 Cervical cancer incidence and mortality in the study groups of Dindigul district cervical screening cluster randomized controlled trial, India (2000–2006)[29]

END POINT	VIA GROUP	CONTROL GROUP	ADJUSTED HAZARD RATIO* (95% CI)
Total number of women	49,311	30,958	–
Number screened	31,343	951	–
Number screen positive	3,088		
Cervical cancer cases	167	158	–
Age-standardized incidence rate	75.2/100,000	99.1/100,000	0.75 (0.59–0.95)
Cervical cancer deaths	83	92	–
Age-standardized mortality rate	38.3/100,000	54.9/100,000	0.65 (0.47–0.89)

*Adjusted for cluster design, age, education, marital status and parity

HPV Testing

HPV DNA testing is the most objective and reproducible of all cervical screening tests. Its sensitivity in detecting CIN 2 and 3 lesions varied from 66–100% and its specificity varied from 62–96%; it had a higher sensitivity, but lower specificity, than cytology in detecting high-grade lesions.[34,40–42] Self-sampling for HPV DNA testing is promising for use in under-resourced areas or for women who are reluctant to participate in screening programs. In low-resource settings, where repeated testing of women at risk for cervical neoplasia is not feasible, a single HPV testing may provide an objective method of identifying women at risk for disease and investing the limited resources. A single HPV test is more effective than cytology in predicting future CIN2 or worse lesions.[43] However, HPV testing is currently more expensive (US$30–60) than other screening tests and requires sophisticated laboratory infrastructure including testing equipment, storage facilities for samples and trained technicians.

A simple, user-friendly, affordable, fast (results within 3 hours) and accurate HPV test (*care*HPV test) suitable for use in low-resource settings has now been evaluated in China and was found to have similar accuracy as that of Hybrid Capture II (HC II) test and significantly higher sensitivity than VIA (90.2% vs.41.4%), but lower specificity (84.2% vs. 94.5%).[44] It is expected to be commercially available in 2011. The availability of rapid, accurate, affordable and simple HPV tests is an essential prerequisite for the wide-spread use of HPV testing for screening.

In a randomized controlled trial in South Africa assessing safety and efficacy of HPV testing based screen-and-treat with cryotherapy intervention, the prevalence of CIN 2 and 3 lesions was reduced by a significant 77% at 6 months and by 73% at 36 months of follow-up as compared to a delayed evaluation ("control") group (Table 5.3); there was a significant 77% reduction in the prevalence of CIN 3 lesions at 36 months follow-up in the intervention group as compared to the control group.[38,39] Screen-and-treat utilizing HPV testing reduced the prevalence of CIN 2 or worse lesions in HIV-negative women by 69% and among HIV-positive women by 80% at 36 months follow-up as compared to the control group.[45] The impact of screening by a single round of HPV testing, VIA or cytology on cervical cancer incidence and mortality was investigated in a cluster randomized controlled trial in Osmanabad District, India, in which 143,000 women aged 30–59 years were randomized into four groups for a single round of screening by trained midwives with either VIA, cytology, HPV testing or to a control group.[10] There was a significant 53% reduction in the incidence rate of stage II or worse stages of invasive cervical cancer and a significant 48% reduction in cervical cancer mortality in the HPV testing group as compared to the control group (Table 5.5). The reduction in cervical cancer mortality observed in the cytology and VIA groups as compared to the control group did not reach statistical significance; during the 8-year follow-up period, 8 of the 24,380 HPV-negative women developed cervical cancer as opposed to 22 of 23,762 Pap smear-negative and 25 of 23,032 VIA-negative women, indicating that HPV testing more accurately identified women at risk for developing cervical cancer.

New Paradigms

Screening in developed countries involves repeated rounds at yearly (e.g. Germany, United States), three-yearly (e.g. France, Norway) or five-yearly (Finland, United Kingdom) intervals involving sexually active women across a wide age range beginning from early 20s to late 60s. The conventional diagnostic and treatment algorithms following a positive cytology screening test in western health care settings include three visits for colposcopy, diagnostic confirmation, and treatment. Such regimes, which are labour intensive and rely on

TABLE 5.5 Comparative efficacy of three different cervical screening tests in reducing cervical cancer mortality in a randomized controlled trial in Osmanabad district, India[10]

VARIABLE	HPV GROUP (N = 34,126)	PAP SMEAR GROUP (N = 32,058)	VIA GROUP (N = 34,074)	CONTROL (ROUTINE CARE) GROUP (N = 31,488)
Women screened	27,192	25,549	26,765	–
Test–positive women	2,812	1,787	3,733	–
Women with CIN 2 and 3 lesions	245	262	195	–
Women diagnosed with cervical cancer 2000–2007 (rate per 100,000 person-years)	127 (47.4)	152 (60.7)	157 (58.7)	118 (47.6)
Women with stage II or more advanced cancer (rate per 100,000 person-years)	39 (14.5)	58 (23.2)	86 (32.2)	82 (33.1)
Hazard ratio (95% CI)	*0.47 (0.32–0.69)*	*0.75 (0.51–1.10)*	*1.04 (0.72–1.49)*	*1.00*
Women dying from cervical cancer 2000–2007 (rate per 100,000 person-years)	34 (12.7)	54 (21.5)	56 (20.9)	64 (25.8)
Hazard ratio (95% CI)	*0.52 (0.33–0.83)*	*0.89 (0.62–1.27)*	*0.86 (0.60–1.25)*	*1.00*

CI: confidence interval; HPV: human papillomavirus; VIA: visual inspection with acetic acid; CIN: cervical intraepithelial neoplasia.

Rates and hazard ratios for the comparison between each intervention group and control group have been adjusted for age.

well-functioning clinical, laboratory, and referral systems, are not feasible, and multiple visits following screening will result in substantial nonparticipation by women in developing countries.

In recent years, new paradigms have been proposed to maximise participation of women in screening and treatment and to improve cost-effectiveness and efficiency.[30] These include a single life-time screening targeted at women aged 30–59 or 30–49 years[9,10] with emphasis on covering a large proportion of target women with a highly sensitive test, a "single visit approach" following positive screen when colposcopy, directed biopsies, and treatment with cryotherapy or LEEP are provided in the same sitting[9,10,32] and a single visit "screen and treat" approach when screen-positive women, without evidence of invasive cancer, are treated with cryotherapy or cold coagulation in the same screening session, without triaging procedures such as colposcopy and biopsy.[20,32,38,46] Screening tests such as visual tests (VIA and VILI) or fast HPV testing (*care*HPV test) provide immediate results making the single visit approach much more feasible. A major concern with "screen-and-treat" cervical cancer prevention strategies is that a large number of women without precursor lesions will undergo cryotherapy/cold coagulation, although there are no data to suggest that over-treatment is harmful; on the other hand, it may provide some marginal benefit by protecting women against future HPV infection and by reducing cervical ectopy and targeting the transformation zone where cervical neoplasia occur. Current evidence suggests that screen-and-treat interventions are safe, are well accepted by women and are effective in preventing cervical neoplasia.

Cervix Screening among HIV-Positive Women

HIV-infected women have a higher prevalence, incidence, and persistence of HPV infection and experience a higher incidence, persistence, and progression of CIN. They have a higher frequency of high-grade lesions and larger, extensive lesions than HIV-negative women. The currently available screening tests such as cytology and VIA are less accurate and treatment methods for CIN are less effective in preventing cervical neoplasia and yielded suboptimal results with high recurrence rates in HIV-infected women. Recent evidence from a randomized trial in South Africa indicates that HPV testing followed by treatment of HPV-positive women with cryotherapy using a "screen-and-treat" approach is an effective method to reduce high-grade CIN in HIV-positive women in LMIC; a significant 80% reduction in CIN 2 or worse lesions following HPV screening and treatment as compared to the control group was observed in this study (Table 5.6).[45] Highly active anti-retroviral therapy (HAART) increases the life expectancy of HIV-positive women, but has little beneficial effect on the natural history of cervical neoplasia. Thus, it is likely that more of these women will develop cervical cancer unless effective intervention is available. Repeated screening, using new screening tests such as HPV testing, close surveillance and repetitive treatment are necessary to prevent cervical neoplasia among HIV-positive women.[47-49]

Efficacy, Safety and Acceptability of Field Based Treatments for CIN in Developing Countries

Cryotherapy, provided by nurses, and LEEP, provided by newly trained doctors, in field conditions in India, Peru, Thailand, and South Africa have been found to be safe, acceptable, and effective and cured 85–90% of women with CIN.[20,38,46,50-56] These experiences are similar to the results reported from developed countries where these procedures were carried

TABLE 5.6 Magnitude of reduction in cervical intraepithelial neoplasia grade 2 or 3 (CIN 2 and 3) lesions at 36 months after human papillomavirus (HPV) DNA or visual inspection with acetic acid (VIA) based 'screen and treat' approach among human immunodeficiency virus (HIV) infected women in South Africa[45]

CHARACTERISTIC	HPV SCREEN AND TREAT (N = 270)	VIA SCREEN AND TREAT (N = 279)	DELAYED EVALUATION CONTROL GROUP (N = 265)
Cumulative cases of CIN 2 and 3 lesions	4	18	36
Rate ratio (95% CI)	0.20 (0.06–0.69)	0.51 (0.29–0.89)	1.0

out by experienced doctors in hospital settings. Cervical cryotherapy is also reported to significantly reduce newly acquired high-risk HPV infection in HIV-negative women, but not in HIV-positive women.[57]

COST-EFFECTIVE SCREENING APPROACHES IN LOW-RESOURCE SETTINGS

The cost-effectiveness of a variety of cervical-cancer screening strategies in India, Kenya, Peru, South Africa, and Thailand were assessed using computer-based models and the most cost-effective strategies were those requiring fewest visits, resulting in improved follow-up testing and treatment.[58] Screening women once in their lifetime at the age of 35 years, with a one- or two-visit screening strategy involving VIA or HPV testing reduced the lifetime risk of cancer by approximately 25 to 36% and cost less than $500 per year of life saved. Relative risk of cancer declined by an additional 40% with two screenings (at 35 and 40 years of age), resulting in a cost per year of life saved that was less than each country's per capita gross domestic product; this is a very cost-effective result, according to the Commission on Macroeconomics and Health.

Breast Cancer Screening Programs

Breast cancer accounted for an estimated 1,384,000 cases and 458,300 deaths in the world around 2008 and LMIC accounted for a little more than half of this burden.[3] The incidence rate of breast cancer varies around eight-fold across the world, indicating large differences in the distribution of underlying risk factors[4]. Breast cancer incidence and mortality rates are rising in LMICs of Latin America, Middle East and Asia (Figures 5.3 and 5.4), whereas changes in underlying risk factors, advent of mammography screening and improvements in

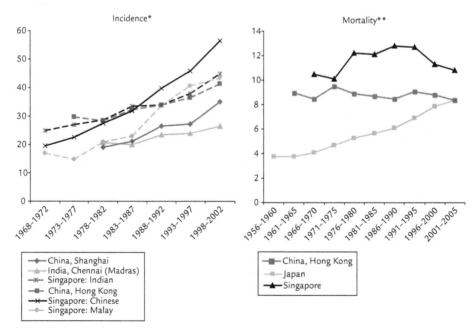

FIGURE 5.3 Trends in age standardized breast cancer incidence and morality rates in selected Asian countries. *International Agency for Research on Cancer. Cancer Incidence in Five Continents Volumes I to IX. Available at: http://ci5.iarc.fr/CI5i-ix/ci5i-ix.htm **World Health Organization. Mortality database. Available at: http://www who int/whosis/en/

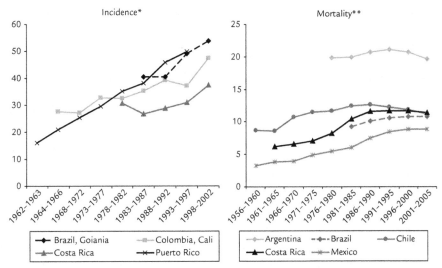

FIGURE 5.4 Trends in age standardized breast cancer incidence and morality rates in selected Latin American countries. *International Agency for Research on Cancer. Cancer Incidence in Five Continents Volumes I to IX. Available at: http://ci5.iarc.fr/CI5i-ix/ci5i-ix.htm **World Health Organization. Mortality database. Available at: http://www.who.int/whosis/en/

treatment have resulted in either stable or declining incidence rates and declining mortality in high income countries. Substantial improvements in survival have been observed in developed countries since 1970, where the five-year survival exceeds 85% whereas survival in low income countries is less than 50%[6,59,60] (Table 5.2). The poor survival in LMICs reflects the advanced clinical stages at presentation and the inadequate access to appropriate treatment.

Screen film mammography is the most widely used breast cancer screening method in the world. Ultrasonography, magnetic resonance imaging, core biopsy, and fine aspiration cytology (FNAC) are increasingly used in the diagnostic evaluation of those with mammographic abnormalities. Diagnostic mammography, ultrasonography, and FNAC ("triple diagnosis") are useful in the evaluation of women presenting with early breast lumps.

The process of acquiring information about the efficacy of breast cancer screening with mammography was initiated in 1963 and a number of randomized controlled trials, conducted in five different countries over a 20-year period, provided the scientific basis for mammography screening. There is sufficient evidence from randomized trials that screening women aged 50–69 years with mammography reduces their mortality from breast cancer; the best current estimate of the average reduction is 25%; the reduction in mortality from breast cancer in women aged 50–69 years who accept an invitation to screening has been estimated at around 35%.[2] There is only limited evidence for this effect in women aged 40–49 years, in whom the reduction is estimated to be 19% or less. Population-based, organized mammographic screening was first introduced in Iceland in 1987, followed by Sweden, Netherlands, Canada, and Finland. Currently breast cancer screening programs are operational in at least 22 developed countries.

A mammography breast cancer screening program is a complex multidisciplinary undertaking and its success depends on the quality of the individual components and involves substantial resources, which are not within the reach of most LMICs. Large-scale mammography screening is ongoing in Singapore, Hong Kong SAR, Taiwan, Republic of Korea,

Uruguay, and Chile (whose per capita gross national annual income exceeds $US10,000), as well as urban areas of Brazil and Argentina. Opportunistic mammography screening is less common in other Asian and Latin American countries

Breast cancer is the most common malignancy among women in Singapore, accounting for 30% of all female cancers, with an age-standardized rate of 55 per 100,000 per year, and where annually about 1100 new cases are diagnosed and approximately 270 women die from it. Following large-scale opportunistic mammography since the 1980s, Singapore initiated the first population-based screening program incorporating quality assurance and practice guidelines in Asia in 2002, offering two-view mammography biennially for women aged 50–69 years with the objective of achieving 70% coverage and a 25–30% reduction in mortality.[61,62] In the pilot phase of the program, screen-positivity rate was 9.5% and the invasive cancer detection rate was 4.5 per 1000 screened women. Current coverage is around 60% in women aged 50–59 and 35% among those aged 60–69 years old. Following large-scale improvements in early diagnosis and treatment and the introduction of the program, breast cancer mortality rates have slowly started to decline since 1995. In fact, Singapore is the only country in Asia which has shown a decline in mortality for breast cancer (Figure 5.3). In the Republic of Korea, Clinical Breast Examination (CBE) and mammographic screening are provided once in two years for women aged 40–69 years, but the coverage is less than 20% per annum.[63] In spite of large scale opportunistic mammographic screening in the Republic of Korea, Hong Kong SAR, and Taiwan, where at least a quarter of women aged 50 to 69 years have received screening, breast cancer mortality rates are on the rise.

Breast cancer mortality rates are currently stable in Mexico, Brazil and Costa Rica whereas a slow decline has been observed in Argentina and Chile reflecting the impact of opportunistic early detection (coverage around 25 to 50% of the women aged 50 to 69 years) and improved treatments (Figure 5.4). There is no large-scale breast cancer screening in any of the other Asian, African and Latin American countries.

Research Initiatives on Alternative Screening Technologies

The fact that mammographic screening is not feasible in low-resource countries has prompted the assessment of breast self examination (BSE) and CBE as alternative screening approaches. There are no population-based programs that solely rely on CBE or BSE as screening methods. Attention is now focussed on evaluating ultrasonography as a screening modality in LMICs.[64]

CBE involves systematic visual examination and palpation of breast by a health care provider to detect suspicious lumps and other abnormalities suggestive of breast cancer. The reported frequency of breast cancer diagnosis, stage, interval cancers, and breast cancer mortality were similar in the Canadian National Breast Screening Study that compared CBE plus mammography to CBE alone in women aged 50 to 59 years; these findings compared favorably with other trials of mammography alone.[65,66]

Although CBE and BSE are important components of routine breast care in all countries, the evidence does not support the use of CBE and BSE in population-based organized screening programs involving asymptomatic women at this time, due to the fact that data from countries with very limited resources are lacking.

A large cluster randomized trial of CBE in the Philippines to assess the effect of five annual CBE carried out by trained nurses on breast cancer mortality was terminated after the first round of screening due to the refractory attitude of the population with respect to clinical follow-up and the cultural and logistic barriers to seeking diagnosis and treatment.[67]

There are currently two on-going randomized trials in India evaluating the role of CBE in reducing breast cancer mortality.[68,69] The cluster randomized controlled trial in

Mumbai, initiated in 1998 and involving 150,000 women aged 30 to 64 years, is evaluating the efficacy and cost-effectiveness of five rounds of biennial CBE in reducing breast cancer deaths.[68,69] Half of the participants are randomized to receive CBE and the other half to usual care and health education, as well as VIA once in two years. After three rounds of CBE screening, a significant early detection of breast cancers in the intervention group has been observed.[69]

Another randomized trial involving 120,000 women initiated in 2006 in Trivandrum district, India is currently evaluating three rounds of CBE at three-year intervals. The first round of intervention has been completed and the preliminary results suggest that 5% of women were referred with a lump, that 50% of those complied with referral for diagnostic investigations and that a significant proportion of cases were detected in early stages (stages I or II A).

A recent cost-effectiveness simulation study in India indicated an estimated cost-effectiveness ratio (CER) of 1135 international dollars per life year gained among women aged 40–60 years offered CBE every 5 years and CER increased to $1341 for biennial CBE (age 40–60 years); the corresponding estimated reductions in breast cancer mortality were 8.2% and 16.3%, respectively.[70] CBE performed annually from ages 40 to 60 was predicted to have similar results as biennial mammography screening for reducing breast cancer mortality which incurs only half the net costs. The main factors affecting cost-effectiveness were breast cancer incidence, stage distribution, and cost savings on prevented palliative care. The study concluded that the estimated cost-effectiveness of CBE screening for breast cancer in India compares favorably with that of mammography in developed countries, although the introduction of screening in India would be challenging, given the competing health priorities and economic conditions.

BSE involves educating and motivating women to systematically self inspect their breasts for lumps and other abnormalities at regular intervals. A large randomized trial involving 266 064 women in Shanghai to receive either BSE instruction, reinforcement and encouragement, or instructions on the prevention of lower back pain reported 135 breast cancer deaths in the BSE instruction group and 131 in the control group after 10 years of follow-up (relative risk [RR] = 1.04; 95% CI, 0.82–1.33).[71] Although the number of invasive breast cancers diagnosed in the two groups was about the same, women in the instruction group had more breast biopsies and more benign lesions diagnosed than women in the control group. In the U.K. Trial of Early Detection of Breast Cancer, two districts invited more than 63,500 women aged 45 to 64 years to educational sessions about BSE. After 10 years of follow-up, there was no difference in mortality rates in these two districts compared with four centres without organized BSE education (RR = 1.07; 95% CI, 0.93–1.22).[72] A meta-analysis of trials of BSE training showed that BSE was associated with considerably more women seeking medical advice and having biopsies, but was not an effective method of reducing breast cancer mortality.[73]

Colorectal Screening Programs in LMICs

Colorectal cancer (CRC) is the third most common cancer world-wide accounting for 1,234,000 cases and 609,000 deaths annually around 2008 (Table 5.1).[3] It is less common in people aged less than 50 years. There is more than 30-fold difference in the risk of CRC across the world, with the highest risk being in developed high-income countries.[4] There has been significant increase in the incidence of CRC in some LMICs such as Argentina, Brazil, Uruguay, Chile and Thailand, among others, due to rapid socio-economic development and western style dietary changes, in recent years. However, incidence rates are still less than 8 per 100,000 in many developing countries and consequently, a mass screening policy for CRC is not recommended in most LMICs Africa, Latin America and Asia n view of the limited resources and low risk of CRC.[74]

Five-year survival rates vary from 4% to 44% in LMICs indicating the vast potential for early diagnosis and treatment (Table 5.2).[6] Survival rates are significantly improved when the disease is detected early and treated appropriately. Thus, early clinical diagnosis and prompt treatment among symptomatic people are important to improve prognosis and reduce mortality in LMIC.

Noninvasive faecal occult blood tests (FOBT) are widely used to screen participants in CRC screening programs and they have been shown in clinical trials and in programmatic settings to be simple to use and resulted in an approximate 16% decrease in colorectal cancer mortality.[75] The immunochemical (iFOBT) test, in contrast to the guaiac (gFOBT) test, requires no restrictions on diet or medication. Sigmoidoscopy, colonoscopy and imaging investigations, such as double contrast barium enema, are used to triage FOBT positive subjects. Effective screening can reduce incidence by detecting and removing precancerous lesions in adenomatous polyps and reduce mortality by detecting cancers limited to the mucosa. The benefit of screening is greatest when targeted at populations of greatest risk, such as those aged 50 years and more, those with a family history of bowel cancer or polyps and those with inflammatory bowel disease and adenomas. Organized CRC screening programs in many developed countries are still in the early stages of their development and there is considerable opportunity to incorporate quality assurance to ensure efficiency from the beginning.

Currently, opportunistic FOBT based screening is widely practiced in Singapore, Republic of Korea, Hong Kong SAR, Taiwan, Argentina, Brazil, Chile, Costa Rica, Mexico and Uruguay. It is estimated that a quarter of persons aged 50–69 years in Singapore have been covered by FOBT screening; among those aged 50 and 70, only 1 in 9 men and 1 in 13 women have undergone a colonoscopy at least once. There is considerable early clinical diagnosis activity and the treatment services have significantly improved in Singapore. Consequently, the CRC mortality declined in men from 19 per 100,000 in 1995 to 14 per 100,000 in 2005 (Figure 5.5) and from the peak value of 14 per 100,000 to 10 per 100,000 in women, respectively.

Annual iFOBT has been offered to individuals aged 50 years and above as part of the national screening program since 2004 in the Republic of Korea. Colonoscopy or double contrast barium enema is used to triage FPBT-positive persons. The program targets around 5 million persons and coverage was around 16% in 2006. A national program in Taiwan targets 1.3 million persons aged 50 to 69 years with annual FOBT. Thailand has recently organised a provincial CRC screening program using iFOBT and colonoscopy triage in Lampang as the pilot phase to inform and upscale screening in the country. CRC mortality has stabilized since 1995 in Latin American countries such as Argentina, Brazil, Chile, Costa Rica and Mexico where there are large scale case finding using colonoscopy and sigmoidoscopy (Figure 5.6).

Oral Cancer Screening in LMICs

Oral cancer accounts for 264,000 new cases and 128,000 deaths annually (Table 5.1). A high incidence is observed in the Indian subcontinent, East Asia, eastern Europe, and parts of Latin America, which account for more than two-thirds of the global burden. The major risk factors are for oral cancer are use of tobacco and/or alcohol in any form and it is very rare among those who do not use any of these substances.

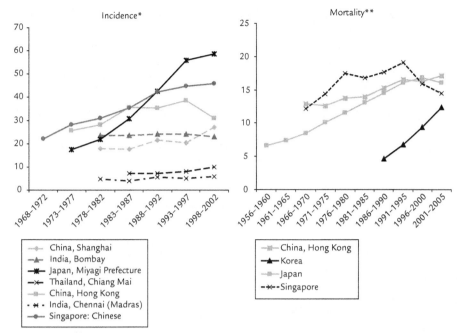

FIGURE 5.5 Trends in age standardized colorectal cancer incidence and morality rates in men in selected Asian countries. *International Agency for Research on Cancer. Cancer Incidence in Five Continents Volumes I to IX. Available at: http://ci5.iarc.fr/CI5i-ix/ci5i-ix.htm **World Health Organization. Mortality database. Available at: http://www who int/whosis/en/

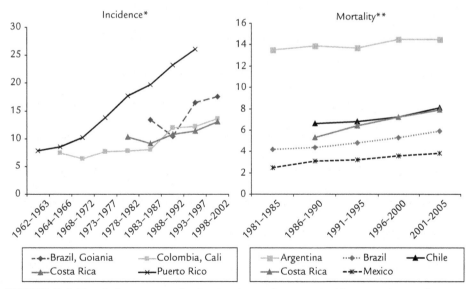

FIGURE 5.6 Trends in age standardized colorectal cancer incidence and morality rates in men in selected Latin American countries. *International Agency for Research on Cancer. Cancer Incidence in Five Continents Volumes I to IX. Available at: http://ci5.iarc.fr/CI5i-ix/ci5i-ix.htm **World Health Organization. Mortality database. Available at: http://www who int/whosis/en/

Oral cancer has a long preclinical detection phase consisting of well documented potentially malignant disorders (PMD). These PMD include homogeneous leukoplakia, nonhomogeneous leukoplakia, verrucous leukoplakia, erythroplakia, oral submucous fibrosis, lichen planus and oral fibrosis due to systemic sclerosis and traumatic ulcers, among others, and very early preclinical invasive cancers presenting as painless, small ulcers or nodular lesions or growths. These changes can be easily visualized and are clinically detectable through careful visual inspection and palpation of the oral mucosa. The malignant transformation of the PMD can be prevented by appropriate interventions such as avoiding exposure to tobacco use and alcohol drinking and in selected instances by excision of the lesions. Early, localized oral cancers (<4 cms) with no spread to the regional lymph nodes can be effectively treated and cured with single modality treatments, such as surgery or radiotherapy, with no functional or cosmetic defects resulting in five-year survival rates exceeding 80%. Thus, death from oral cancer can be avoided by early detection and appropriate treatment and acceptable cosmesis, as well as quality of life ensured.

Visual inspection and palpation of the oral cavity under adequate light is the most widely used screening test for oral neoplasia. Its sensitivity ranged from 40 to 93% and specificity ranged from 50–99% to detect PMDs and early asymptomatic oral cancers.[76–79] The reference diagnostic standard for oral mucosal lesions that are suggestive of PMD or cancer is tissue biopsy and microscopic examination. A digital atlas depicting and describing PMDs as well as early cancers and related differential diagnosis can be accessed in the internet.[80] This atlas is a useful learning tool and clinical aid for primary care practitioners, dentists, nurses, and health workers when providing visual screening.

Current evidence indicates that adjunctive screening tests based on toludine blue intravital staining, chemiluminescence, tissue fluorescence imaging, tissue fluorescent spectroscopy, salivary analysis and cytology, do not allow the providers to overcome the limitation of visual and tactile screening and use of these devices and techniques may be associated with an increased risk of false-positive tests.[81] There is insufficient evidence to recommend their routine use and well-designed, large-scale cross-sectional studies involving sufficient numbers of asymptomatic high-risk individuals in the general population with appropriate reference standard for final diagnosis are required to document their clinical utility in improving the performance of visual and tactile examinations. A randomized controlled trial in Taiwan did not support the routine use of toludine blue staining.[82]

The efficacy and cost-effectiveness of oral visual screening in reducing oral cancer mortality has been addressed in the context of a randomized trial.[83,84] Subjects aged 35 years and above in 13 geographical clusters in Trivandrum district, South India were randomized to receive three rounds of oral visual inspection by trained health workers (7 clusters, 96,517 subjects) or to a control group (6 clusters, 95,536 individuals). In all, 87,645 (91%) eligible subjects in the intervention group were screened at least once (33,343 screened once only, 24,210 twice and 29,102 three times), and 5145 were screened positive, of whom 3218 (63%) complied with referral for diagnosis.[83] There was a significant 34% reduction in oral cancer mortality among users of tobacco and/or alcohol in the intervention group compared to the control group.

An expert panel of the American Dental Association (ADA) recently concluded that community-based visual screening may decrease oral cancer-specific mortality among people who use tobacco, alcohol or both, based on the evidence from the above described randomized trial.[85] They recommended that clinicians should look for signs of PMDs or early-stage cancers while performing routine visual and tactile screening in all subjects, but particularly in those who use who use tobacco or alcohol or both. The panel also concluded that the life saving benefits for subjects with treatable lesions was more important than the potential harms incurred by those with benign or nonprogressive lesions.

There are no large-scale on-going national oral cancer screening programs other than in Taiwan and Cuba. The Cuban national oral visual screening program is on-going since 1984 and an evaluation carried out in 1994 indicated that 12–26% of the target population has been screened annually and only less than 30% of screen-positive individuals complied with referral.[86] Consequently, the program was reorganized in 1996 with target age raised from 15 years to 35 years, screening intervals raised from 1 to 3 years in order to improve coverage and the referral system was revamped. No further formal evaluation has been carried out since, but there has been no reduction in oral cancer mortality rates in Cuba over the last three decades.[5] The outcomes from the Cuban program emphasizes that screening programs without efficient policies and organization for invitation and coverage of appropriate target groups, referral systems and information flow should be discouraged.

▓ CONCLUSION

Cancer screening programs do not exist in most of the LMICs and large countries such as China, India, Indonesia, Nigeria and South Africa, among others. In countries where they do exist, they are still evolving and being reorganized. Mortality reduction is becoming evident after reorganization of Pap smear screening programs in some LMICs such as Chile, Costa Rica, and Mexico. Pap smear screening is still the most widely existing screening for cervical cancer. The challenges in providing good quality cytology screening have prompted the search for alternative screening approaches. Although VIA is the most feasible technique for premenopausal women in low-income countries, HPV testing is the most promising alternative screening test, in view of its high accuracy, with the development of an affordable and rapid HPV test for LMICs. Screen-and-treat strategies using HPV testing or VIA not only cure prevalent disease, but also reduce the risk of developing cancer over time in populations without access to routine, repeat cervical screening.

Breast cancer screening programs are few and CRC and oral cancer screening programs are even fewer. Evidence for the efficacy and cost-effectiveness of CBE in reducing the incidence of node positive and advanced breast cancer and reduced mortality from rigorously conducted randomized trials in high-risk LMICs is essential before population-based CBE screening programs can be recommended. Meanwhile, measures to improve awareness about detecting breast lumps and seeking early diagnosis and treatment are important for breast cancer control. Upper middle-income countries with high and increasing risk of CRC and well-developed health systems may consider introducing iFOBT based screening programs with colonoscopy triage in selected regions and expand step by step. LMIC with a high burden of oral cancer, such as India, may consider visual screening of tobacco/alcohol users through routine health services complimentary to primary prevention efforts.

It is worthwhile to note that the countries with the successful and large programs have a per capita GNI exceeding $US5000. Most of the existing programs do not have comprehensive and all inclusive information systems. The incidence data from existing long-standing population based cancer registries, as well as routine mortality data, have contributed to the evaluation of effectiveness of screening in those countries where screening programs exist, underscoring the importance of such information systems. Existing health service infrastructure, human resources and meagre health service investments in many low- and medium-resource countries preclude the possibility of introducing and sustaining effective screening programs in the near future. Substantial investments in improving population and professional awareness, health care infrastructure, human resources and information systems will be required to improve early detection and treatment of cancers and the eventual introduction screening programs in LMICs.

▪ SUMMARY

The objective of cancer screening is to reduce cancer mortality and improve quality of life by detection and treatment of persons with early cancers or precancerous lesions. Despite the high burden of breast, cervix, oral cavity and large bowel cancer, screening programs do not exist in many low- and medium income countries (LMICs) due to resource constraints and less priority that cancer receives. In few countries where they do exist, they are still evolving. Cytology is the most widely used cervical screening test. Given the difficulties in achieving good quality cytology screening, alternative approaches based on HPV testing and visual inspection with acetic acid (VIA) and new paradigms such as reduced frequency of screening and screen-and treat- approaches have been evaluated. While VIA is the most feasible technique in low-income countries, HPV testing is the most promising alternative screening test, due to its high sensitivity, objectivity and negative predictive value for cervical neoplasia. Breast cancer control is a priority given its increasing incidence and mortality in LMICs. Mammography screening is complex and resource intensive and not feasible in LMICs. Evidence for the efficacy of clinical breast examination (CBE) in reducing breast cancer mortality from randomized trials in LMICs is essential before CBE screening programs can be recommended. Meanwhile, measures to improve breast awareness and early diagnosis and treatment are important for breast cancer control. Middle-income countries with high risk of colorectal cancer and well-developed health systems may consider introducing immunochemical fecal occult blood test (iFOBT) screening with colonoscopy triage. LMICs with a high burden of oral cancer, such as India, may consider visual screening of tobacco/alcohol users through routine health services. Substantial investments in improving awareness, health care infrastructure, human resources and information systems will be required for the eventual introduction screening programs in LMICs.

▪ REFERENCES

1. IARC Working Group on the Evaluation of Cancer. *Cervix cancer screening.* Lyon: IARC Press; 2005. http://search.library.duke.edu/search?id=DUKE003507831.

2. IARC Working Group on the Evaluation of Cancer-Preventive Strategies., Vainio H, Bianchini F, International Agency for Research on Cancer. *Breast cancer screening.* Lyon, France: IARC Press; 2002: xiii, 229 p.

3. Ferlay J, Shin HR, Bray F, Forman D, Mathers C, Parkin DM. GLOBOCAN 2008 v1.2, cancer incidence and mortality worldwide: IARC CancerBase no. 10 [internet]. 2010. Available from: http://globocan. iarc.fr, accessed 07/02/2012.

4. Curado MP, International Agency for Research on Cancer., International Association of Cancer Registries. *Cancer incidence in five continents, volume IX.* Lyon :Geneva: International Agency for Research on Cancer; Distributed by WHO Press, World Health Organization; 2008:lx, 837 p.

5. World Health Organization. Mortality database. http://www.who.int/whosis/en/.

6. Sankaranarayanan R, Swaminathan R, Brenner H, et al. Cancer survival in Africa, Asia, and Central America: A population-based study. *Lancet Oncol.* 2010;11(2):165–173.

7. Munoz N, Castellsague X, de Gonzalez AB, Gissmann L. Chapter 1: HPV in the etiology of human cancer. *Vaccine.* 2006;24 Suppl 3:S3/1–10.

8. Clifford GM, Gallus S, Herrero R, et al. Worldwide distribution of human papillomavirus types in cytologically normal women in the international agency for research on cancer HPV prevalence surveys: A pooled analysis. *Lancet.* 2005;366(9490):991–998.

9. Sankaranarayanan R, Esmy PO, Rajkumar R, et al. Effect of visual screening on cervical cancer incidence and mortality in Tamil Nadu, India: A cluster-randomized trial. *Lancet*. 2007;370(9585):398–406.

10. Sankaranarayanan R, Nene BM, Shastri SS, et al. HPV screening for cervical cancer in rural India. *N Engl J Med*. 2009;360(14):1385–1394.

11. Ronco G, Giorgi-Rossi P, Carozzi F, et al. Efficacy of human papillomavirus testing for the detection of invasive cervical cancers and cervical intraepithelial neoplasia: A randomized controlled trial. *Lancet Oncol*. 2010;11(3):249–257.

12. Parkin DM, Whelan SL, Ferlay J, Raymond L, Young J. Cancer incidence in five continents, volume VII. Lyon, France: International Agency for Research on Cancer. 1997.

13. Parkin DM, Whelan SL, Ferlay J, Teppo L, Thomas DB. Cancer incidence in five continents, volume VIII. Lyon, France: International Agency for Research on Cancer. 2002.

14. Kwak MS, Choi KS, Spring BJ, Park S, Park EC. Predicting the stages of adoption of cervical cancer screening among Korean women. *Prev Med*. 2009;49(1):48–53.

15. Yoo KY. Cancer control activities in the republic of Korea. *Jpn J Clin Oncol*. 2008;38(5):327–333.

16. Kim YT. Current status of cervical cancer and HPV infection in Korea. *J Gynecol Oncol*. 2009; 20(1):1–7.

17. Koong SL, Yen AM, Chen TH. Efficacy and cost-effectiveness of nationwide cervical cancer screening in Taiwan. *J Med Screen*. 2006;13 Suppl 1:S44–S47.

18. Chen YY, You SL, Chen CA, et al. Effectiveness of national cervical cancer screening programme in Taiwan: 12-year experiences. *Br J Cancer*. 2009;101(1):174–177.

19. Deerasamee S, Srivatanakul P, Sriplung H, et al. Monitoring and evaluation of a model demonstration project for the control of cervical cancer in Nakhon Phanom province, Thailand. *Asian Pac J Cancer Prev*. 2007;8(4):547–556.

20. Gaffikin L, Blumenthal PD, Emerson M, Limpaphayom K, Royal Thai College of Obstetricians and Gynaecologists (RTCOG)/JHPIEGO Corporation Cervical Cancer Prevention Group [corrected]. Safety, acceptability, and feasibility of a single-visit approach to cervical-cancer prevention in rural Thailand: A demonstration project. *Lancet*. 2003;361(9360):814–820.

21. Nessa A, Hussain MA, Rahman JN, Rashid MH, Muwonge R, Sankaranarayanan R. Screening for cervical neoplasia in Bangladesh using visual inspection with acetic acid. *Int J Gynaecol Obstet*. 2010;111(2):115–118.

22. Lazcano-Ponce E, Palacio-Mejia LS, Allen-Leigh B, et al. Decreasing cervical cancer mortality in Mexico: Effect of papanicolaou coverage, birthrate, and the importance of diagnostic validity of cytology. *Cancer Epidemiol Biomarkers Prev*. 2008;17(10):2808–2817.

23. Murillo R, Almonte M, Pereira A, et al. Cervical cancer screening programs in Latin America and the Caribbean. *Vaccine*. 2008;26 Suppl 11:L37–L48.

24. Sepulveda C, Prado R. Effective cervical cytology screening programmes in middle-income countries: The Chilean experience. *Cancer Detect Prev*. 2005;29(5):405–411.

25. Robles SC, Periago MR. Guanacaste, Costa Rica: A landmark for cervical cancer prevention. *Rev Panam Salud Publica*. 2004;15(2):73–74.

26. Fonseca LA, Ramacciotti Ade S, Eluf Neto J. Mortality trends from uterine cervical cancer in the city of Sao Paulo from 1980 to 1999. *Cad Saude Publica*. 2004;20(1):136–142.

27. Zeferino LC, Pinotti JA, Jorge JP, Westin MC, Tambascia JK, Montemor EB. Organization of cervical cancer screening in Campinas and surrounding region, Sao Paulo state, Brazil. *Cad Saude Publica*. 2006;22(9):1909–1914.

28. Arrossi S, Ramos S, Paolino M, Sankaranarayanan R. Social inequality in pap smear coverage: Identifying under-users of cervical cancer screening in Argentina. *Reprod Health Matters*. 2008;16(32):50–58.

29. Sankaranarayanan R, Budukh AM, Rajkumar R. Effective screening programmes for cervical cancer in low- and middle-income developing countries. *Bull World Health Organ*. 2001;79(10):954–962.

30. Alliance for Cervical Cancer Prevention (ACCP). Planning and implementing cervical cancer prevention and control programs: A manual for managers. Seattle: ACCP. 2004.

31. Sankaranarayanan R, Wesley R. A practical manual on visual screening for cervical neoplasia. Lyon, France: IARC Press. 2003;IARC Technical Publication No. 41.

32. World Health Organization (WHO). Comprehensive cervical cancer control: A guide to essential practice. Geneva: WHO. 2006.

33. Blumenthal PD, Lauterbach M, Sellors JW, Sankaranarayanan R. Training for cervical cancer prevention programs in low-resource settings: Focus on visual inspection with acetic acid and cryotherapy. *Int J Gynaecol Obstet*. 2005;89 Suppl 2:S30–S37.

34. Sankaranarayanan R, Gaffikin L, Jacob M, Sellors J, Robles S. A critical assessment of screening methods for cervical neoplasia. *Int J Gynaecol Obstet*. 2005;89 Suppl 2:S4–S12.

35. Murillo R, Luna J, Gamboa O, et al. Cervical cancer screening with naked-eye visual inspection in Colombia. *Int J Gynaecol Obstet*. 2010;109(3):230–234.

36. Sarian LO, Derchain SF, Naud P, et al. Evaluation of visual inspection with acetic acid (VIA), lugol's iodine (VILI), cervical cytology and HPV testing as cervical screening tools in Latin America. This report refers to partial results from the LAMS (latin AMerican screening) study. *J Med Screen*. 2005;12(3):142–149.

37. Sangwa-Lugoma G, Mahmud S, Nasr SH, et al. Visual inspection as a cervical cancer screening method in a primary health care setting in Africa. *Int J Cancer*. 2006;119(6):1389–1395.

38. Denny L, Kuhn L, De Souza M, Pollack AE, Dupree W, Wright TC,Jr. Screen-and-treat approaches for cervical cancer prevention in low-resource settings: A randomized controlled trial. *JAMA*. 2005;294(17):2173–2181.

39. Denny L, Kuhn L, Hu CC, Tsai WY, Wright TC,Jr. Human papillomavirus-based cervical cancer prevention: Long-term results of a randomized screening trial. *J Natl Cancer Inst*. 2010;102(20):1557–1567.

40. Naucler P, Ryd W, Tornberg S, et al. Human papillomavirus and papanicolaou tests to screen for cervical cancer. *N Engl J Med*. 2007;357(16):1589–1597.

41. Mayrand MH, Duarte-Franco E, Rodrigues I, et al. Human papillomavirus DNA versus papanicolaou screening tests for cervical cancer. *N Engl J Med*. 2007;357(16):1579–1588.

42. Bulkmans NW, Berkhof J, Rozendaal L, et al. Human papillomavirus DNA testing for the detection of cervical intraepithelial neoplasia grade 3 and cancer: 5-year follow-up of a randomised controlled implementation trial. *Lancet*. 2007;370(9601):1764–1772.

43. Shi JF, Belinson JL, Zhao FH, et al. Human papillomavirus testing for cervical cancer screening: Results from a 6-year prospective study in rural China. *Am J Epidemiol*. 2009;170(6):708–716.

44. Qiao YL, Sellors JW, Eder PS, et al. A new HPV-DNA test for cervical-cancer screening in developing regions: A cross-sectional study of clinical accuracy in rural China. *Lancet Oncol*. 2008;9(10):929–936.

45. Kuhn L, Wang C, Tsai WY, Wright TC, Denny L. Efficacy of human papillomavirus-based screen-and-treat for cervical cancer prevention among HIV-infected women. *AIDS*. 2010;24(16):2553–2561.

46. Blumenthal PD, Gaffikin L, Deganus S, et al. Cervical cancer prevention: Safety, acceptability, and feasibility of a single-visit approach in Accra, Ghana. *Am J Obstet Gynecol*. 2007;196(4):407.e1–e8; discussion 407.e8–e9.

47. De Vuyst H, Lillo F, Broutet N, Smith JS. HIV, human papillomavirus, and cervical neoplasia and cancer in the era of highly active antiretroviral therapy. *Eur J Cancer Prev*. 2008;17(6):545–554.

48. Maiman M. Management of cervical neoplasia in human immunodeficiency virus-infected women. *J Natl Cancer Inst Monogr*. 1998;(23)(23):43–49.

49. Sahasrabuddhe VV, Bhosale RA, Joshi SN, et al. Prevalence and predictors of colposcopic-histopathologically confirmed cervical intraepithelial neoplasia in HIV-infected women in India. *PLoS One*. 2010; 5(1):e8634.

50. Sankaranarayanan R, Keshkar V, Kothari A, Kane S, Fayette JM, Shastri S. Effectiveness and safety of loop electrosurgical excision procedure for cervical neoplasia in rural India. *Int J Gynaecol Obstet*. 2009;104(2):95–99.

51. Nene BM, Hiremath PS, Kane S, Fayette JM, Shastri SS, Sankaranarayanan R. Effectiveness, safety, and acceptability of cryotherapy by midwives for cervical intraepithelial neoplasia in Maharashtra, India. *Int J Gynaecol Obstet*. 2008;103(3):232–236.

52. Rema P, Suchetha S, Thara S, Fayette JM, Wesley R, Sankaranarayanan R. Effectiveness and safety of loop electrosurgical excision procedure in a low-resource setting. *Int J Gynaecol Obstet.* 2008;103(2):105–110.

53. Luciani S, Gonzales M, Munoz S, Jeronimo J, Robles S. Effectiveness of cryotherapy treatment for cervical intraepithelial neoplasia. *Int J Gynaecol Obstet.* 2008;101(2):172–177.

54. Ngoma T, Muwonge R, Mwaiselage J, Kawegere J, Bukori P, Sankaranarayanan R. Evaluation of cervical visual inspection screening in Dar es Salaam, Tanzania. *Int J Gynaecol Obstet.* 2010;109(2):100–104.

55. Muwonge R, Manuel Mda G, Filipe AP, Dumas JB, Frank MR, Sankaranarayanan R. Visual screening for early detection of cervical neoplasia in Angola. *Int J Gynaecol Obstet.* 2010;111(1):68–72.

56. Chamot E, Kristensen S, Stringer JS, Mwanahamuntu MH. Are treatments for cervical precancerous lesions in less-developed countries safe enough to promote scaling-up of cervical screening programs? A systematic review. *BMC Womens Health.* 2010;10:11.

57. Taylor S, Wang C, Wright TC, Denny L, Tsai WY, Kuhn L. Reduced acquisition and reactivation of human papillomavirus infections among older women treated with cryotherapy: Results from a randomized trial in South Africa. *BMC Med.* 2010;8:40.

58. Goldie SJ, Gaffikin L, Goldhaber-Fiebert JD, et al. Cost-effectiveness of cervical-cancer screening in five developing countries. *N Engl J Med.* 2005;353(20):2158–2168.

59. Ries LAG, Harkins D, Krapcho M, et al. SEER cancer statistics review, 1975–2003. Bethesda, MD: National Cancer Institute. 2006.

60. Sant M, Allemani C, Santaquilani M, et al. EUROCARE-4. Survival of cancer patients diagnosed in 1995–1999. Results and commentary. *Eur J Cancer.* 2009;45(6):931–991.

61. Yeoh KG, Chew L, Wang SC. Cancer screening in Singapore, with particular reference to breast, cervical and colorectal cancer screening. *J Med Screen.* 2006;13 Suppl 1:S14–S19.

62. Jara-Lazaro AR, Thilagaratnam S, Tan PH. Breast cancer in Singapore: Some perspectives. *Breast Cancer.* 2010;17(1):23–28.

63. Yoon NH, Lee HY, Kwak MS, et al. Comparison of satisfaction with cancer screening at mobile van and static sites: National cancer screening program in Korea. *Jpn J Clin Oncol.* 2009;39(3):169–174.

64. Galukande M, Kiguli-Malwadde E. Rethinking breast cancer screening strategies in resource-limited settings. *Afr Health Sci.* 2010;10(1):89–92.

65. Miller AB, To T, Baines CJ, Wall C. Canadian national breast screening study-2: 13-year results of a randomized trial in women aged 50–59 years. *J Natl Cancer Inst.* 2000;92(18):1490–1499.

66. Miller AB, To T, Baines CJ, Wall C. The Canadian national breast screening study: Update on breast cancer mortality. *J Natl Cancer Inst Monogr.* 1997;(22)(22):37–41.

67. Pisani P, Parkin DM, Ngelangel C, et al. Outcome of screening by clinical examination of the breast in a trial in the Philippines. *International Journal of Cancer.* 2006;118(1):149–154.

68. Dinshaw K, Mishra G, Shastri S, et al. Determinants of compliance in a cluster randomised controlled trial on screening of breast and cervix cancer in Mumbai, India. 1. Compliance to screening. *Oncology.* 2007;73(3–4):145–153.

69. Mittra I, Mishra GA, Singh S, et al. A cluster randomized, controlled trial of breast and cervix cancer screening in Mumbai, India: Methodology and interim results after three rounds of screening. *Int J Cancer.* 2010;126(4):976–984.

70. Okonkwo QL, Draisma G, der Kinderen A, Brown ML, de Koning HJ. Breast cancer screening policies in developing countries: A cost-effectiveness analysis for India. *J Natl Cancer Inst.* 2008;100(18): 1290–1300.

71. Thomas DB, Gao DL, Ray RM, et al. Randomized trial of breast self-examination in Shanghai: Final results. *J Natl Cancer Inst.* 2002;94(19):1445–1457.

72. Ellman R, Moss SM, Coleman D, Chamberlain J. Breast self-examination programmes in the trial of early detection of breast cancer: Ten year findings. *Br J Cancer.* 1993;68(1):208–212.

73. Hackshaw AK, Paul EA. Breast self-examination and death from breast cancer: A meta-analysis. *Br J Cancer.* 2003;88(7):1047–1053.

74. Lambert R, Sauvaget C, Sankaranarayanan R. Mass screening for colorectal cancer is not justified in most developing countries. *Int J Cancer.* 2009;125(2):253–256.

75. Hewitson P, Glasziou P, Watson E, Towler B, Irwig L. Cochrane systematic review of colorectal cancer screening using the fecal occult blood test (hemoccult): An update. *Am J Gastroenterol.* 2008;103(6):1541–1549.

76. Warnakulasuriya KA, Ekanayake AN, Sivayoham S, et al. Utilization of primary health care workers for early detection of oral cancer and precancer cases in Sri Lanka. *Bull World Health Organ.* 1984;62(2): 243–250.

77. Warnakulasuriya KA, Nanayakkara BG. Reproducibility of an oral cancer and precancer detection program using a primary health care model in Sri Lanka. *Cancer Detect Prev.* 1991;15(5):331–334.

78. Mehta FS, Gupta PC, Bhonsle RB, Murti PR, Daftary DK, Pindborg JJ. Detection of oral cancer using basic health workers in an area of high oral cancer incidence in India. *Cancer Detect Prev.* 1986;9(3–4):219–225.

79. Mathew B, Sankaranarayanan R, Sunilkumar KB, Kuruvila B, Pisani P, Nair MK. Reproducibility and validity of oral visual inspection by trained health workers in the detection of oral precancer and cancer. *Br J Cancer.* 1997;76(3):390–394.

80. Ramadas K, Lucas E, Thomas G, et al. A digital manual for the early diagnosis of oral neoplasia. Available from: http://screening.iarc.fr/atlasoral.php.

81. Patton LL, Epstein JB, Kerr AR. Adjunctive techniques for oral cancer examination and lesion diagnosis: A systematic review of the literature. *J Am Dent Assoc.* 2008;139(7):896–905; quiz 993–4.

82. Su WW-, Yen AM-, Chiu SY-, Chen TH-. A community-based RCT for oral cancer screening with toluidine blue. *Journal of Dental Research.* 2010;89(9):933–937.

83. Sankaranarayanan R, Ramadas K, Thomas G, et al. Effect of screening on oral cancer mortality in Kerala, India: A cluster-randomized controlled trial. *Lancet.* 2005;365(9475):1927–1933.

84. Subramanian S, Sankaranarayanan R, Bapat B, et al. Cost-effectiveness of oral cancer screening: Results from a cluster randomized controlled trial in India. *Bull World Health Organ.* 2009;87(3):200–206.

85. Rethman MP, Carpenter W, Cohen EE, et al. Evidence-based clinical recommendations regarding screening for oral squamous cell carcinomas. *J Am Dent Assoc.* 2010;141(5):509–520.

86. Frenandez Garrote L, Sankaranarayanan R, Lence Anta JJ, Rodriguez Salva A, Maxwell Parkin D. An evaluation of the oral cancer control program in Cuba. *Epidemiology.* 1995;6(4):428–431.

CHAPTER 6

BEHAVIORAL, SOCIAL, AND CULTURAL ASPECTS OF EPIDEMIOLOGIC STUDIES IN LOW- AND MIDDLE-INCOME COUNTRIES AND IN SPECIAL POPULATIONS

ROBERT M. CHAMBERLAIN

IDENTIFYING SPECIAL POPULATIONS FOR EPIDEMIOLOGIC RESEARCH

Why special populations?: A "special population" is usually a subpopulation within a larger population, and has features that make it unique in some way. A special population allows for a focused epidemiologic study that takes advantage of homogeneity of the special feature.

Unique Features of Special Populations: Social, Cultural, Behavioral, and Political

A subpopulation is a segment of a larger population, usually defined by geography or other criteria. Epidemiologists have been conducting special population research for a very long time, but not often identifying it with the more modern term: special population. For example, epidemiologic studies of breast cancer risk have been conducted on the special populations of Ashkenazi Jewish women[1,2] and Japanese women in California.[3] Early population-based epidemiologic studies of prostate cancer identified a higher incidence in African American men,[4] and subsequent studies have often focused on this special population.[4-8]

One of the principal advantages of special populations to epidemiologic research is the increased numbers of higher risk individuals that can be studied within the confines of a research budget.

Special populations can also share a unique environment of exposures; including dietary practices, smoking, sun exposure, and so forth. Special population studies that focus on these exposures, combined with genetic characteristics are now identified by the term "eco-genetics." The classic study of breast cancer among women in Japan, Hawaii and California,[9] would be considered an eco-genetic study, although it did not measure specific genes, nor specific environmental risks. As a descriptive study, it showed a higher incidence of breast cancer among Japanese women in California than in Hawaii or Japan. These women were considered similar in their genetics, yet their exposures to western lifestyles were greater in California. Today, eco-genetic studies are much more sophisticated, using SNP analysis, GWAS, and using well-developed anthropomorphic and dietary measures.

■ CANCER INCIDENCE AND MORTALITY: BY CANCER SITE, AGE, SEX

Cancer incidence and mortality are not uniform across large populations, although we use rates calculated on the general population for an entire province, state or country. Until recently, age and sex were our only reliable predictors of many types of cancer. Large geographic populations are usually heterogeneous in their age and sex distributions, as well as many other risk characteristics. Identifying higher risk subpopulations has long been the strong suit of chronic disease epidemiologists, and their work has been the basis for the development of prevention strategies, such as mammography targeted to women in certain age groups. Careful epidemiologic analysis has also been the basis for the development of cancer risk models[10] that incorporate several risk factors to estimate the risk of individuals in subpopulations who can benefit from intensive preventive interventions such as chemoprevention or prophylactic mastectomy.

Epidemiologists working on projects in low and middle income countries should be alert to special circumstances that can bias even the most standard measures that underlie rates for cancer incidence and mortality. Often these biases are unknown to outside researchers and are not described in the footnotes of published tables. For example, in many areas of the developing world birthdates are not well documented, and there may be good reasons why people report incorrect ages even when they know otherwise. For example, in Ghana certain heath services have been free to residents who are 70 and older. Therefore, cancer incidence and mortality rates rise abruptly in this age group because of patients in their 60s who claim to be 70 or older in order to benefit from government-provided treatment. This benefit is well known by most adults and certainly all medical providers in Ghana, but it would not appear as a footnote of a published table or be generally known to outsiders. Consequently, outside researchers should develop a familiarity with the local culture and customs of an area, and develop trusted relationships with local informants of all types, ranging from doctors and folk healers, to taxi drivers. Otherwise biases will remain hidden, that otherwise might explain unexpected research results.

■ A BRIEF HISTORY OF CANCER EPIDEMIOLOGY IN INTERNATIONAL SETTINGS, SPECIAL POPULATIONS, AND FUTURE TRENDS

Phase 1: The Discovery Phase. Approximately 1920—Present

Cancer epidemiologic relationships are discovered by careful observation, usually by physicians working in the underdeveloped world and in special populations in the developed world.

Examples of developing world: Burkett's lymphoma, bladder cancer/shistosomiasis, liver cancer/hepatitis.

Examples in US special populations: Occupational groups and minority communities: dust and asbestos exposures/lung cancer, PCBs, etc.

Phase 2: The Documentation Phase. Approximately 1950—Present

Epidemiologic documentation, often from hospital tumor registries in both developing and developed world. Reliable national statistics were first developed in northern Europe and particularly in Scandinavia where the populations were precisely documented with identification numbers and almost universal access to medical services. Other developed countries, such as the United States, developed cancer data systems based on regional registries (SEER) that represented the general population. In low and middle income countries, regional population-based cancer registries have been developed in defined geographic areas such as those in Gharbiah in the Nile Delta and in the city of Aswan, Egypt. Such population-based registries have been developed with the technical training and funding provided by the International Agency for Research on Cancer (IARC) which publishes international data in print and on the web.[11] In addition to the measurement of time trends in incidence and mortality, this documentation from cancer registries was and is used politically in developed and less developed countries, to successfully justify increased governmental and foundation support to prioritize resources for cancer prevention, detection, treatment, training in medicine and public health, and public education.

Phase 3: Public Health Intervention Phase. Approximately 1970—Present

Epidemiologic and tumor registry data used to justify screening and early detection programs, such as breast screening and prostate screening.

Phase 4: Identification of Vulnerable Subpopulations. Approximately 1990—Present

Better hospital and population-based registry data make it possible to identify segments of the population such as triple negative breast cancer in African American women,[12,13] high-risk prostate in African American men,[14] and rural residents in Egypt with pesticide and herbicide exposures.[15,16]

Phase 5: Epidemiologic Registry or Population Data for Identification of High-Risk Participants for Research. Approximately 1995 to the Present

Cancer prevention trials may focus healthy participants of a certain age and/or sex in a general population, such as the Shanghai breast cancer prevention trial using breast self-examination.[17] Even with a special population, some of these prevention trials have required thousands of participants, such as the Prostate, Lung, Colorectal, and Ovarian Cancer Screening (PLCO) Trial, Study of Tamoxifen and Raloxifene (STAR) Trial, Women's Health Initiative and others.[18-20] Chemoprevention or screening trials in a special population of cancer survivors aimed at detecting recurrence or second primary tumors can be more efficient because the special population is more susceptible to cancer.

UNIQUE GENETICS, EXPOSURES, AND LIFESTYLE

Special population studies can advance our knowledge about the genetic components of carcinogenesis, by focusing on groups that have a predisposition to certain cancers. For example, racial and ethnic minority populations generally share common genetic features and these can best be studied epidemiologic studies of special populations. For a simple example, the higher incidence of prostate cancer among African Americans in a large population study is more difficult and costly to investigate when only a small segment of the larger population is African American. However, when the study is focused entirely on this special population, it is possible to generate more statistical power more efficiently at less cost. It is also more likely that if genetic subtypes exist within the special population, these can be elucidated.

Another example is gall bladder cancer, which is rare worldwide, has a high incidence among Peruvians of European ancestry, but not among the native or admixed European-native population.[21] This clinical observation is not well described or understood, but special population studies could unlock the answer. Another example of the strength of international studies of special populations might be the comparison of prostate cancer among African Americans and men living in West Africa. Because a very high proportion of African Americans have ancestry in western Africa, comparison studies might identify unique genetic components that contribute to the disease.

Epidemiologists sometimes wish to describe certain rare cancers that have low incidence in their home countries. Because these cancers are rare they are often not definitively diagnosed either clinically or by pathology. An example is inflammatory breast cancer. In 2000, an epidemiologic study was begun by a group of scientists at the NCI (United States), with collaborators in Egypt, Tunisia, and the University of Michigan. The objective was to accrue and characterize patients in North Africa where inflammatory breast cancer (IBC) was reported to be much higher than in western countries.[22–24] Clinicians in Egypt and Tunisia reported that IBC was 10 to 15% of all breast cancer in hospital registries, therefore presenting a research opportunity not available in the United States.

■ ACCESS TO COLLABORATORS, SPECIAL POPULATIONS, AND DATA IN LMI COUNTRIES

Access to Collaborators: Planning epidemiologic research projects in LMI countries requires access to local resources such as approvals of government ministries, IRBs, hospital authorities, and most important, local scientific and medical collaborators. Local collaborators are usually aware of the barriers to access that are often difficult for outsiders to identify. Their advice about research design acceptability, data collection, local staffing, social norms, medical politics, turf boundaries, payments, and other matters is essential to outside researchers.

Identifying potential local collaborators in LMI countries: Epidemiologists from universities, cancer centers and other organizations in the developed countries usually develop their studies in LMI countries by identifying potential local collaborators who are sometimes epidemiologists, but usually they are medical clinicians. This process of identification can be accomplished through professional networking with colleagues in the developed and LMI countries. Typically, the numbers of potential cancer study collaborators is small in most LMI countries, so the task is not too formidable.

Cancer specialists in LMI countries are usually general surgeons, surgical oncologists, medical oncologists, radiation oncologists and pathologists. Generally, they have clinical practices that are based in university or government hospitals, military facilities, private practices, and often more than one. Many senior physicians earn the majority of their income from private practice, since university and government salaries are typically low. With few exceptions, these physicians have little formal training in epidemiology, even when they have completed advanced medical training abroad in developed countries. In this regard, they are somewhat similar to their clinical colleagues in developed countries. Consequently, recruiting local medical collaborators requires a tactful orientation to the purpose and design of epidemiologic studies. Fortunately, some potential collaborators have participated in clinical treatment trials that may impart valuable experience in some aspects of epidemiologic research such as IRB approvals, eligibility of subjects, and statistical considerations in design. In addition, some LMI countries are developing hospital and population-based cancer incidence registries and these impart some knowledge of descriptive epidemiology to local physicians. Most important, these registries impart a paradigm that is a sea change for physicians and others in LMI countries: that epidemiologic research almost never benefits today's patients, but is an investment for the benefit of future patients and for prevention.

Epidemiologists in LMI Countries: LMI countries are generally lacking in epidemiologists. Ministries of Health are the first place to look for epidemiologists or for someone with the title of epidemiologist. The background and training of these people is highly variable. Many are physicians who had one or two epidemiology courses in medical school, but some have Master's degrees in public health which provided them considerable training in epidemiology. Cancer registrars in LMI countries often have received training in descriptive epidemiology. In most LMI countries these epidemiologists focus on infectious diseases, as they do in developed countries. Nonetheless, they can be valuable allies in cancer studies. Failing to identify and interact with these local epidemiologists is usually a mistake, because they usually know important information that will be useful in setting up a study in cancer epidemiology. Furthermore, if they are ignored there could be negative consequences resulting from professional jealousy, failure to follow protocol within a Ministry of Health or local health department, and other reasons.

The Epidemiologic Perspective among LMI-Country Collaborators: In the preliminary phases of building partnerships, local collaborators are rarely unequivocal in their commitment to an epidemiologic project and to the future scientific partnership. And the reasons are many. First, most epidemiologic studies do not directly benefit the human subjects and this is sometimes baffles clinicians. Clinicians generally have a higher regard for hospital-based tumor registry treatment outcome studies, because these can improve practice and guide health policy. Second, epidemiologic studies usually have long-term future benefits, rather than immediate benefits, for special populations in LMI countries. However, most clinician collaborators will appreciate the benefits of down-staging cancer as this is a high priority in LMI countries. And they appreciate that special population studies can identify characteristics of higher risk individuals who could be targeted for screening with the very limited available resources, such as mammography. And third, descriptive studies can have major impact on cancer incidence when primary prevention is practical and cheap, as in the reduction of bladder cancer or liver cancer incidence by public health interventions in schistosomiasis and hepatitis. These outcomes are especially relevant to potential collaborators, policy makers, and gatekeepers in government health ministries.

Benefits for LMI-Country Collaborators: Perhaps the least discussed and often most contentious benefit is professional recognition and credit to the collaborators. Just as in the developed counties, professional recognition comes in many forms. Foremost among these is the publication of results in the peer-reviewed scientific literature. Medical professionals and scientists in LMI countries usually have fewer funds and opportunities to participate in publishable research that is valued for the prestige and other rewards it conveys. However, it is difficult in any new collaboration, to determine in advance, who might deserve a place on the list of authors of various publications that might result. In negotiating the roles and obligations of collaborators in any new research project it is imperative to communicate clearly. Since English is the international lingua franca of science, it is especially important to have a sequential record of both written and oral communication when English is not the first language of all participants. Following any meeting, the oral discussion and agreements should be summarized and sent to all participants. This is important because scientists from different cultures may have different assumptions and expectations. In some LMI countries, everyone involved in a study, no matter how small their role, expects to be included as an author, often in order of rank or seniority. In most developed countries the standards are based on contributions to the research and role in writing. When discussions are about manuscripts for publication, a manuscript proposal document should be drafted, briefly describing the topic, data, author list, role of each author, persons to be acknowledged, probable journal(s), and date the first draft is expected. All participants should acknowledge the document and know that it is a working document that might be re-drafted several times, as roles and circumstances change, before the manuscript is finally submitted for publication. In this manner, arguments and misunderstandings, that are potential threats to collaborations within the research project, can be minimized. Collaborators and others in LMI countries may not be aware of the various requirements for authorship required by many scientific journals, and when these are made known to everyone they can be used to resolve issues of undeserved authorship. In addition, if the LMI country's government or hospital administrators expect to have approval or embargo power over data or manuscripts, this must be known in advance and discussed. It is not unusual for gatekeepers in LMI countries to quarantine research results they consider detrimental to the image of the country or reputation of a hospital or to require that the manuscript be modified. These issues must be resolved, ideally during the planning of the study.

In addition to scientific publications, special reports should be anticipated and prepared. Progress reports, final reports and executive summaries are often necessary and/or desirable to local supporters, gatekeepers, IRBs, and funding agencies. Because scientific publications usually become available many months or even years after the completion of a study, special summary reports during and immediately after completion of the research, will fulfill a variety of purposes. These reports can contain summary scientific findings and make suggestions and recommendations to improve local conditions such as screening and targeted diagnosis for cancer downstaging. These special reports can be adapted by the Ministry of Health, hospitals and local health agencies in their own reports and newsletters. Such reports make it possible to feature the local research collaborators and these can be valuable them in achieving their local goals and improve the climate for future research.

▪ SPECIAL RESEARCH BUDGETING CONSIDERATIONS IN LMI COUNTRIES

Money is one of the least discussed and understood component of epidemiologic studies in LMI countries. This is because money has both practical and cultural connotations. Budget discussions should parallel scientific discussions during project planning and periodically during the project implementation. Experienced epidemiologic researchers from universities in developed countries are usually experts at this, but this experience is often lacking in LMI countries. Nonetheless, the cost of each aspect of a project must be accurately estimated and the knowledge of the local collaborators is critical. For example, budgeting for skilled interviewers, DNA extraction, –80 freezer storage, and other items is critical. Yet many of these items are budgeted, based on the flimsiest guesses, because no one has done a local study in the particular LMI country. To avoid embarrassment and satisfy expectations, the local collaborators may be tempted to provide seemingly confident estimates of the cost of various items. To help ensure the credibility of a budget, it can be reviewed by disinterested parties who may be knowledgeable, such as hospital administrators, social service providers, and lab managers.

Cultural Perceptions of Money: It is most important for all collaborators to understand that the cultural aspects of money may be very different. In some cultures, senior and upper-class people do not consider it appropriate to discuss the practical aspects of money. These matters are more suited to merchants, accountants and bookkeepers in these societies. Women in particular, may be excluded from discussions about money. Therefore, scientists from developed countries where money is openly discussed, should be careful when, where, and with whom they can discuss the monetary aspects of research. Cultural norms can be very powerful, and must be understood in order to have functional collaborations and avoiding conflicts about budgets and expenditures. This is another reason why gaining knowledge of the LMI country, its social class structure, medical traditions, and culture can prevent problems in epidemiologic research.

Budgeting Funds to Support Collaborators: Another consideration is whether the local LMI collaborators will be paid, and how much. As mentioned previously, few academic physicians and other scientists can survive on their university hospital or medical school income. In some LMI countries, most to their income will be earned in their private clinics and hospitals, pathology labs, and consulting. Sometimes their service at the university will be unpaid. Consequently, university department chairs, deans, and administrators might have little power to influence their faculties and this can come as a surprise to university-based researchers from developed countries. The point of this is to consider whether a particular collaborator should be compensated with salary from a research budget and whether it should be paid through his or her university or separately. Private discussions must resolve these matters.

Budgeting Funds to Support Staff: Another budgeting consideration is how salary should be paid for technicians and others who will function in the epidemiologic research project. In order to gain their commitment and enthusiasm for the project, they should know that their salaries are being supported, in part, from the budget of the project. Otherwise, they may consider this as unappreciated additional work. In many LMI countries these technicians are overburdened with their regular duties, and should be hired to work overtime or on weekends, in order to complete the research work in a timely and careful manner. The quality control and observation of their work should be regularly scheduled and culturally appropriate.

Nonstandard Budget Items: Lastly, budgets for research projects in LMI countries may require many items that would be nonstandard, particularly by research administrators in developed countries. For example, female interviewers might require a car with a male driver in order to complete home interviews, a petty cash fund might be needed to pay various small cash tips and fees that are necessary and expected, and certain unavailable equipment might need to be imported and require "expediting fees." Equipment, such as lab apparatus and computers, can be a particularly troublesome item when it cannot be rented locally. Unusual items such as generators may be needed to maintain lab equipment and freezers in LMI countries where electrical service is unreliable. If equipment is imported or purchased locally with external research funds from a US university there may be requirements that it be inventoried as off-site property of the university and with the impractical requirement that it be returned to campus when the project is completed. These issues can become complicated and delay budget approvals and payments at every turn. When the research funds originate in the United States for example, the investigators are likely to spend a great deal of time and effort justifying these costs. It is advised that these nonstandard costs be carefully written into the budget justification at the proposal stage of the research project.

▥ ACCESS TO SPECIAL POPULATIONS

As in the developed world, special populations in LMI countries may be socially and economically disadvantaged. In some instances it is easy to identify members of a special population, but unless eligibility criteria are simple and clear, this can present problems, wasted resources, and delays. The concept of research may be completely alien to individuals in special population groups and this is likely to reduce participation unless issues of trust, benefit, anonymity and other issues can be addressed. Epidemiologists are usually adept at this and often they enlist the endorsements of leaders or respected individuals in these communities. Identifying the members of special populations can be easier when they are already organized or identified as a group, such as workers in an industry, recipients of pensions, or patients at a clinic or hospital. Sometimes it is essential that subjects receive some incentive or compensation for their participation and this should be anticipated in budgeting the project.

Special populations in LMI countries may be defined occupationally or in areas near high-risk areas such as certain industries, dump sites, and other hazards. Exposure studies can be especially problematic in LMI countries because the results may point to blameful industries that provide employment to the industry's workers and livelihood to the surrounding neighborhood and community. Furthermore, government agencies responsible for controlling these hazards may actually attempt to block epidemiologic studies that would potentially expose their ineffectiveness.

Cancer organ sites that have sexual connotations or imply sexual behavior can be particularly sensitive in LMI countries. It is not unusual for women with cancer to hide this from their families and the community because it can imply a stigma that will make their daughters less desirable marriage partners. This may account, in part, for much late-stage presentation of beast, ovarian and cervical cancers. Epidemiologists who plan studies of these cancers must be especially sensitive to the social and cultural barriers to data collection and to the social stigma that could affect participants.

In summary, epidemiologists working with special populations will benefit by taking time to learn about all aspects of a LMI country, especially the culture, social norms, customs, health beliefs, the health care systems. Learning some of the native language, idioms, and expressions, will always enhance goodwill and show evidence of respect and caring; key components in interpersonal communication that reduce barriers for research.

▥ ACCESS TO DATA

In developing most epidemiologic studies, the identification and use of existing data is desirable. In LMI countries, existing data may be incomplete, unreliable, and substandard in many ways, just as it may be in developed countries. If existing data are essential to a study, then a complete evaluation may require site visits and discussions with data personnel. Stories are legion among epidemiologists who have visited LMI hospitals with incomplete medical records in disarray, molded and infested with insects and rodents. Cancer registries may have time gaps of several years when funding was unavailable. Tumors may or may not have been verified by pathology reports, and conversely pathology lab data may be completely void of patient characteristics. Furthermore, hospital registries are rarely digitized and often incompatible with one another. Environmental exposure data may be imputed, rather than measured. The important lesson from these tales is not to accept the assurances of high quality by the local data-keepers, knowing that they have many motivations to gloss over imperfections.

SUMMARY

Research access in LMI countries, in all aspects, is strongly influenced by lay and professional social norms, culture, traditions, and communication. Local professional collaborators work in the milieu of their culture where patterns of communication may be marked by politeness, where direct questioning and unpleasant issues are avoided. It should be recognized that the social norms of every culture have an influence, regardless of the dispassionate professional standards of objectivity, sharing, and disclosure. Epidemiologic researchers from the developed countries will be less frustrated with methodological imperfections, schedule delays, and other barriers, if they anticipate these issues and remain flexible and willing to make on-site adaptations. The more aware we are of this phenomenon, the better our collaborative research in LMI countries will be. Lastly, the interpersonal relationships that develop between collaborators in these settings usually develop into enjoyable friendships that bring their own rewards.

REFERENCES

1. Struewing JP, Abeliovich D, Peretz T, et al. The carrier frequency of the BRCA1 185delAG mutation is approximately 1% in Ashkenazi Jewish individuals. *Nat Genet*. 1995;11(2):198–200.
2. Struewing JP, Hartge P, Wacholder S, et al. The risk of cancer associated with specific mutations of BRCA1 and BRCA2 among Ashkenazi Jews. *N Engl J Med*. 1997;336(20):1401–1408.
3. Buzin CH, Tang SH, Cunningham JM, et al. Low frequency of p53 gene mutations in breast cancers of Japanese-American women. *Nutr Cancer*. 2001;39(1):72–77.
4. Platz EA, Rimm EB, Willett WC, Kantoff PW, Giovannucci E. Racial variation in prostate cancer incidence and in hormonal system markers among male health professionals. *J Natl Cancer Inst*. 2000; 92(24):2009–2017.
5. Gueye SM, Zeigler-Johnson CM, Friebel T, et al. Clinical characteristics of prostate cancer in African Americans, American whites, and Senegalese men. *Urology*. 2003;61(5):987–992.
6. Drake BF, Lathan CS, Okechukwu CA, Bennett GG. Racial differences in prostate cancer screening by family history. *Ann Epidemiol*. 2008;18(7):579–583.
7. Husaini BA, Reece MC, Emerson JS, Scales S, Hull PC, Levine RS. A church-based program on prostate cancer screening for African American men: Reducing health disparities. *Ethn Dis*. 2008;18(2 Suppl 2):S2–179–184.
8. Giri VN, Egleston B, Ruth K, et al. Race, genetic West African ancestry, and prostate cancer prediction by prostate-specific antigen in prospectively screened high-risk men. *Cancer Prev Res (Phila)*. 2009;2(3): 244–250.
9. Ziegler RG, Hoover RN, Pike MC, et al. Migration patterns and breast cancer risk in Asian-American women. *J Natl Cancer Inst*. 1993;85(22):1819–1827.
10. Gail MH, Brinton LA, Byar DP, et al. Projecting individualized probabilities of developing breast cancer for white females who are being examined annually. *J Natl Cancer Inst*. 1989;81(24):1879–1886.
11. Ferlay J, Shin HR, Bray F, Forman D, Mathers C, Parkin DM. GLOBOCAN 2008 v1.2, cancer incidence and mortality worldwide: IARC CancerBase no. 10 [internet]. 2010. Available from: http://globocan.iarc.fr, accessed 07/02/2012.
12. Lund MJ, Butler EN, Hair BY, et al. Age/race differences in HER2 testing and in incidence rates for breast cancer triple subtypes: A population-based study and first report. *Cancer*. 2010;116(11):2549–2559.
13. Stark A, Kleer CG, Martin I, et al. African ancestry and higher prevalence of triple-negative breast cancer: Findings from an international study. *Cancer*. 2010;116(21):4926–4932.

14. McDougall JA, Li CI. Trends in distant-stage breast, colorectal, and prostate cancer incidence rates from 1992 to 2004: Potential influences of screening and hormonal factors. *Horm Cancer.* 2010;1(1):55–62.

15. Dey S, Hablas A, Seifeldin IA, et al. Urban-rural differences of gynaecological malignancies in Egypt (1999–2002). *BJOG.* 2010;117(3):348–355.

16. Dey S, Soliman AS, Hablas A, et al. Urban-rural differences in breast cancer incidence by hormone receptor status across 6 years in Egypt. *Breast Cancer Res Treat.* 2010;120(1):149–160.

17. Thomas DB, Gao DL, Ray RM, et al. Randomized trial of breast self-examination in Shanghai: Final results. *J Natl Cancer Inst.* 2002;94(19):1445–1457.

18. Andriole GL, Levin DL, Crawford ED, et al. Prostate cancer screening in the prostate, lung, colorectal and ovarian (PLCO) cancer screening trial: Findings from the initial screening round of a randomized trial. *J Natl Cancer Inst.* 2005;97(6):433–438.

19. Vogel VG, Costantino JP, Wickerham DL, Cronin WM, Wolmark N. The study of tamoxifen and raloxifene: Preliminary enrollment data from a randomized breast cancer risk reduction trial. *Clin Breast Cancer.* 2002;3(2):153–159.

20. Fouad MN, Corbie-Smith G, Curb D, et al. Special populations recruitment for the women's health initiative: Successes and limitations. *Control Clin Trials.* 2004;25(4):335–352.

21. Lazcano-Ponce EC, Miquel JF, Munoz N, et al. Epidemiology and molecular pathology of gallbladder cancer. *CA Cancer J Clin.* 2001;51(6):349–364.

22. Lo AC, Kleer CG, Banerjee M, et al. Molecular epidemiologic features of inflammatory breast cancer: A comparison between Egyptian and US patients. *Breast Cancer Res Treat.* 2008;112(1):141–147.

23. Lo AC, Georgopoulos A, Kleer CG, et al. Analysis of RhoC expression and lymphovascular emboli in inflammatory vs non-inflammatory breast cancers in Egyptian patients. *Breast.* 2009;18(1):55–59.

24. Soliman AS, Banerjee M, Lo AC, et al. High proportion of inflammatory breast cancer in the population-based cancer registry of Gharbiah, Egypt. *Breast J.* 2009;15(4):432–434.

CHAPTER 7

ETHICAL ISSUES IN CANCER EPIDEMIOLOGIC STUDIES

STEVEN S. COUGHLIN

Several important ethical issues are discussed in this chapter, including the protection of privacy and confidentiality, informed consent, the need for review by an institutional review board or other research ethics committee, the balancing of risks and potential benefits, issues arising in studies of vulnerable populations, and the obligations that cancer epidemiologists have to communities and to individual research subjects. The professional obligations identified in this chapter, including the need to be sensitive to cultural differences, are based upon widely recognized ethical principles such as respect for the autonomy of persons, beneficence, and justice. Epidemiologists who undertake cancer studies, including research conducted in low- and middle-income countries and in special populations, have ethical and professional obligations to maximize the potential benefits of research studies to participants and to the communities in which the research is undertaken, and to minimize risks and potential harms. Other obligations include ensuring that the benefits and burdens of epidemiologic research are distributed in an equitable fashion.

Epidemiologic studies of cancer, including international collaborative studies conducted in low- and middle-income countries, raise a number of ethical issues that have been addressed in ethics guidelines such as those developed and recently updated by the Council for International Organizations of Medical Sciences.[1] Several of these ethical issues are discussed in this chapter including the protection of privacy and confidentiality, informed consent, the need for review by an institutional review board or other research ethics committee, the balancing of risks and potential benefits, issues arising in studies of vulnerable populations, and the obligations that cancer epidemiologists have to communities and to individual research subjects. The professional obligations identified in this chapter, such as the need to be sensitive to cultural differences, are based upon widely recognized ethical principles such as respect for the autonomy of persons, beneficence, and justice. Because cancer epidemiologic studies often utilize data collected as part of cancer registries, ethical issues pertaining to cancer registries are also discussed in this chapter. This review of ethical issues arising in cancer epidemiologic studies focuses on studies with an observational design and does not deal with challenging issues that arise in some intervention studies and clinical trials such as what standard of care should be provided to research participants in impoverished, medically under-served communities and what happens to those individuals and communities once a clinical trial is over.[2–4]

It is not possible to adequately consider the potential benefits of cancer epidemiologic research conducted in special populations and in low- and middle-income countries, or the balance of potential benefits and risks or potential harms, without delving deeply into the scientific rationale for such studies, a topic expertly addressed by the authors of other chapters in this volume. It is worthwhile noting here, however, that cancer epidemiology is an important part of cancer control which aims to reduce the burden and suffering from cancer by preventing exposure to risk factors, early detection, effective treatment, and palliative care.[5–7] Several causes of cancer which have particular relevance to low- and middle-income countries have been identified through epidemiologic and clinical research. Examples include adenocarcinoma of the liver due to chronic infection with hepatitis B, bladder cancer due to *Schistosoma haematobium* infection, *Helicobacter pylori* infection and gastric cancer, and cervical cancer due to persistent infection with human papillomavirus. Epidemiological studies are also vital to understanding environmental and occupational causes of cancer (for example, cancer of lung or other site that may be prevented by reducing or eliminating exposure to risk factors).

In order to lay a foundation for the discussion that follows, I begin with an overview of the ethical context of cancer research in international settings.

■ THE ETHICAL CONTEXT OF CANCER RESEARCH IN INTERNATIONAL SETTINGS

Epidemiologists who undertake cancer studies, including research conducted in low- and middle-income countries and in special populations, have ethical and professional obligations to maximize the potential benefits of research studies to participants and to the communities in which the research is undertaken, and to minimize risks and potential harms. Minimizing risks and potential harms in such settings generally requires being sensitive to cultural differences. For example, researchers or their collaborators should be knowledgeable about the local political structure, language, and customs, including local moral systems.[2] Other obligations include not causing harm, respecting the autonomy of persons who participate in studies, and ensuring that the benefits and burdens of epidemiologic research are distributed in an equitable fashion.[1,8–10]

Ethical concerns about the need to maximize benefits from international health research and ensure a just distribution of benefits must be viewed within the context of marked global disparities in health, sanitation, nutrition, housing, income, and other resources. Substantial inequities in health status and socioeconomic factors occur both within countries and internationally.[11]

Epidemiologists working in international settings may encounter difficult ethical dilemmas. For example, how should standards of health care be applied in international studies? A frequently expressed concern, which has more frequently been raised in the context of clinical trials than in epidemiologic studies, is the potential for exploitation of research participants or communities when studies are undertaken in resource poor countries by researchers from developed countries. To address such concerns, it is desirable for IRB or research ethics committee review to occur both in the country from which the researchers or funding agency are from and in the host country. Collaborative research with researchers or institutions from the host country and studies employing community advisory boards are also more likely to take into account local perspectives, values, and concerns. In countries where there is inadequate capacity for independent ethical review, ethical review by the external sponsoring country and international agency is necessary.[1]

Researchers and communities are increasingly working together to define new approaches for collaboration and to facilitate important research studies, while at the same time being responsive to community needs and priorities.[2,12] Community advisory boards with representatives from the target community are likely to facilitate many types of health research including studies designed to assess the effectiveness of interventions. Potential stakeholders in international health research include research participants, community representatives, researchers, activists, international agencies, governments, nongovernmental organizations, and sponsors.

■ ETHICAL ISSUES IN CANCER EPIDEMIOLOGY

The results of epidemiologic research studies contribute to generalizable knowledge by elucidating the causes of disease; by combining epidemiologic data with information from other disciplines such as genetics and microbiology; by evaluating the consistency of epidemiologic data with etiological hypotheses; and by providing the basis for developing and evaluating health promotion and prevention procedures.[13] The primary professional roles of epidemiology are the design and conduct of scientific research and the public health application of scientific knowledge. This includes reporting research results and maintaining and promoting health in communities. In carrying out these professional roles, epidemiologists often encounter a number of ethical issues and concerns that require careful consideration. Many of these issues have been addressed in the literature on ethics in epidemiology including international and national ethics guidelines.[1,14–16] Ethics guidelines such as those developed for the International Society for Environmental Epidemiology and the American College of Epidemiology provide useful accounts of epidemiologists' obligations to research participants, society, employers, and colleagues.[14,16] International guidelines for ethical review of epidemiologic studies were developed by the Council of International Organizations of Medical Sciences and recently updated.[1] The CIOMS guidelines draw a distinction between epidemiologic research and routine practice (for example, outbreak investigations and public health surveillance) and consider some of the issues associated with obtaining informed consent in epidemiologic studies. Specific ethical issues arising in epidemiologic research and public health practice that have been highlighted in ethics guidelines include minimizing risks and providing benefits, informed consent, avoiding and disclosing conflicts of interest, obligations to communities, and the institutional review board system.

Minimizing Risks and Providing Benefits

Ethical concerns in epidemiology and public health practice often relate to the obligations of health professionals to acquire and apply scientific knowledge aimed at maintaining and restoring public health while respecting individual rights. Potential societal benefits must often be balanced with risks and potential harms to individuals and communities, such as the potential for stigmatization or invasions of privacy.

Epidemiologists have ethical and professional obligations to maximize the potential benefits of studies to research participants and to society, and to minimize potential harms and risks. In addition, these obligations are legal or regulatory requirements in many countries. In studies that rely upon interview data or existing records, there are no physical risks to the participants. Some emotional distress may be experienced, however, as a result of fear of illness, embarrassment, or concerns over violations of privacy. Dimensions of privacy include the sensitivity of the information and the setting being observed.[17] Social and legal risks that could result from the disclosure of confidential information should be eliminated or minimized by rigorously protecting the confidentiality of health information. Although the risks posed by epidemiologic studies are often minor compared with those that may be associated with clinical trials and other experimental studies, participants in epidemiologic studies may be burdened by a loss of privacy, by time spent completing interviews and examinations, and by possible adverse psychological effects such as enhanced grief or anxiety.[18] Such risks and potential harms can be minimized by careful attention to study procedures and questionnaire design, for example, by limiting the length of interviews or by scheduling them on a date that is less likely to result in adverse psychological effects. Cross-cultural studies and studies of special populations can pose potential risks to groups of individuals and communities. For example, populations defined by race or ethnicity may suffer stigmatization or lowered self-image following the publication of research findings that create or reinforce negative cultural stereotypes. Disparaging information about a group can result in harms such as discrimination in employment, housing, or insurance. It is important to note, however, that the identification of disparities in health or the maldistribution of health services across groups defined by race, ethnicity, or other factors can serve as a basis for health planning and policy making and thereby contribute to improving the health of those who are less well-off in society.

Minimizing risks and potential harms and maximizing potential benefits are particularly important in epidemiologic studies of vulnerable populations. Examples include studies of children, pregnant women, some elderly people, and populations that are marginalized or socioeconomically disadvantaged.

A further obligation is the need to ensure that the burdens and potential benefits of epidemiologic studies are distributed equitably. The potential benefits of epidemiologic research are often societal in nature, such as obtaining new information about the causes of diseases, or identifying health disparities across groups defined by race, ethnicity, socioeconomic status, or other factors.[18] Research participants may receive direct benefits from participation in some studies, such as when a previously unrecognized disease or risk factor is detected during examinations. The provision of ancillary care in health research conducted in low- and middle-income countries is an important topic discussed in recent reports.[2,19] Ancillary care refers to health care needed by research participants but which is not necessary to ensure scientific validity, prevent study-related harms, or address study-related injuries. This can include treatment for conditions discovered during the study procedures and conditions unrelated to the study. Considering how best to meet the ancillary care needs of research participants is of particular concern in studies carried out in low-resource settings such as many developing countries. Epidemiologic studies conducted in low-resource settings frequently identify important unmet health needs including conditions for which treatment is not available with the local health system. The research protocol should specify what health care services will be made available during and after the research and what action the investigators will take, if any, when medical conditions are detected within a study population that are not related to the study but that need treatment.[1]

Cancer epidemiologists conducting research in low- and middle-income countries may have special opportunities to help build research capacity in those countries. For example, by helping representatives of those countries to set their own priorities for research, conducting research that is relevant to local health needs, and helping to train members of the host country in disease surveillance and epidemiologic research methods.[1] As noted by the Nuffield Council on Bioethics,[2] the lack of appropriate infrastructure and local expertise are important constraints to adequately addressing health disparities and developing research capacity may help to maximize the long-term value of the research.

Avoiding and Disclosing Conflicts of Interest

Other ethical issues that arise in the professional practice of epidemiology relate to how best to deal with potential conflicts of interest, in order to maintain public trust in epidemiology and sustain public support for health research. Recent media reports about previously undisclosed conflicts of interest have raised public awareness of the potential for conflicts of interest in clinical research and epidemiology, and about the need for institutions and individual researchers to address such conflicts. Conflicts of interest can affect scientific judgment and harm scientific objectivity. Studies have suggested that financial interests and researchers' commitment to a hypothesis can influence reported research results.[20] To address such concerns, funding agencies and research institutions have taken steps such as adopting new training programs that encourage researchers to avoid or disclose conflicts of interest, and revising or strengthening institutional rules and guidelines. Professional societies and medical associations have also issued policy statements and recommendations about how best to address conflicts of interest in clinical research.[21] Researchers should disclose financial interests and sources of funding when publishing research results. It may also be important to disclose information about potential or actual financial conflicts of interest when obtaining informed consent from research participants. A related issue is that health researchers should avoid entering into contractual agreements that prevent them from publishing results in a timely manner. Communicating research results in a timely manner, without censorship or interference from the funder, is essential for maintaining public trust.

Obligations to Communities

The obligations of epidemiologists to study participants have been highlighted in several reports.[14,16] These obligations include communicating the results of epidemiologic studies at the earliest possible time, after appropriate scientific peer review, so that the widest possible audience stands to benefit from the information. Epidemiologists should strive to carry out studies in a way that is scientifically valid and interpret and report the results of their studies in a way that is scientifically accurate and appropriate. In addition, epidemiologists should respect cultural diversity in carrying out studies and in communicating with members of affected communities. Other obligations to community members and to research participants have been highlighted in ethics guidelines for epidemiologists and public health institutions.[1]

Research conducted in low- and middle-income countries by investigators from more affluent countries raises special concerns about the extent to which the research helps the host country to address its own research priorities. As noted by the Nuffield Council on Bioethics,[2] the process of how individual countries set their own research priorities is a complex process; many countries utilize World Health Organization recommendations that are relevant to their own country. Questions can arise about the extent to which external sponsors, research institutions, or individual researchers are guided by the host country's national priorities when making decisions about what studies to pursue.[22] Epidemiologic studies of prevalent cancers and other cancer prevention and control activities that potentially benefit large segments of the population are much less likely to give rise to such concerns. Specific recommendations for research sponsors, researchers, and IRB members about how best to address host country research priorities are offered in the CIOMS *International Ethical Guidelines for Epidemiological Studies.*[1]

Informed Consent

Provisions for obtaining informed consent are also important. High rates of illiteracy in many resource poor nations may increase the difficulty of obtaining informed consent from research participants.[23] There is often a need to translate informed consent statements into a language other than English. Potential research participants should be provided with information about the study in a language that they can understand and at their level of comprehension.[2] Misunderstandings about research are more likely to occur when researchers and participants speak different languages or when there are no equivalent words or phrases for particular research concepts.[23] Practical steps that may be taken to promote understanding about research, at least in some settings, include providing information through health workers rather than physicians so that participants feel more comfortable discussing and asking questions.[2] The availability of female health workers may be particularly important when the research involves women.

Informed consent provisions in epidemiologic studies ensure that research participants make a free choice and also give institutions the legal authorization to proceed with the research.[24] Investigators must disclose information that potential participants use to decide whether to consent to the study. This includes the purpose of the research, the scientific procedures, anticipated risks and benefits, any inconveniences or discomfort, and the participant's right to refuse participation or to withdraw from the research at any time. Investigators or there collaborators should be knowledgeable about the social and cultural context in which the research will be conducted so that potential research participants can be adequately informed of any aspects of the research that may be of concern to them.[2] In some contexts, research ethics review committees may grant a waiver for the requirement of signed written consent documents. For example, the requirement for signed consent may be waived in certain low-risk studies or in communities where signing a consent form would pose an undue risk to confidentiality. However, the research protocol should specify how it will be documented that the research participants have given their voluntary informed consent such as procedures for witnessing verbal consent.[2]

Informed consent requirements may be waived in exceptional circumstances when obtaining consent is impractical, the risks are minimal, and the risks and potential benefits of the research have been carefully considered by an independent ethics review committee. For example, in some epidemiology studies involving the analysis of large databases of routinely collected information (for example, insurance claims data), it may not be feasible to recontact patients to ask them for their informed consent. Risks and potential harms in such studies may be very low, and risks may be further reduced by omitting personal identifiers from the computer databases. As noted in the CIOMS[1] guidelines, "People have a right to know that their medical records or biological specimens may be used for research. Records and specimens taken in the course of clinical care, or for an earlier study, may be used for research without the consent of the patients/subjects only if an ethical review committee has determined that the research poses minimal risk, that the rights or interests of the patients will not be violated, that their privacy and confidentiality or anonymity are assured, and that the research is designed to answer an important question and would be impracticable if the requirement for informed consent were to be imposed." When collecting and storing human biological samples for future epidemiologic research, investigators should obtain the voluntary informed consent of the individual donor or their legal guardian.

Some cancer epidemiologic studies target vulnerable groups such as children, the elderly, persons with diminished mental capacity, or persons who are seriously ill or near the end of their life. Such individuals are considered vulnerable because of their increased potential for risks or harms or their decreased capacity for understanding or because of their dependence upon health care providers. They may also be dependent upon other family members.

Children need parental consent for most research oriented activities and are often considered minors until the age of 18 or older. Legal definitions of age of consent vary across countries and across jurisdictions within individual countries. Parents are the traditional advocates and decision-makers of children.[25] Nevertheless, the autonomy of all potential research participants must be respected and so, in some countries, assent is usually required for children who are old enough to provide assent.

It sometimes has been argued that research involving children is ethically not permissible if it does not directly benefit the individual child. It has been argued, for example, that no research ought to be performed on children unless there is the possibility of direct benefit, because children are not capable of giving informed consent.[26] Others have convincingly argued, however, that children should be allowed to participate in research, even if they do not stand to benefit directly, provided the research poses no or only minimal risk and parental permission is obtained. In deciding whether or not to allow children to be included in research studies, both the risks and the negative consequences of not conducting research on children must be considered.[25]

In studies of older persons, ethical issues related to obtaining informed consent often take on greater significance. Although persons with diminished autonomy are entitled to special protections, such as obtaining surrogate consent for their participation in research from a close relative, the need for personal autonomy to be respected does not diminish with advancing years.

Indigenous populations and other special populations may also be considered to be vulnerable. Minority groups are readily identifiable subsets of the population that can be distinguished by racial, ethnic, or cultural heritage. Subpopulations often exist within such minority groups that have unique geographic or national origins and important cultural differences. Other vulnerable groups in society include individuals who are socioeconomically disadvantaged or marginalized.

Special considerations for obtaining informed consent may arise in epidemiologic studies of socioeconomically deprived people. People who have limited access to health care may misunderstand an invitation to participate in a study as an opportunity to receive medical care. In addition, they may be reluctant to refuse participation when the researcher is viewed as someone in a position of authority, such as a physician or university professor. Socioeconomically deprived people may also be more motivated to participate in studies involving financial incentives for participation. Researchers and members of IRBs or research ethics committees must carefully weigh incentives for participation in research to avoid incentives that may be manipulative or coercive. In different countries, research ethics committees have often considered payment for travel or lost earnings due to time away from work and the receipt of healthcare during research to be reasonable forms of compensation[2]. However, researchers and IRB members must carefully consider research protocols and procedures for obtaining informed consent in situations where potential participants are seriously ill and do not have alternative sources of treatment.

The important issues that arise in international research conducted by researchers from countries such as the United States and Great Britain in developing countries have also received considerable attention.[1,27] The ongoing debate over the trans-cultural applicability of standards for informed consent and other ethical precepts that have become widely accepted in the United States and Europe revolves around the merits and weaknesses of arguments based upon ethical relativism. Relativists argue that culturally sensitive standards are needed for obtaining the informed consent of research participants when studies are undertaken in other societies. Others point out the need for some minimal set of universally applicable safeguards to protect the welfare and rights of individuals who are the target of health research, such as when researchers from developed countries undertake studies in less developed countries. These important issues are addressed in international guidelines for medical research and in the Nuffield Council on Bioethics[2] report on *The Ethics of Research Related to Healthcare in Developing Countries*. In some cultures, it may be necessary to obtain the assent and cooperation of community leaders or heads of households, although this should not replace the requirement of obtaining the informed consent of each individual participant. In some communities or cultures, individuals may not feel comfortable refusing to participate in research that their community leader or head of household has assented to; this potential concern requires special attention by researchers.[2] Although provisions for obtaining informed consent in cross-cultural studies may be complicated by language barriers and cultural differences, persons in other cultures do not as a general rule have diminished capacities for understanding consent requirements.

Privacy and Confidentiality

The custodian of a database and investigators who receive data for research must establish secure safeguards to protect the confidentiality of the data.[1] One important way in which public health researchers reduce potential harms and risks to participants in epidemiologic studies is by rigorously protecting the confidentiality of their health information. Specific measures taken by researchers to protect the confidentiality of health information include keeping records under lock and key, limiting access to confidential records, discarding personal identifiers from data collection forms and computer files whenever feasible, and training staff in the importance of privacy and confidentiality protection.[18] Other measures that have been employed to safeguard health information include encrypting computer databases, limiting geographic detail, and suppressing cells in tabulated data where the number of cases in the cell is small. As part of informed consent, potential research participants should be informed about the limits to the investigators' ability to safeguard confidentiality and the possible consequences of breaches of confidentiality.[1]

Closely related to confidentiality requirements are provisions for data security. Study materials and databases may contain confidential data which needs to be secure over long periods of time. For longitudinal studies, standards and methods need to be developed and followed for the secure preservation of data. General principles for the adequacy of data protection methods are outlined in the CIOMS[1] guidelines.

Institutional Review Boards and Research Ethics Committees

The purpose of research ethics committees or institutional review boards (IRBs) is to ensure that studies involving human research participants are designed to conform with relevant ethical standards and that the rights and welfare of participants are protected. Human-subjects review by such committees ensures that studies have a favorable balance of potential benefits and risks, that participants are selected equitably, and that procedures for obtaining informed consent are adequate. In international collaborative research, research ethics committee or IRB review should occur both in the country from which the researchers or funding agency are from and in the host country.[1] As noted in the CIOMS guidelines, the health authorities of the host country and the national or local ethics review committee should strive to ensure that the proposed research is responsive to the health needs and priorities of the host country and that it meets the required ethical standards. IRBs or comparable research ethics committees now exist in most countries around the world and there have been continuing efforts to ensure that all countries have adequate mechanisms in place to ensure the protection of human subjects who participate in research. In countries where there is inadequate capacity for independent ethical review, ethical review by the external sponsoring country and international agency is necessary.[1] The World Health Organization has established operational guidelines for ethics committees that review biomedical research. Efforts to sustain or build capacity for research ethics committee review in low- and middle-income countries was discussed by CIOMS and the Nuffield Council on Bioethics.[1,2] In addition to review by an IRB or research ethics committee, some studies also require community review and approval of studies. In the United States, for example, a Native American tribal council must formally approve any research conducted within tribal jurisdiction.[1]

Despite the important role played by research ethics committees and IRBs, researchers have sometimes expressed concern about the obstacles that human-subjects review can create. In some countries, human-subjects review has been streamlined with the use of standardized forms and review processes or by centralizing review by research ethics committees. As previously mentioned, one of the important issues considered by research ethics committees and by individual researchers is the adequacy of provisions for obtaining the informed consent of study participants.

Some observational studies (for example, those utilizing publicly available or anonymous data) may not require prior review by and IRB or research ethics committee under the regulations of the local jurisdictions.[1] Cancer epidemiologists should confer with the research ethics review committee to determine requirements in the country in which the research is to be conducted.

These are just some of the ethical issues addressed in ethics guidelines developed for epidemiologists and other public health professionals. Other issues addressed in the guidelines include those pertaining to scientific misconduct, intellectual property and data sharing, and publication of research findings.

■ ETHICAL ISSUES IN CANCER SURVEILLANCE

An expanding body of literature has considered the important ethical issues that arise in such areas of public health practice as disease surveillance and program evaluation.[8,28,29] In further specifying ethical norms in particular contexts, it is important to draw distinctions between epidemiologic research and public health practice activities. For example, requirements for submitting research protocols to an IRB do not necessarily apply to routine disease surveillance conducted as part of public health practice.[30]

Surveillance can be defined as the ongoing, systematic collection, analysis, and interpretation of outcome-specific data, with the timely dissemination of these data to those responsible for preventing and controlling disease or injury.[31] A fundamental public health activity is to measure and monitor changes in health status, risk factors, and health service access and utilization. The effective dissemination of information is as important as data collection and analysis; the collected information must have a demonstrated utility.[32]

United States federal regulations which deal with issues such as IRB review and informed consent requirements mostly address biomedical research.[30] These regulations

define research as a systematic investigation, including development, testing, and evaluation designed to develop or contribute to generalizable knowledge. In applying the federal
regulations for protecting participants in public health research, United States agencies have
sometimes distinguished health research and nonresearch public health practice activities
by considering the primary intent of the activity. For example, the primary intent of cancer
research is to generate or contribute to generalizable knowledge. Cancer surveillance projects are likely to be nonresearch when they involve the regular, ongoing collection and analysis of health-related data, conducted to monitor the frequency and distribution of cancer in
the population. Surveillance projects may have a research component when they involve the
collection and analysis of health-related data conducted either to generate knowledge that
is applicable to other populations and settings or to contribute to general knowledge about
the health condition. In determining whether cancer surveillance projects conducted in low-
or middle-income countries are research or nonresearch (and perhaps exempt from review
by an IRB or research ethics committee), researchers should consult with the appropriate
authorities and agencies in the host country and in their own country. As noted by CIOMS,[1]
the "generalizable knowledge" definition of research works better for medical research than
for distinguishing between research and practice in epidemiology. Thus, careful judgment is
needed to determine whether an activity should be classified as research or practice.

Codes of ethics and ethics guidelines have been developed for cancer registry professionals.[33-36] Topics dealt with in the ethics codes and guidelines include provisions for
maximizing the societal benefits of cancer registries and minimizing risks and potential
harms to patients, requirements for protecting confidentiality and privacy, and responding
to requests for use of registry data.

Cancer registry data have several potentially beneficial uses including the efficient allocation of limited resources to provide maximum benefits to communities. Determining
appropriate resource allocation may be achieved by identifying services that are most
needed in specific populations through the evaluation of the accessibility and availability
of healthcare services.[34,35] This can allow for the targeting of intervention programs such
as cervical screening in a particular geographic area or among underserved members of a
community. Cancer registry data may also detect elevated cancer rates and identify regional
or national patterns of cancer risk. Registries often provide data to qualified researchers for
clinical or epidemiologic research into the causes of cancer. Local cancer registries such as
those associated with individual hospitals help healthcare administrators and providers to
monitor the quality, effectiveness, and appropriateness of cancer services at a healthcare
facility or in the community.[34,35,37] Cancer services in a community or region can be compared with local, regional, or national data, including trends in cancer services.

Confidentiality issues in cancer registration have also been addressed by the North
American Association of Central Cancer Registries (NAACCR) and the International
Association of Cancer Registries (IACR).[33,38] The NAACCR standards, for example,
include standards for confidentiality and disclosure of data and confidentiality policies
and procedures relating to data collection and management.[38] These policies and procedures include the registry's responsibilities to protect its data from unauthorized access
and release, standards for policies and procedures for data security, and standards for policies and procedures for release of registry data. The IACR Guidelines on Confidentiality in
the Cancer Registry[33] explain how confidentiality safeguards protect the right to privacy.
Guidelines for the maintenance of confidentiality are needed primarily to provide adequate
safeguards for the individual's right to privacy, so that identifiable information on persons
registered with cancer does not reach unauthorized third parties, while at the same time
preserving the right of the individual, and that of other community members, to benefit

from the knowledge on cancer causation, prevention, treatment, and survival that can be obtained from cancer registration and research.

▓ SUMMARY

Cancer epidemiologic studies are needed to address the more than 70% of all cancer deaths worldwide that occur in low- and middle-income countries and to help alleviate human suffering.[7] Due to increases in cancer deaths associated with cigarette smoking and obesity, and declines in deaths from infectious diseases, the cancer burden is growing in many poorer countries. Designing and conducting such studies will require careful attention to the rights and welfare of the persons who are included in the studies. Potential stakeholders in international health research include research participants, community representatives, researchers, activists, international agencies, governments, nongovernmental organizations, and sponsors. In international studies on cancer epidemiology, it is desirable for IRB or research ethics committee review to occur both in the country from which the researchers or funding agency are from and in the host country. Collaborative research with researchers or institutions from the host country and studies employing community advisory boards are also more likely to take into account local perspectives, values, and concerns. Researchers and communities are increasingly working together to define new approaches for collaboration and to facilitate important research studies, while at the same time being responsive to community needs and priorities. Community advisory boards with representatives from the target community are likely to facilitate many types of health research including those aimed at understanding cancer etiology or prevention.

▓ ACKNOWLEDGMENTS

The findings and conclusions in this article are those of the author and do not necessarily represent the official position of the Department of Veterans Affairs.

▓ REFERENCES

1. Council for International Organizations of Medical Sciences (CIOMS), World Health Organization. International ethical guidelines for epidemiological studies. Geneva: CIOMS. 2009.
2. Nuffield Council on Bioethics. *The ethics of research related to healthcare in developing countries.* London: Nuffield Council on Bioethics; 2002.
3. World Medical Association. Declaration of Helsinki, ethical principles for medical research involving human subjects, 6th revision. Seoul: World Medical Organization. 2008.
4. Holm S, Harris J. The standard of care in multinational research. In: Emanuel EJ, Grady C, Crouch RA, Lie RK, Miller FG, Wendler DD, eds. *The oxford textbook of clinical research ethics.* New York: Oxford University Press; 2008.
5. Sankaranarayanan R, Boffetta P. Research on cancer prevention, detection and management in low- and medium-income countries. *Ann Oncol.* 2010;21(10):1935–1943.
6. Ngoma T. World health organization cancer priorities in developing countries. *Ann Oncol.* 2006;17 Suppl 8:viii9–viii14.
7. Coughlin SS, Ekwueme DU. Breast cancer as a global health concern. *Cancer Epidemiol.* 2009;33(5): 315–318.
8. Coughlin SS, American Public Health Association. *Ethics in epidemiology and public health practice: Collected works.* Washington, DC: American Public Health Association; 2009.
9. Porter JDH, Stephens C, Kessel A. Ethical issues in international health research and epidemiology. In: Coughlin SS, Beauchamp TL, Weed DL, eds. *Ethics and epidemiology.* New York: Oxford University Press; 2009:227–244.

10. Lee LM. Public health ethics theory: Review and path to convergence. *J Law Med Ethics*. 2012; 40(1):85–98.

11. Anand S, Peter F, Sen A. Public health, ethics and equity. New York: Oxford University Press. 2004.

12. UNAIDS. Creating effective partnerships for HIV prevention trials: Report of a UNAIDS consultation, Geneva 20–21 June 2005. *AIDS*. 2006;20(6):W1–W11.

13. Lilienfeld AM, Lilienfeld DE. *Foundations of epidemiology, 2nd edition*. New York: Oxford University Press; 1980.

14. American college of epidemiology ethics guidelines. *Ann Epidemiol*. 2000;10(8):487–497.

15. Beauchamp TL, Cook RR, Fayerweather WE, et al. Ethical guidelines for epidemiologists. *J Clin Epidemiol*. 1991;44 Suppl 1:151S–169S.

16. Soskolne CL, Light A. Towards ethics guidelines for environmental epidemiologists. *Sci Total Environ*. 1996;184(1–2):137–147.

17. Glanz K, Rimer BK, Lerman C. Ethical issues in the design and conduct of community-based intervention studies. In: Coughlin SS, Beauchamp TL, Weed DL, eds. *Ethics and epidemiology*. New York: Oxford University Press; 2009:103–127.

18. Coughlin S. Ethically optimized study design in epidemiology. In: Coughlin SS, Beauchamp TL, eds. *Ethics and epidemiology*. New York: Oxford University Press; 1996:145, 155 p.

19. Participants in the 2006 Georgetown University Workshop on the Ancillary-Care Obligations of Medical Researchers Working in Developing Countries. The ancillary-care obligations of medical researchers working in developing countries. *PLoS Med*. 2008;5(5):e90.

20. Seigel D. Clinical trials, epidemiology, and public confidence. *Stat Med*. 2003;22(21):3419–3425.

21. AAMC Task Force on Financial Conflicts of Interest in Clinical Research. Protecting subjects, preserving trust, promoting progress II: Principles and recommendations for oversight of an institution's financial interests in human subjects research. *Acad Med*. 2003;78(2):237–245.

22. London AJ. Responsiveness to host community health needs. In: Emanuel EJ, Grady C, Crouch RA, Lie RK, Miller FG, Wendler DD, eds. *The oxford textbook of clinical research ethics*. New York: Oxford University Press; 2008:737–745.

23. Marshall PA. Public health research and practice in international settings: Special ethical concerns. In: Jennings B, Kahn J, Mastroianni A, Parker LS, eds. *Ethics and public health: Model curriculum*. Association of Schools of Public Health; 2003:85–96.

24. Beauchamp TL. Moral foundation. In: Coughlin SS, Beauchamp TL, Weed DL, eds. *Ethics and epidemiology*. New York: Oxford University Press; 2009:22, 52 p.

25. Leikin S. Ethical issues in epidemiologic research with children. In: Coughlin SS, Beauchamp TL, eds. *Ethics and epidemiology*. New York: Oxford University Press; 1996:199, 218 p.

26. Ramsey P. Children as research subjects: A reply. *Hastings Cent Rep*. 1977;7(2):40–42.

27. Macklin R. *Against relativism: Cultural diversity and the search for ethical universals in medicine*. New York: Oxford University Press; 1999:xii, 290 p.

28. Gostin LO. Health information: Reconciling personal privacy with the public good of human health. *Health Care Anal*. 2001;9(3):321–335.

29. Fairchild AL, Bayer R. Public health. ethics and the conduct of public health surveillance. *Science*. 2004;303(5658):631–632.

30. Snider DE, Jr, Stroup DF. Defining research when it comes to public health. *Public Health Rep*. 1997; 112(1):29–32.

31. Thacker SB, Berkelman RL. Public health surveillance in the United States. *Epidemiol Rev*. 1988; 10:164–190.

32. Wetterhall SF, Pappaioanou M, Thacker SB, Eaker E, Churchill RE, Centers for Disease Control (CDC). The role of public health surveillance: Information for effective action in public health. *MMWR Morb Mortal Wkly Rep*. 1992;41 Suppl:207–218.

33. Coleman MP, Muir CS, Menegoz F. Confidentiality in the cancer registry. *Br J Cancer*. 1992; 66(6):1138–1149.

34. Chen VW. The right to know vs. the right to privacy. *J Registry Management*. 1997;125:7.

35. Stiller CA. Cancer registration: Its uses in research, and confidentiality in the EC. *J Epidemiol Community Health*. 1993;47(5):342–344.
36. Muir CS, Demaret E. Cancer registration: Legal aspects and confidentiality. In: Jensen OM, Parkin DM, MacLennan R, Muir CS, Skeet RG, eds. *Cancer registration: Principles and methods*. Lyon, France: IARC Scientific Publications; 1991:199–207.
37. Coughlin S, Clutter GG, Hutton M. Ethics in cancer registries. *J Registry Management*. 1999; 26(1):5–10.
38. Seiffert JE, ed. *Standards for cancer registries, vol. 3: Standards for completeness, quality, analysis, and management of data*. NP: North American Association of Central Cancer Registries; 1994.

2

Methodological Principles in Conducting International Studies

CASE-CONTROL STUDIES OF CANCER IN LOW- AND MIDDLE-INCOME COUNTRIES: OPPORTUNITIES AND CHALLENGES

FARIN KAMANGAR,
KYLE ESDAILLE, FARHAD ISLAMI

INTRODUCTION

Retrospective case-control studies conducted in low- and middle-income countries (LMIC) have played a major role in identifying or establishing causes of cancer. Notable examples include identification of carcinogens that are highly common in geographic areas within LMIC, such as the liver fluke *Opisthorchis viverrini*, a main cause of cholangiocarcinoma in Thailand, or bidi, a tobacco product that is known to cause oropharyngeal cancers in India. More broadly, etiologic factors for nearly all cancers have been studied in LMIC. A PubMed search of "case-control AND Cancer AND China" in December 4, 2011, resulted in 3018 entries. Adding Brazil, Egypt, India, Iran, and Thailand to the list resulted in 4650 entries. While not all of these entries necessarily reflect case-control studies of cancer and there may be several publications from individual case-control studies, the search results indicate substantial numbers of case-control studies of cancer conducted in LMIC. Such studies have generated new hypotheses, established important associations, led to the identification of new etiologic factors, established consistency of association across populations, or have provided clues to effect modification.

In this chapter, we (1) review several salient examples of cancer causes initially discovered, or later established, through case-control studies in LMIC; (2) highlight some potential opportunities for further cancer research using case-control studies in these countries; (3) discuss some scientific advantages and unique opportunities for conducting case-control studies in LMIC; (4) discuss the potential challenges of conducting case-control studies in LMIC; and (5) discuss some important methodologic and design issues, as well as practical considerations for such studies.

▨ EXAMPLES OF PREVIOUS CONTRIBUTIONS TO CANCER EPIDEMIOLOGY

As mentioned previously, many examples of excellent and important studies in LMIC can be found. We offer a few in Table 8.1. Some of these associations, such as that of Epstein-Barr Virus and Burkitt's lymphoma, were initially accepted through studying case-series, rather than conducting case-control studies. When odds ratios are quite high, one might conclude an association exists, even in the absence of a formal control group. However, case-control studies further formalize the association and are able to provide a quantitative estimate of the odds ratio.

Bidi: Several case-control studies in India have established bidi, a tobacco product chiefly made in India, as an important risk factor for oropharyngeal cancers.[1-4] A meta-analysis of epidemiologic studies has shown a three-fold increased risk of oral cancers in bidi smokers.

Cantonese-style salted fish: Case-control studies in China have strongly contributed to the recognition of Cantonese-style salted fish as a risk factor for nasopharyngeal cancers.[5-8]

Maté: Case-control studies in Brazil, Argentina, Uruguay, and Paraguay have provided strong evidence for a three-fold increased risk of esophageal squamous cell carcinoma associated with drinking maté.[9-13] Possible reasons include high temperature of these drinks that can cause epithelial damage or their high content of carcinogenic polycyclic aromatic hydrocarbons.[14]

Epstein-Barr virus: Case-control studies in China and other East-Asian countries have shown a strong association between EBV and nasopharyngeal cancers.[15-17]

Opium use: Several case-control studies in Iran have shown an increased risk of cancers of the esophagus,[18,19] larynx,[20] and bladder.[21] An increased risk of cancer due to chronic opium use has now been confirmed in a large cohort study.[22]

Cigarette smoking: There are a number of case-control studies in LMIC that have shown the association between cigarette smoking and many cancer types. As an example, data from eight case-control studies conducted in eight countries, including Thailand, Philippines, Morocco, Brazil, Peru, Paraguay, Colombia, and Spain, nearly all considered LMIC, showed an approximate two-fold increased risk of cervical cancer in HPV-positive women who smoke cigarettes.[23]

Liver flukes: Studies in Thailand have shown liver flukes, such as *Opisthorchis viverrini*, to be strong risk factors for cholangiocarcinomas of the biliary tract.[24,25] Northern Thailand,

TABLE 8.1 Examples of carcinogenic factors identified with the aid of case-control studies in LMIC

CARCINOGENIC FACTOR	CANCER SITE
Bidi	Oral cavity and pharynx
Cantonese-style salted fish	Nasopharynx
Maté	Esophagus (squamous cell carcinoma)
Opium	Multiple organs
Ebstein-Barr virus	Nasopharynx
Tobacco smoking	Cervix (in HPV-positive women)
Opisthorchis viverrini and *Clonorchis sinensis*	Cholangiocarcinoma

where infestation with *O. viverrini* is endemic, is a high-risk area for cholangiocarcinoma. *Chlonorcis Cinesis* is another liver fluke shown in case-control studies to be associated with cholangiocarcinoma.[26]

▓ FUTURE RESEARCH OPPORTUNITIES

There is little doubt that case-control studies in LMIC will continue to elucidate more causes of cancer in the future. Better economic prospects in countries like China and India, which has led to availability of more funds for research, easier access to information via internet, and increasing numbers of students from LMIC that study epidemiology either in high-income countries or in their own native country, all indicate that the number of epidemiologic studies, including case-control studies, will increase in the future. Next we mention two examples of studies that can be done in the future.

The cost of full-genome sequencing is declining sharply, and it is anticipated to be less than $1000 by the year 2015.[27] Low-cost genome sequencing may be able to identify rare somatic mutations that are strongly associated with risk of cancer. Since such mutations are rare, studies may need large numbers of cases and controls to identify such mutations. LMIC, where the majority of the population of the world live, could provide many such cases and controls. Large sequencing facilities are already established in countries such as China.

Certain areas of Iran and China have very high rates of esophageal squamous cell carcinoma, the reasons for which are largely unknown.[28] It is possible that a yet unknown strong risk factor be responsible for such rates.[29] If so, small case-control studies are the most effective way to find such a risk factor. Studies with 60 cases and 60 controls have over 90% power to detect carcinogens that are present in 20% of controls and 50% of cases (odds ratio = 4). If one study does not find the risk factor, given the small sample size and low cost, one can quickly examine other exposures.

▓ SCIENTIFIC ADVANTAGES AND UNIQUE OPPORTUNITIES

There are multiple scientific reasons that case-control studies in LMIC can play a unique role in studying causes of cancer. As detailed next, these include higher prevalence of certain exposures, higher prevalence of some cancers, assessment of consistency of association and effect modification, potentials for higher internal validity and higher response rate, and increasing sample size via conducting multicenter studies (Table 8.2).

Some exposures are much more common in LMIC than in high-income countries, thus making studies of these exposures in relation to cancer feasible. For example, opium consumption is very common in certain areas of Afghanistan and Iran, thus allowing for studies of this exposure in relation to cancer.[18,19,30] Other highly common exposures of this nature include infestation with *S. hematobium, O. viverrini,* or *C. cinesis,* exposure to aflatoxin, drinking maté, smoking bidi, smoking a hookah, chewing of nass and betel quid, local and regional diets, and genetic polymorphisms that are common in certain ethnic groups.

Another reason to conduct case-control studies in LMIC is higher prevalence or different epidemiologic patterns of cancers in such countries. For example, incidence rates of esophageal squamous cell carcinoma are extremely high in Linxian, China, and Golestan Province of Iran.[31,32] Likewise, studying liver cancer in certain areas of China and cervical cancer in many LMIC is of interest.

Investigating consistency of association or effect modification can be an important motivation for doing case-control studies in LMIC. Consistency, as in the case of HPV 16

TABLE 8.2 Some potential advantages of and challenges for conducting cancer case-control studies in LMIC

ADVANTAGES

More extensive exposures or higher prevalence of exposures to some carcinogens

Higher prevalence or different epidemiologic patterns of some cancers

Investigating consistency of association or effect modification identified in developed countries

Potential increase in the range (heterogeneity) of exposure of interest in multicenter studies

Potentially higher homogeneity in other exposures, including confounding factors

Potentially higher response rates

Increase in sample size and power in pooled analyses

Lower cost

Potentially lower bureaucratic hurdles when efficient collaborators are involved

CHALLENGES

Finding the right collaborator and well-trained personnel

Political instability, wars, revolutions, and domestic strife

Availability of required infrastructure and facilities

Accurate translation of the study protocol and questionnaire (when they are designed in another language)

Transfer of biological samples

Finding the appropriate controls (in particular when cases come from a large geographic area due to scarcity of cancer treatment centers)

and cervical cancer, is reassuring.[33] By contrast, differences in results, if due to effect modification, might lead to new lines of research. For example, in most western countries, a large fraction of esophageal squamous cell carcinomas are attributed to tobacco smoking and alcohol consumption, but these two risk factors have a relatively low importance in high-risk areas of China and Iran.[19,34] Also, in western countries esophageal squamous cell carcinomas incidence rates are approximately three-fold higher in men than in women, but rates are similar for men and women in high-risk areas of China and Iran.[35] These differences make studying esophageal squamous cell carcinomas in China and Iran very intriguing.

Sometimes case-control studies in LMIC are preferred because of homogeneity of population, which may lead to higher internal validity of results. For example, if we study the role of a virus that infects 20–80% of the rural population of a Chinese Province, there is enough heterogeneity of exposure to study the virus, yet other factors in the population, such as diet and cultural practice, may be more homogeneous than what is seen in Europe.

There are usually higher response rates in case-control studies in LMIC, especially in remote areas, because people of these areas are less exposed to research and thus are not saturated with requests for participation in research. For example, in case-control studies conducted on risk factors of Esophageal Squamous Cell Carcinoma in Iran, nearly all cases and the large majority of the randomly selected controls agreed to participate.[19] However, to ensure a high response rate, one needs to obtain support from local leadership, ask culturally appropriate questions, and avoid culturally unpleasant procedures.

Another motivation for conducting case-control studies in LMIC is to increase sample size and power by performing combined analysis of data. Such studies may also help in increasing range of exposure, when there are differences in range of exposure across countries. In collaboration with local research teams, International Agency for Research on Cancer has conducted a number of such multinational studies in LMIC. Examples include smoking and cervical cancer,[23] HPV and cervical cancer,[33] HPV and oral cancer,[36] and maté and esophageal cancer.[9]

▦ POTENTIAL LOGISTICAL ADVANTAGES

When it comes to logistical issues, it is usually easier to conduct studies in high-income countries, as there are more funds, better infrastructure, and more people trained to conduct research. However, there may be some potential logistical advantages to conducting case-control studies in LMIC too.

One important advantage of conducting case-control studies in LMIC is lower cost of conducting studies. This could be of substantial benefit if the studies are multinational and the study is partly funded by high-income countries.

Another advantage could be lower bureaucratic hurdles when the right person is leading the studies. It is our experience, and the experience of most of our colleagues, that in general there are more hurdles and more bureaucracy in LMIC; however, with the right collaborators in these countries, there is a potential for moving the projects even faster than in high-income countries. This is to some extent because many regulations are left vague in low-income countries and, depending on the leader or collaborator, this may result in a fast pace of developing the study, or a very slow one.

▦ CHALLENGES

Perhaps the most important challenge of conducting case-control studies in LMIC, especially in low-income countries, is finding well-trained personnel who understand the logic of epidemiologic case-control studies, are able to translate questionnaires and ask questions in appropriate ways, understand the methods of handling biological samples, are able to conduct data entry and keep electronic files, and are able to communicate well and share data appropriately. Such problems arise in part because research training is less of a priority in low-income countries; many of those who are well-trained migrate to higher-income countries; and those who choose to stay in their native country often live in more privileged, large urban areas, not in the remote research fields.

Political instability, wars, revolutions, and domestic strife are potential threats to successful conduct and completion of studies, particularly in low-income countries and when the recruitment of cases may take a long time. For example, the 1979 revolution of Iran precluded scientists from completing case-control studies of opium use and esophageal cancer.[18]

Another major challenge, particularly in remote areas of low-income countries, is availability of infrastructure and facilities. For example, one needs to make sure that there is a stable power supply if biological samples are to be collected and stored in the field and that there are enough −70°C freezers when needed.

If questionnaires are designed by scientists from other countries, ensuring that translations are done accurately is important.

Transfer of biological samples, particularly DNA, to other countries has sometimes been an issue for some countries, including India and China. However, such problems, often politically motivated, can be avoided by having the right collaborators and obtaining the permissions in advance.

Two limitations of case-control studies in LMIC—control selection and biases in exposure assessment—merit special consideration and are discussed separately next.

▦ CONTROL SELECTION IN LMIC

Case-control studies are, in theory, more efficient versions of cohort studies. The idea is that from a theoretical cohort, we choose all or a representative sample of all cases and a random sample of all controls, usually one to four times as a many as cases. This way, we have nearly the same statistical efficiency as though we had studied an entire cohort but at a much lower cost. While this theoretical framework is realized in case-control studies nested within cohort studies, in retrospective case-control studies it is very difficult to find the appropriate base from which the cases have been selected, to randomly select the controls, and to obtain the required information from them. An excellent discussion of the principles of control selection, types of controls, and design options has been provided elsewhere,[37–39] so we will not elaborate on them there. However, selecting controls in LMIC may be particularly challenging.

In many low-resource countries, there are usually few centers that can treat cancer patients, usually in the capital city. Therefore, the study base may be the entire country. However, even a random sample of the country is often not comparable with cases, referrals depend on the wealth of the patients, their proximity to the referral center, age and sex of the patients (in some places men and younger individuals are more likely to seek treatment), and culture of the people (in some areas, they may accept death as the fate of the disease and never go to the center). In other instances, the referral base is even less clear. For example, due to high incidence of the esophageal cancer in Linxian, China, there are centers in the area that specialize in surgery of esophageal cancer. Patients from several neighboring provinces refer to those centers, and it becomes extremely difficult to obtain a clear sense of the base.

Epidemiologists conducting case-control studies in LMIC have used a variety of approaches to select controls, including both hospital-based controls[40–42] and population-based controls.[4,43,44] Where there is a chance to define the base population and enroll all or random sample of cases arising from this base population, it is preferred to enroll population-based controls. Where this is not feasible, one might need to use clinic-based or hospital-based controls, selected from diseases that are not expected to be associated with risk factors with the cancer studied.[37–39]

▦ POTENTIAL BIASES AND MISCLASSIFICATION IN EXPOSURE DATA

Case-control studies are subject to several sources of bias and misclassification of exposure data. Reporting bias (including recall bias) and interviewer bias are all among the potential biases. Also nondifferential misclassification due to random errors in recall or poor record keeping is possible.

Some of these problems may be more pronounced in some ways in LMIC. Because of a lack of resources, it is more likely that patient records have been kept poorly in low-resource countries. In these countries, people are less likely to report on exposures that are forbidden by law, culture, or religion. This is partly because keeping confidentiality of the results may be more difficult. For case-control studies, if case data are collected by the physician but the control data are collected by others who travel to the neighborhood of case patients, there may be a bias in data collection.

■ ISSUES TO CONSIDER WHEN CONDUCTING CASE-CONTROL STUDIES IN LMIC

Each study and each geographic location is unique. Low- and middle-income countries, while having some common features, vary substantially. Challenges in China, Iran, and Tanzania are not similar, and challenges one might face when conducting a study in Beijing may not be the same as those conducted in a remote area of China. However, based on our experience and that of others, there are some general rules that help. In particular, make sure

1. to find the right local study leader or collaborator, a person who knows how to navigate the system in his/her country; can obtain the confidence and support of the local leaders and local population; can communicate with multinational colleagues effectively; and is knowledgeable about elements of research.

2. that trained personnel are available who are capable of helping with design of the questionnaires, selection of controls, administering the questionnaires, collecting and handling the biological samples, entering data into databases, translating information, trouble-shooting for equipment when needed, analyzing data, and writing papers. It is important to train researchers about biases most commonly encountered in case-control studies, including interviewer bias and recall bias, and to make sure such biases are minimized. If such personnel are not available, training is a key issue.

3. to provide adequate incentives, such as opportunities for future education and higher salaries, and coauthorship in the resulting papers for the trained personnel to continue their work in their country.

4. that study procedures and questionnaires are acceptable to the local population. Extensive consultation with local political and religious leaders, local universities, and federal government would be very important.

5. to provide incentives for the population to enroll in the study, such as providing them with the results of their cholesterol or blood pressure. It is also important to maintain the relationship with people by disseminating some salient results of the study.

6. that there are ways to identify the base from which cases arise, and to find appropriate controls. It is also important that an acceptable proportion of all cases of disease enter the study. This is mostly done via obtaining the confidence of the people and that of local health providers. Providing incentives to local health providers may be of importance too.

7. that the minimum required facilities, such as power supply, freezers, and medical equipment, are available.

8. that when questionnaires are translated from another language, they are back-translated and compared with the original language.

9. that agreements are in place to transfer data and biological samples.

10. that when the study is conducted over a few years, the biological samples are stored in two locations. In the case of multinational studies, half may be transferred to another country, so that if one center loses the samples to domestic strife, loss of power, or other causes, the other centers retain the remaining samples.

11. that if the study is multinational, research teams meet, at least annually, and have regular conference calls. Such meetings encourage a faster pace of study, help in diagnosing and solving potential problems, and will help in minimizing misunderstandings.

12. that agreements are in place for sources of funding, design of the study, coauthorship, and publications.

■ RETROSPECTIVE CASE-CONTROL STUDIES VIS-À-VIS COHORT STUDIES IN LMIC

Conducting cohort studies in LMIC poses even a much larger challenge than conducting case-control studies in these countries. Contributing to these factors are low research budget in LMIC, which hampers funding the cohort over long periods of time; political instability, which may make follow-up difficult; and immigration of the trained personnel, which requires finding and training additional personnel. For these reasons, case-control studies have been done more frequently in LMIC, particularly in African countries, where political stability has been an issue.

Nevertheless, cohort studies have certain methodologic advantages such as a more clear population base and therefore better control selection, being less subject to recall bias and interviewer bias, and the ability to collect more accurate data that are less subject to misclassification. In addition, cohort studies could potentially study a large number of exposures and outcomes, could test several hypotheses, and subsequently result in many scientific publications. For these reasons, over the past 30 years, several cohort studies have been established in the more stable LMIC such as in China and Iran. Some of these cohorts were initially randomized trials, the subjects of which were later followed as a cohort. Such cohort studies have provided unique opportunities to study exposures in relation to overall mortality, cardiovascular diseases, and cancer. For a more detailed discussion of this subject, please see Chapter 9.

■ CONCLUSIONS

Case-control studies in low- and middle-income countries have helped us in discovering etiologic factors for cancers such as bidi, *O. viverrini*, and opium use. They have also helped in establishing consistency of associations, in increasing sample size, and in learning about effect modifications. Given the economic rise of many low- and middle-income countries, the number of case-control and other epidemiologic studies in these countries will likely increase in the future. Collaborations between high-income countries and LMIC are important in furthering our knowledge of epidemiology of cancer.

■ SUMMARY

Case-control studies in low- and middle-income countries (LMIC) have substantially contributed to our knowledge of causes of cancer. Some cancer risk factors found in these studies are bidi, maté, opium, Epstein-Barr virus, and *O. viverrini*. Such studies are likely to continue to further our knowledge of risk factors of cancer, particularly because many countries currently in LMIC, such as China and India, are economically on the rise and the number of scientists and facilities for doing research in these countries is increasing. Studying unique exposures and locally common cancers will continue. In addition, multinational partnerships are likely to increase in number to provide more powerful studies. This chapter provides a short overview of accomplishments of case-control studies in LMIC, highlights some potential opportunities for further cancer research using case-control studies in these countries, and discusses certain methodological and logistical considerations that increase the likelihood of successful completion of these studies.

■ REFERENCES

1. Sankaranarayanan R, Duffy SW, Padmakumary G, Day NE, Krishan Nair M. Risk factors for cancer of the buccal and labial mucosa in Kerala, southern India. *J Epidemiol Community Health*. 1990;44(4):286–292.

2. Sankaranarayanan R, Duffy SW, Padmakumary G, Day NE, Padmanabhan TK. Tobacco chewing, alcohol and nasal snuff in cancer of the gingiva in Kerala, India. *Br J Cancer.* 1989;60(4):638–643.

3. Sankaranarayanan R, Duffy SW, Day NE, Nair MK, Padmakumary G. A case-control investigation of cancer of the oral tongue and the floor of the mouth in southern India. *Int J Cancer.* 1989;44(4):617–621.

4. Dikshit RP, Kanhere S. Tobacco habits and risk of lung, oropharyngeal and oral cavity cancer: A population-based case-control study in Bhopal, India. *Int J Epidemiol.* 2000;29(4):609–614.

5. Jia WH, Luo XY, Feng BJ, et al. Traditional Cantonese diet and nasopharyngeal carcinoma risk: A large-scale case-control study in Guangdong, China. *BMC Cancer.* 2010;10:446.

6. Yu MC. Nasopharyngeal carcinoma: Epidemiology and dietary factors. *IARC Sci Publ.* 1991;(105)(105):39–47.

7. Yu MC, Ho JH, Lai SH, Henderson BE. Cantonese-style salted fish as a cause of nasopharyngeal carcinoma: Report of a case-control study in Hong Kong. *Cancer Res.* 1986;46(2):956–961.

8. Yuan JM, Wang XL, Xiang YB, Gao YT, Ross RK, Yu MC. Preserved foods in relation to risk of nasopharyngeal carcinoma in Shanghai, China. *Int J Cancer.* 2000;85(3):358–363.

9. Castellsague X, Munoz N, De Stefani E, Victora CG, Castelletto R, Rolon PA. Influence of mate drinking, hot beverages and diet on esophageal cancer risk in South America. *Int J Cancer.* 2000;88(4):658–664.

10. De Stefani E, Munoz N, Esteve J, Vasallo A, Victora CG, Teuchmann S. Mate drinking, alcohol, tobacco, diet, and esophageal cancer in Uruguay. *Cancer Res.* 1990;50(2):426–431.

11. De Stefani E, Fierro L, Mendilaharsu M, et al. Meat intake, "mate" drinking and renal cell cancer in Uruguay: A case-control study. *Br J Cancer.* 1998;78(9):1239–1243.

12. Pintos J, Franco EL, Oliveira BV, Kowalski LP, Curado MP, Dewar R. Mate, coffee, and tea consumption and risk of cancers of the upper aerodigestive tract in southern Brazil. *Epidemiology.* 1994;5(6):583–590.

13. Rolon PA, Castellsague X, Benz M, Munoz N. Hot and cold mate drinking and esophageal cancer in Paraguay. *Cancer Epidemiol Biomarkers Prev.* 1995;4(6):595–605.

14. Kamangar F, Schantz MM, Abnet CC, Fagundes RB, Dawsey SM. High levels of carcinogenic polycyclic aromatic hydrocarbons in mate drinks. *Cancer Epidemiol Biomarkers Prev.* 2008;17(5):1262–1268.

15. Mutalima N, Molyneux E, Jaffe H, et al. Associations between Burkitt lymphoma among children in Malawi and infection with HIV, EBV and malaria: Results from a case-control study. *PLoS One.* 2008;3(6):e2505.

16. Carpenter LM, Newton R, Casabonne D, et al. Antibodies against malaria and Epstein—Barr virus in childhood burkitt lymphoma: A case-control study in Uganda. *Int J Cancer.* 2008;122(6):1319–1323.

17. Parkin DM, Garcia-Giannoli H, Raphael M, et al. Non-Hodgkin lymphoma in Uganda: A case-control study. *AIDS.* 2000;14(18):2929–2936.

18. Ghadirian P, Stein GF, Gorodetzky C, et al. Oesophageal cancer studies in the Caspian littoral of Iran: Some residual results, including opium use as a risk factor. *Int J Cancer.* 1985;35(5):593–597.

19. Nasrollahzadeh D, Kamangar F, Aghcheli K, et al. Opium, tobacco, and alcohol use in relation to oesophageal squamous cell carcinoma in a high-risk area of Iran. *Br J Cancer.* 2008;98(11):1857–1863.

20. Mousavi MR, Damghani MA, Haghdoust AA, Khamesipour A. Opium and risk of laryngeal cancer. *Laryngoscope.* 2003;113(11):1939–1943.

21. Hosseini SY, Safarinejad MR, Amini E, Hooshyar H. Opium consumption and risk of bladder cancer: A case-control analysis. *Urol Oncol.* 2010;28(6):610–616.

22. Khademi H, Malekzadeh R, Pourshams A, et al. Opium use and mortality in golestan cohort study: Prospective cohort study of 50,000 adults in Iran. *BMJ.* 2012;344:e2502.

23. Plummer M, Herrero R, Franceschi S, et al. Smoking and cervical cancer: Pooled analysis of the IARC multi-centric case—control study. *Cancer Causes Control.* 2003;14(9):805–814.

24. Parkin DM, Srivatanakul P, Khlat M, et al. Liver cancer in Thailand. I. A case-control study of cholangiocarcinoma. *Int J Cancer.* 1991;48(3):323–328.

25. Itoh M, Pairojkul C, Thamawit W, et al. Association of antibodies to opisthorchis viverrini with hepatobiliary disease in northeastern Thailand. *Am J Trop Med Hyg.* 1994;51(4):424–429.

26. Choi D, Lim JH, Lee KT, et al. Cholangiocarcinoma and clonorchis sinensis infection: A case-control study in Korea. *J Hepatol.* 2006;44(6):1066–1073.

27. Church GM. Genomes for all. *Sci Am*. 2006;294(1):46.

28. Kamangar F, Chow WH, Abnet CC, Dawsey SM. Environmental causes of esophageal cancer. *Gastroenterol Clin North Am*. 2009;38(1):27–57, vii.

29. Kamangar F, Malekzadeh R, Dawsey SM, Saidi F. Esophageal cancer in northeastern Iran: A review. *Arch Iran Med*. 2007;10(1):70–82.

30. Aliasgari MA, Kaviani A, Gachkar L, Hosseini-Nassab SR. Is bladder cancer more common among opium addicts? *Urol J*. 2004;1(4):253–255.

31. Ke L. Mortality and incidence trends from esophagus cancer in selected geographic areas of China circa 1970–90. *Int J Cancer*. 2002;102(3):271–274.

32. Mahboubi E, Kmet J, Cook PJ, Day NE, Ghadirian P, Salmasizadeh S. Oesophageal cancer studies in the Caspian littoral of Iran: The Caspian cancer registry. *Br J Cancer*. 1973;28(3):197–214.

33. Muñoz N, Bosch FX, de Sanjosé S, et al. Epidemiologic classification of human papillomavirus types associated with cervical cancer. *N Engl J Med*. 2003;348(6):518.

34. Tran GD, Sun XD, Abnet CC, et al. Prospective study of risk factors for esophageal and gastric cancers in the linxian general population trial cohort in China. *Int J Cancer*. 2005;113(3):456–463.

35. Islami F, Kamangar F, Aghcheli K, et al. Epidemiologic features of upper gastrointestinal tract cancers in northeastern Iran. *Br J Cancer*. 2004;90(7):1402–1406.

36. Herrero R, Castellsague X, Pawlita M, et al. Human papillomavirus and oral cancer: The international agency for research on cancer multicenter study. *J Natl Cancer Inst*. 2003;95(23):1772–1783.

37. Wacholder S, McLaughlin JK, Silverman DT, Mandel JS. Selection of controls in case-control studies. I. principles. *Am J Epidemiol*. 1992;135(9):1019–1028.

38. Wacholder S, Silverman DT, McLaughlin JK, Mandel JS. Selection of controls in case-control studies. III. design options. *Am J Epidemiol*. 1992;135(9):1042–1050.

39. Wacholder S, Silverman DT, McLaughlin JK, Mandel JS. Selection of controls in case-control studies. II. types of controls. *Am J Epidemiol*. 1992;135(9):1029–1041.

40. De Stefani E, Correa P, Oreggia F, et al. Black tobacco, wine and mate in oropharyngeal cancer. A case-control study from Uruguay. *Rev Epidemiol Sante Publique*. 1988;36(6):389–394.

41. Szymanska K, Matos E, Hung RJ, et al. Drinking of mate and the risk of cancers of the upper aerodigestive tract in Latin America: A case-control study. *Cancer Causes Control*. 2010;21(11):1799–1806.

42. Zaridze D, Borisova E, Maximovitch D, Chkhikvadze V. Alcohol consumption, smoking and risk of gastric cancer: Case-control study from Moscow, Russia. *Cancer Causes Control*. 2000;11(4):363–371.

43. Sun X, Chen W, Chen Z, Wen D, Zhao D, He Y. Population-based case-control study on risk factors for esophageal cancer in five high-risk areas in China. *Asian Pac J Cancer Prev*. 2010;11(6):1631–1636.

44. Abnet CC, Kamangar F, Islami F, et al. Tooth loss and lack of regular oral hygiene are associated with higher risk of esophageal squamous cell carcinoma. *Cancer Epidemiol Biomarkers Prev*. 2008;17(11):3062–3068.

COHORT STUDIES IN LOW- AND MIDDLE-INCOME COUNTRIES

STEPHANIE MELKONIAN, YU CHEN, HABIBUL AHSAN

INTRODUCTION TO COHORT STUDIES

In a cohort study concerned with ascertaining disease etiology, investigators begin by identifying a group, or cohort, of apparently healthy individuals free of the disease outcome of interest.[1] This cohort is divided into subjects that are either exposed or unexposed to the potential risk factor of interest. These individuals are then followed over time and observed for the incidence of disease or mortality in relation to exposure status as well as other measured risk factors and lifestyle, behavioral or personal characteristics.

While case-control studies are often preferred for investigating rare outcomes, such as cancer, cohort studies have several advantages and are often considered the "gold standard" for observational epidemiologic research, in the absence of a feasible randomized design. Cohort studies can be utilized prospective analysis of associations between predictors and outcomes and a more thorough collection of information regarding a participant's exposure status. Prospective data collection on information on exposure, potential confounders, and effect-modifiers reduces the likelihood of misclassification of these factors dependent on the outcomes, since the collection is done prior to the disease occurrence, allowing more reliable data management and quality control.[2] Cohort studies are useful in that they allow for the simultaneous observation of multiple outcomes related to the exposure in question. Finally, associations derived from cohort studies demonstrate the appropriate temporal sequence between the exposure and the outcome.[3] Therefore, while determining causality remains difficult within the context of observational research, establishing temporality provides investigators with one of the hallmark characteristics of causality between an exposure and an outcome.

Despite its numerous advantages, however, cohort study designs have various drawbacks. As previously stated, cohort studies are often not appropriate or feasible for the study of rare outcomes, as large sample sizes are required for sufficient statistical power. The prospective analysis of large samples requires a great deal of time and allocation of monetary resources. Researchers must also take into consideration that the efficacy of cohort studies is generally maximized when the time between exposure and disease manifestation is relatively short.

In addition to logistical concerns regarding the execution of a cohort analysis, researchers must also consider the various opportunities for bias within the context of a cohort design. First, as with any observational study, researchers must be careful to take into account possible confounders of the relationship between the risk factor and outcome of interest. Often these confounders take the form of unmeasured variables. It is likely that in the process of data collection via, for example, questionnaires, physical measurements or laboratory methods, that the investigator does not take into account a variable (whether it is environmental, occupational or genetic) that is related to the exposure or the outcome.[4] This can lead the investigator to a biased conclusion regarding the association between the predictor and outcome.

Researchers must also be concerned with the effects of nonparticipation and loss to follow-up. It is possible that those individuals that were ineligible to participate, or are lost to follow-up over the course of the study period, are in some ways systematically different than participants in the study population. If this is the case, then the results may not be generalizable to other populations. If the loss to follow-up is related to both the exposure and the disease of interest, biases could be introduced that may further affect internal validity of the study.

The advantages and disadvantages of the cohort study design may be altered given its context. International settings provide both unique challenges and opportunities for conducting observational studies in epidemiology. The following sections will discuss various aspects of cohort studies and their utility and challenges within the context of developing nations.

Utility of Cohort Studies In Low- and Middle-Income Countries

There are several unique advantages and disadvantages to conducting cohort studies in low- and middle-income countries. Several of the obstacles facing researchers, such as high cost, difficulties in patient follow-up and inability to control for genetic heterogeneity can be addressed by conducting cohort studies internationally. Developing countries often present unique opportunities to study influences of distinctive risk factors on diseases outcomes that otherwise cannot be investigated in other populations.

Cost Efficiency

One of the primary disadvantages of a traditional cohort study is the high cost associated with compiling a sufficiently large cohort for observation, and subsequently the cost attributed to repeated follow-ups and retention of study subjects over the duration of the study period[5]. The cost of a cohort study can easily be in the millions of dollars, significantly limiting their feasibility. This limitation is particularly true in cases where the outcome is of low disease incidence. Outcomes like cancer occur in only a small proportion of the entire population; therefore researchers may still not be able to derive stable estimates of incidence based on this data due to insufficient numbers of cases. Like cohort studies in developed countries, challenges remain in following individuals over an extended period of time and capturing truly incident cases of disease. Despite these limitations, cohort studies of cancer in developing countries often provide unique settings in exploring cancer etiology.

While outcomes like cancer are still relatively rare in low- and middle-income countries, international settings potentially provide a unique opportunity for conducting more efficient cohort studies. An investigator may choose a particular country or region in which to conduct a cohort study because it has a higher incidence of the disease or a higher prevalence of the exposure in question, allowing for a more efficient data collection on new cases of disease, and more stable estimates of disease incidence. Not only are costs reduced by more efficient data collection, but it is also likely that in low- and middle-income countries, costs associated with training study staff, assembling and maintaining the cohort and utilization of local resources may also be reduced when compared to more developed nations.[6] Costs associated with participant retention or follow-up may be lower due to a more stable population since, in low resource areas, study participants are less likely to be lost during follow-up due to movement out of the community and study area. Follow-up methods that use existing health care or insurance system may also reduce costs and loss to follow-up. For instance, Beasley et al followed more than 22,000 Chinese civil servants in Taiwan to study the relationship between hepatitis B virus and liver cancer. Using data from mandatory health and life insurance, loss to follow-up was minimized, with a complete record for detection of disease.[7] Low- and middle-income countries are also known to have unique exposures associated with disease outcomes that may not be found with the same prevalence in more developed countries. Finally, it is also likely that participation rates in developing countries will be higher, as often times the study provides the community with a convenient source of medical care that is generally lacking in remote areas.[8] For example, a recent study aimed at identifying the effects of cardiovascular risk factors on an occupational cohort within the Thai population, had response rates of over 95% in the first two rounds of follow-up. This is a considerably more favorable response than the approximately 70% response rate seen in the Framingham heart study, perhaps the most well known cohort study conducted in the United States.[9]

Unique Environmental, Occupational and Nutritional Risk Factors

Another advantage of cohort studies is the potential for expanding the range of risk factors being studied. Low- and middle-income countries have distinctive environmental and nutritional exposures that may be otherwise difficult to investigate. For example, it has been noted that several developing nations around the world, including India, Bangladesh, Taiwan, China, Mexico, Argentina and Chile have drinking water supplies naturally contaminated with levels of arsenic higher than the World Health Organization's national standard for those countries.[10-19] Understanding the association between arsenic and various health outcomes is made difficult due to low levels of arsenic contamination in most countries. Naturally occurring arsenic with a wide range of possible exposure values, such as those found in the developing nations listed above, allows for researchers to not only more accurately assess the relationship between arsenic exposure and various health outcomes, but also allows for the observation of a dose response relationship between exposure and outcome, if it exists.

The occupational range within developing nations is another unique opportunity for researchers. Low- and middle-income countries often have work environment that differs greatly in its content from more developed nations. For example, developing nations are more likely to have more individuals engaged in labor centric occupations including farmers, day laborers and factory workers. While these occupations exist in more developed nations, there are much higher proportions of individuals engaged in these activities in low- and middle-income countries. Individuals that comprise the population within these occupations have unique exposures to certain risk factors such as fertilizers, pesticides, chemical agents, excessive sun exposure and other hazardous materials and exposures that could potentially have large effects on rates of disease and mortality. One example of this is the exposure to endotoxins and its relation to lung cancer incidence. A study conducted in Shanghai China utilized approximately ten years of data between 1989 and 1998 from a large, well characterized cohort of 267,000 female textile workers. The results of this study suggests that long-term and high level exposure to endotoxin appears to actually reduce the risk of lung cancer, even taking into account smoking status.[20] A study of this size and with this amount of statistical power would be difficult to assemble in an area where there did not exist a high prevalence of female workers with exposure to this factor. With such a large female population working in the textile industry and concentrated to a relatively specific region, conducting this type of study within this cultural context was a highly efficient method for detecting an association between the factor in question and the disease outcome.

Nutritional and dietary patterns also vary greatly by country. Ecologic studies comparing disease rates in populations with the population per capita consumption of specific dietary factors has been an important way to study international variation in disease, and formulate hypotheses regarding the role of diet in disease incidence.[21] While these population level analyses provide only weak evidence for causation,[22] they do allow researchers to see international variation in dietary patterns and highlight areas potentially important for understanding the diet/disease association.

Accurately measuring exposure to dietary patterns has been difficult in epidemiologic research. Results are often impacted by the over or under reporting of exposure to, or consumption of, certain nutrients and food groups. However, in settings with limited access to processed foods, researchers may be able to measure dietary intakes more accurately with a better reliability, and to make links between certain dietary patterns and disease incidence. Conducting nutritional epidemiologic studies in low or middle income countries can provide researchers with specific advantages. Often religious or ethnic groups can have specific dietary patterns. Groups that consume an unusual or atypical diet provide the opportunity to more specifically study the association between diet and disease.

One example of this is the association between meat consumption and colorectal cancer incidence. Ecological studies have suggested high geographic variation in the link between higher per capita consumption of red meat and higher incidence of colorectal cancer. Studying this association, however, has been difficult due to inaccurate measures of dietary intake. In an attempt to control better for difficulties in accurately measuring meat consumption, several analyses have attempted to determine this relationship in vegetarian groups.[23] A collaborative analysis of five prospective studies of vegetarians in the United States, United Kingdom, and Germany used a combined series of 76,000 individuals to investigate the association between vegetarian diets and colorectal cancer incidence.[24] Unfortunately, a limitation of these studies is the inability for researchers to determine the accuracy with which individuals report abstinence from consumption of red meat. Therefore, if researchers conduct this study in an area with low levels of meat consumption generally (for example, an area with a large population of Hindus, who abstain from eating red meat), then they can benefit in two ways: (1) there can be more certainty regarding the accuracy of the data. If meat consumption is generally rare, there will be less variation in response and it will be more likely that individuals are correctly classified as individuals that abstain from consuming red meat and (2) they can sample a population that is otherwise rare.

Nutritional, environmental and occupational variation across countries is one avenue through which conducting cohort studies in low- and middle-income countries can contribute to discovering novel associations between risk factors and disease outcomes. However, another important consideration within the context of cohort studies in developing nations is their unique disease profiles.

Infectious Origins of Disease and the Epidemiologic Transition

The term "epidemiologic transition" signifies a shift in the paradigm of disease. Patterns in mortality transition from being high in infants and children to predominantly affecting the aging population. Infectious disease states, that previously impacted all age groups, give way to more degenerative and chronic diseases affecting the most elderly individuals in the population.[25] It is generally accepted that this transition is brought on by a phase of development marked by increases in the population growth rates caused by secular trends in development of medical technologies and innovation in disease treatment, therapy and preventions.[26] With a rapidly aging population, and minimal risk of infectious disease, a majority of epidemiologic research conducted in developed nations focuses on chronic diseases incidence and mortality and outcomes such as coronary heart disease, diabetes, and various cancers.

However, many developing nations are still in the midst of this transition. At any given time different countries, and perhaps even different regions in those countries, are at different states of this epidemiologic transition. This provides researchers an opportunity to study certain infectious causative agents that may no longer be feasibly investigated in more developed nations. Also, in the coming decades it is likely that the global burden of disease will change in several ways. Low- and middle-income countries will probably adopt a more western lifestyle; as a result it is likely that cancer and chronic disease patterns in these countries will begin to approximate those of more developed nations.[25] Investigators can take advantage of this transition by observing the change in disease profiles over time which can help clarify the role of environmental versus occupational versus genetic risk factors for disease. Recently, researchers have begun address the lack of data regarding noncommunicable diseases in low- and middle-income nations. A recent study examining the distribution of hyperglycemia and related cardiovascular disease risk factors in a population-based sample in Uganda described the prevalence of likely diabetes, hypertension, and obesity in a population previously not described in relation to these kinds of chronic risk factors.[27] Researchers suggest that the description of the transition from communicable to noncommunicable disease is critical particularly as mortality rates from communicable diseases decline and populations in these countries begin to age and become more susceptible to risk factors associated with chronic disease.[27]

Genetic Factors with Homogenous Ancestry

Determining an association in the context of a cohort study requires that certain conditions are met. Researchers must be able to select an unbiased, population based sample for their study, accurately assess their exposures and their outcomes, and thoroughly collect as much information as possible regarding other co-occurring risk factors that may modify or confound the relationship between the exposure and outcome of interest. As previously stated, an important source of potential bias in cohort studies is the difficulty in accounting for unmeasured or unobservable variables in the study population. Researchers cannot fully account for all potential confounders, however, and these unmeasured risk factors will impact study results. Recently, the importance of understanding individual disease susceptibility based on genetic variation has become an important factor to consider in epidemiologic research. In highly genetically heterogeneous populations, such as the United States, most observational epidemiologic studies cannot sufficiently take into account the interindividual variability due to genetic heterogeneity.

Consideration of genetic variability and its contribution to disease has become a more prominent issue in epidemiologic research.[28] Various studies attempt to take this into account by conducting genetic analysis on a limited sub cohort of their population. However, a more efficient way to control for unmeasured genetic variation is to select a population that is relatively genetically homogenous. In conducting a cohort study internationally, researchers have the opportunity to focus their analyses on a group of individuals that are not only exposed to similar lifestyle, dietary, environmental and occupational exposures, but also have a relatively stable genetic composition, in turn limiting the potential for unmeasured variation and bias due to population stratifications.[28]

Generalizability

Within the context of cohort studies, and generally within observational epidemiology, study validity is extremely important. There are two key types of validity, internal and external. Internal validity is the degree to which the observed association is accurate for the group of individuals being studied. In other words, it relates to the extent to which we can accurately state that the predictor, or risk factor, actually caused the observed outcome within our study population[1]. Internal validity is threatened by all sources of systematic errors, including selection biases, measurement errors dependent on exposure or disease status, unmeasured or measured confounding, all these may influence causal inference; the degree to which we can attribute the variation in disease to the variation in the risk factor in question.

However, individuals that utilize epidemiologic findings in real world settings, such as policy makers and public health officials, are often more concerned with the external validity, or generalizability, of the findings to the target population, or various populations across time.[29] Generalizability relies on a variety of factors including the consistency of study participant recruitment and selection processes, the representative nature of participant subjects and staff and consistency of implementation across time and settings. Naturally, a concern in observational research conducted internationally is the external validity of the findings. Are the results of this study conducted in one country, with its own exposure and risk factor profile, generalizable to another population? Unfortunately, generalizability across international populations is still a highly debated issue. The extent to which we can use results from one study to make decisions about policy in another country is not clear. However, replication of results in various settings will provide a more clear understanding of the generalizability and utility of study results. It should be noted that the focus on populations with more homogeneous risk factors for disease of interest should in general enhance the internal validity of the study. The purpose of most cohort studies is to study associations between exposure and disease rather than absolute rates of disease. If the internal validity of the study is maintained, then measures of association typically are unbiased and are generalizable even if the cohort is not a random sample of a defined underlying population.[2,5,24,29,30] For instance, the smoking-disease associations found in the British Doctors Study have shown to be generalizable to other populations.[31,32] Analyses of interaction among risk factors can be used to examine generalizability of associations across different subgroups within the study population.

Nested Case-Control and Case-Cohort Studies

For answering research questions from a cohort study requiring resource consuming laboratory assays or data collection/generation often more efficient study designs nested within the total cohort are applied. Two such efficient strategies include: nested case-control[1] and case-cohort designs.[1,33] Nested case-control studies utilize all (or some defined set of) cases in the cohort and a group of controls selected from the cohort who are matched to the cases on length of follow-up and optionally other covariates. In nested case-control studies, controls are selected concurrently as cases develop, and this sampling procedure is called incidence density sampling. By matching on the follow-up time between cases and controls, the ratio of exposed to unexposed number of controls represents, on average, the ratio of exposed to unexposed person-time for the total cohort. This allows the odds ratio derived from the nested case-control study to estimate the incidence rate ratio for the exposure-disease relationship in the full cohort. On the other hand, case-cohort studies utilize all (or some defined set of) cases in the cohort and a group of subjects randomly selected from the baseline cohort (subcohort) as controls. The subcohort (including those who develop disease) is representative of the total cohort, and case-cohort studies can be analyzed with appropriate weighting to estimate the rate ratio for the exposure-disease relationship in the total cohort. These studies have advantages in being efficient and cost effective compared to full cohort analyses as they use a fraction of the sample of the full cohort study. In addition, nested case-control and case-cohort studies preserve the prospective nature of a cohort study in maintaining the temporal relationship of exposure and disease as well as avoid recall and other biases affecting standard case-control studies.

Both study designs are often considered in modern molecular epidemiologic studies investigating biomarkers as exposure variables. In general, case-cohort design has the strength that the data on subcohort could be used for different case groups. In addition, the subcohort is representative of the overall cohort, and therefore the data can be used to study determinants of biomarkers that can be generalizable to the overall cohort. However, for the subcohort to be validly representative of the overall cohort, the number of subjects included should be substantial, usually including >10% of randomly selected subjects from the overall cohort. If batch effects, storage time, and freeze-thaw cycles are critical for the measurements of the biomarkers, careful planning to analyze subsets of subcohort and cases with some matching within the case-cohort studies will be needed[34]. An example of case-cohort study is studies on insulin, glucose, insulin resistance in relation to cancer in the Alpha-Tocopherol, Beta-Carotene Cancer Prevention (ATBC) Study, which included 29,133 male smokers in Finland. Investigators compared serum levels of insulin and glucose in incident cases of colorectal cancer,[35] pancreatic cancer,[36] and prostate cancer[37] with the levels in the same set of subcohort that included 400 randomly selected subjects. The data on subcohort were used repeatedly in the studies of different cancers. In the setting of developing countries, the choice for the study designs is particularly critical when the resources are limited. Investigators often would like to optimize study designs such that the same data can be used to investigate multiple research questions. In addition, the opportunity of assessing correlates or determinants of the biomarker is valuable as often it is the first time to study the biomarkers of interest in the population. For instance, in the Health Effects of Arsenic Longitudinal Study (HEALS), conducted in Bangladesh in order to determine the association between arsenic exposure in drinking water with health outcomes, investigators aimed to evaluate gene-environment interaction in cardiovascular disease (CVD) using a case-cohort study with CVD cases occurred in the overall cohort during the follow-up and a random 10% of the overall cohort as the subcohort. Genotyping on more than 300 single polymorphisms in 10 genes related to arsenic methylation, oxidative stress, and vascular inflammation was planned. Because the subcohort, consisting of about 1200 subjects, is representative of the overall cohort, investigators measured carotid intima media thickness using ultrasound system as an early sub-clinical marker for atherosclerosis for the subcohort. This way investigators can study gene-arsenic interaction in both clinical endpoints of CVD in the overall case-cohort study as well as gene-arsenic interaction in levels of atherosclerosis, indicated using IMT, in the subcohort. The genotyping data in the subcohort can be utilized cost-effectively for both purposes. In addition, the IMT data on subcohort can be used to study other risk factors of IMT in the population. A similar example can be seen in the Atherosclerosis Risk in Communities (ARIC) study, in which case-cohort studies were conducted to study associations of c-reactive protein with both stroke[38] and coronary heart disease.[39]

Nested case-control studies, on the other hand, often involve detailed matching between cases and controls on follow-up time and dates at sample collection as well as potential confounding factors such as age and sex. Cases and their matched controls are usually analyzed together to avoid batch effects. Further matching on sample storage time and freeze-thaw cycles can be easily incorporated in the selection of controls. These matching can often reduce substantial differential and nondifferential measurement errors and thus improve efficiency and validity of the study. In addition, in international consortia that combine cases from cohort studies, nested case-control study is often preferred. This is especially true when the outcome of interest is rare, and the number of cohorts involved in the pooling project is large. Because each cohort contributes only some cases, it would be more efficient if a limited number of controls are selected, compared with case-cohort studies with a subcohort consisting of 10% of the individual cohort. In addition, given the heterogeneity of different cohorts, matching controls with cases on potential confounding factors may improve study efficiency. For instance, using a nested case-control study design, the Cohort Consortium Vitamin D Pooling Project of Rarer Cancers (VDPP) brought together 10 cohorts to conduct a prospective study of the association between vitamin D status, measured as serum concentrations of 25-hydroxyvitamin D (25(OH)D), and the development of 7 rarer cancer sites: endometrial, esophageal, gastric, kidney, non-Hodgkin lymphoma, ovarian, and pancreatic cancers.[40]

Taken together, if the goal is to study multiple biomarkers for a given outcome, and the measurements are sensitive, nested case-control studies may be preferred. On the other hand, if the goal is to investigate a biomarker in relation to multiple outcomes, case-cohort studies may be considered, provided that the measurements are not sensitive for batch effects or careful planning is done in advance to handle batch effects. Although both study designs allow estimating rate ratios, it should be noted that recent literature suggests that individual risks and prediction measures can be conducted with appropriate reweighting in case-cohort studies, while matching variables could not be included in the individual risk estimation in the finely matched nested case-control design.[41]

■ SPECIAL ISSUES RELATED TO THE COMPONENTS OF COHORT STUDIES IN LOW-INCOME COUNTRIES

Cohort studies conducted within the context of low- and middle-income countries often have special issues associated with components of cohort study design. Issues relating to hypothesis generation, selection of local collaborators and partner institutions, defining of a sampling frame and ethical considerations regarding informed consent all take on new implications within the context of epidemiologic research conducted internationally.

Formulation of Hypotheses

Descriptive or correlational studies are particularly useful in identifying international variation in disease related incidence or mortality. This variation can be due to characteristics such as age distributions, gender, race, marital status, social class, occupation, diet and other lifestyle factors. This information is often then used in conjunction with existing clinical, laboratory or epidemiologic data regarding mortality or other disease outcomes to further investigate international variation. Often, international variance in disease incidence allows researchers to develop likely hypotheses regarding associations between predictive risk factors and disease outcomes. International variation can point to differences in genetic susceptibility as well as pertinent lifestyle factors such as diet, physical activity level, and environmental or occupational risk factors as key predictors of the outcome of interest. As previously discussed in this section, utilizing low- and middle-income countries is one way to identify unique risk factors that may be linked with the disease outcome of interest. Once this hypothesis is generated, researchers must then turn their focus to the practical aspects of implementing a cohort study design in these populations.

Selection of Study Site, Collaborators and Partner Institutions

A primary challenge in assembling a cohort is establishing appropriate collaborators and partner institutions to aid in the practical aspects of data collection and management at the study site. Because cohort studies are longitudinal and require consistent collection of follow-up data and continued contact with participants over time, it is important that researchers carefully consider local collaboration at the study site.

Formulation of the hypothesis is only the first step in the initiation of an observational study. After identifying the appropriate scientific question, researchers must then select the appropriate study site. While it is critical that the study population meets the requirements for being able to answer the research question, investigators must also consider logistical issues regarding transportation and commuting in and out of the study site. The study site must be accessible for both participants as well as local members of the research team.

Ideally, local collaborators in the context of a cohort study will be familiar with longitudinal data collection and community based interventions or trials, with a particular emphasis on complete and accurate follow up methods. Therefore, investigators must be careful to select institutions and co-investigators based on their specific needs. For example, it would be inappropriate to utilize an institution focused primarily on molecular or genetic epidemiologic studies in the context of a community based intervention. Because the validity of a prospective cohort study relies heavily on minimizing attrition and maintaining accurate and consistent follow up data collection, the establishment of a cohesive network of investigators at the study site is critical to the success of the study. One example of this type of collaboration is the development of the International Centre for Diarrhoeal Disease Research, Bangladesh (ICDDR, B), which is a nonprofit international research, training and service institution based in Dhaka, Bangladesh (http://www.icddrb.org/). The purpose of this center is to establish a meaningful partnership between various research groups in order to promote realistic and cost effective solutions of major problems in international health (http://www.icddrb.org/). In utilizing a mix of national and international staff from various fields including public health officials, laboratory scientists, clinicians, nutritionists, epidemiologist and demographers, the ICDDR,B is able to develop and share knowledge regarding important issues in international health.

Sampling Frames

In addition to choosing appropriate local collaborators, investigators must select an appropriate study population. For prospective analyses, a sampling frame is generally a list, either real or theoretical- of the population from which the study sample should be drawn.[42] Alternatively, in the absence of a list of potential participants, sampling frames can be defined by geographic regions or enumeration areas. An important underlying assumption of a population based cohort study is that the sample ultimately used for analysis is representative of the population, as it is defined through the sampling frame.

The Health Effects of Arsenic Longitudinal (HEALS), conducted in Bangladesh in order to determine the association between arsenic exposure in drinking water, and the incidence of premalignant skin lesions, provides a good example of this kind of sampling frame construction. With the collaboration of local officials and government agencies, the investigators were able to identify a region within Bangladesh that not only provided a wide dose range of arsenic exposure through drinking well concentrations, but also included a large enough population of socioculturally homogeneous individuals from which to draw the study sample. Once the study site was identified, researchers worked to establish a study base-first enumerating the entire population in the study area by ascertaining their arsenic exposure and sociodemographic characteristics.

Once the concentrations of each well in the area were described, a total of 65,876 men and women from the study area were identified. Individuals that fulfilled the inclusion criteria constituted the primary pool for the cohort study. A working list of these potential participants was created for use in recruitment, taking into account several considerations-including the need for a wide exposure distribution. From here, the study team ultimately recruited 11,746 individuals for inclusion in the study population.[43] Ultimately, constructing the sampling frame is a critical part of the cohort study design in that it provides researchers with the framework from which to select a representative sample of the population of interest.

Informed Consent

Ethical concerns, particularly the issue of informed consent, are also prominent features of conducting cohort studies in low and middle income countries. Informed consent in clinical and community based epidemiologic research has been universally accepted as a precondition for scientific investigations that involve human participants.[44] National and international guidelines that outline specific requirements for obtaining informed consent have been developed.[44] Despite these developments, however, the application of the guidelines are particularly challenging within international settings. Researchers conducting observational epidemiologic investigations must be careful to take these challenges into consideration.

The notion of informed consent is one that is based on primarily western notions of respect for personal autonomy.[45] Within this context, informed consent is viewed as an ethical ideal and a necessary social process within the context of scientific research. However, the process of informed consent has some underlying assumptions that often may be challenging to meet, if possible at all, within low- and middle-income developing nations.

One of the primary challenges is that of communication. Research participants in an international setting may have difficulties understanding the consent documents for a variety of reasons. Firstly, it is likely that language barriers may hinder communication between the researchers and the participants. Translations of consent documents may not be exact-and these translations may fail to fully communicate the research process with sufficient detail or in the exact manner as originally intended. Likewise, in developing nations, it is likely that the study population, in general, has low levels of literacy and educational attainment, making the scientific concepts detailed in the consent forms difficult to communicate and verbal consent procedures necessary. Requirements for written consent may be further complicated by low levels of trust for medical institutions often seen in developing nations where there is less familiarity with western biomedical and behavioral research methods. Finally, there is elevated concern that individuals within resource poor areas are vulnerable populations and more easily coerced into participation, by study staff, local leaders, or necessity for medical care.

Subject Identification and Data Collection Approach

Several data collection methods have been developed for use in cohort studies including self-administered questionnaires, web-based and mail-in surveys and telephone interview methods. These methods, though widely used in developed nations, are often not always feasible in low- and middle-income settings. Often, due to lack of accessibility of certain technologies (including phone and internet access) in-person interviewing is frequently the only feasible method of data collection in low resource nations. While these methods have their own challenges (i.e. they require more man power and study resources) they provide a unique opportunity to collect more valid and complete data, as well as providing researchers the chance to collect clinical assessment data concurrently with baseline survey data. This allows for the more valid assessment of cross-sectional associations.

Data Management and Informatics

While the implementation of automated or web-based data management systems are becoming more feasible in low resource settings, challenges still remain in establishing these data management techniques in developing nations. Data management necessitates the collaboration and cooperation of local partners and institutions in order to promote consistent data collection techniques as well as trust between study staff and local participants.

Exposure Measurement

Cohort study design relies on the accurate identification of exposed and unexposed individuals. Methods for exposure assessment vary greatly depending on the study and the risk factor in question. General population based studies may choose to measure a variety of possible risk factors at the outset by using questionnaires, laboratory tests, physical measurements and medical procedures. Based on this information, each of the participants can then be categorized into their appropriate exposure group. Risk factor assessment can also be accomplished through historical records; however, this method limits researchers to information available based on past data collections and limits the number of risk factors that can be assessed and historical exposure data may often only available at the group level. Researchers must also decide which exposure time point is most important. Exposure to risk factors can change over time and depending on the factor being studied the most relevant predictor can be past exposure, current exposure, cumulative exposure, or peak exposure.

As previously discussed in this section, cohort studies within low- and middle-income settings are often useful for the measurement of unique risk factors stemming from dietary patterns, occupational risk factors and environmental exposures. However, risks associated with these exposures are generally small. For example, dietary patterns vary by country and region of the world, and therefore studying the effect of diet on disease outcome is useful in identifying novel associations within an international context. However, exposure assessments for risk factors like diet are difficult. Food frequency questionnaires (FFQs) have been relatively well validated in certain populations, including several within the United States. However, the same questionnaire cannot be implemented in studies in countries with drastically differing dietary profiles. Developing these kinds of questionnaires for different settings requires extensive piloting and validation within the study population, which will be discussed later in this section.

Follow-up Process

Follow-up of study participants is arguably the most important aspect of a cohort study. Validity and reliability of study results depend on minimizing attrition of participants over time and performing consistent and accurate assessment of follow-up measures. Longitudinal studies that span many years, however, present logistical issues; for instance, it becomes difficult to locate participants in the study over time, and people are likely to move and lose interest in participating. These challenges can often be overcome in the context of low- and middle-income countries because participants may be less likely to move out of the study area and therefore be easier to track consistently over the study follow-up periods.

Endpoint Assessment

While the assessment of discrete outcomes such as mortality is often considered to be straightforward, there are several challenges in the evaluation of specific disease endpoints, particularly within the context of developing nations. An important obstacle in the assessment of various disease endpoints is that the advanced medical procedures necessary for measurement of these outcomes is not yet in place in several developing nations. Generally, however, with the addition of some minor improvements to the existing systems, the major medical center in the study area may be made responsible for the collection of this data. Therefore, it is again important that the research staff and local institutions establish collaborate in order to ensure accurate and timely data collection regarding study endpoints.

However, there are some unique advantages to endpoint assessment in these settings. In low income countries, if feasible, investigators may take the model of providing free basic health care through the study clinic established for study purpose. Not only does this enhance the ability to detect several simple endpoints, but it alleviates the reliance on medical systems that do not have detailed and easily accessible documentation of health information. Investigators must also keep in mind, however, the ethical issues implicit in conducting a study that involves assessment of disease endpoints- namely the need to treat conditions diagnosed as a part of the research protocol.

Questionnaire Designs

Accuracy and reliability of exposure assessment, participant follow-up, and endpoint assessment are naturally linked to the accuracy of the measures utilized for data collection. As previously discussed, questionnaires are often used as the primary method for collecting data regarding baseline exposures in the study population, as well as assessing disease outcomes during follow up. In order for these questionnaires to be functional within the context of a cohort analysis, particularly in studies conducted internationally, they must be well validated within the population from which the study group is derived.

Validation

Validation is an important step in utilizing a questionnaire for exposure and outcome assessment.[46] Although an instrument may be well validated within one population, it does not necessarily follow that it is appropriate for use in its current form in another population. In general, survey instruments need to be validated in their target population prior to implementation in the context of the study so as to ensure that the questionnaire is not only measuring what the researchers intended, but also that the results can be utilized in a similar population in the future. Often this is accomplished through pilot testing.

Piloting

A pilot test is a preliminary test of the data collection tools that have been derived for use in the study and generally conducted in order to identify, and ultimately eliminate, potential problems with the instrument. This allows researcher to make adjustments and modifications prior to the initiation of data collection in the study population.

Pilot testing involves simulating the actual data collection process on a much smaller scale in order to get feedback regarding whether or not the instrument being developed is likely to work in the study setting and is appropriate for the selected study population.[1] In a typical pilot study, a smaller group of individuals, similar in characteristics to those chosen as a part of the study cohort are administered the same questionnaire meant for the study population.

Pilot testing is meant to detect a wide range of potential problems with a study instrument and to identify questions that study subjects may find ambiguous or difficult to understand. Also, the process can identify questions that can make study subjects uncomfortable and therefore less likely to respond.

Overall, piloting is meant to improve the way in which an instrument or survey is administered. This is an extremely relevant point for researchers conducting cohort studies internationally in developing nations. A primary concern is the translation of the instrument into the native language. There may be issues with certain words or concepts that cannot be accurately translated and can potentially lead to the ascertainment of incorrect information. Back-translation should be conducted to identify errors. Cultural norms also play an important role during the piloting of survey instruments as a question that may be appropriate to ask in one context can be inappropriate in another. Ultimately, the piloting process, particularly within the context of developing nations, is an important aspect of the cohort study design

Quality Control and Oversight of Field Work

Maintaining the quality of study data is an important aspect of conserving study validity and generalizability. It is critical to train and sensitize local study staff to the importance of quality control measures in regards to the study data with a particular focus on the consistency in data collection techniques and adherence to study protocol. There are several ways to ensure quality control of study data—including frequent field visits to the study site and the implementation of a separate study staff at various stages of study implementation solely in charge of quality control.

Liaisons with Local Government and Health Organizations

The importance of establishing local collaboration was discussed earlier in this section. While local collaboration is critical in successfully conducting a cohort study in developing nations, investigators in these settings need to be careful to maintain a balance between obtaining support from local government and health organizations and not compromising the quality of the study data by allowing these organizations to interfere too much in the scientific process.

▦ DISSEMINATION AND POLICY IMPLICATIONS

During the process of conducting a cohort study, researchers must be aware of the continued need to inform both study participants, as well as public health officials and policy makers of the ongoing results of study analyses. Public health officials and policy makers rely on this information to make informed decisions about health programs and interventions. In cases where study findings can inform health behaviors and choices of study participants, it is also imperative that they are kept informed of important findings regarding associations between exposure and disease status. Therefore, researchers must be aware of the continued need to disseminate study findings and integrate this process into the planning of the cohort study from its initiation.

Implications of Cohort Studies in Low- and Middle-Income Countries

Low- and middle-income countries provide a unique and interesting perspective for conducting observational epidemiologic research. There are several advantages to these types of studies, both scientific and social, and ample opportunity for expansion into other aspects of epidemiologic and scientific research. In particular, data collected from these cohorts may be used to further knowledge in the area of genomics and disease prevention.

Biobanking and Genomics

To date, cohort studies conducted within the context of low- and middle-income countries have focused on purely observational research questions and data collection methods have been limited to survey based designs. However, broadening the scope of these studies will make them increasingly relevant as epidemiologic research focuses more on genetic and molecular risk factors of disease, in addition to the environmental, occupational and behavioral factors now being examined. Large cohorts can set the stage for an informative nested case control study for the examination of associations between genetic variants and disease outcome, as well as potential interactions with environmental cofactors, within that same population. Therefore, future international cohorts can be an important resource for expanding the breadth of available genetic data for analysis.

Prevention

A general goal of epidemiologic research is to identify modifiable risk factors in the population for the purposes of preventing disease. Because health care systems in these low and middle-income countries are not well established, cohort studies conducted in these settings should look beyond simply the observational question at hand. Often times, with the unique exposures seen in low- and middle-income countries, researchers have the opportunity to intervene in a very real way. For example, the Health Effects of Longitudinal Research Study, as previously mentioned, was initiated in 2000 to prospectively evaluate the effects of naturally occurring arsenic in the drinking supply of a small region in Bangladesh. This study, among many conducted in low- and middle-income countries, has linked arsenic in drinking water to the incidence of premalignant skins lesions in the population. Based on this information, researchers involved in the HEALS study were able to intervene by labeling wells with high arsenic concentration and informing the members of the community of its risks.

International Consortia

One of the limitations of cohort analysis is the necessity for large numbers to provide the amount of statistical power needed to detect significant effects in rare outcomes. Consortia are a way for investigators to pool data resources regarding certain risk factors and disease outcomes to provide greater power to existing analyses. Therefore, when developing and initiating a cohort study internationally researchers should concurrently consider involvement in an international consortium at the outset to aid in standardizing protocol and data collection techniques.

One example of this type of collaboration is the Asia Cohort Consortium (ACC). The ACC was initiated as a mechanism for understanding the relationship between genetics, environmental exposures and the etiology of various diseases through the establishment of an at least one million person cohort from various countries around the world including China, India, Japan, Korea, Malaysia, Singapore, Taiwan, and the United States (http://www.asiacohort.org/Pages/About.aspx). The ACC addresses the scientific need to establish the complete pattern of susceptibility and resistance to disease, and to define disease more finely by recruiting and tracking large numbers of individuals from diverse areas. These individuals are characterized based on genetics, as well as behavioral and environmental characteristics. This collaboration allows researchers to share and compile results, standardize methodologies, and replicate important findings.

Social Empowerment and Economic Stimulation

There are also several direct and indirect economic and social benefits of conducting cohort studies in developing nations. Aside from the obvious scientific benefits related to characterizing novel risk factor/disease associations, conducting these cohort studies in low- and middle-income settings have additional advantages that are important to consider. As previously discussed, the success of a cohort study conducted internationally relies on the cooperation of local institutions in the study area. In addition to cooperation from medical and research institutions, however, data collection often relies on a locally organized research staff generally of individuals from in or around the study area. This stimulates the local economy by creating several new jobs. In addition to these direct benefits to the local economy, cohort studies conducted in these settings serve as a model for the community by bringing to the forefront issues of health, thus allowing individuals to recognize important roles in maintaining community health and taking part in promoting awareness of relevant health issues.

■ CONCLUSIONS

Low- and middle-income countries include a wide range of nations with dramatic variations in available resources, rates of economic growth, political conditions, health care services, and stages of the epidemiologic transition from infectious disease to chronic disease conditions. Because of these circumstances, these countries represent interesting opportunity to investigate unique disease risk factors and health outcomes. Indeed, several challenges face researchers in these environments; however, important knowledge can be gained by conducting thorough and large-scale cohort based investigations. These investigations will potentially lead to resource and population specific solutions for major public health issues.

■ SUMMARY

Conducting cohort studies in low- and middle-income countries provide a unique landscape for the rigorous investigation of risk factors and prevention of diseases. Despite difficulties researchers will often face due to lack of resources and cultural barriers to research in some of these populations, the gain in knowledge especially for research questions that are not addressable by case-control or cross-sectional studies will be imperative in understanding the public health landscape of developing nations. In addition to full cohort analyses, nested case-control and case-cohort sampling allows efficient investigations of research questions involving resource-consuming assays. These countries have unique nutritional, anthropometric, genomic, and environmental risk profiles yet their relatively homogenous distributions within a country or group of countries facilitate translation of cohort study findings. Collaboration and formation of consortia will be exceedingly important in this type of research in order to overcome obstacles related to long-term follow-up and maintenance of study protocol. Given that the overwhelming majority of worldwide mortality and morbidity happen in low- and middle-income countries and this proportion will continue to rise with economic development of these countries, sound epidemiological investigations to understand the risk factors and prevention avenues for these populations are urgently needed. These population-specific research findings are needed for formulating developing country health policy rather than extrapolating these key decisions solely based on the findings from studies in the developed nations. This chapter outlines the key components of designing and conducting cohort studies in low- and middle-income countries, as well as the challenges and opportunities associated with these components.

■ REFERENCES

1. Rothman KJ, Greenland S, Lash TL. *Modern epidemiology.* Philadelphia: Wolters Kluwer Health/ Lippincott Williams & Wilkins; 2008:x, 758 p.
2. Willett WC, Colditz GA. Approaches for conducting large cohort studies. *Epidemiol Rev.* 1998;20(1): 91–99.
3. Ahrens W, Pigeot I, SpringerLink (Online service). *Handbook of epidemiology.* Berlin, Heidelberg: Springer-Verlag Berlin Heidelberg; 2005.
4. Yang W, Zilov A, Soewondo P, Bech OM, Sekkal F, Home PD. Observational studies: Going beyond the boundaries of randomized controlled trials. *Diabetes Res Clin Pract.* 2010;88 Suppl 1:S3–S9.
5. Szklo M. Population-based cohort studies. *Epidemiol Rev.* 1998;20(1):81–90.
6. Holmes MD, Dalal S, Volmink J, et al. Non-communicable diseases in sub-Saharan Africa: The case for cohort studies. *PLoS medicine.* 2010;7(5):e1000244.
7. Beasley RP, Hwang LY, Lin CC, Chien CS. Hepatocellular carcinoma and hepatitis B virus. A prospective study of 22 707 men in Taiwan. *Lancet.* 1981;2(8256):1129–1133.
8. Van Ommeren M. Validity issues in transcultural epidemiology. *Br J Psychiatry.* 2003;182:376–378.
9. Vathesatogkit P, Woodward M, Tanomsup S, et al. Cohort profile: The electricity generating authority of Thailand study. *Int J Epidemiol.* 2012;41(2):359–365.
10. Chen Y, Factor-Litvak P, Howe GR, et al. Arsenic exposure from drinking water, dietary intakes of B vitamins and folate, and risk of high blood pressure in Bangladesh: A population-based, cross-sectional study. *Am J Epidemiol.* 2007;165(5):541–552.
11. Haque R, Mazumder DN, Samanta S, et al. Arsenic in drinking water and skin lesions: Dose-response data from West Bengal, India. *Epidemiology.* 2003;14(2):174–182.
12. Hopenhayn-Rich C, Biggs ML, Kalman DA, Moore LE, Smith AH. Arsenic methylation patterns before and after changing from high to lower concentrations of arsenic in drinking water. *Environ Health Perspect.* 1996;104(11):1200–1207.
13. Mazumder DN, Haque R, Ghosh N, et al. Arsenic in drinking water and the prevalence of respiratory effects in West Bengal, India. *Int J Epidemiol.* 2000;29(6):1047–1052.
14. Parvez F, Chen Y, Argos M, et al. Prevalence of arsenic exposure from drinking water and awareness of its health risks in a Bangladeshi population: Results from a large population-based study. *Environ Health Perspect.* 2006;114(3):355–359.

15. Smith AH, Arroyo AP, Mazumder DN, et al. Arsenic-induced skin lesions among atacameno people in northern Chile despite good nutrition and centuries of exposure. *Environ Health Perspect.* 2000;108(7):617–620.

16. Tondel M, Rahman M, Magnuson A, Chowdhury IA, Faruquee MH, Ahmad SA. The relationship of arsenic levels in drinking water and the prevalence rate of skin lesions in Bangladesh. *Environ Health Perspect.* 1999;107(9):727–729.

17. Chen CL, Hsu LI, Chiou HY, et al. Ingested arsenic, cigarette smoking, and lung cancer risk: A follow-up study in arseniasis-endemic areas in Taiwan. *JAMA.* 2004;292(24):2984–2990.

18. Hopenhayn-Rich C, Biggs ML, Fuchs A, et al. Bladder cancer mortality associated with arsenic in drinking water in Argentina. *Epidemiology.* 1996;7(2):117–124.

19. Diaz-Barriga F, Santos MA, Mejia JJ, et al. Arsenic and cadmium exposure in children living near a smelter complex in San Luis Potosi, Mexico. *Environ Res.* 1993;62(2):242–250.

20. Astrakianakis G, Seixas NS, Ray R, et al. Lung cancer risk among female textile workers exposed to endotoxin. *J Natl Cancer Inst.* 2007;99(5):357–364.

21. Riboli E, Kaaks R. The EPIC project: Rationale and study design. European prospective investigation into cancer and nutrition. *Int J Epidemiol.* 1997;26 Suppl 1:S6–S14.

22. Asher MI, Stewart AW, Mallol J, et al. Which population level environmental factors are associated with asthma, rhinoconjunctivitis and eczema? Review of the ecological analyses of ISAAC phase one. *Respir Res.* 2010;11:8.

23. Truswell AS. Meat consumption and cancer of the large bowel. *Eur J Clin Nutr.* 2002;56 Suppl 1:S19–S24.

24. Key TJ, Fraser GE, Thorogood M, et al. Mortality in vegetarians and nonvegetarians: Detailed findings from a collaborative analysis of 5 prospective studies. *Am J Clin Nutr.* 1999;70(3 Suppl):516S–524S.

25. Gaziano TA, Bitton A, Anand S, Abrahams-Gessel S, Murphy A. Growing epidemic of coronary heart disease in low- and middle-income countries. *Curr Probl Cardiol.* 2010;35(2):72–115.

26. OMRAN AR. The epidemiologic transition: A theory of the epidemiology of population change. *Milbank Q.* 2005;83(4):731.

27. Maher D, Waswa L, Baisley K, Karabarinde A, Unwin N, Grosskurth H. Distribution of hyperglycaemia and related cardiovascular disease risk factors in low-income countries: A cross-sectional population-based survey in rural Uganda. *Int J Epidemiol.* 2011;40(1):160.

28. Burton PR, Tobin MD, Hopper JL. Key concepts in genetic epidemiology. *Lancet.* 2005; 366(9489):941.

29. Calle EE, Rodriguez C, Jacobs EJ, et al. The American Cancer Society cancer prevention study II nutrition cohort: Rationale, study design, and baseline characteristics. *Cancer.* 2002;94(9):2490.

30. Dawber TR. *The Framingham study: The epidemiology of atherosclerotic disease.* Cambridge, Mass.: Harvard University Press; 1980:viii, 257 p.

31. Doll R, Hill AB. The mortality of doctors in relation to their smoking habits: A preliminary report. *BMJ: British Medical Journal.* 2004;328(7455):1529.

32. Doll R, Peto R, Hall E, Wheatley K, Gray R. Mortality in relation to consumption of alcohol: 13 years' observations on male British doctors. *BMJ: British Medical Journal.* 1994;309(6959):911.

33. Prentice RL. A case-cohort design for epidemiologic cohort studies and disease prevention trials. *Biometrika.* 1986;73(1):1–11.

34. Rundle AG, Vineis P, Ahsan H. Design options for molecular epidemiology research within cohort studies. *Cancer epidemiology, biomarkers & prevention: a publication of the American Association for Cancer Research, cosponsored by the American Society of Preventive Oncology.* 2005;14(8):1899.

35. Limburg PJ, Stolzenberg-Solomon RZ, Vierkant RA, et al. Insulin, glucose, insulin resistance, and incident colorectal cancer in male smokers. *Clinical Gastroenterology and Hepatology.* 2006;4(12):1514.

36. Stolzenberg-Solomon RZ, Graubard BI, Chari S, et al. Insulin, glucose, insulin resistance, and pancreatic cancer in male smokers. *JAMA: the journal of the American Medical Association.* 2005;294(22):2872.

37. Albanes D, Weinstein SJ, Wright ME, et al. Serum insulin, glucose, indices of insulin resistance, and risk of prostate cancer. *J Natl Cancer Inst.* 2009;101(18):1272.

38. Nambi V, Hoogeveen RC, Chambless L, et al. Lipoprotein-associated phospholipase A2 and high-sensitivity C-reactive protein improve the stratification of ischemic stroke risk in the atherosclerosis risk in communities (ARIC) study. *Stroke.* 2009;40(2):376–381.

39. Ballantyne CM, Hoogeveen RC, Bang H, et al. Lipoprotein-associated phospholipase A2, high-sensitivity C-reactive protein, and risk for incident coronary heart disease in middle-aged men and women in the atherosclerosis risk in communities (ARIC) study. *Circulation.* 2004;109(7):837–842.

40. Helzlsouer KJ. Overview of the cohort consortium vitamin D pooling project of rarer cancers. *Am J Epidemiol.* 2010;172(1):4.

41. Ganna A, Reilly M, de Faire U, Pedersen N, Magnusson P, Ingelsson E. Risk prediction measures for case-cohort and nested case-control designs: An application to cardiovascular disease. *Am J Epidemiol.* 2012;175(7):715.

42. Kelsey JL, Whittemore AS, Evans A,S., Thompson WD. *Methods in observational epidemiology.* New York: Oxford University Press; 1996:viii, 432 p.

43. Ahsan H, Chen Y, Parvez F, et al. Health effects of arsenic longitudinal study (HEALS): Description of a multidisciplinary epidemiologic investigation. *Journal of exposure science & environmental epidemiology.* 2006;16(2):191.

44. Corrigan O. Empty ethics: The problem with informed consent. *Sociol Health Illn.* 2003;25(7):768.

45. Jepson RG, Hewison J, Thompson AGH, Weller D. How should we measure informed choice? the case of cancer screening. *J Med Ethics.* 2005;31(4):192.

46. Cade JE, Burley VJ, Warm DL, Thompson RL, Margetts BM. Food-frequency questionnaires: A review of their design, validation and utilisation. *Nutrition Research Reviews.* 2004;17(01):5.

CHAPTER 10

MOLECULAR EPIDEMIOLOGY IN LOW- AND MIDDLE-INCOME COUNTRIES

HONGBING SHEN AND HONGXIA MA

■ INTRODUCTION

Conventional epidemiology has been very successful in identifying environmental and lifestyle factors that increase or reduce risk of specific cancers, and this information may lead to cancer prevention strategies. The investigations linking smoking and lung cancer are perhaps best known and have led to widespread and successful cancer prevention initiatives and policy changes.[1,2] However, in conventional epidemiological research, the cause (exposure) is correlated with the outcome (a disease) in populations, but without detailed exploration of the biological mechanisms or data from individuals that could better establish cause and effect. Therefore, despite the extensive use of questionnaires and interview-based approaches in conventional epidemiologic studies, the etiology of many types of diseases including cancer is still poorly understood. Molecular epidemiology is the integration of molecular biology and traditional epidemiology in the study of populations, an approach that overcomes many limitations of conventional epidemiology and elucidates disease causation by identifying specific pathways and molecules and genes that influence disease risk.

The phrase "molecular epidemiology" was introduced in 1973 by Kilbourne in an article entitled "The molecular epidemiology of influenza."[3] The term became better known with the publication of "Molecular Epidemiology: Principles and Practice" by Schulte and Perera, in which molecular epidemiology was defined as "the incorporation of molecular, cellular, and other biologic measurements into epidemiologic research."[4] Subsequently, molecular epidemiology was more specifically elaborated as "a science that focuses on the contribution of potential genetic and environmental risk factors, identified at the molecular level, to the etiology, distribution and prevention of disease within families and across populations."[5] From then on, there has been a steady growth in the use of the term in the scientific literature, with more than 45000 articles published by 2011.

The objectives of molecular epidemiology are broad and mainly focus on the assessment of the biologic basis for associations, by using biologic measurements to assess exposure, effects of exposure, and susceptibility. In this way, the epidemiologists may help open up the "black box" of causation by examining the events that intermediate between exposure and disease occurrence or progression. That is to say, molecular biology clarifies the process of disease development, and it thus has a promising role in furthering our understanding of disease detection, treatment prediction, and prognosis.

Molecular epidemiology has a wide range of applications in disease research. In cancer, for example, it can be applied to the following areas:[6] (1) To increase the accuracy of exposure assessment to a potential environmental carcinogen. Environmental exposures, including lifestyle, infections, radiation, natural and man-made chemicals, and occupation, are major causes of human cancer. However, the precise contribution of specific risk factors and their interaction continues to be difficult to elucidate. In response to this need, molecular cancer epidemiology promises to provide special biomarkers to refine exposure assessment. (2) To discover fundamental mechanisms in the induction of cancer. Molecular cancer epidemiology focuses not only on risk factors, but also on the whole process from exposure to the occurrence of cancer. Therefore, it involves the use of biomarkers of exposure and effect in studies of exogenous or endogenous agents and/or host factors that play a role in causing cancer. (3) To identify genetic and/or acquired susceptibility factors that contribute to the risk of cancer. For example, it has been estimated that tobacco smoke is responsible for 87% of all lung cancers,[7] yet only a fraction of smokers develop lung cancer, suggesting that there is inter-individual variation in genetic susceptibility to smoking exposure in the general population. Molecular epidemiologic studies have identified some susceptibility markers that have been used to identify populations with a high-risk of cancer. (4) To predict cancer outcome in exposed populations. During the last decade there has been a huge expansion in the number of molecular epidemiology studies, with respect to both association studies of disease risk and studies of prognosis and treatment response. Cancer predisposition, treatment response, and prognosis are interrelated at the genetic level (Figure 10.1), and the use of biomarkers to predict a patient's risk of disease, treatment response or prognosis is one step toward improved, personalized approaches for cancer prevention, screening and treatment selection.[8]

Molecular epidemiology has developed quickly and achieved a lot in prevention and control of disease across the world. However, low- and middle-income countries lag

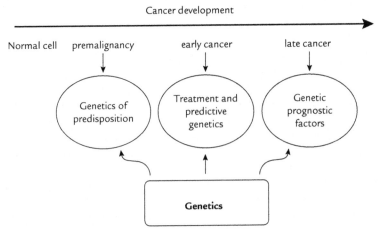

FIGURE 10.1 Interrelatedness of the biology behind the predisposition, treatment (drug and/or radiotherapy) response, and outcome in cancer.[8]

behind, and few have a significant capability in carrying out the studies of molecular epidemiology, due to a lack of trained molecular epidemiologists and a pervasive shortage of appropriate equipment and reagents. Many low- and middle-income countries are undergoing the epidemiologic transition. Despite the high prevalence of communicable disorders in these areas, the burden of chronic diseases, including cancer, is rapidly increasing. Naturally, the disparities in disease risk, combined with poor access to epidemiological data, research, treatment, and disease control and prevention, combine to result in significantly worse survival rates in low- and middle-income countries for a range of specific malignancies. Therefore, there is an urgent need to develop epidemiology capabilities in low- and middle-income countries to provide useful strategies for disease prevention, detection, diagnosis, treatment, and palliation. Furthermore, the wide variety of dietary, lifestyle, and environmental exposures, as well as the genetic variation among people in these countries, can provide valuable new information on factors that contribute to cancer or that protect against it.

In China, molecular epidemiology emerged in early 1980s in the context of infectious diseases and had a slow development during the early 1990s, with less than 10 reports annually. However, the number of research studies on molecular epidemiology has almost doubled each year since then. Establishment of the first molecular epidemiological study group in 1997 by the Fourth Epidemiology Council of China was a remarkable event in this process. Developing over the past three decades, and particularly rapidly in recent years, molecular epidemiology in China now has a relatively complete system of theories and methods. Notable advances have been achieved in the control and prevention of diseases through studies of molecular epidemiology in China. For example, a series of toxicological and molecular epidemiological studies were conducted to investigate the effect of benzene on health by researchers at the Chinese Academy of Preventive Medicine (CAPM) (1973–1986) and subsequently by collaboration between the CAPM and the National Cancer Institute (NCI) in the United States. The findings suggested that risk of leukemia and lymphoma among benzene-exposed workers was significantly increased, and elevated risks for leukemia were present not only at higher exposure but also among workers exposed to less than 10 ppm. According to these results, the benzene permissible level was decreased to 1.8 ppm (6 mg/m), and benzene-induced leukemia is now treated as an occupational cancer in China.[9]

DEFINITION OF BIOMARKERS

Studies have shown that carcinogenesis is a prolonged process that involves multiple biological changes. During the last decade, many biomarkers that are frequently associated with abnormal biological events have been integrated into molecular epidemiological studies to clarify the biological progress of cancer. In 1982, Perera and Weinstein proposed the concept "molecular cancer epidemiology" as a new paradigm for cancer research that incorporated biomarkers into epidemiologic studies to assess individual exposure, dose, preclinical effects and susceptibility to carcinogens.[10] The official NIH definition of a biomarker is: "a characteristic that is objectively measured and evaluated as an indicator of normal biologic processes, pathogenic processes, or pharmacologic responses to a therapeutic intervention." In molecular cancer epidemiology, biomarkers have been widely used to assess exposure to potential environmental hazards, to gain insight into disease mechanisms and to understand acquired or inherited susceptibility. Therefore, use of biomarkers covers the whole spectrum from hazard exposure to disease pathogenesis and may offer improved understanding of the pathway between exposure measures and the health outcome. Major objectives of biomarker research in cancer epidemiology can be summarized into the following aspects:[6]

1. To discover fundamental mechanisms in the induction of cancer.
2. To increase the accuracy of exposure assessment to a potential environmental carcinogen.
3. To identify genetic and/or acquired susceptibility factors that contribute to the risk for cancer.
4. To predict cancer outcome in exposed populations.

Biomarkers used for molecular cancer epidemiology can be usually categorized into at least three classes: markers of exposure, markers of early response/effect, and markers of susceptibility (Figure 10.2).[11] These classes of biomarkers are discussed in more detail below.

Markers of Exposure

Environmental exposures are a major cause of human cancer; however, the precise mechanism of specific exposure in cancer continues to be difficult to elucidate. One of the primary challenges of molecular cancer epidemiology, therefore, is to improve exposure assessment. Exposure markers can characterize changes in endogenous substrates resulting from the effects of exogenous factors with greater validity and precision. Markers of exposures have two subcategories: markers of internal dose and markers of biologically effective dose. Environmental chemicals, or their metabolites in human tissues, body fluids, or exhaled air, have been used to measure exposure, and are termed markers of internal dose. Examples include chemical substances (dioxins, polychlorinated biphenyls, aromatic amines, polycyclic aromatic hydrocarbons (PAH), aflatoxins, heavy metals) and products of their metabolism, nutrients (vitamins and microelements), and infectious agents (viruses, *Helicobacter pylori*).[12] Meanwhile, carcinogen-DNA and carcinogen-protein adducts have been widely measured in human biological samples; these have been referred to as biomarkers of "biologically effective dose."[13] DNA adducts are especially well recognized as biomarkers of exposure to various environmental, life style, or occupational chemical carcinogens and have been shown to be modified through various interventions.[14] The presence and persistence of carcinogen-DNA adducts are early markers of biological response to exposure and particularly reflect the processes of metabolism of carcinogens (their activation and

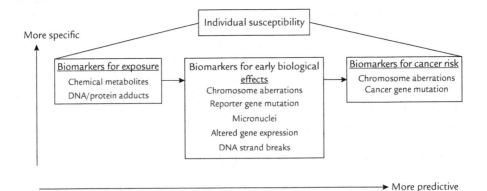

FIGURE 10.2 Scheme of biomarkers for genetic toxicology and susceptibility in investigation.[11]

detoxification), DNA repair, and biologically effective dose. Such studies are typically used to investigate protein and DNA adducts of the carcinogenic components of tobacco smoke, such as tobacco-specific-nitrosamine (TSN)-adduct and PAH-adduct. Likewise, the role of the aflatoxin-DNA and aflatoxin-hemoglobin adducts that are associated with aflatoxin carcinogenicity has been identified in liver cancer.

Markers of Effect

Markers of effect are intermediate biomarkers that measure early biological events that take place in the progress from exposure to cancer development and reflect the cumulative exposure to a variety of environmental factors. Typical events include chromosomal alterations (CA), sister chromatid exchange, micronuclei, measures of cellular or tissue toxicity, changes in DNA, RNA and protein expression, and alterations in functions relevant to carcinogenesis (e.g. DNA repair, immunological response, etc.).[15] Among these biomarkers of effect, CA may be the gold standard, and the mechanisms of CA formation by a variety of environmental toxic substances are relatively well understood.[11] Additionally, there is a growing interest in the study of relationships among carcinogenic exposures, risk of cancer at specific sites, and mutational spectra in relevant cancer genes (i.e. oncogenes and tumor-suppressor genes), such as the *ras* gene family, the *myc* family, *erb B1*, *int-2/hst-1* and the *p53* tumor suppressor gene. The most illustrative example of carcinogen-specific molecular markers is the mutation spectra in the human *p53* gene. Research studies have indicated that mutation of *p53* is involved in hepatocellular cancer in South Africa and China, and a high proportion of patients in these areas with high aflatoxin exposure have the characteristic G:C somatic mutation in codon 249 of the *p53* gene.[16,17]

Markers of Susceptibility

Epidemiological studies have demonstrated that 90–95% of malignant tumors are related to environmental and lifestyle factors, such as smoking, infectious agents, exogenous hormones, obesity, low physical activity, professional carcinogens, ultraviolet and ionizing radiation, and alcohol consumption. However, a particular exposure does not result in the same degree of risk in all individuals, suggesting that inter-individual variation in genetic susceptibility to disease exists in the general population. The most common markers of susceptibility are variations in specific genes that confer increased or decreased risk of human cancer. Until now, a great deal of interest has been devoted to the so-called "high-penetrance" susceptibility genes, that is, those with a high probability of cancer in mutation carriers, such as *p53*, *Rb*, *BRCA1* and *BRCA2*. High-penetrance mutations are usually identified by studying families at high risk of specific cancers or multiple cancer syndromes. Since the prevalence of such mutations in the population is rare, they account for only a small percentage of the general cancer risk.[18] In contrast, the situation is quite different in the case of the so-called "low-penetrance" genes, such as metabolic and DNA repair genes, in that a much lower proportion of carriers are diagnosed with cancer. Such genes are characterized by single nucleotide polymorphisms (SNPs) whose frequency in the healthy population may be high. Although the association between such polymorphisms and cancer is very low (typically <1.5-fold increased risk), their high frequency in the general population (typi­cally >5%) makes their major impact on the population attributable risk of cancer much greater.[19,20] Most of the gene polymorphisms identified through cancer epidemiology pertain to metabolic enzymes involved in phases I or II of chemical metabolism, DNA repair, inflammatory response, cell adhesion, or vascular growth.

In studies of molecular cancer epidemiology, many types of biospecimen can be collected and used to detect biomarkers that cover the whole range of biological materials, including DNA, RNA, proteins, lipids, cellular and tissue materials, biochemical building blocks of macromolecules, metabolites, hormones, markers of infections, inflammation, immune responses, as well as their modifications.[21] For example, blood can be stored as such or centrifuged to separate red blood cells (RBCs), plasma, serum, or buffy coat (i.e. white blood cells, WBCs). RBCs are a source of hemoglobin, which can be used for the measurement of adducts. The use of WBCs for the measurement of adducts will be described later in an example. WBCs in general are a source of DNA that can be used, for example, for the genotyping of subjects. Urine can be collected to measure metabolites or be centrifuged to collect exfoliated bladder cells (to measure DNA adducts for example). Buccal washes or swabs are another important source and are relatively easy to obtain in epidemiological studies. Furthermore, different samples may require different collection, storage and processing protocols in order to maintain stability. For example, at $-20°C$ urine is stable; at $-70°C$ DNA, serum, and most hormones, and most vitamins are stable, although cell viability (if not cryopreserved) is limited; at $-120°C$ hormones, carotenoids and other nutrients are stable.[22]

Although biomarkers can be used as meaningful and indispensable tools for investigation into environmental mutagenesis and cancer risk assessment, some challenges to epidemiological research still need to be addressed. First, most biomarker-based studies rely on only one biomarker to indicate exposure and to predict health problems, and this may be insufficient. This challenge can be better addressed by using several appropriate biomarkers that indicate exposure to specific mutagenic agents and the biological effects from such exposure on health risk. Using biomarkers that clearly represent biological events along the pathway from exposure to cancer may be especially helpful. Second, selection of tissues may affect the usefulness of biomarkers and the results of an investigation. Easily available surrogate cells, such as peripheral blood lymphocytes, are often used in assays instead of target cells such as lung and liver cells, but the major questions persist as to whether the biological events observed in surrogate cells also occur in target cells and whether the observed events predict cancer.[11] Third, external conditions, such as the duration of sample storage and freeze-thaw cycles, can alter levels of some biomarkers and reduce the accuracy of their assays. For instance, some biomarkers, such as levels of lipoprotein A, total and high-density lipoprotein cholesterol, free prostate-specific antigen, progesterone, estradiol, hepatitis virus C RNA concentrations, and salivary IgA, have been shown to change during sample storage. Likewise, studies have shown that cycles of freezing and thawing impact measures of lipoprotein A, anticardiolipin antibodies, endogenous antioxidants, hepatitis C viral RNA quantification, epidermal growth factor receptor, and tissue inhibitor of metalloproteinase-1.[23] Last, sample processing is one of most important steps for the test of biomarkers, which can produce a variety of banked specimens for future purposes. Efficient and effective processing ensures that the appropriate components of the samples can be retrieved after the storage and that the highest yield of those components is achieved.[24]

Studies have evaluated the effect of sample processing, shipment, and storage on the performance of conventional and nucleic acids-based tests and showed that optimal results depend on correct sample processing, minimal transport time and lowest possible storage and shipping temperatures. However, it is noteworthy that unfavorable conditions, such as increased temperatures, a weak infrastructure, and a shortage of adequately trained staff in many low- and middle-income countries, make it difficult to follow proper procedures for sample processing, shipping, and storage. Handling methods of biological samples from the time of collection to the analysis in low-resource settings can affect the quality of the specimens and the validity of the results of studies in low- and middle-income countries.

All these issues need be addressed in the standard process protocol and carried out through scientific quality assurance as an integral part of the successful molecular epidemiologic study in these countries.

▦ STUDY DESIGN AND RESEARCH METHODS

Molecular epidemiological studies often focus on exploring gene-environment interactions, and some of the methods of conventional epidemiology are commonly used. The two types of study use the same designs and require the same critical approach regarding selection or information bias, the comparability of groups that are recruited (cases and controls, exposed and unexposed), the presence of potential confounding, and statistical power. The nested case–control study design and special designs conceived for genetic epidemiology are frequently used. The following discussion will focus on two main study designs in molecular epidemiology: case-control study and cohort study.

The case-control study is often used to assess associations between disease and potential risk factors by taking separate samples of diseased cases and of disease-free controls. Information may be collected for both cases and controls on genetic, social, behavioral, environmental or other determinants of disease risk. Case-control studies can be hospital- or population-based depending on how cases are collected. The hospital-based case-control study is the most widely used method in molecular epidemiology, because the hospital setting makes it easy to get participants' agreement to provide biological specimens such as blood samples or fresh tumor tissue. Controls will also be much more receptive concerning their participation, since they are already in hospital. This design allows the efficient collection of a large number of samples in a relatively short period.[25] In contrast, population-based case-control studies attempt to identify all cases occurring in a predefined population during a particular time period, and controls are a random sample of the source population from which the cases arose. However, the disadvantage is that it is difficult to get population lists and to identify and enroll subjects.[26]

Although the speed and cost advantages of case-control methodology may have greatly contributed to identifying risk factors for cancer, some inherent biases in observational studies are still a challenge; these include confounding, selection bias, information bias, and lack of validity and precision of exposure and disease measures. Whilst it is possible to collect information on confounders, exposure assessment is usually a problem, particularly if retrospective collection of information for a long time preceding disease is needed. Furthermore, population stratification is a particularly important type of confounding in the era of the Human Genome Project and extensive studies of genes and disease may identify differences in allele frequencies between cases and controls that are due to systematic differences in ancestry rather than to true associations of genes with disease.[27]

Problems faced by case-control studies in low- and middle-income countries, which include small sample size and lack of power to show statistical significance, difficulties in control selection, and variations in accuracy of laboratorial methods, have at times resulted in inconclusive results and a lack of biological plausibility.[21] Many studies on genetic polymorphisms and cancer give conflicting results and need to be validated by larger studies in different populations. Meanwhile, the experimental error in some assays may be larger than many epidemiologists would expect. For example, for DNA adducts measured by P^{32}-postlabelling, the coefficient of variation is at least 30%.[28]

There are variations on the case-control study approach, such as the case-only study and the family-based case-control study. Case-only designs remove the control component from variance, and achieve the same statistical power as a study with a larger number of controls per case. A case-only study is a choice when the main objective is estimation of the joint effect or interaction of environment and genetic factors; however, one is unable to examine the separate effects of environmental exposure or genetic polymorphisms with this approach.[29] Family-based case-control studies have also been proposed to evaluate effects of gene polymorphisms on cancer; these use relatives, such as parents or siblings, as "matched controls." Families of a diseased member are recruited, and data on environmental exposures and biological samples are collected from all family members. The challenge is to collect individual data on gene polymorphisms and environmental exposures and other covariates on all family members in a sample size large enough to allow detection of interactions.[30]

Case-control studies are commonly used for molecular epidemiologic studies, but cohort studies are considered a more rigorous tool for making causal inferences in observational epidemiology.[31] In a cohort study, biological samples are collected from the cohort members at baseline and stored, and the individuals are then followed up over time for outcome regarding health, morbidity, and mortality. Cohort studies that succeed in achieving a high degree of adherence by participants can avoid the problems of misclassification of exposure status and the uncertain temporal relationship between biomarkers and disease risk that hamper traditional case-control studies. However, two main challenges in cohort studies are to define a well-established population exposed to an environmental carcinogen and to convince participants to provide biological samples. The small number of subjects who may agree to be involved in the study can induce selection bias, which might compromise the internal validity of the study and limit the generalization of the estimated associations.[25] Furthermore, some problems, such as the lengthy time and high expense, also limit the application of cohort studies in molecular epidemiology in low- and middle-income countries.

Two methodologically distinct cohort study designs, the case-cohort study and the nested case-control studies, offer logistic efficiency over a full cohort analyses and are typically used for molecular epidemiologic studies. In the case-cohort design, cases are sampled from all incident cases, as is done in conventional case-control studies; however, the controls are sampled from the initial cohort members (the population at risk at the start of the risk period) regardless of their future disease status.[32] This design allows accurate estimation of the risk ratio without the need for the rare-disease assumption. The major advantage of this design is that one reference group (controls), who are a random subset of the baseline cohort, can be used for comparison to multiple different case groups arising from the cohort. For the nested case-control design, cases of a disease that occur in a defined cohort are selected and a specified number of matched controls are selected from those in the cohort who have not developed the disease by the time of disease occurrence in the case.[33] The nested case-control design potentially offers impressive reductions in the cost and effort of data collection and analysis compared with the full cohort approach, and at the price of only a relatively minor loss in statistical efficiency. Another major advantage of the nested case-control design is the matching of controls to cases on follow-up duration between biological sample collection and disease development.[34]

▪ STUDY STRATEGY AND EXAMINATION ASSAYS

Rapid developments in biology and molecular technology have led to innovations in assay methods that are reshaping the field of molecular epidemiology in low- and middle-income countries. Assay methods of particular interest include:

1. Functional assays of susceptibility for early molecular epidemiology studies. Some functional assays are applied in early molecular epidemiologic studies to evaluate

susceptibility to carcinogenesis, such as the host-cell reactivation assay (measuring cellular ability to remove adducts from plasmids transfected into in vitro lymphocyte cultures by expression of damaged reporter genes), the mutagen sensitivity assay (evaluating the frequency of chromatid breaks induced by challenge mutagens in cultured lymphocytes in vitro as an integrated biomarker of mutagen sensitivity and an indirect measure of DRC), and Comet assay (measuring DNA breakage in single cells using a chemical or physical mutagen challenge.[35-37] Longitudinal evaluation of these functional assays, rather than cross-sectional analysis, is the ideal; however, this is difficult to achieve in practice, because repositories often do not have sequential samples that have been collected longitudinally from the same individuals, nor do they have prediagnostic samples collected in a way that ensures viability of the lymphocytes. In addition, we need to know how well these functional data (derived from surrogate lymphocytic tissue) reflect events at the level of the target tissue, and the issues of "inconsistence" or "reverse causality" are a constant challenge.[38]

2. Candidate gene association study (CGAS). Due to the relative simplicity of acquiring patient samples and genotype data, CGAS is the most common method for investigating associations between human genetic variations and the phenotypes they produce. This approach attempts to test a priori hypotheses that specific genes are associated with disease risk. Typically, the genes involved in the disease should be known from prior studies of pathophysiology, cancer biology, and other experimental or in vitro data.[39] Laboratory methods usually used in CGAS for known polymorphisms include gel electrophoresis-based genotyping methods, such as polymerase chain reaction (PCR), coupled with restriction fragment-length polymorphism analysis, allele-specific amplification, and oligonucleotide ligation. Because CGAS is a hypothesis-driven approach, it allows for targeted evaluation of selected alleles in study populations relevant to the hypothesis. Within the targeted candidate genes, this approach may confer inferential advantages in comparison with untargeted screening strategies such as genome-wide association studies, where coverage is spread across the whole genome and typically does not specifically target functional SNPs.[39] However, some issues in selecting SNPs to evaluate in CGAS cannot be ignored. First, many genes are probably involved in the development of complex diseases, including cancer, but the functions of some genes may not have been well characterized, thus precluding their investigation. Second, many early candidate gene studies were underpowered because of small samples or other study design issues. Initial positive findings were rarely replicated in subsequent larger scale studies. It has been reported that only 10% of published research papers investigating SNPs in relation to cancer risk have been validated by further study.[40] Third, the effects of candidate genes are moderate and often depend upon interactions among the risk alleles of several genes in a pathway or with other environmental risk factors; however gene–gene and gene–environmental interactions remain a challenge for researchers.[41]

3. Genome-wide association study (GWAS). With the advances in high-throughput technology and genome-wide association methods, the genome-wide association study (GWAS) has become a powerful tool for investigating the genetic basis of common diseases. The principle is to genotype a number of common genetic variants that are spaced across the genome and can act as proxies for ungenotyped variants, due to coinheritance of neighboring variants on a chromosomal segment.[42] This approach moves beyond known genes in known pathways to identify unanticipated genes that contribute to risk. Several commercial products are available from some companies, such as Affymetrix and Illumina, that offer the potential to assay hundreds of thousands of SNPs simultaneously genome-wide.[43] According to the National Human Genome Research Institute, about 950 articles of

GWAS have been published until June 2011, which reported over 4 thousands of genetic SNPs or loci associated with more than 200 diseases or traits in human, including diabetes, hypertension and cancer, etc., physiological indicators such as body mass index (BMI) and blood lipid levels, physiological traits such as height and hair color, as well as behaviors such as smoking addiction (www.genome.gov/gwastudies). Just in the first five months of 2007, a wave of GWAS emerged and covered four genome-wide scans for Type 2 Diabetes loci,[44-47] three scans for breast cancer loci,[48-50] three scans for Crohn disease,[51-53] and scans for prostate cancer[54,55] and cardiovascular disease.[56] These studies have not only replicated previously known associations (e.g., TCF7L2 for Type 2 Diabetes), but also found novel trait loci. Finding important variants of GWAS is essential for understanding the biological processes underlying cancer pathogenesis, improving predictive models of cancer risk, offering hints for developing new treatments and identifying modifiable nongenetic exposures. The achievements are mainly due to the relatively large study sample sizes for screening, multi-stage designs and well-performed replications, stringent statistical significance levels (usually $< 10^{-7}$) to limit false positive results, robust genotyping platforms, and quality control of the data. However, despite the celebrated achievements, only a small proportion of genetic heritability can be explained by the GWAS findings and thus there are many concerns on GWAS that are being debated. One of the most daunting is the difficulty moving from identification of statistical associations to elucidating the functional basis of the link between a genomic region and the trait of interest.[57] Meanwhile, GWA studies identify loci, but not specific genes, and identification of actual causative loci will require deep resequencing methods and fine mapping approaches.

Accumulative evidence have highlighted that ethnic heterogeneity of disease susceptibility may be substantial, and it is necessary to carry out more GWAS in multiple populations. However, in the past 5 years, the success of GWAS is not equally enjoyed by all the populations and countries, with the majority of GWAS being performed in Caucasian populations. The achievements of GWAS from Caucasian populations can provide the theoretical foundation for related studies and thus foster development of molecular epidemiology in low- and middle-income countries. Furthermore, extending analyses to samples from populations with differing mutational and demographical histories, such as populations from some low- and middle-income countries in Asia, Africa, and Latin America, can offer new opportunities to detect additional susceptibility loci,[58] to generate ethnic specific patterns of cancer markers[59] and to identify other genetic or environmental factors with which they might interact.

Although few GWA studies have been conducted in low- and middle-income countries because of the challenges posed by high costs and the need for sophisticated technology, the past two years did witness dramatically accelerated activities of GWAS in low- and middle-income countries including China. For example, a number of GWAS relevant to common cancers, such as lung cancer,[60] gastric cancer,[61] breast cancer,[58] esophageal cancer,[62,63] hepatocellular carcinoma,[64] nasopharyngeal darcinoma,[65] and pancreatic cancer,[63] have been completed in Chinese population, which not only discover novel loci, but also provide the valuable data for transethnic comparative studies.

■ PROGRESS OF CANCER MOLECULAR EPIDEMIOLOGY

Thus far, considerable progress has been made in the validation and application of biomarkers that are directly related to carcinogenesis progress. Molecular epidemiology has become a major field of cancer research and has provided evidence related to inter-individual variation in human cancer risk, gene-environment interactions, and host susceptibility factors in the multistage process of carcinogenesis.

▓ INVESTIGATION OF GENE-ENVIRONMENT AND GENE-GENE INTERACTION

Although the majority of cancer epidemiology studies focus on associations with exposure to potential causative "environmental agents" or disease outcome, the interaction between environmental agents and genetic factors has become a hot point of research, not only in high-income counties but in low- and middle-income countries as well. Many cancers have a complex etiology, where one or more environmental risk factors interact with genetic background, age, sex, sociodemographic status and other factors. As we know, not all smokers get lung cancer and not all women with an inherited BRCA1 and BRCA2 mutation develop breast cancer. Some studies from China have investigated gene-environment interactions in a various of cancers and demonstrated new findings, such as significant interactions between WRN leu1074Phe and age at menarche in breast cancer,[66] CYP1B1 1294G allele and cigarette smoking in colorectal cancer,[67] polymorphisms of IL-12A and IL-12B and parity in cervical cancer,[68] and RsaI polymorphism of CYP2E1 and ever-smoking in stomach cancer.[69] In addition, there are other studies focusing on gene–gene, and gene–gene–environment interactions as well as gene–hormone–environment interaction, etc. All these studies will help improve our understanding of cancer etiology.

▓ THE DISCOVERY OF NOVEL MARKERS FOR MOLECULAR CANCER EPIDEMIOLOGY

Recently, with development of high-throughput technologies and theoretical advances in biology, several new and exciting biomarkers have become available for epidemiologic studies. Panels that incorporated different kinds of biomarkers, from blood cells, exfoliated cells, tissues and body fluids, have been widely used in epidemiological studies to improve our knowledge of the causes of specific human cancers.[70] In 2005, a study in Nature indicated that miRNA profiling can separate tumor and nontumor tissues, and the profiles are tumor-specific.[71] It was also found that the information gained from miRNA profiling might provide more accurate classification of cancer subtypes than using the expression profiles of proteins. From then on, more studies focusing on miRNAs profiling in different cancer tissues emerged. Two research groups, from the USA and China, respectively, reported that miRNAs exist in blood circulation stably and can serve as blood-based markers for cancer detection, a finding that showed great promise of a novel noninvasive biomarker for diagnosis of cancer and other diseases.[72,73]

▓ THE ETHNIC DIFFERENCE OF GENETIC SUSCEPTIBILITY OF COMMON CANCERS

With the emergence of more and more molecular epidemiological studies in low- and middle income countries, ethnic differences in genetic susceptibility of common cancers have become a special issue. Although polymorphisms in susceptibility genes are diffuse in the healthy population, their frequency varies with ethnicity. Variation in genotype frequencies across diverse populations may affect the number of individuals at increased risk for a disease, and population substructure imbalances may create spurious differences in genotype frequencies of the compared groups in gene-disease association studies.[74] For example, polymorphisms of the *CYP1A1* gene are more frequent in subjects of Asian descent than in Caucasians, whilst a special *CYP1A1* polymorphism is only found in subjects in African descent.[75] A study in a Chinese population investigated variations within *CASP8* and found a six-nucleotide deletion within the *CASP8* promoter (-652 6N Ins/Del, rs3834129) that is associated with decreased risk for different cancers, including cancer of the breast.[76] Further analysis demonstrated that this SNP -652 6N Ins/Del polymorphism exhibited considerable heterozygosity in multiple ethnic groups; frequencies of the 6N del allele are 50% in sub-Saharan Africans, 60% in individuals of European ancestry, 40.9% in Hispanics, and 21.7% in Asians.[76] These reports have suggested that ancestry influences the impact of gene variants on disease risk. Therefore, molecular epidemiological studies conducted in low- and middle-income countries that contain populations of different ancestry may help find special genetic markers of diseases for a special population and may enhance measures to control diseases in these countries.

■ CHALLENGES AND OPPORTUNITIES

Economic improvement and advances in biotechnology provide new opportunities for molecular epidemiologic studies in low- and middle-income countries; however, many challenges still must be addressed and resolved.

■ TRAINING IN MOLECULAR EPIDEMIOLOGY

Molecular epidemiology research capabilities must be strengthened in low- and middle-countries, and researchers in these countries must be properly trained to allow cancer research programs of molecular epidemiology to develop. This can be achieved, in part, through collaborative research, which not only allows scientists in low- and middle-income countries to learn new research skills, but also allows scientists from high-income nations to better understand local scientific capabilities and customs. It is also important to develop programs to train new molecular epidemiologists in low- and middle-income countries and regions, improve the interactions between scientists from low- and middle-income countries and high-income countries, and support education programs for mid-career scientists of low- and middle-income countries. Luckily, with the help of high-income countries, some plans have been made to supply regional training courses in molecular epidemiology. For example, an International Molecular Epidemiology Task Force was established in 1993 with the mission to facilitate the development and implementation of programs in molecular epidemiology in all regions of the world and to promote advanced biotechnology transfer for scientific research and its integration into epidemiology, medicine and public health for disease prevention. In 1993, a molecular genetics course was held in Mexico and included lectures on molecular epidemiology and its applications. Full training courses in molecular epidemiology, which included laboratory experiments and instruction in basic epidemiologic methods, were held in Saudi Arabia and China in 1994. At present, the research capabilities of molecular epidemiology in low- and middle-income countries have been improved to a certain degree; however, training is still necessary for the reason that a big gap in molecular epidemiology research still exists between high-income and low- and middle-income countries.

■ FAIR AND EFFECTIVE COLLABORATIONS

The success of epidemiology research in low- and middle-income countries also depends on fostering fair and effective collaborations between investigators from high-income and low- and middle-income countries. It is important for investigators to transfer knowledge and scientific skills to scientists of collaborating low- and middle-income countries whenever possible. Equitable credit should also be negotiated and given to both sets of researchers in the form of shared authorships and presentations at international scientific conferences. Such international efforts require the development and implementation of standards, which can be applied across populations to assure that accurate comparisons can be made.[77] Recently, collaborative large-scale studies have increased in several centers and countries, thereby providing good opportunities for the development of molecular epidemiology in low- and idle-income countries.

▦ ETHICAL ISSUES

Epidemiologic ethics focus on the research-related issues of informed consent, balancing of risks and benefits, protection of privacy, data storage and handling, data sharing, and conduct of research. These are issues that have been regulated by the National Research Act of 1974 and more recently by the Health Insurance Portability and Accountability Act (HIPAA), and that have been addressed in ethical guidelines put forth by the American College of Epidemiology (http://www.acepidemiology.org/policystmts/Ethics-Guide.htm).[77] Some problems of ethics in molecular cancer epidemiology have been encountered in low- and middle-income countries. One of the most difficult questions concerns informed consent, which includes two important principles: understanding and autonomy. For understanding, the information should be given in clear and understandable language fit for the age and education of the target group. Autonomy of a person requires a voluntary consent for a specific study. Many authors regard the right of people to decide what their tissue and DNA is used for as an important one,[79,80] and it is important to retain the right for study participants to withdraw their consent. However, some studies in low- and middle-income countries have been performed without informed consent or any overview by ethical committees—either these committees were never fully established, or the subjects were uninformed of their rights and therefore were coerced into study participation.[77] Data and samples have also been collected from people without consent of the government or local scientists. However, it is very important for scientists to follow international ethical regulations when conducting population-based studies, not only because it is necessary to allow researchers from low- and middle-income countries to obtain recognition for contributions, but also because failure to follow these regulations can prevent subjects from participating in future studies. Complete transparency, involving explanations of research protocols and objectives, can help address this issue in low- and middle-income countries.

▦ SUMMARY

In this chapter, we introduce the development and application of molecular epidemiology in low- and middle-income countries and provide an overview of the opportunities and challenges in future. Low- and middle-income countries are carrying a disproportionate share of the global disease burden, but most of them are lack of the technology, resources, and capacity to participate in researches of molecular epidemiology. In the genomics era, some low- and middle-income countries begin to reevaluate their role in molecular epidemiology research and explore the unique opportunities that arise from the vast natural and genomic diversity that they embody. Although some great progresses have been achieved in these countries, such as China, making substantial contributions to our understanding of disease etiology, there are still many challenges and problems for the development of molecular epidemiology in low- and middle-income countries. Increased communication and collaboration between all epidemiologists—regardless of national income—is an excellent first step to increase the capacities of low- and middle-income countries to control disease.

■ REFERENCES

1. Doll R, Hill AB. Smoking and carcinoma of the lung; preliminary report. *Br Med J*. 1950;2(4682): 739–748.
2. Wynder EL, Graham EA. Landmark article may 27, 1950: Tobacco smoking as a possible etiologic factor in bronchiogenic carcinoma. A study of six hundred and eighty-four proved cases. *JAMA*. 1985;253(20):2986–2994.
3. Kilbourne ED. The molecular epidemiology of influenza. *J Infect Dis*. 1973;127(4):478–487.
4. Schulte PA, Perera FP. *Molecular epidemiology: Principles and practices*. San Diego: Academic Press; 1993:xx, 588 p.
5. Dorman J. Molecular epidemiology and DNA technology transfer: A program for developing countries. In: Dorman J, ed. *Standardization of epidemiological studies of host susceptibility*. New York: Plenum Press; 1994:241, 251 p.
6. Albertini RJ. Mechanistic insights from biomarker studies: Somatic mutations and rodent/human comparisons following exposure to a potential carcinogen. *IARC Sci Publ*. 2004;(157)(157):153–177.
7. Parkin DM, Pisani P, Lopez AD, Masuyer E. At least one in seven cases of cancer is caused by smoking. Global estimates for 1985. *Int J Cancer*. 1994;59(4):494–504.
8. Savas S, Liu G. Genetic variations as cancer prognostic markers: Review and update. *Hum Mutat*. 2009;30(10):1369–1377.
9. Li G, Yin S. Progress of epidemiological and molecular epidemiological studies on benzene in China. *Ann N Y Acad Sci*. 2006;1076:800–809.
10. Perera FP, Weinstein IB. Molecular epidemiology and carcinogen-DNA adduct detection: New approaches to studies of human cancer causation. *J Chronic Dis*. 1982;35(7):581–600.
11. Au WW. Usefulness of biomarkers in population studies: From exposure to susceptibility and to prediction of cancer. *Int J Hyg Environ Health*. 2007;210(3–4):239–246.
12. Wild CP. Environmental exposure measurement in cancer epidemiology. *Mutagenesis*. 2009;24(2): 117–125.
13. Poirier MC. Chemical-induced DNA damage and human cancer risk. *Nat Rev Cancer*. 2004;4(8): 630–637.
14. Santella RM. DNA damage as an intermediate biomarker in intervention studies. *Proc Soc Exp Biol Med*. 1997;216(2):166–171.
15. Boffetta P. Biomarkers in cancer epidemiology: An integrative approach. *Carcinogenesis*. 2010;31(1): 121–126.
16. Bressac B, Kew M, Wands J, Ozturk M. Selective G to T mutations of p53 gene in hepatocellular carcinoma from southern Africa. *Nature*. 1991;350(6317):429–431.
17. Hsu IC, Metcalf RA, Sun T, Welsh JA, Wang NJ, Harris CC. Mutational hotspot in the p53 gene in human hepatocellular carcinomas. *Nature*. 1991;350(6317):427–428.
18. Narod SA, Foulkes WD. BRCA1 and BRCA2: 1994 and beyond. *Nat Rev Cancer*. 2004;4(9):665–676.
19. Ponder BAJ. Cancer genetics. *Nature*. 2001;411(6835):336–341.
20. Taioli E. Biomarkers of genetic susceptibility to cancer: Applications to epidemiological studies. *Future Oncol*. 2005;1(1):51–56.
21. Wild C, Vineis P, Garte SJ, Wiley online library. *Molecular epidemiology of chronic diseases*. Chichester, England; Hoboken, NJ: J. Wiley; 2008:xiv, 368 p.
22. Ahrens W, Pigeot I, SpringerLink (Online service). *Handbook of epidemiology*. Berlin, Heidelberg: Springer-Verlag Berlin Heidelberg; 2005.
23. Rundle AG, Vineis P, Ahsan H. Design options for molecular epidemiology research within cohort studies. *Cancer epidemiology, biomarkers & prevention: a publication of the American Association for Cancer Research, cosponsored by the American Society of Preventive Oncology*. 2005;14(8):1899.

24. Holland NT, Smith MT, Eskenazi B, Bastaki M. Biological sample collection and processing for molecular epidemiological studies. *Mutat Res.* 2003;543(3):217–234.

25. Wunsch Filho V, Zago MA. Modern cancer epidemiological research: Genetic polymorphisms and environment. *Rev Saude Publica.* 2005;39(3):490–497.

26. Rebbeck TR, Ambrosone CB, Shields PG. *Molecular epidemiology: Applications in cancer and other human diseases.* New York: Informa Healthcare; 2008:xi, 302 p.

27. Freedman ML, Reich D, Penney KL, et al. Assessing the impact of population stratification on genetic association studies. *Nat Genet.* 2004;36(4):388–393.

28. Phillips DH, Castegnaro M. Standardization and validation of DNA adduct postlabelling methods: Report of interlaboratory trials and production of recommended protocols. *Mutagenesis.* 1999;14(3):301–315.

29. Brennan P. Gene-environment interaction and aetiology of cancer: What does it mean and how can we measure it? *Carcinogenesis.* 2002;23(3):381–387.

30. Goldstein AM, Andrieu N. Detection of interaction involving identified genes: Available study designs. *J Natl Cancer Inst Monogr.* 1999;(26)(26):49–54.

31. Greenland S. Interpreting time-related trends in effect estimates. *J Chronic Dis.* 1987;40 Suppl 2:17S–24S.

32. Sato T. Risk ratio estimation in case-cohort studies. *Environ Health Perspect.* 1994;102 Suppl 8:53–56.

33. Langholz B, Thomas DC. Nested case-control and case-cohort methods of sampling from a cohort: A critical comparison. *Am J Epidemiol.* 1990;131(1):169–176.

34. Ernster VL. Nested case-control studies. *Prev Med.* 1994;23(5):587–590.

35. Singh NP, Danner DB, Tice RR, Brant L, Schneider EL. DNA damage and repair with age in individual human lymphocytes. *Mutat Res.* 1990;237(3–4):123–130.

36. Hsu TC, Johnston DA, Cherry LM, et al. Sensitivity to genotoxic effects of bleomycin in humans: Possible relationship to environmental carcinogenesis. *Int J Cancer.* 1989;43(3):403–409.

37. Athas WF, Hedayati MA, Matanoski GM, Farmer ER, Grossman L. Development and field-test validation of an assay for DNA repair in circulating human lymphocytes. *Cancer Res.* 1991;51(21):5786–5793.

38. Spitz MR, Bondy ML. The evolving discipline of molecular epidemiology of cancer. *Carcinogenesis.* 2010;31(1):127–134.

39. Jorgensen TJ, Ruczinski I, Kessing B, Smith MW, Shugart YY, Alberg AJ. Hypothesis-driven candidate gene association studies: Practical design and analytical considerations. *Am J Epidemiol.* 2009;170(8): 986–993.

40. Schmidt C. SNPs not living up to promise; experts suggest new approach to disease ID. *Journal of the National Cancer Institute.* February 7, 2007;99(3):188–189.

41. Kraft P, Raychaudhuri S. Complex diseases, complex genes: Keeping pathways on the right track. *Epidemiology.* 2009;20(4):508–511.

42. Manolio TA. Collaborative genome-wide association studies of diverse diseases: Programs of the NHGRI's office of population genomics. *Pharmacogenomics.* 2009;10(2):235–241.

43. Ragoussis J. Genotyping technologies for genetic research. *Annu Rev Genomics Hum Genet.* 2009;10: 117–133.

44. Diabetes Genetics Initiative of Broad Institute of Harvard and MIT, Lund University, and Novartis Institutes of BioMedical Research, Saxena R, Voight BF, et al. Genome-wide association analysis identifies loci for type 2 diabetes and triglyceride levels. *Science.* 2007;316(5829):1331–1336.

45. Scott LJ, Mohlke KL, Bonnycastle LL, et al. A genome-wide association study of type 2 diabetes in Finns detects multiple susceptibility variants. *Science.* 2007;316(5829):1341–1345.

46. Sanghera DK, Ortega L, Han S, et al. Impact of nine common type 2 diabetes risk polymorphisms in Asian Indian Sikhs: PPARG2 (Pro12Ala), IGF2BP2, TCF7L2 and FTO variants confer a significant risk. *BMC Med Genet.* 2008;9:59.

47. Zeggini E, Weedon MN, Lindgren CM, et al. Replication of genome-wide association signals in UK samples reveals risk loci for type 2 diabetes. *Science.* 2007;316(5829):1336–1341.

48. Easton DF, Pooley KA, Dunning AM, et al. Genome-wide association study identifies novel breast cancer susceptibility loci. *Nature.* 2007;447(7148):1087–1093.

49. Hunter DJ, Kraft P, Jacobs KB, et al. A genome-wide association study identifies alleles in FGFR2 associated with risk of sporadic postmenopausal breast cancer. *Nat Genet.* 2007;39(7):870.

50. Stacey SN, Manolescu A, Sulem P, et al. Common variants on chromosomes 2q35 and 16q12 confer susceptibility to estrogen receptor-positive breast cancer. *Nat Genet.* 2007;39(7):865.

51. Hampe J, Franke A, Rosenstiel P, et al. A genome-wide association scan of nonsynonymous SNPs identifies a susceptibility variant for crohn disease in ATG16L1. *Nat Genet.* 2007;39(2):207.

52. Libioulle C, Louis E, Hansoul S, et al. Novel crohn disease locus identified by genome-wide association maps to a gene desert on 5p13.1 and modulates expression of PTGER4. *PLoS Genet.* 2007;3(4):e58.

53. Rioux JD, Xavier RJ, Taylor KD, et al. Genome-wide association study identifies new susceptibility loci for crohn disease and implicates autophagy in disease pathogenesis. *Nat Genet.* 2007;39(5):596–604.

54. Gudmundsson J, Sulem P, Steinthorsdottir V, et al. Two variants on chromosome 17 confer prostate cancer risk, and the one in TCF2 protects against type 2 diabetes. *Nat Genet.* 2007;39(8):977–983.

55. Yeager M, Orr N, Hayes RB, et al. Genome-wide association study of prostate cancer identifies a second risk locus at 8q24. *Nat Genet.* 2007;39(5):645–649.

56. McPherson R, Pertsemlidis A, Kavaslar N, et al. A common allele on chromosome 9 associated with coronary heart disease. *Obstet Gynecol Surv.* 2007;62(9):584.

57. Frazer KA, Murray SS, Schork NJ, Topol EJ. Human genetic variation and its contribution to complex traits. *Nat Rev Genet.* 2009;10(4):241–251.

58. Zheng W, Long J, Gao YT, et al. Genome-wide association study identifies a new breast cancer susceptibility locus at 6q25.1. *Nat Genet.* 2009;41(3):324–328.

59. Wu C, Hu Z, Yu D, et al. Genetic variants on chromosome 15q25 associated with lung cancer risk in Chinese populations. *Cancer Res.* 2009;69(12):5065–5072.

60. Hu Z, Wu C, Shi Y, et al. A genome-wide association study identifies two new lung cancer susceptibility loci at 13q12.12 and 22q12.2 in Han Chinese. *Nat Genet.* 2011;43(8):792–796.

61. Shi Y, Hu Z, Wu C, et al. A genome-wide association study identifies new susceptibility loci for non-cardia gastric cancer at 3q13.31 and 5p13.1. *Nat Genet.* 2011;43(12):1215–1218.

62. Wang LD, Zhou FY, Li XM, et al. Genome-wide association study of esophageal squamous cell carcinoma in Chinese subjects identifies susceptibility loci at PLCE1 and C20orf54. *Nat Genet.* 2010;42(9):759–763.

63. Wu C, Hu Z, He Z, et al. Genome-wide association study identifies three new susceptibility loci for esophageal squamous-cell carcinoma in Chinese populations. *Nat Genet.* 2011;43(7):679–684.

64. Zhang H, Zhai Y, Hu Z, et al. Genome-wide association study identifies 1p36.22 as a new susceptibility locus for hepatocellular carcinoma in chronic hepatitis B virus carriers. *Nat Genet.* 2010;42(9):755–758.

65. Bei JX, Li Y, Jia WH, et al. A genome-wide association study of nasopharyngeal carcinoma identifies three new susceptibility loci. *Nat Genet.* 2010;42(7):599–603.

66. Wang Z, Xu Y, Tang J, et al. A polymorphism in Werner syndrome gene is associated with breast cancer susceptibility in Chinese women. *Breast Cancer Res Treat.* 2009;118(1):169–175.

67. Fan C, Jin M, Chen K, Zhang Y, Zhang S, Liu B. Case-only study of interactions between metabolic enzymes and smoking in colorectal cancer. *BMC Cancer.* 2007;7:115.

68. Chen X, Han S, Wang S, et al. Interactions of IL-12A and IL-12B polymorphisms on the risk of cervical cancer in Chinese women. *Clin Cancer Res.* 2009;15(1):400–405.

69. Gao C, Takezaki T, Wu J, et al. Interaction between cytochrome P-450 2E1 polymorphisms and environmental factors with risk of esophageal and stomach cancers in Chinese. *Cancer Epidemiol Biomarkers Prev.* 2002;11(1):29–34.

70. Perera FP, Weinstein IB. Molecular epidemiology: Recent advances and future directions. *Carcinogenesis.* 2000;21(3):517–524.

71. Lu J, Getz G, Miska EA, et al. MicroRNA expression profiles classify human cancers. *Nature.* 2005;435(7043):834–838.

72. Mitchell PS, Parkin RK, Kroh EM, et al. Circulating microRNAs as stable blood-based markers for cancer detection. *Proc Natl Acad Sci U S A.* 2008;105(30):10513–10518.

73. Chen X, Ba Y, Ma L, et al. Characterization of microRNAs in serum: A novel class of biomarkers for diagnosis of cancer and other diseases. *Cell Res.* 2008;18(10):997–1006.

74. Thomas DC, Witte JS. Point: Population stratification: A problem for case-control studies of candidate-gene associations? *Cancer epidemiology, biomarkers & prevention: a publication of the American Association for Cancer Research, cosponsored by the American Society of Preventive Oncology.* 2002;11(6):505.

75. Taioli E, Crofts F, Trachman J, Demopoulos R, Toniolo P, Garte SJ. A specific African-American CYP1A1 polymorphism is associated with adenocarcinoma of the lung. *Cancer Res.* 1995;55(3):472–473.

76. Sun T, Gao Y, Tan W, et al. A six-nucleotide insertion-deletion polymorphism in the CASP8 promoter is associated with susceptibility to multiple cancers. *Nat Genet.* 2007;39(5):605–613.

77. Rastogi T, Hildesheim A, Sinha R. Opportunities for cancer epidemiology in developing countries. *Nat Rev Cancer.* 2004;4(11):909–917.

78. Foxman B, 2002 Epidemiology Society Leadership Group. Challenges of epidemiology in the 21st century: Comments from the leaders of several epidemiology associations. *Ann Epidemiol.* 2005;15(1):1–4.

79. Andrews LB. Harnessing the benefits of biobanks. *J Law Med Ethics.* 2005;33(1):22–30.

80. Trouet C. New European guidelines for the use of stored human biological materials in biomedical research. *J Med Ethics.* 2004;30(1):99–103.

CHAPTER 11

METHODOLOGICAL ISSUES IN INTERNATIONAL MULTICENTRIC STUDIES, INCLUDING THE ROLE OF CONSORTIA IN INTERNATIONAL CANCER EPIDEMIOLOGY

FARHAD ISLAMI AND PAOLO BOFFETTA

IMPORTANCE OF CANCER RESEARCH IN LOW- AND MEDIUM-RESOURCE COUNTRIES

Conducting cancer studies in low- and medium-resource countries is important for several reasons, including the following:

1. Low- and medium-resource countries consist of the majority of the world's population. It has been estimated that more than half of 12.4 million incident cases and two third of 7.6 million cancer deaths worldwide in 2008 occurred in low- and medium-resource countries.[1] The age structure of the population in most of low- and medium resource countries shows a large proportion of young people. In many those countries, improvement in sanitation has reduced the incidence of infection-related health outcomes, and life expectancy at birth has dramatically increased in the recent decades.[1] Therefore, we can expect a rapid increase in the number of elderly people in those countries in next few decades, and consequently, a substantial increase in the number of new cancer cases, as cancer is more common among the elderly.

2. In order to conduct efficient cancer prevention and control programs, information on patterns of cancer incidence and major etiologic factors of cancers is required. As a result of more limited resources in many of low- and medium-resource countries, appropriate diagnostic and therapeutic facilities may not be easily accessible for the majority of the population; this increases the importance of cancer prevention in those countries. Nevertheless, limited information on cancer epidemiology and risk factors is available from a substantial number of low- and medium-resource countries. Although the risk factors that have been identified in high-resource countries will also be carcinogenic in other areas, the magnitude of association and distribution of risk factors/cofactors may be considerably varied. For

example, heavy alcohol drinking is one of major risk factors of esophageal squamous cell carcinoma in low-incidence areas, but only very small proportion of the cancer cases has been attributed to alcohol drinking in high-incidence areas of China and Iran.[2,3] For hepato-cellular carcinoma, hepatitis virus C is a more prominent risk factor in western world, while hepatitis virus B is more important in low- to medium-source countries[4]. Furthermore, exposure to aflatoxin is more common in certain low- and medium-resource countries, while alcoholic cirrhosis and nonalcoholic fatty liver disease is more prevalent in western populations.[4] Cancer studies in low- and medium-resource countries not only can be help-ful in identifying major risk factors of cancers but also permit examination of previously known associations in various populations.

3. Many populations in low- and medium resource countries experience fairly rapid transitions in lifestyle.[5,6] The newly emerging problems in those populations, such as low physical activity, obesity, and tobacco epidemic, may rapidly increase the occurrence of cancer.[5-7] The use of tobacco, a major risk factor for several cancers, in low- and medium resource countries has increased rapidly during the past few decades.[6] Carcinogenic effects of tobacco usually appear clinically after several years. With aging of the currently young/middle-aged smoking populations in low- and medium-resource countries, the burden of tobacco-related cancers is estimated to increase considerably in near future. Such a trend may also be observed with several other potential risk factors of cancer, such as overweight. As an example, tobacco smoking has already become a major risk factor for mortality in China.[7] It has been estimated that by 2030, more than 80% of tobacco deaths will be in developing countries.[8]

▪ IMPORTANCE OF INTERNATIONAL MULTICENTER CANCER STUDIES

In order to obtain sufficient study power to investigate etiologic factors of cancer appropri-ately, having proper study size is an essential issue. With low study power, the results could be misleading. In particular, investigation of interactions between two or more risk factors usually needs large sample sizes. Providing resources to conduct large studies by a single research center, particularly in low- and medium-resource countries, can be challenging. This can be particularly difficult with regard to cohort studies, because population-based cohort studies are usually need a large sample size and long-term follow-up. The number of available cancer cases in a specific time period may be another problem. In case of rare can-cers, it may take a long time to recruit sufficient number of cases in one study center/area.

Conducting collaborative multicenter studies is one of the effective ways to overcome such problems. Researchers can collect research material in several centers. By sharing the material, a big sample size can be achieved. Furthermore, researchers can share their expe-rience in design and conduct of studies, which can be helpful in improving the quality of research. As discussed earlier, international multicenter studies can permit researchers to investigate their study hypotheses, as well as heterogeneity in the associations, in differ-ent populations. International research institution may also be more interested in getting involved in well-designed collaborative studies, rather than in small- to moderate-sized single center studies. Similarly, collaborative studies may be more likely to receive local or international resources.

Table 11.1 lists several international collaborative studies that have been conducted in at least three countries and have some publications indexed in the PubMed database, excluding the studies on treatment only (treatment trials). Some studies are overlapped; for example, an international study on several cancers in eastern and central Europe[9] is also included in other epidemiologic and genetic studies.[10,11] Although the list may not be

TABLE 11.1 International studies on cancer epidemiology and etiology‡

NAME OF STUDY	DESIGN	CANCER SITE/TYPE*	COUNTRY
MULTIPLE ORGANS			
IARC Central and Eastern Europe Study[9,12]	CCS	Lung, oral cavity, pharynx, larynx, esophagus, and kidney	Czech Republic, Hungary, Poland, Romania, Russia, Slovenia, and United Kingdom
European study on risk factors for rare cancers of unknown etiology[13]	CCS	Gall bladder, extrahepatic bile ducts, small intestine, bone, male breast, eye melanoma, and mycosis fungoides	Denmark, France, Germany, Italy, Latvia, Portugal, Spain, Sweden, and United Kingdom
Asia Pacific Cohort Studies Collaboration (APCSC)[14]	Cohort	Multiple	Australia, China, Hong Kong, Japan, New Zealand, Singapore, South Korea, Taiwan, and Thailand
European Prospective Investigation into Cancer and Nutrition study (EPIC)[15]	Cohort	Multiple	Denmark, France, Germany, Greece, Italy, Netherlands, Spain, Sweden, and United Kingdom
Cohort Consortium Vitamin D Pooling Project of Rarer Cancers[16]	Nested CCS	Multiple	China, Finland, and United States
A study on clinical epidemiology of childhood cancer in Central America and Caribbean countries[17]	CCS	Multiple	Costa Rica, Cuba, Dominican Republic, El Salvador, Guatemala, Honduras, and Nicaragua
The International Childhood Cancer Cohort Consortium (I4C)[18]	Cohort	Multiple	Australia, China, Denmark, France, Israel, Norway, Spain, United Kingdom, and United States
European study on cancer mortality among welders[19]	Cohort	Multiple	Denmark, England, Finland, France, Germany, Italy, Norway, Scotland, and Sweden
An international study on cancer mortality in workers exposed to chlorophenoxy herbicides and chlorophenols[20]	Cohort	Multiple	Australia, Canada, Denmark, Finland, Italy, Netherlands, New Zealand, Sweden, and United Kingdom
European study on cancer mortality in workers exposed to styrene in rubber and plastics industry[21]	Cohort	Multiple	Denmark, Finland, Italy, Norway, Sweden, and United Kingdom

Study	Study type	Cancer type	Countries
European study on workers employed in the vinyl chloride industry[22]	Cohort	Multiple	Italy, Norway, Sweden, and United Kingdom
IARC multicenter study on silica workers[23]	Cohort	Multiple	Australia, China, Finland, South Africa, and United States
An international study on workers exposed to phenoxy herbicides, chlorophenols, and dioxins[24]	Cohort	Multiple	Australia, Canada, Denmark, Finland, Germany, Italy, Netherlands, New Zealand, Sweden, United Kingdom, and United States
IARC-coordinated European cohort study among asphalt workers[25]	Cohort	Multiple	Denmark, Finland, France, Germany, Israel, Netherlands, and Norway
An international study on cancer risk among radiation workers in the nuclear industry[26]	Cohort	Multiple	Australia, Belgium, Canada, Finland, France, Hungry, Japan, South Korea, Lithuania, Slovak Republic, Spain, Sweden, Switzerland, United Kingdom, and Unites States
International consortium for research on the health effects of radiation[27]	CCS	Childhood leukemia and thyroid cancer	Belarus, Russia, and Ukraine
European study on occupational exposures and cytogenetic changes and chromosomal aberrations in relation to cancer[28]	Cohort	Multiple	Denmark, Finland, Italy, Norway, and Sweden
An international study on secondary cancers[29]	CCS	Multiple	Australia, Canada, Denmark, Finland, Iceland, Norway, Scotland, Singapore, Slovenia, Sweden, and Spain
Breast Cancer Linkage Consortium (BCLC)[30]	Cohort	Multiple (in breast or ovarian cancer families with BRCA2)	Canada, Finland, France, Germany, Iceland, Netherlands, Spain, Sweden, Switzerland, United Kingdom, and United States
European Network of Genetic and Genomic Epidemiology (ENGAGE Consortium)[31]	Cohort	Multiple	Australia, Canada, Estonia, Finland, Germany, Iceland, Latvia, Netherlands, Norway, Spain, Sweden, and United Kingdom
A multicenter prospective study on cancer[32,33]	Cohort	Multiple	Italy, Sweden, and United States

(continued)

TABLE 11.1 (Continued)

NAME OF STUDY	DESIGN	CANCER SITE/TYPE*	COUNTRY
Hereditary Breast Cancer Clinical Study[34,35]	Cohort	Multiple (in breast or ovarian cancer families with BRCA1 or BRCA2)	Austria, Canada, France, Israel, Italy, Norway, Poland, Sweden, United Kingdom, and United States
International BRCA1 and BRCA2 Carrier Cohort Study (IBCCS)[36]	Cohort	Multiple (in breast or ovarian cancer families with BRCA1 or BRCA2)	**Austria, Belgium, France, Germany, Hungary, Iceland, Italy, Netherlands, Spain, Sweden, Denmark, and United Kingdom**
An international study on Cancer in patients on dialysis for end-stage renal disease[37]	Cohort	Multiple	Australia, New Zealand, United States, and 36 European countries
An International Cohort Study of Cancer in Systemic Lupus Erythematosus[38]	Cohort	Multiple	Canada, Iceland, South Korea, Sweden, United Kingdom, and United States
International Cancer Genome Consortium (ICGC)[39]	CCS	>50 cancer type/subtype	Australia, Canada, China, Czech Republic, France, Germany, India, Italy, Japan, Latvia, Netherlands, Norway, Romania, Russia, Spain, Sweden, United Kingdom, and United States
A collaborative analysis of data from 19 genome-wide association studies[40]	CCS	Prostate, breast, lung, colorectum, melanoma, and pancreas	Australia, China, Denmark, Finland, France, Germany, Greece, Italy, Netherlands, Spain, Sweden, United Kingdom, and United States
Middle East Cancer Consortium (MECC)[41,42]	Cancer registry	Multiple	Cyprus, Egypt, Israel, Jordan, Palestinian Authority, and Turkey
International Collaborative Study on Genetic Susceptibility to Environmental Carcinogens (GSEC)[43]	CCS	Lung, skin, breast, bladder, colon, head and neck, prostate, and some other cancers	Australia, Belgium, Finland, France, Germany, Italy, Japan, Norway, Slovenia, Spain, Sweden, Taiwan, United Kingdom, and United States
Human Micronucleus project (HUMN)[44,45]	Cohort	Multiple	Belgium, Bulgaria, Croatia, Italy, Japan, Poland, Slovakia, Sweden, Taiwan, and Yugoslavia

Study	Type	Cancer site(s)	Countries
A genome-wide study on several cancers[46]	CCS	Lung, urinary bladder, prostate, cervix, breast, colorectum, endometrium, kidney, multiple myeloma, ovary, pancreas, stomach, Skin (melanoma, basal cell, and squamous cell), thyroid	Belgium, Canada, China, Czech Republic, Denmark, France, Germany, Hungary, Iceland, Israel, Italy, Japan, Netherlands, Norway, Poland, Romania, Russia, Singapore, Slovakia, Slovenia, South Korea, Spain, Sweden, Taiwan, United Kingdom, and United States
Breast and Prostate Cancer Cohort Consortium[47]	CCS	Breast and prostate	Denmark, Finland, France, Germany, Greece, Italy, Netherlands, Spain, Sweden, United Kingdom, and United States
FEMALE BREAST AND REPRODUCTIVE SYSTEM			
WHO Collaborative Study of Neoplasia and Steroid Contraceptives[48]	CCS	Female breast and reproductive system	Kenya, Mexico, and Thailand
Asia Breast Cancer Consortium[49]	CCS	Breast	China, Hong Kong, Japan, and United States
Breast Cancer Family Registries (BCFR)[50]	Registry	Breast (cancer cases and their family)	Australia, Canada, and United States
Breast Cancer Association Consortium (BCAC)[51]	CCS	Breast	Australia, Denmark, Finland, Germany, Poland, South Korea, Spain, Thailand, United Kingdom, and United States
A genome-wide association study on breast cancer[52]	CCS	Breast	Australia, Denmark, Finland, Germany, Poland, South Korea, Spain, Thailand, United Kingdom, and United States
International Breast Cancer Screening Network (IBSN)[53] [First: the International Breast Cancer Screening Database Project]	Screening	Breast	Australia, Belgium, Canada, Denmark, Finland, France, Germany, Greece, Israel, Japan, Hungary, Iceland, Ireland, Italy, Luxembourg, Netherlands, New Zealand, Norway, Portugal, Spain, Sweden, Switzerland, United Kingdom, United States, and Uruguay
An international study on risk factors of breast cancer[54]	CCS	Breast	Brazil, Greece, Japan, Slovenia, Taiwan, United States, Wales, and Yugoslavia
European Community Multicenter Study on Antioxidants, Myocardial Infarction, and Breast Cancer (EURAMIC)[55]	CCS	Breast	Germany, Ireland, Netherlands, Spain, and Switzerland

(continued)

TABLE 11.1 (Continued)

NAME OF STUDY	DESIGN	CANCER SITE/TYPE*	COUNTRY
Consortium of Investigators of Modifiers of BRCA1 and BRCA2 (CIMBA)[56]	CCS	Breast	Australia, Austria, Canada, Czech Republic, Denmark, France, Finland, Germany, Greece, Iceland, Israel, Italy, Netherlands, Russia, Spain, Sweden, United Kingdom, and United States
Ovarian Cancer Association Consortium (OCAC)[57]	CCS	Ovary	Australia, Belgium, Canada, Denmark, Finland, Germany, Iceland, Netherlands, Poland, United Kingdom, and United States
A study on the association between ovarian cancer and candidate SNPs[58]	CCS	Ovary	Australia, Denmark, England, Germany, Poland, and Unites States
Epidemiology of Endometrial Cancer Consortium[59]	CCS	Endometrium	Australia, Canada, China, Greece, Italy, Netherlands, Norway, Poland, Sweden, and United States
IARC Human Papillomavirus Prevalence Surveys Study[60]	Screening	Cervix	Argentina, Chile, China, Colombia, Guinea, Mongolia, Nigeria, Poland, South Korea, Spain, Thailand, Vietnam,
IARC Multicentre Study Group on Cervical Cancer Early Detection[61]	Screening	Cervix	Burkina Faso, Congo, Guinea, India, Mali, and Niger
IARC Multicenter Cervical Cancer Study[62,63]	CCS	Cervix	Algeria, Brazil, Colombia, India, Mali, Morocco, Paraguay, Peru, Philippines, Spain, and Thailand
New Independent States of the Former Soviet Union and the Latin American Screening Study[64]	Cohort	Cervix	Belarus, Latvia, and Russia
URINARY TRACT AND MALE REPRODUCTIVE SYSTEM			
International Renal-Cell Cancer Study[65]	CCS	Kidney	Australia, Denmark, Germany, Sweden and United States
International Consortium of Bladder Cancer (ICBC)[66]	CCS	Urinary bladder	China, France, Hungry, Italy, Spain, Sweden, United Kingdom, and United States

Study	Type	Cancer site	Countries
An international study on bladder cancer[67]	CCS	Urinary bladder	Denmark, France, Germany, Greece, Italy, and Spain
International Consortium for Prostate Cancer Genetics (ICPCG)[68]	CCS	Prostate	Australia, Canada, Finland, France, Germany, Norway, Sweden, United Kingdom, and United States
The International ACTANE (Anglo/Canadian/Texan/Australian/Norwegian/EU Biomed) Consortium[69]	CCS	Familial prostate cancer	Australia, Canada, Norway, United Kingdom, and United States
Prostate Cancer Association Group to Investigate Cancer Associated Alterations in the Genome (PRACTICAL consortium)[70]	CCS	Prostate	Australia, Canada, Finland, Germany, Switzerland, United Kingdom, and United States
A genome-wide association study on prostate cancer[71]	CCS	Prostate	Australia, Canada, Finland, Germany, Switzerland, United Kingdom, and United States
HRP Multicenter Study of Prostate Cancer and Vasectomy[72]	CCS	Prostate	China, Nepal, and South Korea
International Testicular Cancer Linkage Consortium[73]	CCS	Familial testicular cancer	Australia, Canada, Czech Republic, Denmark, France, Germany, Hungry, Ireland, Netherlands, New Zealand, Norway, Switzerland, United Kingdom, and United States

RESPIRATORY TRACT AND UPPER GASTROINTESTINAL SYSTEM

Study	Type	Cancer site	Countries
International Lung Cancer Consortium (ILCCO)[74]	CCS	Lung	Canada, China, Czech Republic, Denmark, France, Germany, Hungary, Iceland, Israel, Italy, Japan, Netherlands, Norway, Poland, Romania, Russia, Singapore, Slovenia, South Korea, Spain, Taiwan, United Kingdom, and United States
IARC multicenter study on the role of markers of individual susceptibility to lung cancer among non-smokers[75]	CCS	Lung	France, Germany, Italy, Poland, Romania, Russia, and Sweden

(continued)

TABLE 11.1 (Continued)

NAME OF STUDY	DESIGN	CANCER SITE/TYPE*	COUNTRY
An international study on genetic factors of independence to smoking[76]	CCS	Lung	Italy, United Kingdom, and United States[a]
An international study on genetic factors of independence to smoking[77]	CCS	Lung	Iceland, Netherlands, Spain, and United States[a]
Alcohol related cancer and genetic susceptibility in Europe (ARCAGE)[78]	CCS	Oral cavity, pharynx, larynx, and esophagus	Croatia, Czech Republic, Estonia, France, Germany, Greece, Ireland, Italy, Norway, Spain, and United Kingdom
International head and neck cancer epidemiology consortium (INHANCE)[79]	CCS	Oral cavity, pharynx, and larynx	Argentina, Brazil, Czech Republic, Costa Rica, Croatia, Cuba, Estonia, France, Hungry, India, Ireland, Italy, Japan, Netherlands, Norway, Poland, Puerto Rico, Romania, Russia, Slovakia, Spain, Switzerland, United Kingdom, and United States
An international study on upper aerodigestive tract cancers in South America[80]	CCS	Oral cavity, pharynx, larynx and esophagus	Argentina, Brazil, and Cuba
A study on risk factors for nasopharyngeal carcinoma in Maghrebian countries[81]	CCS	Nasopharynx	Algeria, Morocco, and Tunisia
IARC multicenter study on oral cancer[82]	CCS	Oral Cavity	Australia, Canada, Cuba, India, Italy, Northern Ireland, Poland, Spain, and Sudan
IARC multicenter study in Southwest Europe[83,84]	CCS	Hypopharynx and larynx	France, Italy, Spain, and Switzerland
Barrett's Esophagus and Esophageal Adenocarcinoma Consortium (BEACON)[85]	CCS	Adenocarcinoma of the esophagus and gastric cardia	Australia, Canada, Ireland, Sweden, United Kingdom, and United States
International Gastric Cancer Linkage Consortium (IGCLC)[86]	Case-series	Familial gastric cancer	Canada, Denmark, Germany, Hungry, Pakistan, Portugal, Ukraine, United Kingdom, and United States

NERVOUS SYSTEM

Study	Type	Site	Countries
Interphone Study[87]	CCS	Central nervous system	Australia, Canada, Denmark, Finland, France, Germany, Israel, Italy, Japan, New Zealand, Norway, Sweden and United Kingdom
An international study on mobile phone use and cancer of the central nervous system[88,89]	CCS	Central nervous system	Denmark, England, Finland, Norway, and Sweden
International Case-Control Study of Childhood Brain Tumors[90-92]	CCS	Brain	Australia, Canada, France, Israel, Italy, Spain, and United States
International Case-Control Study of Adult Brain Tumor Risk[93]	CCS	Brain	Australia, Canada, France, Germany, Sweden, and United States
An international consortium on familial glioma, glioma gene (GLIOGENE)[94]	CCS	Familial glioma	Denmark, Israel, Sweden, United Kingdom, and United States
An international study on familial isolated pituitary adenoma[95]	Cohort	Pituitary Adenomas	Argentina, Belgium, Brazil, Czech Republic, France, Italy, Netherlands, Spain, and United States
International *succinate dehydrogenase* Consortium (*SDH* consortium)[96]	CCS	Pheochromocytoma/paraganglioma syndromes	Australia, Canada, France, Germany, New Zealand, United Kingdom, and United States
Non-*succinate dehydrogenase* head and neck paraganglioma Consortium (Non-*SDHx* HNP Consortium)[97]	CCS	Head and neck paragangliomas	Argentina, Austria, Australia, Belgium, Brazil, Chile, China, Denmark, Finland, France, Germany, Greece, Hungary, Iran, Italy, Japan, Netherlands, New Zealand, Poland, Serbia, Spain, Sweden, Switzerland, Turkey, Ukraine, and United States

HEMATOLOGIC

Study	Type	Site	Countries
An European study on Hodgkin's lymphoma (EPILYMPH)[98]	CCS	Hodgkin and Non-Hodgkin lymphoma and multiple myeloma	Czech Republic, France, Germany, Ireland, Italy, and Spain

TABLE 11.1 (Continued)

NAME OF STUDY	DESIGN	CANCER SITE/TYPE*	COUNTRY
International Lymphoma Epidemiology Consortium (InterLymph)[99]	CCS	Lymphoid system	Australia, Canada, Czech Republic, Denmark, England, France, Germany, Ireland, Italy, Sweden, and United States
An international study on risk of cancer following chemotherapy[100]	CCS	Leukemia	Canada, Denmark, Finland, Norway, German Democratic Republic, United Kingdom, Slovenia, and Sweden
OTHER ORGANS			
International Pancreatic Cancer Cohort Consortium (PanScan)[101]	Nested CCS	Pancreas	China, Denmark, Finland, France, Germany, Greece, Italy, Netherlands, Spain, Sweden, United Kingdom, and United States
International Pancreatitis Study[102]	Cohort	Pancreas	Denmark, Germany, Italy, Sweden, Switzerland, and United States
International Colorectal Cancer Genetic Association Consortium[103]	CCS	Colorectum	Canada, Finland, Germany, and United Kingdom
Colorectal Cancer Genetics Consortium (COGENT)[104]	CCS	Colorectum	Australia, Canada, China, Colombia, Czech Republic, Finland, Germany, Hong Kong, Italy, Netherlands, Spain, Sweden, and United Kingdom
An international genome-wide study on colorectal cancer[105]	CCS	Colorectum	Australia, Finland, Germany, Netherlands, Spain, and United Kingdom
An international study on polymorphism in a selected gene and risk of colorectal cancer[106]	CCS	Colorectum	Australia, Finland, Netherlands, Spain, and United Kingdom
International Liver Cancer Study (ILCS)[107]	CCS	Liver	Italy, Gambia, and Thailand

Study	Type	Cancer	Countries
Multicentre International Liver Tumor Study (MILTS)[108]	CCS	Liver	France, Germany, Greece, Italy, Spain, and United Kingdom
Melanoma Genetics Consortium (GenoMEL)[109]	CCS	Melanoma	Australia, Germany, Israel, Italy, Latvia, Netherlands, Poland, Slovenia, Spain, Sweden, United Kingdom, and United States
Genes Environment and Melanoma Study (GEM)[110]	CCS	Melanoma	Australia, Canada, Italy, and United States
An replication international study for the association of selected SNPs with risk of melanoma[111]	CCS	Melanoma	Australia, Sweden, and United Kingdom
A genome-wide study on thyroid cancer[112]	CCS	Thyroid	Iceland, Spain, and United States

Abbreviations: CCS, case-control study; IARC, International Agency for Research on Cancer; SNP, single nucleotide polymorphism; WHO, World Health Organization.

[#] The studies that were conducted in at least 3 countries and a publication of which was identified in the PubMed database (indexed by September 15, 2010) using our selected search terms. The only exception was International Liver Cancer Study (ILCS), from which no publication was found.

* Multiple indicates that data on all or almost all kinds of cancer in the study population have been collected.

[a] This study was also included studies on chronic obstructive pulmonary disease from several other countries.

complete, a large majority of studies are from western Europe and northern America and a few are from low- and medium-resource countries.

■ STRATEGIES TO CONDUCT INTERNATIONAL MULTICENTER STUDIES

There are two major strategies to conduct international multicenter studies: (1) pooling data and samples that were collected separately and (2) conducting an international study with a common protocol. Here we review the usual characteristics and methodological issues for each strategy separately, and then the choice between the two strategies is discussed.

Pooling data: Pooling data and samples from existing studies is relatively easy and can provide substantial research material in a relatively short time. As an example, over 12,000 cases and 17,000 controls were included in INHANCE consortium, a pooled analysis of 33 case-control studies on upper aerodigestive tract (UADT) cancers.[113] The investigators were able to examine several factors that usually are not common, so may not be investigable in many single studies due to lack of enough statistical power, including the association of tobacco and alcohol secession and of marijuana use with risk of UADT.[10,114]

However, the major drawback of pooling data is potential incomparability of the collected material. All studies might not have collected data on same factors. While data on tobacco smoking and alcohol drinking, as major risk factors for UADT, were available from all studies in INHANCE consortium, information on tobacco and alcohol cessation and marijuana use was available from 17, 13, and 5 studies, respectively.[10,114] Moreover, even if data on specific variables are collected, the comprehensiveness of data can be considerably varied. Some studies may collect very detailed information on certain variables, on which little data may be obtained in some other studies. In these situations, merging full data may not be possible. There are two major options to manage this: (1) detailed data may be changed to a concise version; in this case some important aspects of data may be omitted, and (2) studies with tiny data on the variables of interest may be excluded from respective analyses; again, a part of data will be missed. Although the problem may be managed by losing a part of data, a major problem with pooling separately collected data is heterogeneity in the quality of data, which is related to quality of the design and conduct of individual studies. It can be difficult to assess the quality of data in previously conducted studies. In meta-analyses, combining observational studies conducted with various qualities of design to obtain summary relative risks can sometimes be misleading and summary statistics need to be interpreted with caution.[115,116] A similar problem can happen when the quality of data is highly heterogeneous among the pooled studies.

Biologic samples collected in separately conducted studies may also be pooled for achieving bigger sample sizes. A good example is genome-wide association studies, in which DNA is used as the main biologic material. Pooling samples for those studies is usually feasible, because the majority of studies worldwide keep their samples in the situations that fulfill the standards of DNA storage procedures. However, this may not true for more sensitive constituents of biologic samples, such as RNA. Furthermore, collection of samples for certain studies need more sophisticated methods. As an example, in certain studies on viral particles, the risk of contamination of samples at the time of collection should be minimized. For these reasons, many previously collected samples may not be appropriate for certain studies. Finally, if the association between biomarkers and questionnaire data in validation studies or the effect modification of genetic factors on environmental exposures in genome-wide studies is to be investigated, the potential problem of heterogeneity in quality and incompatibility of environmental data may also occur.

Identifying eligible studies: The idea of conducting pooled analyses is generally raised by the experts in the respective field who normally are familiar with the previous work. Further potentially eligible studies may be identified by searching the literature; as the studies of interest have already been conducted, it is very likely that some of their results have been already published. The principal investigators of the identified eligible studies are contacted regarding their willingness for being involved in the pooled study, and if so, regarding their available questionnaire data and/or biologic samples and how the material was collected. The investigators may set some inclusion criteria for studies, including minimum requirements with regard to study design, number of participants, variables included in the questionnaire, and quality of biologic samples. For example, the minimum number of participants in the studies included in a consortium of genome-wide association study on colorectal cancer was 500 cases and 500 controls.[104] After the studies fulfilling the required criteria are identified, a meeting of the principal investigators to discuss the details of the study will be helpful. It should be noted that individual studies in a pooled study may not be included in all projects that will be conducted within the pooled study. For any project within the same pooled study, a separate agreement will be necessary. The inclusion will depend on the availability of the data of interest from individual studies (see the INHANCE study discussed previously as an example) and willingness of the investigators to share their data for any individual project. Furthermore, studies may have to fulfill some criteria to be included in a specific project. For example, among studies included in a consortium of pancreatic cancer studies, only data from prospective studies were considered for studying the association between alcohol drinking and the cancer.[117] After a pooled study is established, further studies may join to the originally pooled studies and involve in later projects.

Organization of the study: Members of pooled epidemiological studies are investigators involved in epidemiological research, including molecular and genetic epidemiology, on cancer(s) of interest. In order to make the study more comprehensive, it is advisable to include scientists from other disciplines.[118] Pooled studies usually consist of several working groups, in which collaborative projects in specific areas of the cancer research of interest are proposed and developed; they direct data analyses and write manuscripts in the respective projects.[113,119] The operational field of working groups will depend on the study questions and hypotheses and on the available material. As an example, working groups in an international consortium on lymphoma constituted of diet and behavioral factors, family studies, genotyping, immunology, infections, occupation, pathology, and sunlight groups,[118] while in a consortium on vitamin D and rarer cancers the working groups were defined by cancer site.[119] Regular meetings (e.g. annual) can be held to exchange inter-disciplinary experience and discuss new initiatives. General statistical analysis plan and quality control procedures may be developed by a group of investigators and are applied and surveyed by working groups in the respective projects. An alternative is to establish statistical and quality control working groups.[119] When one of the centers is much more experienced in conducting international studies, it is plausible that the center coordinates the study. An example is the INHANCE study, which was coordinated by International Agency for Research on Cancer (IARC).[113]

Quality control procedures: As discussed earlier, it is usually difficult to control for the quality of whole study procedure when the studies have been already conducted. However, some general aspects of study design can be inspected, including ethical approval and informed consents, the way that the participants were selected, how questionnaire data was collected (face to face interview versus self-administered questionnaires), and whether or not any validation study was conducted. On the other hand, quality control procedures can be well-organized for laboratory assessments that are done after pooled studies are established. It will be very important for controlling the validity of assessments' results, particularly when more than one laboratory does the analyses. As an example for these procedures, masked reference/standard and masked quality control samples can be provided among the study samples.[119]

Harmonization of collection of data and samples: In order to make the pooled material comparable with together, all collected data and samples in individual studies need to be harmonized. Variables on exposure that are going to be pooled should refer to the same exposure with similar units. Some other variables, such as job classification in occupational studies, might have been categorized using different systems or different versions of the same system (e.g. national systems; ISCO: International Standard Classification of Occupations; or ISIC: International Standard Industrial Classification). Data on the outcome of interest should also be harmonized. When several cancer types are included in a pooled study, the cancers might have been coded using different systems or versions in individual studies (e.g. ICD: International Classification of Diseases, versions 9, 10, or O). The coding in different studies should be converted to an identical system.

Use of data at the local versus central level: Usually, results of the individual studies that are included in pooled analyses have been already published at the local level. Therefore, the new results from pooled analyses usually are at the central level, although the results by study centers are also commonly presented in the publications from pooled studies.

After being harmonized, data from each individual center are sent to the coordinating center, where the data from all centers are merged. Checks for completeness of data and for outliers and inconsistencies will be done in the coordinator center before merging the data. The required variables for any pooled analysis will be sent to the center that will conduct the analysis, where more detailed data management will be performed before data analysis. In general, anonymous data are transferred.

Transfer of samples to central bio-repositories and laboratories: Similar to data, biological samples are transferred to central bio-repositories or the laboratories in which planned assessments are to be done. The samples that cannot be kept at room temperature may be transferred in dry ice, nitrogen tanks, or refrigerator/freezers depending to the required temperature and the facilities provided by transport agents. Special attention should be paid to the quality of samples during the shipments that need a cold chain, particularly in transfers from remote areas with limited access, long-duration transfers, and when the transfer takes place in high-temperature climates. Harmonization of biologic samples at the study center level usually is less complicated than of data. However, at the central level, one of the most important issues is appropriate registration and/or labeling of samples, so that the samples that are coming from different centers and have been labeled differently can be identified and traced during laboratory assessments and when the results are linked to individual data. The central bio-repositories and laboratories should have enough operational and reserve capacity for storing the samples in a safe way. In order to identify and use the samples, they should also have appropriate data banks to record the required information about the samples in the repository.

Strategies for funding: Usually, pooled studies do not have specific resources, and working groups apply for grants to fund specific projects.[118] In order to support coordination and meetings, the executive group may raise funds either independently or in collaboration with working groups. Collaborating centers may also provide a minimal amount of resources (e.g., by contributing to the coordination of working groups).[118]

Long-term sustainability of projects: As research material has already been collected in pooled studies, it is likely that most of the analyses are completed in middle-term provided that resources are available and investigators still willing to participate in the pooled projects. Reaching to an agreement in the beginning of pooled studies or projects regarding detailed responsibilities and benefits of researchers and centers can be helpful in keeping the collaboration for a longer period. Authorship in publications is an example of the such issues. The collaborators should be confident that what will be achieved from the sharing material will be greater than what might be lost as a result of collaboration. For this, respect for the intellectual property and fairness in collaboration is necessary. Mechanisms may be introduced in the pooled studies for reporting any unfair use of the shared material to the executive group, which will make the appropriate decision on the action to be taken.[118]

Studies with common protocols: In this method, all studies use a common protocol. The protocol may be designed specifically for the study or the protocol of a previously conducted study is used in some further studies. Therefore, all or the majority of included studies are conducted after establishment of the multicenter study. These studies are not necessarily conducted at the same time. It is possible that a later study that has used the same protocol joins the original studies in further projects. Although the studies with a common protocol generally take longer than pooling previously collected material, the problem of incompatibility of material is not expected in those studies, and the problem of heterogeneity in the quality of collected data can be overcome by appropriate quality control procedures. However, conducting international studies with common protocol need a very good level of coordination among study centers in all steps of study, including study design, training of staff, data ascertainment, and biologic sample collection and storage.

As an example, IARC conducted three large multicenter studies with common protocols in several, mainly low- and medium-resource, countries on etiologic factors of cervical cancer, cervical cancer screening, and prevalence of cervical HPV infection, which is the main risk factor for the cancer. These studies are examples of very successful international studies on cancer. The association between HPV infection and risk of cancer had been suggested by single studies, but the IARC multicenter case-control study provided very strong evidence for such an association and also detailed information on the association of different subtypes of HPV and of some lifestyle factors with the cancer.[60,62] The IARC screening study has been helpful in identifying new cervical cancer cases in the collaborating centers in India and 5 African countries, but even more important, the experience may be useful for conducting screening programs in other parts of the respective countries or in other low- to medium-resource countries.[61] The IARC study on prevalence of HPV infection in several countries with different resource levels provides information about epidemiology of main carcinogenic HPV subtypes.[60] This information can be helpful in determining the extent of required screening and prevention measures in collaborating areas for HPV-related cancers, including cancers of the cervix, vulva, vagina, penis, anus, oral cavity, and oropharynx and tonsil.[120]

Identifying potential collaborators: Similar to pooled studies, the idea of collaborative studies is proposed by the experts in the respective field, who usually know several other investigators that are capable of conducting studies of interest. Further potential collaborators that work in the same field may be identified by searching the literature.

Organization of the study: Similar to pooled studies, the members of multicenter epidemiological studies are investigators involved in epidemiological research, including molecular and genetic epidemiology. Inclusion of scientists from other disciplines can make the study more comprehensive. The collaborative studies are generally consisted of several working groups, which propose and develop collaborative projects in specific areas of the cancer research. Coordinators of each working group will inform all members of the study about the activities of the group. Regular meetings (e.g. annual) can be held to report the progress of study, exchange inter-disciplinary experience, and discuss new initiatives. An executive group will oversee the whole projects. The group usually is also responsible for the communication among working groups, the organization of general meetings, and the coordination of grant applications. Members of the executive group may be elected for specified durations.

Preparation of common protocols: For new studies, after potential collaborators agreed with the outline of the study, a group of researchers from a center or several centers are assigned to develop a common protocol using the input from all involved investigators. The responsible group is selected by the investigators. However, when one of the centers is much more experienced in conducting international collaborative studies, the center may take care of the development of the protocol. However, as mentioned earlier, this will be done in contact with all investigators, who will give comments and suggestions and finally should approve the protocol. Literature search can be helpful is retrieving updated information on some potentially important issues at the time of study design, including the prevalence of exposures of interest among the general population and magnitude of association between potential risk factors and outcomes of interest in other recent studies. Similarly, study hypotheses may be updated with the latest information.

As studies are to be conducted in different countries with possibly different lifestyles and patterns of exposures to risk factors, protocols should be designed in a manner that the required material is collected in a similar way despite of these variations (see "Harmonization of collection data and samples," below). Although the majority of epidemiological studies are generally designed by epidemiologists, other specialists are usually involved in designing some parts of the protocol; for example, clinicians may define clinical outcomes and diagnostic methods (such as colposcopy) and pathologists provide histological criteria for the outcome of interest.

In general, it is advisable to get the data of interest as much more detailed as possible. For example, cumulative use of tobacco is a more precise indicator for the risk associated with tobacco use than ever/never use. Therefore, collecting data on whole life tobacco consumption is preferred. Some information can be categorized according to the currently accepted criteria, such as blood pressure with regard to hypertension criteria. In such cases, the original values should be recorded, as the criteria may be subject to change in future. When the study is to be conducted in populations with different languages, the investigators should make sure that the materials administered to participants, including questionnaires and consent form, are clearly understandable and have the same meaning to all participants.

All biological samples should be collected and processed in a same way. The factors that may influence the quality of the samples at the time of collection, processing, storage, and transfer should be considered. Examples for collection of samples include fasting status of participants, sampling diurnal time in certain hormonal studies and menstrual time in studies on female reproductive hormones, equipment that is used for sampling (e.g. syringes, saliva collection kits, and any probe) and any additive (e.g. anticoagulants), and the places from which biopsy samples should be collected. Examples for processing include the maximum duration of putting blood samples in room temperature or refrigerators, duration and speed of centrifuge, fixation of cytology and biopsy samples, and use of any additives. The standards for such procedures may be various. For the common protocol, appropriate ones should be chosen based on the study hypotheses, expected laboratory assessments, and feasibility of procedures.

The protocol and its constituents like questionnaires and forms may be prepared in a more commonly used international language (e.g. English) and then be translated to local languages. The manuals documenting the protocol should be clear. In order to check the quality of the translations to local languages, the translated protocols may be translated back to the original language by independent people and compared with the original protocol and checked for any inconsistency. Preparing guidelines for local personnel in respective languages regarding how to conduct the study can be helpful.

Quality control procedures: In contrast to pooled studies, quality control in studies with a common protocol can be conducted prospectively using predefined guidelines. This is one of the main advantages of studies with a common protocol over the pooled studies, provided that the control is well designed and conducted.

The essentials of quality control procedures in multicenter international studies are similar to any other study. However, due to international and multicentric nature of those studies, and consequently the possibility of more heterogeneous conduct of study and application of study protocol than in single center studies, quality control may be more challenging. The quality of study protocol should be controlled when it is designed. Pilot studies may be conducted to check the reproducibility and validity of data before starting the actual study. After being started, quality of all steps of the study should be controlled regularly. The examples are checking for participant eligibility; coding procedures; training of interviewers, technicians, and data entry operators; application of protocol by personnel; completeness of data; data entry packages; data cleanup; quality of equipment data; and routine maintenance of equipment.[121] Using a standard checklist will be helpful in conducting more homogenous quality assessments of different procedures. In order to check the quality of data entry, a part of the data may be entered twice (double entry). Conducting a pilot study on quality control itself is also advisable.

The control may be conducted at different levels, including field level, study center level, and working or executive group level. Quality control reports should be provided regularly (e.g. monthly) by the responsible people in the study field and study center. Investigators from each study center will regularly visit the process in the study field. Members of the working or executive groups may visit each study field and center regularly, for example in a yearly basis.

Harmonization of collection of data and samples: Questionnaire data should be collected in a same way as much as possible. However, pattern of exposure to specific factors may vary in different populations. For example, while cigarette smoking is the most common way of tobacco use worldwide, other types of exposure, including pipe and water-pipe (hookah) smoking and tobacco chewing and sniffing, may be prevalent in some of the populations that are included in collaborative studies. In such situations, it is important to collect data on all types of tobacco. For this, questions about specific tobacco products can be added to the questionnaires. These questions will be administered to populations in which the respective product is commonly used. For any other exposure of interest with similar variations, e.g. the consumption of different alcoholic beverages, such a comprehensive data should be collected.

All study centers should use the same coding systems for any classification, e.g. classifications of occupation and outcome and coding for endoscopy and histopathological findings. Similarly, biologic samples should be collected and processed in a same way (see preceding "Preparation of common protocols"). Storage and transfer of samples should fulfill the requirements proposed in the protocol.

Use of data at the local versus central level: As any multicenter study is bigger than any of its individual collaborating studies, and consequently has higher study power, the use of data at central rather than local level is preferable, because results of whole multicenter study can be theoretically more valid than of the individual studies. However, results of individual studies may be first published at the local level, because local investigators and the sources of local funding may be interested in the results being published first at the local level. In practice, the use of data at the central level may be much more feasible when they have already been fully or partly reported, because a part of collaborators may be reluctant to share their unpublished material for original collective publications.[118]

Similar to pooling separately conducted studies, data from collaborating centers in a study with common protocol will be merged at the coordinating center after checks for completeness of data and for outliers are done. The merged variables necessary for any project within the multicenter study will be transferred to the responsible center.

Transfer of samples to central biorepositories and laboratories: Biological samples are transferred to central bio-repositories. Similar to pooled studies, for the samples that cannot be kept at room temperature the transfer may be done in dry ice, nitrogen tanks, or refrigerator/freezers depending to the facilities provided by transport agents. Again, special attention should be paid to the quality of samples during shipments. In the central repository, the samples from different study centers should be appropriately registered and labeled, so that the samples can be identified and traced easily. The central bio-repositories and laboratories should have enough operational and reserve capacity and appropriate data banks to store the samples in a safe and efficient way. All or a part of the samples may be transferred to the central biorepository. This will depend on the original agreements. When a part of samples is transferred, the remaining of the samples will be kept at the study center. The samples may be transferred once the study is completed. An alternative is to transfer the samples in regular intervals, e.g. time intervals (such as annual transfers) or when the number of samples reached to a specified limit. This method will be much safer if there are some concerns about the maintenance of the storage systems in study centers, e.g. maintenance of deep freezers and nitrogen tanks, continuous availability of electricity and liquid nitrogen, and the reserve capacity in case of any problem for the operational capacity.

Strategies for funding: Usually, studies with common protocol apply for both local and international grants. Although obtaining large-scale grants for international studies has become increasingly challenging, agencies such as Wellcome Trust, the European Commission and the National Institutes of Health remain potential sources. A strategy used in successful collaborations between high-income and low- and middle-income countries consists of applying for funds for technical and economic development rather than scientific research. In many middle-income countries, increasing resources are becoming available for medical research, and applicants participating in international studies often have a competitive advantage.

Long-term sustainability of projects: All or majority of collaborating studies are new studies that may take place, perhaps without major results being available, for several years. Therefore, collaborators should be committed to conduct the study following the standards of the collaborative study and to communicate with other collaborators. Involvement of young motivated researchers from each center, in addition to senior investigators, in the collaborative study and working groups can be helpful in this regard. Another major issue is assured resources to continue the studies, particularly in low-income countries. Finally, as discussed for pooled analyses, agreement on responsibilities and benefits of researchers and centers at the beginning, including authorships, may prevent rising of potential problems later in the course of study.

The choice between the two methods: Besides the availability of resources and logistic consideration, the main determinants of the method of choice are the type of information and samples that are required and the target sample size, which also influence the duration of study. In general, heterogeneity in the type of the obtained information and samples and their collection procedures may hinder the investigation of certain associations in pooled studies or may make the results less valid. If this heterogeneity is not likely to influence the results, the two methods will not have substantial difference in the validity of results. As this is not the case in many instances, conducting studies with common protocols is usually preferred.

In certain situations, however, pooled analysis of previously conducted studies can be very useful. For example, results on the association between human papilloma virus (HPV) and esophageal squamous cell carcinoma (ESCC) were very inconsistent, ranging from strong to no or even inverse associations; the prevalence of HPV in ESCC also ranged from 0% to 70%.[122] The heterogeneity in results might be partly related to geographic variations, contamination of samples when polymerase chain reaction was used for detecting HPV, differences in positivity cutpoints when serological tests were used, and other differences in study design, including insufficient adjustments for other major risk factors of ESCC, including tobacco and alcohol use.[122] A recent study collected serum samples from several large studies conducted in different countries, many of which had collected sufficient data on other risk factors of ESCC.[123] Results of this study can provide strong evidence regarding whether or not there is a strong association between HPV infection and ESCC. A negative finding may preclude this association from high-priority research issues, at least with traditional laboratory assessments, in other studies and consequently may save resource and samples.

Pooling material from previously conducted studies may be the most feasible option for rare cancers. As an example, a multicenter linkage study on familial cancer pooled information and biologic samples from 64 families (63 with at least 3 cases of prostate cancer), while due to rarity of familial prostate cancer, the original studies recruited only a few families.[69] On the other hand, although it may take a longer time until studies with common protocols collect a sufficiently large number of participants with rare cancer, such an approach can also be used. For example, the IARC Central and Eastern Europe Study recruited 361 cases of kidney cancer from several countries using a common protocol,[12] or a study on familial glioma was conducted in 11 centers from 5 countries, with the goal of screening 15,000 newly diagnosed glioma cases for family history of brain tumors to identify 400 informative glioma families for linkage analyses.[94,124] The choice of the study method for rare cancers also follows these general considerations, i.e. studies with common protocols are preferred.

The experience of collaborative study gained in pooled studies may be helpful in developing further studies with common protocols.[118] Finally, there are many international studies that are not directly on cancer outcomes, but there results can be used in cancer studies. Table 11.2 shows a few examples of such studies.

SUMMARY

In this chapter, we first discuss the importance of cancer research and international multi-center studies in low- and medium-resource countries. Then we review major strategies and the relevant methodological issues. Finally, we provide some general guidelines regarding the choice of the strategies in various situations.

TABLE 11.2 Examples of international studies, networks, or procedures whose results may be used in cancer studies

NAME OF STUDY	DESCRIPTION
HapMap Consortium[125]	A genome-wide database of human genetic variation
Environmental Cancer risk, Nutrition and Individual Susceptibility (ECNIS)[126]	A network in Europe to promote *integrating and joint research activities* and *spreading of excellence activities* in environmental carcinogenesis research
The Tobacco and Genetics Consortium[127]	Genome-wide meta-analyses to identify loci associated with smoking behavior
Body Mass Index and All-Cause Mortality Pooling Project[128]	To quantify the risk associated with being overweight or obese and the extent to which the relationship between body mass index and all-cause mortality varies by several other factors
ECP-EURONUT-Intestinal Metaplasia Study[129]	A study on relation between diet and gastric intestinal metaplasia in Croatia, Greece, Italy, Poland, Portugal, and the United Kingdom
DataSchema and Harmonization Platform for Epidemiological Research (DataSHaPER)[130]	To provide a structured approach to the harmonization and pooling of information between studies
Data aggregation through anonymous summary-statistics from harmonized individual-level databases (DataSHIELD)[131]	To provide a simple approach to analyzing pooled data with considering ethico-legal issues

▪ REFERENCES

1. Boyle P, Levin B, International Agency for Research on Cancer., ebrary I. *World cancer report. 2008.* Lyon: IARC Press; 2008.
2. Blot WJ, McLaughlin JK, Fraumeni JF. Esophageal cancer. In: Schottenfeld D, Fraumeni JF, eds. *Cancer epidemiology and prevention.* New York: Oxford University Press; 2006:697–706.
3. Islami F, Kamangar F, Nasrollahzadeh D, Moller H, Boffetta P, Malekzadeh R. Oesophageal cancer in Golestan province, a high-incidence area in northern Iran—a review. *Eur J Cancer.* 2009;45(18): 3156–3165.
4. Jemal A, Center MM, DeSantis C, Ward EM. Global patterns of cancer incidence and mortality rates and trends. *Cancer Epidemiol Biomarkers Prev.* 2010;19(8):1893–1907.
5. Popkin BM. The shift in stages of the nutrition transition in the developing world differs from past experiences! *Public Health Nutr.* 2002;5(1A):205–214.
6. Ezzati M, Lopez AD. Estimates of global mortality attributable to smoking in 2000. *Lancet.* 2003; 362(9387):847–852.
7. Gu D, Kelly TN, Wu X, et al. Mortality attributable to smoking in China. *N Engl J Med.* 2009;360(2): 150–159.
8. World Health Organization. *WHO report on the global tobacco epidemic 2008: The MPOWER package.* Geneva: World Health Organization; 2008.
9. Hung RJ, Hashibe M, McKay J, et al. Folate-related genes and the risk of tobacco-related cancers in central Europe. *Carcinogenesis.* 2007;28(6):1334–1340.
10. Marron M, Boffetta P, Zhang ZF, et al. Cessation of alcohol drinking, tobacco smoking and the reversal of head and neck cancer risk. *Int J Epidemiol.* 2010;39(1):182–196.
11. Hung RJ, McKay JD, Gaborieau V, et al. A susceptibility locus for lung cancer maps to nicotinic acetylcholine receptor subunit genes on 15q25. *Nature.* 2008;452(7187):633–637.

12. Szymanska K, Moore LE, Rothman N, et al. TP53, EGFR, and KRAS mutations in relation to VHL inactivation and lifestyle risk factors in renal-cell carcinoma from central and eastern Europe. *Cancer Lett.* 2010;293(1):92–98.

13. Lynge E, Afonso N, Kaerlev L, et al. European multi-centre case-control study on risk factors for rare cancers of unknown aetiology. *Eur J Cancer.* 2005;41(4):601–612.

14. Woodward M, Barzi F, Martiniuk A, et al. Cohort profile: The Asia pacific cohort studies collaboration. *Int J Epidemiol.* 2006;35(6):1412–1416.

15. Riboli E, Kaaks R. The EPIC project: Rationale and study design. European prospective investigation into cancer and nutrition. *Int J Epidemiol.* 1997;26 Suppl 1:S6–S14.

16. Helzlsouer KJ, VDPP Steering Committee. Overview of the cohort consortium vitamin D pooling project of rarer cancers. *Am J Epidemiol.* 2010;172(1):4–9.

17. Valsecchi MG, Tognoni G, Bonilla M, et al. Clinical epidemiology of childhood cancer in Central America and Caribbean countries. *Ann Oncol.* 2004;15(4):680–685.

18. Brown RC, Dwyer T, Kasten C, et al. Cohort profile: The international childhood cancer cohort consortium (I4C). *Int J Epidemiol.* 2007;36(4):724–730.

19. Simonato L, Fletcher AC, Andersen A, et al. A historical prospective study of European stainless steel, mild steel, and shipyard welders. *Br J Ind Med.* 1991;48(3):145–154.

20. Saracci R, Kogevinas M, Bertazzi PA, et al. Cancer mortality in workers exposed to chlorophenoxy herbicides and chlorophenols. *Lancet.* 1991;338(8774):1027–1032.

21. Kogevinas M, Ferro G, Saracci R, et al. Cancer mortality in an international cohort of workers exposed to styrene. *IARC Sci Publ.* 1993;(127)(127):289–300.

22. Ward E, Boffetta P, Andersen A, et al. Update of the follow-up of mortality and cancer incidence among European workers employed in the vinyl chloride industry. *Epidemiology.* 2001;12(6):710–718.

23. Steenland K, Mannetje A, Boffetta P, et al. Pooled exposure-response analyses and risk assessment for lung cancer in 10 cohorts of silica-exposed workers: An IARC multicentre study. *Cancer Causes Control.* 2001;12(9):773–784.

24. Kogevinas M, Becher H, Benn T, et al. Cancer mortality in workers exposed to phenoxy herbicides, chlorophenols, and dioxins. an expanded and updated international cohort study. *Am J Epidemiol.* 1997;145(12):1061–1075.

25. de Vocht F, Burstyn I, Ferro G, et al. Sensitivity of the association between increased lung cancer risk and bitumen fume exposure to the assumptions in the assessment of exposure. *Int Arch Occup Environ Health.* 2009;82(6):723–733.

26. Cardis E, Vrijheid M, Blettner M, et al. Risk of cancer after low doses of ionising radiation: Retrospective cohort study in 15 countries. *BMJ.* 2005;331(7508):77.

27. International Consortium for Research on the Health Effects of Radiation Writing Committee and Study Team, Davis S, Day RW, et al. Childhood leukaemia in Belarus, Russia, and Ukraine following the Chernobyl power station accident: Results from an international collaborative population-based case-control study. *Int J Epidemiol.* 2006;35(2):386–396.

28. Tinnerberg H, Heikkila P, Huici-Montagud A, et al. Retrospective exposure assessment and quality control in an international multi-centre case-control study. *Ann Occup Hyg.* 2003;47(1):37–47.

29. Scelo G, Boffetta P, Autier P, et al. Associations between ocular melanoma and other primary cancers: An international population-based study. *Int J Cancer.* 2007;120(1):152–159.

30. Cancer risks in BRCA2 mutation carriers. The breast cancer linkage consortium. *J Natl Cancer Inst.* 1999;91(15):1310–1316.

31. Aulchenko YS, Ripatti S, Lindqvist I, et al. Loci influencing lipid levels and coronary heart disease risk in 16 European population cohorts. *Nat Genet.* 2009;41(1):47–55.

32. Lukanova A, Lundin E, Akhmedkhanov A, et al. Circulating levels of sex steroid hormones and risk of ovarian cancer. *Int J Cancer.* 2003;104(5):636–642.

33. Lukanova A, Lundin E, Micheli A, et al. Circulating levels of sex steroid hormones and risk of endometrial cancer in postmenopausal women. *Int J Cancer.* 2004;108(3):425–432.

34. Jernstrom H, Lubinski J, Lynch HT, et al. Breast-feeding and the risk of breast cancer in BRCA1 and BRCA2 mutation carriers. *J Natl Cancer Inst.* 2004;96(14):1094–1098.

35. Ginsburg OM, Kim-Sing C, Foulkes WD, et al. BRCA1 and BRCA2 families and the risk of skin cancer. *Fam Cancer.* 2010;9(4):489–493.

36. Andrieu N, Goldgar DE, Easton DF, et al. Pregnancies, breast-feeding, and breast cancer risk in the international BRCA1/2 carrier cohort study (IBCCS). *J Natl Cancer Inst.* 2006;98(8):535–544.

37. Maisonneuve P, Agodoa L, Gellert R, et al. Cancer in patients on dialysis for end-stage renal disease: An international collaborative study. *Lancet.* 1999;354(9173):93–99.

38. Bernatsky S, Boivin JF, Joseph L, et al. An international cohort study of cancer in systemic lupus erythematosus. *Arthritis Rheum.* 2005;52(5):1481–1490.

39. International Cancer Genome Consortium, Hudson TJ, Anderson W, et al. International network of cancer genome projects. *Nature.* 2010;464(7291):993–998.

40. Elliott KS, Zeggini E, McCarthy MI, et al. Evaluation of association of HNF1B variants with diverse cancers: Collaborative analysis of data from 19 genome-wide association studies. *PLoS One.* 2010;5(5):e10858.

41. Freedman LS, Barchana M, Al-Kayed S, et al. A comparison of population-based cancer incidence rates in Israel and Jordan. *Eur J Cancer Prev.* 2003;12(5):359–365.

42. Bingley A, Clark D. A comparative review of palliative care development in six countries represented by the Middle East cancer consortium (MECC). *J Pain Symptom Manage.* 2009;37(3):287–296.

43. Taioli E. International collaborative study on genetic susceptibility to environmental carcinogens. *Cancer Epidemiol Biomarkers Prev.* 1999;8(8):727–728.

44. Bonassi S, Znaor A, Ceppi M, et al. An increased micronucleus frequency in peripheral blood lymphocytes predicts the risk of cancer in humans. *Carcinogenesis.* 2007;28(3):625–631.

45. Fenech M, Bolognesi C, Kirsch-Volders M, et al. Harmonisation of the micronucleus assay in human buccal cells—a human micronucleus (HUMN) project (www.humn.org) initiative commencing in 2007. *Mutagenesis.* 2007;22(1):3–4.

46. Rafnar T, Sulem P, Stacey SN, et al. Sequence variants at the TERT-CLPTM1L locus associate with many cancer types. *Nat Genet.* 2009;41(2):221–227.

47. Canzian F, Kaaks R, Cox DG, et al. Genetic polymorphisms of the GNRH1 and GNRHR genes and risk of breast cancer in the National Cancer Institute breast and prostate cancer cohort consortium (BPC3). *BMC Cancer.* 2009;9:257.

48. Breast cancer and depot-medroxyprogesterone acetate: A multinational study. WHO collaborative study of neoplasia and steroid contraceptives. *Lancet.* 1991;338(8771):833–838.

49. Long J, Cai Q, Shu XO, et al. Identification of a functional genetic variant at 16q12.1 for breast cancer risk: Results from the Asia breast cancer consortium. *PLoS Genet.* 2010;6(6):e1001002.

50. John EM, Hopper JL, Beck JC, et al. The breast cancer family registry: An infrastructure for cooperative multinational, interdisciplinary and translational studies of the genetic epidemiology of breast cancer. *Breast Cancer Res.* 2004;6(4):R375–R389.

51. Breast Cancer Association Consortium. Commonly studied single-nucleotide polymorphisms and breast cancer: Results from the breast cancer association consortium. *J Natl Cancer Inst.* 2006;98(19):1382–1396.

52. Ahmed S, Thomas G, Ghoussaini M, et al. Newly discovered breast cancer susceptibility loci on 3p24 and 17q23.2. *Nat Genet.* 2009;41(5):585–590.

53. Klabunde CN, Ballard-Barbash R, for the International Breast Cancer Screening Network. Evaluating population-based screening mammography programs internationally. *Semin Breast Dis.* 2007;10(2):102–107.

54. Hsieh CC, Trichopoulos D, Katsouyanni K, Yuasa S. Age at menarche, age at menopause, height and obesity as risk factors for breast cancer: Associations and interactions in an international case-control study. *Int J Cancer.* 1990;46(5):796–800.

55. Kohlmeier L, Simonsen N, van 't Veer P, et al. Adipose tissue trans fatty acids and breast cancer in the European community multicenter study on antioxidants, myocardial infarction, and breast cancer. *Cancer Epidemiol Biomarkers Prev.* 1997;6(9):705–710.

56. Osorio A, Milne RL, Pita G, et al. Evaluation of a candidate breast cancer associated SNP in ERCC4 as a risk modifier in BRCA1 and BRCA2 mutation carriers. Results from the consortium of investigators of modifiers of BRCA1/BRCA2 (CIMBA). *Br J Cancer*. 2009;101(12):2048–2054.

57. Bolton KL, Tyrer J, Song H, et al. Common variants at 19p13 are associated with susceptibility to ovarian cancer. *Nat Genet*. 2010;42(10):880–884.

58. Song H, Ramus SJ, Kjaer SK, et al. Association between invasive ovarian cancer susceptibility and 11 best candidate SNPs from breast cancer genome-wide association study. *Hum Mol Genet*. 2009;18(12):2297–2304.

59. Olson SH, Chen C, De Vivo I, et al. Maximizing resources to study an uncommon cancer: E2C2— epidemiology of endometrial cancer consortium. *Cancer Causes Control*. 2009;20(4):491–496.

60. Franceschi S, Plummer M, Clifford G, et al. Differences in the risk of cervical cancer and human papillomavirus infection by education level. *Br J Cancer*. 2009;101(5):865–870.

61. Muwonge R, Walter SD, Wesley RS, et al. Assessing the gain in diagnostic performance when two visual inspection methods are combined for cervical cancer prevention. *J Med Screen*. 2007;14(3):144–150.

62. Munoz N, Bosch FX, de Sanjose S, et al. Epidemiologic classification of human papillomavirus types associated with cervical cancer. *N Engl J Med*. 2003;348(6):518–527.

63. Louie KS, de Sanjose S, Diaz M, et al. Early age at first sexual intercourse and early pregnancy are risk factors for cervical cancer in developing countries. *Br J Cancer*. 2009;100(7):1191–1197.

64. Syrjanen K, Shabalova I, Naud P, et al. Persistent high-risk human papillomavirus infections and other end-point markers of progressive cervical disease among women prospectively followed up in the new independent states of the former Soviet Union and the Latin American screening study cohorts. *Int J Gynecol Cancer*. 2009;19(5):934–942.

65. McLaughlin JK, Lindblad P, Mellemgaard A, et al. International renal-cell cancer study. I. tobacco use. *Int J Cancer*. 1995;60(2):194–198.

66. Stern MC, Lin J, Figueroa JD, et al. Polymorphisms in DNA repair genes, smoking, and bladder cancer risk: Findings from the international consortium of bladder cancer. *Cancer Res*. 2009;69(17):6857–6864.

67. Fortuny J, Kogevinas M, Chang-Claude J, et al. Tobacco, occupation and non-transitional-cell carcinoma of the bladder: An international case-control study. *Int J Cancer*. 1999;80(1):44–46.

68. Schaid DJ, Chang BL. Description of the international consortium for prostate cancer genetics, and failure to replicate linkage of hereditary prostate cancer to 20q13. *Prostate*. 2005;63(3):276–290.

69. Edwards S, Meitz J, Eles R, et al. Results of a genome-wide linkage analysis in prostate cancer families ascertained through the ACTANE consortium. *Prostate*. 2003;57(4):270–279.

70. Kote-Jarai Z, Easton DF, Stanford JL, et al. Multiple novel prostate cancer predisposition loci confirmed by an international study: The PRACTICAL consortium. *Cancer Epidemiol Biomarkers Prev*. 2008;17(8):2052–2061.

71. Antoniou AC, Rookus M, Andrieu N, et al. Reproductive and hormonal factors, and ovarian cancer risk for BRCA1 and BRCA2 mutation carriers: Results from the international BRCA1/2 carrier cohort study. *Cancer Epidemiol Biomarkers Prev*. 2009;18(2):601–610.

72. Schwingl PJ, Meirik O, Kapp N, Farley TM, HRP Multicenter Study of Prostate Cancer and Vasectomy. Prostate cancer and vasectomy: A hospital-based case-control study in China, Nepal and the Republic of Korea. *Contraception*. 2009;79(5):363–368.

73. Rapley EA, Crockford GP, Easton DF, Stratton MR, Bishop DT, International Testicular Cancer Linkage Consortium. Localisation of susceptibility genes for familial testicular germ cell tumour. *APMIS*. 2003;111(1):128–133; discussion 33–5.

74. Truong T, Hung RJ, Amos CI, et al. Replication of lung cancer susceptibility loci at chromosomes 15q25, 5p15, and 6p21: A pooled analysis from the international lung cancer consortium. *J Natl Cancer Inst*. 2010;102(13):959–971.

75. Boffetta P, Ahrens W, Nyberg F, et al. Exposure to environmental tobacco smoke and risk of adenocarcinoma of the lung. *Int J Cancer*. 1999;83(5):635–639.

76. Saccone NL, Culverhouse RC, Schwantes-An TH, et al. Multiple independent loci at chromosome 15q25.1 affect smoking quantity: A meta-analysis and comparison with lung cancer and COPD. *PLoS Genet.* 2010;6(8):e1001053.

77. Thorgeirsson TE, Gudbjartsson DF, Surakka I, et al. Sequence variants at CHRNB3-CHRNA6 and CYP2A6 affect smoking behavior. *Nat Genet.* 2010;42(5):448–453.

78. Lagiou P, Georgila C, Minaki P, et al. Alcohol-related cancers and genetic susceptibility in Europe: The ARCAGE project: Study samples and data collection. *Eur J Cancer Prev.* 2009;18(1):76–84.

79. Gaudet MM, Olshan AF, Chuang SC, et al. Body mass index and risk of head and neck cancer in a pooled analysis of case-control studies in the international head and neck cancer epidemiology (INHANCE) consortium. *Int J Epidemiol.* 2010;39(4):1091–1102.

80. Szymanska K, Levi JE, Menezes A, et al. TP53 and EGFR mutations in combination with life-style risk factors in tumours of the upper aerodigestive tract from South America. *Carcinogenesis.* 2010;31(6):1054–1059.

81. Feng BJ, Jalbout M, Ayoub WB, et al. Dietary risk factors for nasopharyngeal carcinoma in Maghrebian countries. *Int J Cancer.* 2007;121(7):1550–1555.

82. Herrero R, Castellsague X, Pawlita M, et al. Human papillomavirus and oral cancer: The international agency for research on cancer multicenter study. *J Natl Cancer Inst.* 2003;95(23):1772–1783.

83. Tuyns AJ, Esteve J, Raymond L, et al. Cancer of the larynx/hypopharynx, tobacco and alcohol: IARC international case-control study in Turin and Varese (Italy), Zaragoza and Navarra (Spain), Geneva (Switzerland) and Calvados (France). *Int J Cancer.* 1988;41(4):483–491.

84. Dikshit RP, Gillio-Tos A, Brennan P, et al. Hypermethylation, risk factors, clinical characteristics, and survival in 235 patients with laryngeal and hypopharyngeal cancers. *Cancer.* 2007;110(8):1745–1751.

85. Cook MB, Kamangar F, Whiteman DC, et al. Cigarette smoking and adenocarcinomas of the esophagus and esophagogastric junction: A pooled analysis from the international BEACON consortium. *J Natl Cancer Inst.* 2010;102(17):1344–1353.

86. Oliveira C, Bordin MC, Grehan N, et al. Screening E-cadherin in gastric cancer families reveals germline mutations only in hereditary diffuse gastric cancer kindred. *Hum Mutat.* 2002;19(5):510–517.

87. INTERPHONE Study Group. Brain tumour risk in relation to mobile telephone use: Results of the INTERPHONE international case-control study. *Int J Epidemiol.* 2010;39(3):675–694.

88. Schoemaker MJ, Swerdlow AJ, Auvinen A, et al. Medical history, cigarette smoking and risk of acoustic neuroma: An international case-control study. *Int J Cancer.* 2007;120(1):103–110.

89. Lahkola A, Salminen T, Raitanen J, et al. Meningioma and mobile phone use—a collaborative case-control study in five north European countries. *Int J Epidemiol.* 2008;37(6):1304–1313.

90. Preston-Martin S, Pogoda JM, Mueller BA, et al. Results from an international case-control study of childhood brain tumors: The role of prenatal vitamin supplementation. *Environ Health Perspect.* 1998;106 Suppl 3:887–892.

91. Cordier S, Mandereau L, Preston-Martin S, et al. Parental occupations and childhood brain tumors: Results of an international case-control study. *Cancer Causes Control.* 2001;12(9):865–874.

92. Pogoda JM, Preston-Martin S, Howe G, et al. An international case-control study of maternal diet during pregnancy and childhood brain tumor risk: A histology-specific analysis by food group. *Ann Epidemiol.* 2009;19(3):148–160.

93. Terry MB, Howe G, Pogoda JM, et al. An international case-control study of adult diet and brain tumor risk: A histology-specific analysis by food group. *Ann Epidemiol.* 2009;19(3):161–171.

94. Malmer B, Adatto P, Armstrong G, et al. GLIOGENE—an international consortium to understand familial glioma. *Cancer Epidemiology Biomarkers & Prevention.* 2007;16(9):1730–1734.

95. Daly AF, Vanbellinghen J, Khoo SK, et al. Aryl hydrocarbon receptor-interacting protein gene mutations in familial isolated pituitary adenomas: Analysis in 73 families. *Journal of Clinical Endocrinology & Metabolism.* 2007;92(5):1891–1896.

96. Benn DE, Gimenez-Roqueplo A, Reilly JR, et al. Clinical presentation and penetrance of Pheochromocytoma/Paraganglioma syndromes. *Journal of Clinical Endocrinology & Metabolism.* 2006;91(3):827–836.

97. Boedeker CC, Erlic Z, Richard S, et al. Head and neck paragangliomas in von hippel-lindau disease and multiple endocrine neoplasia type 2. *Journal of Clinical Endocrinology & Metabolism.* 2009;94(6):1938–1944.

98. Fortuny J, de Sanjose S, Becker N, et al. Statin use and risk of lymphoid neoplasms: Results from the European case-control study EPILYMPH. *Cancer Epidemiol Biomarkers Prev.* 2006;15(5):921–925.

99. Vajdic CM, Falster MO, de Sanjose S, et al. Atopic disease and risk of non-Hodgkin lymphoma: An InterLymph pooled analysis. *Cancer Res.* 2009;69(16):6482–6489.

100. Kaldor JM, Day NE, Pettersson F, et al. Leukemia following chemotherapy for ovarian cancer. *N Engl J Med.* 1990;322(1):1–6.

101. Lynch SM, Vrieling A, Lubin JH, et al. Cigarette smoking and pancreatic cancer: A pooled analysis from the pancreatic cancer cohort consortium. *Am J Epidemiol.* 2009;170(4):403–413.

102. Lowenfels AB, Maisonneuve P, Cavallini G, et al. Pancreatitis and the risk of pancreatic cancer. International pancreatitis study group. *N Engl J Med.* 1993;328(20):1433–1437.

103. Houlston RS, Webb E, Broderick P, et al. Meta-analysis of genome-wide association data identifies four new susceptibility loci for colorectal cancer. *Nat Genet.* 2008;40(12):1426–1435.

104. Tomlinson IP, Dunlop M, Campbell H, et al. COGENT (COlorectal cancer GENeTics): An international consortium to study the role of polymorphic variation on the risk of colorectal cancer. *Br J Cancer.* 2010;102(2):447–454.

105. Tomlinson IP, Webb E, Carvajal-Carmona L, et al. A genome-wide association study identifies colorectal cancer susceptibility loci on chromosomes 10p14 and 8q23.3. *Nat Genet.* 2008;40(5):623–630.

106. Pittman AM, Webb E, Carvajal-Carmona L, et al. Refinement of the basis and impact of common 11q23.1 variation to the risk of developing colorectal cancer. *Hum Mol Genet.* 2008;17(23):3720–3727.

107. World Health Organization (WHO). International liver cancer study. http://ilcs.iarc.fr/index.php. Updated 2010.

108. Heinemann K, Willich SN, Heinemann LA, DoMinh T, Mohner M, Heuchert GE. Occupational exposure and liver cancer in women: Results of the multicentre international liver tumour study (MILTS). *Occup Med (Lond).* 2000;50(6):422–429.

109. Bishop DT, Demenais F, Iles MM, et al. Genome-wide association study identifies three loci associated with melanoma risk. *Nat Genet.* 2009;41(8):920–925.

110. Berwick M, Orlow I, Hummer AJ, et al. The prevalence of CDKN2A germ-line mutations and relative risk for cutaneous malignant melanoma: An international population-based study. *Cancer Epidemiol Biomarkers Prev.* 2006;15(8):1520–1525.

111. Duffy DL, Iles MM, Glass D, et al. IRF4 variants have age-specific effects on nevus count and predispose to melanoma. *Am J Hum Genet.* 2010;87(1):6–16.

112. Gudmundsson J, Sulem P, Gudbjartsson DF, et al. Common variants on 9q22.33 and 14q13.3 predispose to thyroid cancer in European populations. *Nat Genet.* 2009;41(4):460–464.

113. Conway DI, Hashibe M, Boffetta P, et al. Enhancing epidemiologic research on head and neck cancer: INHANCE—the international head and neck cancer epidemiology consortium. *Oral Oncol.* 2009;45(9):743–746.

114. Berthiller J, Lee YC, Boffetta P, et al. Marijuana smoking and the risk of head and neck cancer: Pooled analysis in the INHANCE consortium. *Cancer Epidemiol Biomarkers Prev.* 2009;18(5):1544–1551.

115. Shapiro S. Meta-analysis/Shmeta-analysis. *Am J Epidemiol.* 1994;140(9):771–778.

116. Egger M, Schneider M, Davey Smith G. Spurious precision? Meta-analysis of observational studies. *BMJ.* 1998;316(7125):140–144.

117. Michaud DS, Vrieling A, Jiao L, et al. Alcohol intake and pancreatic cancer: A pooled analysis from the pancreatic cancer cohort consortium (PanScan). *Cancer Causes Control.* 2010;21(8):1213–1225.

118. Boffetta P, Armstrong B, Linet M, Kasten C, Cozen W, Hartge P. Consortia in cancer epidemiology: Lessons from InterLymph. *Cancer Epidemiol Biomarkers Prev.* 2007;16(2):197–199.

119. Gallicchio L, Helzlsouer KJ, Chow WH, et al. Circulating 25-hydroxyvitamin D and the risk of rarer cancers: Design and methods of the cohort consortium vitamin D pooling project of rarer cancers. *Am J Epidemiol.* 2010;172(1):10–20.

120. Bouvard V, Baan R, Straif K, et al. A review of human carcinogens—part B: Biological agents. *Lancet Oncol.* 2009;10(4):321–322.

121. Whitney CW, Lind BK, Wahl PW. Quality assurance and quality control in longitudinal studies. *Epidemiol Rev.* 1998;20(1):71–80.

122. Kamangar F, Chow WH, Abnet CC, Dawsey SM. Environmental causes of esophageal cancer. *Gastroenterol Clin North Am.* 2009;38(1):27–57, vii.

123. Cancer Council NSW. The international collaboration on HPV and oesophageal cancer (IntrSCOPE). http://www.cancercouncil.com.au/editorial.asp?pageid=2721. Updated 2011.

124. Robertson LB, Armstrong GN, Olver BD, et al. Survey of familial glioma and role of germline p16INK4A/p14ARF and p53 mutation. *Fam Cancer.* 2010;9(3):413–421.

125. International HapMap Consortium, Frazer KA, Ballinger DG, et al. A second generation human haplotype map of over 3.1 million SNPs. *Nature.* 2007;449(7164):851–861.

126. Vlaanderen J, Vermeulen R, Heederik D, Kromhout H, ECNIS Integrated Risk Assessment Group, European Union Network Of Excellence. Guidelines to evaluate human observational studies for quantitative risk assessment. *Environ Health Perspect.* 2008;116(12):1700–1705.

127. Tobacco and Genetics Consortium. Genome-wide meta-analyses identify multiple loci associated with smoking behavior. *Nat Genet.* 2010;42(5):441–447.

128. National Cancer Institute, U.S. National Institute of Health. Body mass index and all-cause mortality pooling project. http://epi.grants.cancer.gov/bmi/. Updated 2010.

129. Hill MJ. ECP-EURONUT study of diet and intestinal metaplasia. ECP-EURONUT-IM study group. *Eur J Cancer Prev.* 1997;6(2):201–204.

130. Fortier I, Burton PR, Robson PJ, et al. Quality, quantity and harmony: The DataSHaPER approach to integrating data across bioclinical studies. *Int J Epidemiol.* 2010;39(5):1383–1393.

131. Wolfson M, Wallace SE, Masca N, et al. DataSHIELD: Resolving a conflict in contemporary bioscience—performing a pooled analysis of individual-level data without sharing the data. *Int J Epidemiol.* 2010;39(5):1372–1382.

3

Curriculum Requirements in Training Graduate Students

CANCER EPIDEMIOLOGY RESEARCH TRAINING IN LMI COUNTRIES AND SPECIAL POPULATIONS: NEEDS AND OPPORTUNITIES

AMR S. SOLIMAN

ntroduction: Origins of Cancer Epidemiology The field of cancer epidemiology began as early as the 1700s through observational studies of nuns who had high rates of breast cancer and low rates of cervical cancer.[1] The observation of scrotal cancers in chimney sweepers was another early study of a possible link between occupational exposure and cancer development.[1,2]

In the 1900s, the role of infectious disease in cancer epidemiology was the main start for understanding the etiology of certain cancers. Burkitt,[3,4] Beasley,[5-7] and others[8-10] made important early contributions to understanding the possible link between infectious diseases and cancer. Other exposures in addition to infection became evident in the last half of the 20th century. Notable among these were early epidemiologic studies linking cigarette smoking to lung and other cancers.[11-13] This shift also included important questions about inter-individual susceptibility, including prior exposures, genetics, and lifestyle. Research in special populations in the United States—e.g. ethnic minorities—and low- and middle-income (LMI) countries offers unique opportunities to study these factors because of the heterogenenity of the genetics and exposures in special populations. The complexity of cancer epidemiologic research led to development of new analytical biostatistics techniques coupled with the analysis of biospecimens and biomarkers. These developments have required extensive laboratory resources and collaborations with scientists in fields beyond traditional epidemiology such as cytogenetics, molecular biology, genomics, metabolics, systems biology, and others. Today, in high-income (HI) countries, scientists in these fields are often included within the faculties of epidemiology departments.

This section includes five chapters discussing education, current resources, and future opportunities for cancer research training in epidemiology.

▨ HISTORY AND NEEDS FOR TRAINING IN CANCER EPIDEMIOLOGY RESEARCH

Many similarities exist between infectious and chronic disease field epidemiology: formulating and testing of hypotheses, communication with collaborators, setting up or using existing infrastructure for research investigation, planning for future studies, establishing central measures, communication of results, and developing and evaluation of training competencies. In the United States, the origin of systematic field training in epidemiology began with epidemiology field training in infectious disease. This training upgraded the skills of practitioners and researchers and improved the understanding of disease etiology, the spread of epidemics, and techniques of infectious disease surveillance. In particular, The Centers for Disease Control and Prevention (CDC) in Atlanta, Georgia, United States, has a history of a strong epidemiology field training and research program, "Epidemic Intelligence Service" (EIS), which has been in place since 1951. EIS officers serve as public health experts conducting epidemiologic research investigations and surveillance of infectious diseases both nationally and internationally. Over the past 60+ years, over 3000 individuals have worked and trained in this program and gained enormous experience in field epidemiology on both domestic and international fronts.[14]

Systematic training in cancer epidemiology began after the US Congress amended the Public Health Service Act with the National Cancer Act of 1971 to expand the scope and responsibilities of the National Cancer Institute (NCI) of the National Institutes of Health. Cancer training programs began to be funded by the NCI in 1980s as described below.

▨ WHY IS CANCER EPIDEMIOLOGY TRAINING IN SPECIAL POPULATIONS IMPORTANT?

Globalization has paved the way to distant international destinations and increased awareness and interest in health disparities. Many global health programs, including cancer programs, have been initiated at US academic centers and research and medical institutions to promote global health. The NCI launched a new program on global cancer in 2012 to highlight the importance of the field and to strengthen collaborative activities and dissemination of advances in the field of oncology to LMI countries. Thus, whether in HI or LMI countries, educational and learning opportunities in the fields of cancer epidemiology and cancer prevention are increasing. Understanding cancer in LMI countries will have implications for cancer epidemiology research and training and cancer prevention for migrant populations from LMI countries in high-income countries. Moreover, cancer research in special populations will improve our understanding of/insights into gene-environment interactions and may help reduce disparities through prevention and control interventions.

Definition of Special Populations in Cancer Epidemiology

While LMI countries are traditionally referred to as "International," migrant and nonwhite ethnic populations in HI countries are typically referred to as "minority populations." "Special populations" in the United States is a frequently used term in public health and population science research to refer to international and minority populations.[15] Special populations can be defined epidemiologically by geographic, social, and economic characteristics; examples include minority populations, high-risk populations, aged populations, immigrant populations, medically underserved, and cancer survivor populations, both domestically and internationally. In this chapter, special populations are defined as cancer patients in international and minority settings in developed/high-income countries.

The Global Burden of Cancer

The World Cancer Report, issued by the International Agency for Research on Cancer (IARC), documents that cancer rates are set to increase at alarming rates worldwide because of aging and increasing world populations.[16] GLOBOCAN estimated that about 12.7 million cancer cases and 7.6 million cancer deaths occurred in 2008, with 56% of the cases and 64% of the deaths in developing countries.[17] Due to increased longevity and lifestyle risk factors, such as obesity and exposure to environmental carcinogens, industrialized countries are expected to show about a 50% increase in cancer incidence.[18] Expected increase in cancer incidence and mortality in developing countries are not parallel to the needed increase in the workforce in epidemiology to help in future cancer control and prevention in these countries.

Cancer in Low- and Middle-Income Countries

With their unique contrasts in lifestyles, environmental exposures, massive exposure to infectious agents, characteristic familial patterns such as consanguinity, and diverse cancer profiles, LMI countries provide an incomparable, and often neglected, opportunity for studying the mechanisms of environmental carcinogenesis.[19–21] Such studies should eventually lead to the development of novel intervention approaches. Unfortunately, cancer research is difficult to conduct in the LMI countries, due to the lack of population-based registries, poor communication and transportation systems, deficiencies in infrastructure and financial support, and a limited number of trained cancer researchers.[22] These difficulties can be overcome, to the benefit of all, if collaborations in cancer research between the LMI and industrialized nations are extended.

In addition to improving our understanding of health issues in the host countries, cancer research in international settings has shaped public health policies for disease prevention in the United States For example, research on Hepatitis B virus in Taiwan revealed the association between Hepatitis B viral infection and liver cancer[7,23,24] and has shaped the national policy for HBV vaccinations of children in the U.S and other countries.[24] International cancer epidemiology research on the pathogenesis and etiology of Burkitt's lymphoma in Africa and the role of Epstein Barr virus in its development is also a major landmark in the field of cancer epidemiology from international studies.[3,4] In highlighting changing risk in populations by migration and variation in exposures and lifestyle factors by migration from countries of low risk to countries of high risk, the increasing risk for breast cancer among Asian immigrants to the United States is yet another demonstration of the importance of cancer epidemiology research in special populations.[25,26]

Cancer in Minority Populations in the United States

Recent reports from the Surveillance, Epidemiology, and End Results (SEER) database and other reports indicate that cancer incidence, mortality, and survival rates in the United States vary by race and ethnicity.[27–30] The variation in incidence, mortality, and survival highlight the importance of conducting additional studies to clarify the epidemiologic, socioeconomic, medical, behavioral, and biological determinants of these differences among ethnic groups in the United States.[27,29–31]

Numerous examples of important applications and discoveries have helped highlight the need for cancer epidemiology research in minority populations. Research has demonstrated that breast cancer tends to occur at a younger age in African American women compared to white women, and to follow a more aggressive course.[32-36] Hispanics have lower incidence and death rates from all cancers combined and from the four most common cancers (breast, prostate, lung and bronchus, and colon and rectum) compared with non-Hispanic whites.[37-39] However, Hispanics have higher incidence and mortality rates from cancers of the stomach, liver, uterine cervix, and gallbladder, reflecting in part greater exposure to specific infectious agents and lower rates of screening for cervical cancer, as well as dietary patterns and possible genetic factors.[39] Cancer incidence also varies among Hispanics based on their country of origin.[40] Research on Native Americans and Alaskans (AIAN) has shown variable incidence among AINA population according to their region of residence.[41] For all cancer sites combined, AIAN rates are higher than non-Hispanic whites (NHWs) among both males and females in the Northern and Southern plains and among Alaska Native females.[40] AIAN rates are lower than NHW rates in the Southern, the Pacific coast, and the East, and the variations are unlikely to be due to racial misclassification.[40] The universality of cancer is apparent, but cancer site-specific incidence patterns are varied in magnitude and reflect the complexity of multifactorial determinants.

Interventions to reduce health disparities include programs for breast and prostate cancer, early detection programs among ethnic minorities,[42,43] and cancer prevention among physically impaired populations.[44,45] However, recent research has demonstrated numerous obstacles to such interventions. For example, language barriers and limited time with physicians were barriers for cancer information about early detection among Chinese immigrants.[46] The importance of considering the right intervention in the context of the culture of individuals was addressed by Erwin et al., 2010 in studies on Latina women. Country of origin and current geographic residency in the United States were significant determinants of women's perspectives on community-based religious organizations. These factors were also important in women's understanding of anatomy, experiences with the medical system, and access to services to ensure effective cancer control interventions. In other words, programs such as breast and cervical cancer early detection programs cannot be implemented effectively outside the sociopolitical setting of local communities, especially for the most recent immigrant women.[47]

Health care providers and researchers must be educated about culturally sensitive communication skills for effective health information and research among immigrant women.[48]

Epidemiologic Benefits of Linking Minorities and International Studies

Cancer patterns in minorities in the United States show similarities to distinct epidemiologic cancer features in developing countries, and studies of these similarities may improve our understanding of cancer epidemiology, risk factors, and pathways of carcinogenesis. For example, the pattern of breast cancer incidence seen in African American women in the United States (i.e., younger age, more aggressive disease)[32,33] is also seen in developing countries.[49] These patterns may indicate that the young-onset and aggressive pattern seen in developing countries is due to distinct genetic factors as postulated for African Americans,[50] or that African American patterns are due to exposures such as those reported in developing countries.[51] As another example, groups of colorectal cancer patients who do not show familial aggregation of cancers and certain molecular features exist at low frequency in US. white and minority populations as well as in international settings.[52-54] Analysis of differences among these subsets may help shape the development of screening guidelines based on common features of tumors.[53,54] By ascertaining colonic tumors with distinct molecular features—e.g. microsatellite instability on the basis of marked lymphocytic infiltration—the upper age limit for microsatellite testing could be raised to 55 or 60 years without compromising specificity.[54] These comparative studies show many common disease features that need to be further explored.

Differences in cancer incidence and mortality among ethnic and racial groups or between migrant and US populations[55,56] call for research to identify risk factors and tailor prevention and control interventions. Examples of disparities include the higher incidence of breast cancer and its risk factors among US-born Hispanic women compared with foreign-born Hispanics.[57] Protective factors in the home-lands of recent migrants to the United States are also anticipated in this risk difference.[58] Higher risk for prostate cancer among African Americans than whites and possible higher risk for the disease among Africans with West-African ancestry is another example of incidence disparity.[59,60] Limited access to diagnostic facilities and possible therapeutic delay that minorities experience also contribute to gaps in prognosis and outcomes between populations.[61] Taken together, cancer research in special populations can provide opportunities for elucidating etiology, identifying cultural barriers to early detection, and setting the stage for tailored control and prevention.

Target Groups for Cancer Epidemiology Training in Special Populations

Students in Low- and Middle-Income Countries or in the United States in the Fields of Public Health, Medicine, Nursing, and Other Biomedical Sciences

Students in public health, medical schools, nursing, and other health-related and biomedical fields in LMI or high-income countries learn about epidemiology and sometimes cancer epidemiology as part of chronic disease epidemiology education.

In LMI countries and the United States, epidemiology is not a well-recognized field by itself except at graduate level education. In LMI countries, epidemiology is mainly taught in schools of medicine as part of public health education. On a smaller scale, epidemiology is included in some nursing and biomedical institutions in LMI countries. In the few graduate schools or graduate institutes of public health, if available in LMI countries, epidemiology is a recognized field in public health. However, it is important to note that in LMI countries, whether in medical or biomedical education, the main focus of epidemiology instruction is still on infectious disease. With increasing westernization, longevity, better diagnostic facilities, and more awareness and survival of cancer patients in LMI countries, however, chronic disease and cancer should be recognized as an important aspect of epidemiology and public health education.

The type of epidemiological training also needs to change. In addition to traditional didactic teaching via lectures, only a few LMI countries—including Egypt, Uganda, and Ghana—provide field training in public health and epidemiology. The field training is mainly focused on observation, although summer internships may include data collection. Little training is included on research methods or design, data collection or analysis, cultural issues, interviewing, or multidisciplinary or inter-disciplinary research. While resources from cancer hospitals or cancer centers are present in some countries, little or no interaction is available to include such resources in teaching or training of students.

In countries that have adopted a community-based problem-solving teaching approach, public health students may encounter cancer as a part of their education. Those countries recognize the importance of focusing on cancer because of their closer engagements in the field by assessment of disease incidence, working with the community to set up health priorities, and developing interventions. However, because cancer still occurs at a significantly lower incidence than infectious diseases, stigma of cancer in many developing countries still exist, and because cancer status are not known for many patients, field training on cancer is often unsubstantial.

As one notable exception, China has an extensive system for undergraduate and masters' programs in public health, but once again the main focus is on infectious diseases through collaborations with the Centers for Disease Control and Prevention of China. However, cancer is an emerging health problem in China, and steps are on the way for its inclusion in the public health education.[62]

Researchers from Other Fields in High- and Low- and Middle-Income Countries

Cancer epidemiology research is becoming increasingly directed toward multidisciplinary teams. The old days of investigation of epidemics by a single epidemiologist are over. This is happening because of the multifactorial etiology of chronic diseases like cancer. The multidisciplinary nature of cancer epidemiology requires involvement of researchers with different expertise to facilitate the design, implementation, and analysis of complex molecular and genetic cancer epidemiology studies. Researchers involved in such studies include demographers, social scientists, anthropologists, health economists, biostatisticians, oncologists, pathologists, nurses, virologists, nutritionists, and occupational and environmental health scientists. Their experience is needed to formulate hypotheses, share study design, optimize recruitment, analyze biological specimens, integrate field and laboratory results, analyze data, publish the results and plan for future research. The collaboration of researchers from different fields can also add to their own learning experience.

In international cancer epidemiology research studies, cancer epidemiology researchers from high-income countries (which typically fund these collaborations) are in touch with collaborators from the above-listed fields in their home country or in LMI countries. Such collaborations help maximize the success of the design, implementation, and interpretation of the study. Examples include studies on assessment of environmental exposures to chemicals in the etiology of cancer. Without local experts on occupational and environmental health sciences, information on historic exposures, mixtures of chemicals, and changing doses of exposures would have never been available. Another example is the changes in the procedure of diagnosis of inflammatory breast cancer from fine needle aspiration to tissue core biopsy. This revised procedure, suggested by clinical collaborators of studies on the epidemiology of breast cancer in North Africa, has improved the diagnosis of the disease for patients and has also improved access to tissues for the molecular epidemiologic study.[63]

These collaborations between experts in different fields from HI and LMI countries highlight the need for cultural training and sensitivity. Local researchers recognize the best ways of asking sensitive questions in a noninvasive way. For example, in an ongoing case-control study on IBC in North Africa, because of the suspected etiology of mammary tumor virus exposure (MMTV),[64] it was important to ask about study subjects' possible exposure to mice. Local collaborator designed a series of questions to approach study subjects in an indirect way about exposure to mice. The questions started by asking about mice control campaigns in the neighborhood of the study subjects, followed by questions about mice in neighbors' homes, and finally about mice in the study subject's home. Thus, the order of questions could either encourage study subjects to complete the interview or dampen their enthusiasm if they felt that the interview was like a "police interrogation." This kind of cultural sensitivity can have a significant impact on the success of interviewing. Thus, the expertise and advice of local collaborators in LMI countries have a tremendous impact on the success of a given study.

The role of Clinical Health Professionals in HI or LMI Countries (Physicians and Other Professionals in Clinical Practice or Population-Based Prevention) in Cancer Epidemiology

Clinicians in high-income and LMI countries are integral parts of successful multidisciplinary cancer epidemiology studies; therefore, clinicians from LMI countries need to be included in joint cancer epidemiology studies. For example, studies for predicting survivorship in LMI countries can benefit significantly from the experience of participating clinicians who can advise on the best tools to follow cancer patients, reasons for loss to follow-up, and best ways to contact and recruit patients to participate and comply with demanding research and follow-up studies. At the same time, clinicians need to be educated about sound epidemiologic principles to maximize the chances of valid unbiased outcomes. For example, participating clinicians must understand selection and information bias, matching, randomization, confounding, and the ability to generalize the results. Without these skills, the results can be misleading, biased, and un-publishable. For example, it will not be possible to arrive at a representative sample without understanding the general pool of cancer patients at referral cancer centers in terms of income, residence, disease stage at presentation, and referral patterns.

Translating epidemiologic research findings into clinical practice is very important for maintaining the enthusiasm and motivation of clinicians in the epidemiological studies and continuing a reciprocal relationship. Translating cancer epidemiology into cancer prevention and control should consider the local clinical resources and practices in each respective country. Clinical treatment is an individualized process specific to the local country and to even sub-groups with each country. For example, mammography may not be the ideal tool for early detection in many LMI countries.[65] Without epidemiologic data on incidence, age-specific rates, stage of diagnosis of the disease, family history of breast cancer, and possible environmental or genetic factors, mammography might be a poor utilization of resources. In most developing countries where breast cancer incidence is not high and age-specific rates are higher among middle age than older women, applying population-based screening of the general population may not be the best use of resources. It is important to communicate this information to clinicians and policy makers in developing countries and show the importance of understanding the epidemiology of specific cancers before planning for early detection programs or cancer prevention. Even if the early detection tools and equipment are available in a LMI country, available treatment facilities and medications available for the new cancer patients must be identified. If treatment facilities, oncology teams, and medications are not available, identifying the cases and early detection might not be the best benefit for those patients.

Diseases with special and possibly subjective diagnostic clinical criteria such as IBC are also challenging in cancer epidemiology research. Moreover, differences in diagnostic methods and classification of IBC between high-income and LMI countries and different possible risk factors implicated in the disease etiology may interfere with the disease presentation.[66] Studying cases of such disease without standard clinical criteria may lead to misclassification and inaccuracies in conclusions and interpretation of the results.[67]

The understanding of the limited continuous medical education in developing countries highlights the importance of scientific encounters with international collaborators. Junior collaborators involved in international epidemiologic studies are particularly eager to learn about new diagnostic and management protocols, guidelines for treatment and prevention, and new methods for screening. Clinicians in LMI countries may be a great source of identifying high rates of rare cancers in their countries based on clinical observations and impressions. However, these observations need to be documented in proper epidemiologic methods of rates, not just frequency of cases. In the case of young-onset cancer, the population denominator of a large at-risk population young people should raise the questions whether the rate of young-onset cancer is really high or it just seems high due to the younger populations in LMI countries. The same concept applies to the observation noted by many clinicians in many LMI countries about high rates of aggressive tumors in their countries. Without accounting for the total pool of patients, understanding of access to medical care, and accurate documentation of cancer-related mortality, this notion cannot be substantiated.

Overall, collaborators and clinicians in developing countries can be a great resource for streamlining epidemiologic studies and providing innovative ideas to simplify studies, provide sources and good methods for recruitment, interviewing, and logistics of the study. It is extremely important to call on their input, creative ideas, and best practice for the implementation of cancer epidemiology research studies. Because of their familiarity with hospitals, clinics, and communities, in addition to their personal communication with their own patients and other physicians, local clinicians can provide many solutions for improving the efficiency of a study.

Target Beneficiaries of Cancer Epidemiology Training in Special Populations

International Agencies
International agencies interested in health policy and cancer research, prevention, and control [e.g. the World Health Organization (WHO) and the International Agency for Research on Cancer (IARC)] can benefit from cancer epidemiology training in special populations. For example, involvement of trainees in validating cancer registration data in developing countries, migrant populations, and minority populations in high-income countries can improve the quality of data and identify gaps for improvement. Students and trainees can also initiate research studies based on cancer registry data resources.[68–74] Working on hospital registries in developing countries can improve the understanding of cancer distribution, data strengths and limitations, and set the stage for possible population-based cancer registries based on major cancer hospital statistics.[75,76] In minority populations such as Native Americans in the United States, trainees can initiate new ideas such as correcting the under-estimation of cancer and linkage between state registries and special minority population registries.[77]

Governments and Ministries of Health in LMIC
Governments and Ministries of Health in LMI countries can benefit tremendously from joint collaborations in epidemiologic cancer studies. First, these collaborations can initiate or improve the quality of cancer registries in LMI countries. Joint collaborations can also help improve the understanding, handling, and usage of incomplete and inconsistent data registry data. Second, government agencies and health ministries in LMI countries can develop their understanding of the total burden of cancer and its distribution by cancer sites, gender, age groups, stages, diagnostic sites and methods. Third, cancer epidemiology research studies can characterize at-risk populations and cancer clusters based on genetic, environmental, or gene-environment risk. This characterization or profiling can help provide further resources for investigating such clusters and provide treatment and prevention care, along with other social and financial support for these groups.

In particular, research collaboration and training with cancer registries in developing countries can improve the quality of information/data. For example, cancer registries usually collect a short list of standard variables such as age, sex, stage, place of residence, tumor site, date of first diagnosis of cancer and method of diagnosis. Population-based cancer registries are not necessarily designed to provide data for extensive epidemiologic research, but can be used to assess the magnitude of cancer in a population, monitor changes over time, and assess the effect of prevention interventions. However, other information and variables may exist in the medical records where registry data is abstracted that may be added to expand the registry and enhance it for comprehensive cancer research studies. The time and effort needed for their addition should be explored. Evaluation of the benefits of additions to standard registry form or operation must be examined in terms of their research benefits for special studies and for comparison with other registries. For example, in research collaborations of the Middle East Cancer Consortium site in Egypt, hormone receptor data was available in the medical and pathology records, but not in the population-base registry routine data. Because of the need for hormone receptor information in research utilizing the registry data, hormone receptor status became a routine data item for breast cancer cases in the registry after a research study.[72] In addition, the SEER staging for breast cancer is the standard element for international registry. However, SEER staging limits the comparison with datasets using the American Joint Committee on Cancer (AJCC) staging. Research collaboration with the population-based registry of Egypt also initiated the addition of the AJCC staging, which became an additional item in the routine registry afterwards.[72,78]

Populations in LMI Countries

Populations in LMI countries can benefit from epidemiologic studies through increasing their awareness about cancer and identifying hereditary or familial cancer syndrome families. These families can benefit from subsequent screening, early detection, and technology transfer that would have been unavailable without such scientific collaboration between HI and LMI countries. Cancer epidemiology research training can estimate the high-proportions of advance-stage cancers in populations in LMI countries and bring attention to the need for specific types of management, such as palliative care. Cancer epidemiology research in LMI countries can also open opportunities for advancing science and benefiting populations in LMI countries. For example, consanguinity (marriage of close relatives such as first-cousins) is relatively common in LMI countries, especially in some Asian and the Middle Eastern countries.[52,79,80] Studying cancer in those populations can provide valuable insights into cancer genetics, the role of autosomal recessive genes in cancer epidemiology, and cancer risk assessment for populations with consanguineous marriages.[79–82]

Epidemiological studies usually do not provide immediate solutions, and thus there is no immediate benefit to the study participant based on his/her participation. While this concept is usually understood in HI countries, it is generally not the expectation in LMI countries, especially because of the lack of research traditions. Therefore, cancer epidemiology studies should consider providing useful brochures in the native language to provide some immediate benefit to the study participant. While the consent form of the study should maintain the language of no immediate benefit to the participant as a result of participation in the research study, providing services, such as availability of clinics or physicians who are part of the team of the study, can be helpful to the community.

Immigrant Populations in High-Income Countries

Cancer epidemiology research can also create opportunities for understanding the effect of migration on changing cancer profiles. Changing lifestyles caused by migration from one country to another provide examples of the contribution of environmental and lifestyle factors to cancer epidemiology. For example, the classic descriptive study of breast cancer among women in Japan, Hawaii, and California showed a higher incidence of breast cancer among Japanese women in California than in Hawaii or Japan. These women were considered similar in their genetics, yet their exposures to Western lifestyles were greater in California.[25] Similar studies showed that Arab Americans and Americans of Middle Eastern descent have different cancer rates for certain sites than non-Hispanic white populations in the SSER registries in Michigan and California.[83,84] For example, studies conducted in Michigan and California showed that Arab American women living in the United States have a higher risk of thyroid cancer than non-Hispanic white (NHW) women. Arab/Chaldean women in metropolitan Detroit have 57% greater proportion of thyroid cancer as compared to NHW women[83]. Middle Eastern women living in California have a higher incidence of thyroid cancer than NHW women with a risk ratio of 1.3.[84]

Benefits and Skill Development for Students and Collaborators Involved in Field Training in Special Populations

(For additional discussion of this topic, please also read Robert M. Chamberlain's Chapter 6 in Section 1.)

Understanding the academic, clinical, and/or research cultures for special population cancer epidemiology research is an essential initial step for achieving a good learning experience and a productive and long-lasting collaboration. Students need to understand that there are certain principles that they have to master before, during, and after a joint collaboration or training in special populations.

▪ CHARACTERISTICS OF LOW- AND MIDDLE-INCOME COUNTRIES

Before traveling to the LMI country settings, students should learn about the culture of their host country/population, institutions, and collaborators. Prior to training in LMI countries, learning can be achieved through exchanges with faculty and/or students who have travelled to or worked in the same foreign setting or institution. Knowledge about the interest and track record of collaborators, their clinical, research, and/or educational needs, interests and motives, publication portfolio, and their expectation of the collaboration is valuable. If this collaboration is new without a previous track record of collaboration with prior faculty or students from the home institution, searches through publications or internet sites may identify collaborators who could be contacted before traveling to the site in order to learn about the culture of the special population and collaborators.

This preparatory work can save significant time and effort before arriving in the LMI country. It is important to learn about the academic culture of the institution in terms of the hierarchy and seniority systems of the host institution, work hours, national holidays, and full-time or part-time employment of faculty and staff. Understanding the best ways of research navigation is a major part in achieving successful outcomes. Developing and performing epidemiologic studies on cancer might not be best arranged with faculty from departments of epidemiology, even if they exist, but with clinicians and oncologists who typically lead cancer centers or departments in major hospitals in LMI countries. Understanding how nonepidemiologists may help the planning and execution of cancer epidemiologic studies is one of the important cornerstones in successful epidemiologic research studies in LMI countries. Finally, developing relationship with faculty and staff at the collaborating institution may be a valuable asset in accomplishing tasks such as obtaining research permits, renewal of visas, and packaging, preserving, and arrangements shipping biological specimens among many others.

In many LMI countries, political changes are not uncommon and can affect the flow of research studies. Political instability can definitely impact the flow of the study and ability to meet timelines and should be factored in with alternative methods for achieving the study goals.

It should also be noted that in many LMI countries, multiple tribes and ethnic groups exist and many languages may be spoken. There may also be a history of conflict between tribes such as in countries in sub-Saharan Africa, and tribal power may be due to the political history or wealth of certain groups. Those cultural issues should be considered. Furthermore, rooted cultural health beliefs must be understood with respect to health and disease definitions and their variation by ethnic groups in the LMI countries before engagement in cancer epidemiology research. For example, role of hot and cold food for treatment of disease, evil eyes, role of spirits and ghosts in causing or treating diseases such as cancer can vary from one community to another even within a single LMI country.[85–91] Understanding these cultural factors is extremely important for interviewing and capturing of information.

Another important cultural issue that student should be aware of in many LMI countries is the slow pace of activities. Students must be prepared for lowering expectations in terms of what may be achieved during a visit or research period, compared to the same work in high-income countries. The laid-back environment, short and varying work hours, competing personal and academic duties, different structures of clinical and research resources, and time needed for diplomacy and social events will require additional time for achieving the same tasks in high-income country research environments. Students must understand that the interrupted engagement of collaborators in LMI countries does not imply lack of respect or interest in the collaborators from high-income countries; it is a reflection of different work cultures and lifestyles in different research, medical, and academic settings.

▪ PROFESSIONAL AND INSTITUTIONAL CULTURE

Learning about the social culture of collaborators in terms of professional dress code, hosting preferences, and protocols of communication with collaborators by mail, phone, fax, or e-mails is extremely important for achieving the best outcomes of the scientific goals of the study. Students and collaborators can familiarize themselves with these professional and institutional cultural issues by talking to collaborators and staff at the institution and in the country.

Dress code can be particularly important. Students and collaborators from HI countries should inquire about the appropriate dress code inside and outside professional environments. For example, students from western countries who travel to conservative countries in the Middle East should consider a modest dress code, but not the exact code of women in the local community.

While knowledge of many of these topics can be gleaned before traveling to the LMI country, numerous points can also be learned on site and should be left to face-to-face communication. These points may include for example discussion of detailed financial arrangements for the study, institutional overhead rates, and authorship arrangements.

Students who will be conducting field studies in villages must have a local person, preferably a local health unit or center employee, not necessarily at a high rank, from the same village, accompanying them during home visits, approaching participants, and interviewing. If there is a "headman" or a "king" of the village, this person must be approached to support and facilitate the study. The headman or king will usually assign a head nurse or local health professional to be part of the team and facilitate logistic issues during the project.

Because neighbors are usually curious to know the aim of the study and why certain homes are selected for recruitment, it is important to be able to clearly articulate the aims of the study, including why homes are visited, without disclosing confidential information and while protecting the privacy of study participants.

Students involved in research in LMI countries need to be informed about other practical matters: they should carry with them the name, address, phone number/business card of their local sponsor to be given to taxi drivers or police officers if needed, along with the name, phone number, and address of their hotel. They should also check for travel advisory, warning, or banning of travel to specific countries on websites in their home countries, such as the State Department website in the United States. They should register their contact information with their home institution and their home country embassy or consulate in the LMI country and carry the telephone number of the embassy or consulate during their presence in LMI countries in case of emergencies and learn about the any needs for carrying their passports or copies of it while they are in the LMI countries. Students should be aware that traffic, automobile, and motorcycle accidents are major problems in LMI countries and should inquire about the best modes of transportation, such as public buses, taxis, and bicycles and whether they are appropriate for women.

Many of these concerns are also applicable to student research collaboration in minority settings and migrant populations in high-income countries. Students need an understanding of cultural backgrounds of ethnic minorities, cultures of migration and immigrant populations, differences between migrant and subjects born in the new country of migration, and any cultural conflicts between the minorities and mainstream population. It is useful for students to know if they are respected, appreciated, or bothersome in minority cultures.

Trainees of immigrant backgrounds can be particularly helpful in cancer epidemiology research because of their awareness of the cultural and behavioral backgrounds of the community and possible mastery of the native language. However, certain factors must be considered if student trainees are involved in interviewing in migrant population research. The age of the interviewer is important. Relatively young students are sometimes not taken seriously if interviewing older populations. An example was a low response rate resulting from research interviews conducted by a young US-born interviewer from the same ethnic background of a research community mainly because of the young age of the interviewer and her US accent.[78] When the interviewing was conducted by an older nurse from a local community health center who spoke the native language of the community, the response rate was 100%.[78] It should be noted also that students are not trained as interviewers although they may take courses on interviewing and so they are not necessarily the best interviewers in research studies. Even if they speak the language of the community, they may lack certain understanding of cultural background of the community or ethnic groups in the community even if the same language is spoken. For example, interviewing individuals in a Hispanic migrant community may require a special understanding of the community and its utilization of health care through neighborhood clinics, not just the ability to speak Spanish.

Clinicians who are involved in cancer epidemiology research in minority settings in their home country need to learn about cultural issues in the community. Understanding cancer stigmas in certain minority and migrant communities or their skepticism about mainstream medical systems are important for the success of cancer epidemiology and prevention research. The preference for community clinics staffed by physicians from the same ethnic groups over regular general population clinics may be a determining factor in recruiting participants in cancer epidemiology and/or cancer prevention research studies. Lack of interest and skepticism about participation in clinical and/or prevention trials or preference for same-sex physicians in some cultures are all important insights for clinical collaborators who participate in cancer epidemiology research studies in ethnic minority or migrant populations in HI countries.

One example will help explicate this point: A study explored barriers to cervical cancer screening among immigrants in Ontario, Canada and found that access to a primary care physician and a female doctor are important cultural factors that would increase screening rates.[92] Another way to remove barriers for improving breast cancer knowledge and promoting screening behaviors is the understanding that the immigrant populations may not used electronic media or print[93] but rely on community-based discussion groups.[94]

▦ SKILLS DEVELOPED BY STUDENTS CONDUCTING CANCER EPIDEMIOLOGY RESEARCHING IN SPECIAL POPULATIONS

The learning experience for students conducting research in special populations can be immense and can be grouped into three major areas: epidemiologic methods, health systems, and logistics of research.

▦ EPIDEMIOLOGIC METHODS

Cancer centers in LMI countries are usually overloaded with cancer patients because of increasing number of cancer cases, better awareness about cancer, and better access to diagnostic and treatment facilities. In these busy clinics, it is always a challenge to introduce an epidemiologic study and request attention for recruitment of patients and interviewing during the busy clinical schedule. Identifying a research setting, personnel, and time to consent, recruit, and interview patients, and possibly collect biological specimen will require the development of special skills and creativity.[95]

Increased understanding of epidemiologic methods can be achieved through different experiences in cancer epidemiology research in LMI countries. These learning experiences include study design, recruitment of study subjects, control selection, understanding bias, randomization, questionnaire development, and data and biological specimen collection.[95]

Exposure to such research will teach students how to be creative in developing alternative study designs and thinking in ways different from classic textbook epidemiology, without compromising appropriate epidemiological principles. Students will develop increased cultural and social skills by learning how to deal with different cultures for studies in LMI countries where the culture of research and/or volunteering for research studies may not exist.

Examples of untraditional ways of recruiting controls in case-control studies in LMI countries may include "visitor controls" who are not relatives of the cancer patients. Because of the relatively long period of hospital stay of cancer patients during the preoperative and postoperative periods and the large family size in many LMI countries, recruiting visitors' controls may be possible.[96-98] An important point that should be considered in control selection in LMI countries is any preexisting (known or unknown) medical conditions of controls. Undiagnosed medical condition may interfere with the comparison with the cancer patients in the case group and ways should be considered to check preexisting conditions among controls in LMI countries.

Students conducting research in LMI countries can utilize the advantage of the variability of environmental exposures as well as populations with exceptionally high environmental exposures that might be related to cancer. In finding differences between cancer patients and noncancer controls, these settings can enhance the efficiency of cancer epidemiology research studies. In addition, many LMI countries experience the double burden of communicable and noncommunicable diseases and can be an ideal research setting for studying cancers with infectious etiology. Variation in nutritional status in LMI countries with different scales ranging from malnutrition to obesity can present ideal settings for studying the relationship between cancer and nutrition.

Other research skill that may be enhanced in LMI countries is dealing with incomplete and inconsistent data. Medical records in LMI countries present many challenges, and students should be prepared to deal with them. First, medical records may not be organized or archived or kept for very long because of limited storage space or because many medical settings see no value in keeping the records on the assumption that the majority of patients die. Second, multiple medical records for the same patient may exist in different departments of a cancer center or hospital. Third, lack of sufficient demographic or patient identifiers, incomplete or identical names of different patients, and limited clinical information may constitute significant challenges to epidemiologic research. Some LMI countries have begun instituting a social security number system that will help future research studies. Other countries have health insurance numbers, social support numbers, and other similar identifiers that can help link patient information between different departments. With emerging new technologies for electronic medical records and informatics, this is a promising research area for students and researchers to explore creative ways to improve the quality of medical records, linkage between hospitals and departments, and maximizing the efficiency of research in LMI countries, considering the limited resources and lack of electronic tools for medical records of linkage of medical departments.

For designing epidemiologic questionnaire to capture socioeconomic, occupational, and lifestyle factors, consulting the local collaborators and reviewing publications from previous surveys and national studies can be of significant help. Cultural sensitivity in developing the questionnaires, setting up the order of questions and developing questions for sensitive issues should also be developed in collaboration and consultation with the local clinicians and researchers. Translation of questionnaires from English for example to the local language of the LMI country should be conducted locally in the country, not in high-income countries, by professional translators.

Clinical and medical review forms for cancer epidemiology research should be developed in collaboration with the local clinicians and researchers at the LMI country research site. Clinicians can suggest user-friendly forms and the best way to deliver them to capture the needed information.

▪ HEALTH SYSTEMS

Cancer epidemiology research offers important opportunities for learning about health systems of the host LMI countries. For example, understanding the demographic and clinical characteristics of the patient population in the hospital or cancer center will help avoid selection bias and verify the possibility of generalization of the results to the general population. It is imperative to understand the diagnostic and treatment facilities for patients before their arrival at a tertiary cancer center in the LMI country and how this referral may increase or decrease access to cases with late-stage presentation. In other words, patients seen at tertiary cancer centers may not be representative of all social and economic classes of patients and stages of the disease, and may only represent a selected group of patients. Studies from Tanzania showed that patients' economic and residential characteristics are major factors in determining whether or not patients can seek treatment at the major cancer center of the country. Only patients who can afford to get to the cancer center or live nearby can get treatment at the major and only cancer center of the country.[75]

Different types of health care systems exist in LMI countries. Some LMI countries have national health systems, others have private care systems, while many have mix of both national insurance and private systems. Understanding the types of health systems in the country and the research institution will be very important for patient recruitment, representation, and the ability to make inferences on specific groups of patients or the general population of patients in the country. In addition, in many developing countries, traditional healers are one of the main providers of cancer care. Their role in cancer care in the LMI country may influence referrals to cancer hospitals or hindering that referral and biasing the sample of the study.[99]

▦ RESEARCH LOGISTICS

While email communication with collaborators in LMI countries has increased significantly over the past several years, students should be aware that government hospitals in many LMI countries lack individual computers for individual faculty and staff and also lack access to high-speed internet. This point should be considered when collaborators in LMI countries are asked to use websites to upload study forms, data entry, or large-size files. Advanced technology might not be the optimal technology for success of cancer epidemiologic studies in LMI countries. Researchers must consider what is practical and familiar to the local investigators before providing high tech, expensive software for data entry or data management that may require significant training of the local research team. In many cases, low-tech tools for study management and follow-up in LMI countries may be more practical than advanced sophisticated program.

Obtaining sufficient and viable biological specimens is one of the most challenging tasks in cancer epidemiology research in LMI countries. For example, obtaining paraffin-embedded tumor tissues is significantly easier than obtaining fresh frozen tissues. However, with paraffin-embedded tissues, the method of formalin-fixation may not be adequate for obtaining viable DNA. Another possible hurdle in such studies is the reluctance of collaborators to share their paraffin blocks for research outside the home country. Provision of standard protocols from high-income countries for preparing paraffin blocks may optimize the success of obtaining valid tissues. With regard to obtaining tumor tissues for cases diagnosed outside the study hospitals, it is often customary for patients to bring their slides from the diagnosing hospital or pathology laboratory to the study hospital. Personal communication of the study clinicians and pathologists with the hospital or laboratory where the biopsy was done is extremely important for having a complete set of tissues.

Occasionally, collection and shipping of biological specimens from LMI countries to HI countries will be required. Consequently, students need to be aware of the need for research permits and letters from the host institution for shipping specimens. Packaging of specimens, shipping in dry ice or liquid nitrogen, airline rules and regulations, and permits needed at the port of entry in the high-income country may be further requirements. In the United States, for example, CDC has different types of permits that are needed for importing different biological specimens and whether they include infectious agents or not. When biological specimens are part of the study, time necessary for applying, processing, and obtaining such permits should be considered.

Students who will begin a research study in LMI countries must inquire if they need a research permit in the country. Some countries, like Brazil, require a research permit before conducting a research study, and it is important to understand each country's policy regarding researchers and students. Whether the visit of the researcher from high-income countries to LMI for research and/or training is considered an employment or not should be considered during the visa application process. Many LMI countries have specific definitions of what could be considered "employment" and applying for the right visa classification can save many unforeseen problems and violations.

Obtaining an institutional review board (IRB) or ethical committee approvals for cancer epidemiology research in LMI countries is an important task that is different in many respects from the situation in high-income countries. Federal funding agencies in the United States and other high-income countries require ethical approvals and assurances from the collaborating institutions in LMI countries before allowing joint research studies with LMI countries and releasing funding for studies. Moreover, federal agencies in the United States require approvals of the local IRB committee in the foreign country; in addition, the foreign institutions must have a Federal Wide Assurance (FWA) certification from the Office for Human Research Protections (OHRP). Certification of IRB and FWA committees of foreign institutions can be obtained by institutions from LMI countries after their leadership team read certain online modules and answer specific questions. Further information is available on the website of OHRP: http://www.hhs.gov/ohrp/

Because of lack of research resources and traditions in many LMIC, there are plenty of untapped research ideas that could be discovered while students are implementing their original research project. While students may be traveling to LMI countries to conduct a specific research project, they should also be open to discovery of new interesting research ideas that may be encountered or discovered during the conduction of their original research project. For example, during our research on the epidemiology of IBC in North Africa,[63,66,67,100] we uncovered a higher rate of chronic mastitis compared to the rate of the disease in HI countries, which in turn led to identification of possible risk factors of the disease. New ideas that come during the investigation of other research project may open the door for interesting and innovative research studies.

■ MANAGEMENT SKILLS

Logistics of planning, pilot testing, and managing international epidemiologic studies and dealing with diverse teams are rich learning experiences. The unique experience in inter-personal communication and attracting the host country's collaborators to join and continue the interest into a cancer epidemiology study is challenging. This is especially the case as most LMI countries have limited number of trained cancer epidemiologists in cancer centers or hospitals.

Building the team also is a long process. It begins with building the trust, finding common points of interests, and speaking a common language. It is important to keep up the motivation of the local collaborators in the epidemiologic study, especially in collaborations with clinicians and oncologists who do not see an immediate application of epidemiology to their work. It is important to continue to explore and maintain a funding source for the study, maintain a reciprocal relationship, and sustain a long-term track of collaboration and publications. This process will include motivating the international collaboration through a mix of training, publications, and financial incentives. The level of motivation will vary based on the level of the collaborator and the stage of their career. Additionally, collaborators and students from high-income countries who collaborate with partners from LMI countries must clarify data ownership expectations. Getting access, analyzing, and publishing from data or specimens from LMI countries should not deprive the local collaborators from their own intellectual properties and ownership rights.

Once the student has returned to his or her home institution, it is crucial that students continue the communication with the gate keepers in the community of the LMI countries and minority/ immigrant populations in HI countries and provide regular feedback of the progress of the study, print notes summarizing the study progress, and how the students can be contacted in case of future questions or follow-up.

▪ SUMMARY

There is a growing need for cancer epidemiology research training in LMI countries. The impact of globalization on the increasing incidence rates of chronic diseases, including cancer, in LMI countries and the interest of students in global health add to the need for training in cancer epidemiology research in LMI countries. Understanding the special needs and considerations for conducting cancer epidemiology research in LMI countries will reduce the barriers and increase the probability of success. The training of students should include assessment of needs and the importance of their learning and skill development in special population research. Institutional and community agencies benefit in many ways from student involvement in their locations, including new ideas and needs uncovered by student projects. Finally, in the process of mentoring international students, leaders and staff of local institutions and agencies may also increase their epidemiologic skills.

▪ REFERENCES

1. Ramazzini B, Hippocrates., Porzio L. *Bern. ramazzini ... de morbis artificum diatriba accedunt lucae antonii portii in hippocratis librum de veteri medicina paraphrasis nec non ejusdem dissertatio logica.* Ultrajecti: Apud Guilielmum van de Water; 1703:[12], 9–340, [14], 60, [6] p.-[12], 9–340, [14], 60, [6] p.

2. Seffrin JR, Gerberding JL, Boyle P. *The cancer atlas.* Atlanta, Ga.: American Cancer Society; 2007: 128 p.–128 p.

3. Burkitt DP, Wright DH. *Burkitt's lymphoma.* Edinburgh: Livingstone; 1970:xi, 251 p.-xi, 251 p.

4. Burkitt DP. The discovery of Burkitt's lymphoma. *Cancer.* 1983;51(10):1777–1786.

5. Beasley RP, Hwang LY. Hepatocellular carcinoma and hepatitis B virus. *Semin Liver Dis.* 1984;4(2): 113–121.

6. Beasley RP, Hwang LY, Lin CC, Ko YC, Twu SJ. Incidence of hepatitis among students at a university in Taiwan. *Am J Epidemiol.* 1983;117(2):213–222.

7. Beasley RP, Hwang LY, Stevens CE, et al. Efficacy of hepatitis B immune globulin for prevention of perinatal transmission of the hepatitis B virus carrier state: Final report of a randomized double-blind, placebo-controlled trial. *Hepatology.* 1983;3(2):135–141.

8. zur Hausen H. Papillomaviruses—to vaccination and beyond. *Biochemistry (Mosc).* 2008;73(5):498–503.

9. Steben M, Duarte-Franco E. Human papillomavirus infection: Epidemiology and pathophysiology. *Gynecol Oncol.* 2007;107(2 Suppl 1):S2–S5.

10. Brenner H, Bode G, Boeing H. Helicobacter pylori infection among offspring of patients with stomach cancer. *Gastroenterology.* 2000;118(1):31–35.

11. WYNDER EL, GRAHAM EA. Tobacco smoking as a possible etiologic factor in bronchogenic carcinoma; a study of 684 proved cases. *J Am Med Assoc.* 1950;143(4):329–336.

12. Herbst RS, Heymach JV, Lippman SM. Lung cancer. *N Engl J Med.* 2008;359(13):1367–1380.

13. DOLL R, HILL AB. Smoking and carcinoma of the lung; preliminary report. *Br Med J.* 1950;2(4682): 739–748.

14. Centers for Disease Control and Prevention (CDC). Office of surveillance, epidemiology, and laboratory services. Scientific Education and Professional Development Program Office Web site. http://www.cdc.gov/osels/scientific_edu/index.html2010.

15. NationalCancerInstitute(U.S.).Specialpopulationsnetworks.DefinitionsWebsite.http://cancercontrol.cancer.gov/spn/about/def.html. Published Sept. 22, 2006. Updated 2006.

16. Boyle P, Levin B, International Agency for Research on Cancer., ebrary I. *World cancer report. 2008.* Lyon: IARC Press; 2008.
17. Ferlay J, Shin HR, Bray F, Forman D, Mathers C, Parkin DM. GLOBOCAN 2008 v1.2, cancer incidence and mortality worldwide: IARC CancerBase no. 10 [internet]. . 2010. Accessed 07/02/2012.
18. Cooney KA, Gruber SB. Hyperglycemia, obesity, and cancer risks on the horizon. *JAMA.* 2005;293(2):235–236.
19. Magrath I, Litvak J. Cancer in developing countries: Opportunity and challenge. *J Natl Cancer Inst.* 1993;85(11):862–874.
20. Rastogi T, Hildesheim A, Sinha R. Opportunities for cancer epidemiology in developing countries. *Nat Rev Cancer.* 2004;4(11):909–917.
21. Schottenfeld D, Beebe-Dimmer JL. Advances in cancer epidemiology: Understanding causal mechanisms and the evidence for implementing interventions. *Annu Rev Public Health.* 2005;26:37–60.
22. Brundtland GX. Global burden sharing. *Integration.* 1994;(40)(40):11–13.
23. Beasley RP, Hwang LY, Lee GC, et al. Prevention of perinatally transmitted hepatitis B virus infections with hepatitis B virus infections with hepatitis B immune globulin and hepatitis B vaccine. *Lancet.* 1983;2(8359):1099–1102.
24. Beasley RP. Hepatitis B virus. the major etiology of hepatocellular carcinoma. *Cancer.* 1988;61(10):1942–1956.
25. Ziegler RG, Hoover RN, Pike MC, et al. Migration patterns and breast cancer risk in Asian-American women. *J Natl Cancer Inst.* 1993;85(22):1819–1827.
26. Wu AH, Ziegler RG, Pike MC, et al. Menstrual and reproductive factors and risk of breast cancer in Asian-Americans. *Br J Cancer.* 1996;73(5):680–686.
27. Clegg LX, Li FP, Hankey BF, Chu K, Edwards BK. Cancer survival among US whites and minorities: A SEER (surveillance, epidemiology, and end results) program population-based study. *Arch Intern Med.* 2002;162(17):1985–1993.
28. Weir HK, Thun MJ, Hankey BF, et al. Annual report to the nation on the status of cancer, 1975–2000, featuring the uses of surveillance data for cancer prevention and control. *J Natl Cancer Inst.* 2003;95(17): 1276–1299.
29. Eheman C, Henley SJ, Ballard-Barbash R, et al. Annual report to the nation on the status of cancer, 1975–2008, featuring cancers associated with excess weight and lack of sufficient physical activity. *Cancer.* 2012;118(9):2338–2366.
30. American Cancer Society. Cancer facts & figures 2012. Atlanta, GA: American Cancer Society. 2012.
31. Swan J, Edwards BK. Cancer rates among American Indians and Alaska natives: Is there a national perspective. *Cancer.* 2003;98(6):1262–1272.
32. Marie Swanson G, Haslam SZ, Azzouz F. Breast cancer among young African-American women: A summary of data and literature and of issues discussed during the summit meeting on breast cancer among African American women, Washington, DC, September 8–10, 2000. *Cancer.* 2003;97(1 Suppl):273–279.
33. Bernstein L, Teal CR, Joslyn S, Wilson J. Ethnicity-related variation in breast cancer risk factors. *Cancer.* 2003;97(1 Suppl):222–229.
34. Chlebowski RT, Chen Z, Anderson GL, et al. Ethnicity and breast cancer: Factors influencing differences in incidence and outcome. *J Natl Cancer Inst.* 2005;97(6):439–448.
35. Bauer KR, Brown M, Cress RD, Parise CA, Caggiano V. Descriptive analysis of estrogen receptor (ER)-negative, progesterone receptor (PR)-negative, and HER2-negative invasive breast cancer, the so-called triple-negative phenotype: A population-based study from the California cancer registry. *Cancer.* 2007;109(9):1721–1728.
36. Carey LA, Perou CM, Livasy CA, et al. Race, breast cancer subtypes, and survival in the Carolina breast cancer study. *JAMA.* 2006;295(21):2492–2502.
37. Howe HL, Wu X, Ries LA, et al. Annual report to the nation on the status of cancer, 1975–2003, featuring cancer among U.S. Hispanic/Latino populations. *Cancer.* 2006;107(8):1711–1742.
38. Trapido EJ, Burciaga Valdez R, Obeso JL, Strickman-Stein N, Rotger A, Perez-Stable EJ. Epidemiology of cancer among Hispanics in the United States. *J Natl Cancer Inst Monogr.* 1995;(18)(18):17–28.

39. O'Brien K, Cokkinides V, Jemal A, et al. Cancer statistics for Hispanics, 2003. *CA Cancer J Clin.* 2003;53(4):208–226.

40. Pinheiro PS, Sherman RL, Trapido EJ, et al. Cancer incidence in first generation U.S. Hispanics: Cubans, Mexicans, Puerto Ricans, and new Latinos. *Cancer Epidemiol Biomarkers Prev.* 2009;18(8):2162–2169.

41. Wiggins CL, Espey DK, Wingo PA, et al. Cancer among American Indians and Alaska natives in the united states, 1999–2004. *Cancer.* 2008;113(5 Suppl):1142–1152.

42. Rutledge W, Gibson R, Siegel E, et al. Arkansas special populations access network perception versus reality—cancer screening in primary care clinics. *Cancer.* 2006;107(8 Suppl):2052–2060.

43. Husaini BA, Reece MC, Emerson JS, Scales S, Hull PC, Levine RS. A church-based program on prostate cancer screening for African American men: Reducing health disparities. *Ethn Dis.* 2008;18(2 Suppl 2): S2–179–84.

44. Sadler GR, Gunsauls DC, Huang J, et al. Bringing breast cancer education to deaf women. *J Cancer Educ.* 2001;16(4):225–228.

45. Choe S, Lim RS, Clark K, Wang R, Branz P, Sadler GR. The impact of cervical cancer education for deaf women using a video educational tool employing American Sign Language, open captioning, and graphics. *J Cancer Educ.* 2009;24(1):10–15.

46. Todd L, Hoffman-Goetz L. Predicting health literacy among English-as-a-second-language older Chinese immigrant women to Canada: Comprehension of colon cancer prevention information. *J Cancer Educ.* 2011;26(2):326–332.

47. Erwin DO, Trevino M, Saad-Harfouche FG, Rodriguez EM, Gage E, Jandorf L. Contextualizing diversity and culture within cancer control interventions for Latinas: Changing interventions, not cultures. *Soc Sci Med.* 2010;71(4):693–701.

48. Vahabi M. Breast cancer and screening information needs and preferred communication medium among Iranian immigrant women in Toronto. *Health Soc Care Community.* 2011;19(6):626–635.

49. Cheng SH, Tsou MH, Liu MC, et al. Unique features of breast cancer in Taiwan. *Breast Cancer Res Treat.* 2000;63(3):213–223.

50. Jones BA, Kasl SV, Howe CL, et al. African-American/white differences in breast carcinoma: P53 alterations and other tumor characteristics. *Cancer.* 2004;101(6):1293–1301.

51. Levine PH, Pogo BG, Klouj A, et al. Increasing evidence for a human breast carcinoma virus with geographic differences. *Cancer.* 2004;101(4):721–726.

52. Soliman AS, Bondy ML, Levin B, et al. Colorectal cancer in Egyptian patients under 40 years of age. *Int J Cancer.* 1997;71(1):26–30.

53. Soliman AS, Bondy ML, El-Badawy SA, et al. Contrasting molecular pathology of colorectal carcinoma in Egyptian and western patients. *Br J Cancer.* 2001;85(7):1037–1046.

54. Jass JR. Clinical significance of early-onset "sporadic" colorectal cancer with microsatellite instability. *Dis Colon Rectum.* 2003;46(10):1305–1309.

55. Pfeiffer RM, Mitani A, Matsuno RK, Anderson WF. Racial differences in breast cancer trends in the United States (2000–2004). *J Natl Cancer Inst.* 2008;100(10):751–752.

56. Gomez SL, Clarke CA, Shema SJ, Chang ET, Keegan TH, Glaser SL. Disparities in breast cancer survival among Asian women by ethnicity and immigrant status: A population-based study. *Am J Public Health.* 2010;100(5):861–869.

57. Keegan TH, John EM, Fish KM, Alfaro-Velcamp T, Clarke CA, Gomez SL. Breast cancer incidence patterns among California Hispanic women: Differences by nativity and residence in an enclave. *Cancer Epidemiol Biomarkers Prev.* 2010;19(5):1208–1218.

58. John EM, Phipps AI, Davis A, Koo J. Migration history, acculturation, and breast cancer risk in Hispanic women. *Cancer Epidemiol Biomarkers Prev.* 2005;14(12):2905–2913.

59. Drake BF, Lathan CS, Okechukwu CA, Bennett GG. Racial differences in prostate cancer screening by family history. *Ann Epidemiol.* 2008;18(7):579–583.

60. Giri VN, Egleston B, Ruth K, et al. Race, genetic West African ancestry, and prostate cancer prediction by prostate-specific antigen in prospectively screened high-risk men. *Cancer Prev Res (Phila).* 2009;2(3):244–250.

61. Ashing-Giwa KT, Padilla GV, Tejero JS, Kim J. Breast cancer survivorship in a multiethnic sample: Challenges in recruitment and measurement. *Cancer.* 2004;101(3):450–465.

62. Bangdiwala SI, Tucker JD, Zodpey S, et al. Public health education in India and China: History, opportunities, and challenges. *Public Health Rev.* 2011;33:204–24.

63. Lo AC, Kleer CG, Banerjee M, et al. Molecular epidemiologic features of inflammatory breast cancer: A comparison between Egyptian and US patients. *Breast Cancer Res Treat.* 2008;112(1):141–147.

64. Levine PH, Mesa-Tejada R, Keydar I, Tabbane F, Spiegelman S, Mourali N. Increased incidence of mouse mammary tumor virus-related antigen in Tunisian patients with breast cancer. *Int J Cancer.* 1984;33(3):305–308.

65. Harford JB. Breast-cancer early detection in low-income and middle-income countries: Do what you can versus one size fits all. *Lancet Oncol.* 2011;12(3):306–312.

66. Schairer C, Soliman AS, Omar S, et al. Assessment of diagnosis of inflammatory breast cancer cases at two cancer centers in Egypt and Tunisia. *Cancer Medicine.* ; 2013. Accessed at: http://onlinelibrary.wiley.com/doi/10.1002/cam4.48/pdf.

67. Soliman AS, Banerjee M, Lo AC, et al. High proportion of inflammatory breast cancer in the population-based cancer registry of Gharbiah, Egypt. *Breast J.* 2009;15(4):432–434.

68. Lehman EM, Soliman AS, Ismail K, et al. Patterns of hepatocellular carcinoma incidence in Egypt from a population-based cancer registry. *Hepatol Res.* 2008;38(5):465–473.

69. Felix AS, Soliman AS, Khaled H, et al. The changing patterns of bladder cancer in Egypt over the past 26 years. *Cancer Causes Control.* 2008;19(4):421–429.

70. Fedewa SA, Soliman AS, Ismail K, et al. Incidence analyses of bladder cancer in the Nile Delta region of Egypt. *Cancer Epidemiol.* 2009;33(3–4):176–181.

71. Attar E, Dey S, Hablas A, et al. Head and neck cancer in a developing country: A population-based perspective across 8 years. *Oral Oncol.* 2010;46(8):591–596.

72. Dey S, Soliman AS, Hablas A, et al. Urban-rural differences in breast cancer incidence in Egypt (1999–2006). *Breast.* 2010;19(5):417–423.

73. Dey S, Soliman AS, Hablas A, et al. Urban-rural differences in breast cancer incidence by hormone receptor status across 6 years in Egypt. *Breast Cancer Res Treat.* 2010;120(1):149–160.

74. Herzog CM, Dey S, Hablas A, et al. Geographic distribution of hematopoietic cancers in the Nile Delta of Egypt. *Ann Oncol.* 2012;23(10):2748–2755.

75. Peters LM, Soliman AS, Bukori P, Mkuchu J, Ngoma T. Evidence for the need of educational programs for cervical screening in rural Tanzania. *J Cancer Educ.* 2010;25(2):153–159.

76. Burson AM, Soliman AS, Ngoma TA, et al. Clinical and epidemiologic profile of breast cancer in Tanzania. *Breast Dis.* 2010;31(1):33–41.

77. Johnson JC, Soliman AS, Tadgerson D, et al. Tribal linkage and race data quality for American Indians in a state cancer registry. *Am J Prev Med.* 2009;36(6):549–554.

78. Peterson L, Soliman A, Ruterbusch JJ, Smith N, Schwartz K. Comparison of exposures among Arab American and non-Hispanic white female thyroid cancer cases in metropolitan Detroit. *Journal of Immigrant and Minority Health.* 2011;13(6):1033–1040.

79. Shami SA, Qaisar R, Bittles AH. Consanguinity and adult morbidity in Pakistan. *Lancet.* 1991; 338(8772):954.

80. Denic S, Frampton C, Nicholls MG. Risk of cancer in an inbred population. *Cancer Detect Prev.* 2007; 31(4):263–269.

81. Rudan I, Rudan D, Campbell H, et al. Inbreeding and risk of late onset complex disease. *J Med Genet.* 2003;40(12):925–932.

82. Assie G, LaFramboise T, Platzer P, Eng C. Frequency of germline genomic homozygosity associated with cancer cases. *JAMA.* 2008;299(12):1437–1445.

83. Schwartz KL, Kulwicki A, Weiss LK, et al. Cancer among Arab Americans in the metropolitan Detroit area. *Ethn Dis.* 2004;14(1):141–146.

84. Nasseri K. Thyroid cancer in the Middle Eastern population of California. *Cancer Causes Control.* 2008;19(10):1183–1191.

85. Rubel AJ, Haas MR. Ethnomedicine. In: Sargent CF, Johnson TM, eds. *Medical anthropology: Contemporary theory and method.* New York: Praeger Publishers; 1990:131–131.

86. Scrimshaw SC, Hurtado E. Anthropological involvement in the Central American diarrheal disease control project. *Soc Sci Med.* 1988;27(1):97–105.

87. Topley M. Chinese traditional etiology and methods of cure in Hong Kong. In: Leslie CM, ed. *Asian medical systems: A comparative study.* Berkeley, CA: University of California Press; 1976:243, 265 p.–243, 265 p.

88. Reichel-Dolmatoff G, Reichel-Dolmatoff A. *The people of Aritama; the cultural personality of a Colombian Mestizo village.* London: Routledge & K. Paul; 1961:482 p.–482 p.

89. Beals AR. Strategies of resort to curers in south India. In: Leslie CM, ed. *Asian medical systems: A comparative study.* Berkeley, CA: University of California Press; 1976:184, 200 p.–184, 200 p.

90. Freed SA, Freed RS. Spirit possession as illness in a North Indian village. In: Middleton J, ed. *Magic, witchcraft, and curing.* Garden City, NY: Natural History Press; 1967:295, 320 p.–295, 320 p.

91. Scrimshaw SC. Culture, behavior, and health. In: Merson MH, Black RE, Mills AJ, eds. *International public health: Diseases, programs, systems, and policies.* Gaithersburg, MD: Aspen Publishers; 2001:53, 78 p.–53, 78 p.

92. Lofters AK, Moineddin R, Hwang SW, Glazier RH. Predictors of low cervical cancer screening among immigrant women in Ontario, Canada. *BMC Womens Health.* 2011;11:20.

93. Nguyen GT, Shungu NP, Niederdeppe J, et al. Cancer-related information seeking and scanning behavior of older Vietnamese immigrants. *J Health Commun.* 2010;15(7):754–768.

94. Calderon JL, Bazargan M, Sangasubana N, Hays RD, Hardigan P, Baker RS. A comparison of two educational methods on immigrant Latinas breast cancer knowledge and screening behaviors. *J Health Care Poor Underserved.* 2010;21(3 Suppl):76–90.

95. Soliman AS, Schairer C. Considerations in setting up and conducting epidemiologic studies of cancer in middle- and low-income countries: The experience of a case control study of inflammatory breast cancer in North Africa in the past 10 years. *Cancer Medicine.* 2012;1(3):338–349.

96. Ngelangel CA. Hospital visitor-companions as a source of controls for case-control studies in the Philippines. *Int J Epidemiol.* 1989;18(4 Suppl 2):S50–S53.

97. Mendonca GA, Eluf-Neto J, Andrada-Serpa MJ, et al. Organochlorines and breast cancer: A case-control study in Brazil. *Int J Cancer.* 1999;83(5):596–600.

98. Mendonca GA, Eluf-Neto J. Hospital visitors as controls in case-control studies. *Rev Saude Publica.* 2001;35(5):436–442.

99. O'Brien KS, Soliman AS, Annan K, Lartey RN, Awuah B, Merajver SD. Traditional herbalists and cancer management in Kumasi, Ghana. *J Cancer Educ.* 2012;27(3):573–579.

100. Lo AC, Georgopoulos A, Kleer CG, et al. Analysis of RhoC expression and lymphovascular emboli in inflammatory vs. non-inflammatory breast cancers in Egyptian patients. *Breast.* 2009;18(1):55–59.

CHAPTER 13

CANCER EPIDEMIOLOGY IN SCHOOLS OF PUBLIC HEALTH AND MEDICAL SCHOOLS: CULTURE, INFRASTRUCTURE, AND CURRICULA

AMR S. SOLIMAN

■ CURRENT STATUS OF CURRICULA AND PROGRAMS FOR TRAINING IN CANCER EPIDEMIOLOGY IN SCHOOLS OF PUBLIC HEALTH

In the United States

Public health education in the United States is administered and delivered by schools and programs of public health through the Association of Schools of Public Health (ASPH), which was established in 1953. In the United States, programs of public health originally emerged from schools of medicine or de novo programs.[1] Over the past few decades the number of schools of public health has increased significantly; as of 2010, there were 49 accredited schools of public health and 84 programs in public health, up from 24 schools in 1989. The accreditation process of the schools and programs is conducted by the Council on Education for Public Health (CEPH), which reviews different aspects of each school and program activities on periodic basis and renew or issue a new accreditation.

Programs of public health are usually focused on one or more areas of public health while schools of public health typically include departments or divisions of epidemiology, health behavior and health education, health management and policy, biostatistics, and environmental/occupational health. Some schools have departments/divisions for maternal and child health, nutrition, tropical medicine/international health, and over the past few years, global health. The names of the department/division may vary from one school to another and some of the names of the departments/divisions mentioned are included in one department.

Applications to schools and programs in public health have clearly increased in the past 10–12 years from 19,953 applications in 2000 to 49,227 applications in 2010. Epidemiology is the one of the most popular departments with largest number of applications and the one with the top percentage of students in schools of public health. In 2010, the top two programs that admitted students in schools of public health were in health policy (19%) and epidemiology (18%). The next popular departments were health behavior and health education (14%), environmental health (11%), and biostatistics (6%).

The degrees offered by schools of public health vary, but Master of Public Health (MPH) is the largest program, accounting for 59% of admitted students in 2009–2010. Other programs include Master of Sciences (MS) (9% of students) and doctor of philosophy (PhD) (8% of students). Other master and doctoral programs account for the remaining 24% of all admitted students.

The MPH program is most common in the United States and spans a period of one to two years depending on the background of students (e.g., prior medical degree), prerequisites, and other factors. The MPH program is mainly a multidisciplinary professional degree offered by schools of public health and some medical schools in the United States.

Women represent the majority of public health students in the United States; about 71% of students in schools of public health are females and 29% males, reflecting a trend of more women in public health education and future work force. About 77% of students are US citizens while about 23% of students are foreign nationals. Ethnic backgrounds of students vary by state and school, region of the schools and student interest. Average ethnic backgrounds of students in all schools combined are: 6.9% Hispanic, 0.6% American Indian, 15.8% Asian, 12.4% Black/African Americans, 0.2% Pacific Islanders, and about 64% white students. Full time students (9 credit hours or more) constitute about 68% of all students with a range of 31–100%.

The curricula of schools of public health for MPH students range from 42–60 credit hours. While the majority of the programs require students to be physically on campus of schools to attend classes, a new trend of online-courses and distance education, as well as certificate nondegree programs, has recently emerged. Variation in core courses (15–25 credit hours), electives, (Breadth, Integration, and Capstone) (BIC) requirements vary in terms of required nondepartmental required courses to the integration, team teaching, and practicum or capstone requirements.

A wide range exists in terms of required courses and practicum or internship. For epidemiology students in the MPH programs, there are usually core required courses in epidemiologic methods, biology/pathobiology, environmental health, biostatistics, behavioral science, health management or policy, and a statistical analysis package. Cancer epidemiology, if offered, is among the elective courses.

Because schools try to give an overview of both infectious and chronic diseases, students in most public health programs are required to take a variable load of chronic disease courses. Depending on the available faculty in each program, their backgrounds and interest, and teaching loads, cancer courses may or may not be offered. However, most established schools of public health do offer courses in cancer epidemiology with variable degree of depth and focus. The caliber of education, training, and research for cancer in each program also depends on the presence of a comprehensive or designated cancer center on campus. The presence of a comprehensive cancer center on campus significantly increases the interest, teaching and learning about cancer epidemiology because it requires a strong core of faculty and activities in population science, health behavior research, and cancer outreach education. This obligation consequently requires research, education, and training grants through a core of active faculty who teach and mentor students in cancer epidemiology.

As of 2011, there are 44 Comprehensive Cancer Centers and 22 Designated Cancer Centers. Cancer centers acquiring the last 2 status classification represent 4% of all cancer centers in the United States Most comprehensive cancer centers are on medical campuses or affiliated with Schools of Public Health.

Table 13.1 shows listing of the variety of cancer courses and courses that include a cancer component in the schools and programs of public health in the United States as listed on each school's website.

TABLE 13.1 Schools and programs in the United States with courses on cancer epidemiology or courses-related to cancer

INSTITUTION	DEGREE		COURSE TITLE (CREDIT HOURS) COURSES-CONTAINING CANCER TOPICS	FIELD TRAINING HOURS OR CREDITS
	MPH	PHD		
Boston University	Yes	Yes	Cancer Epidemiology (4); Cancer Prevention as a Public Health Problem (4); Nutritional Epidemiology (4); Reproductive Epidemiology (4); Confronting Non-Communicable Diseases in the Developing World: The Burden, Costs & Health Systems Challenges (4); Evidence-Based Program Design for Reproductive Health (4); The Biology of Public Health (4)	112
Brigham Young University	Yes	No	Infectious & Chronic Disease Prevention and Control (3)	300
California State University, Fullerton	Yes	No	Chronic Disease Epidemiology (3)	240
Capella University (Online)	Yes	Yes	Chronic & Infections Disease Epidemiology (6, PhD course)	Unknown
Case Western Reserve University	Yes	No	Obesity & Cancer: Views from Molecules to Health Policy (3); Integrative Cancer Biology (3); Chronic Disease Epidemiology (3); Cancer Epidemiology (1–3)	160
Central New York (SUNY Upstate Medical University & Syracuse University)	Yes	No	Chronic Disease Epidemiology (3); Maternal & Child Health Epidemiology (3)	200
Claremont Graduate University	Yes	No	Theoretical Foundations in Health Promotion & Education (4); Emerging Chronic & Infectious diseases (4)	200–400
Colorado School of Public Health (University of Colorado & Colorado State University)	Yes	Yes	Cancer Prevention and Control (2); Public Health Surveillance (2); Chronic Disease Epidemiology (3); Selected Topics in Nutritional Epidemiology (2)	120
Columbia University	Yes	Yes	Cancer Epidemiology (3); Chronic Disease Epidemiology (3); Environmental Epidemiology (3); Field Methods in Epidemiology (3)	280
Drexel University	Yes	Yes	Cancer Epidemiology (3); Epidemiology for Public Health Practice (3); Occupational & Environmental Cancers (3); Human Genetics (3)	120
East Carolina University	Yes	No	Cancer Epidemiology (3)	240

University			Courses	Number
East Tennessee State University	Yes	Yes	Epidemiology of Chronic Diseases (3); Cancer Epidemiology (3)	300–340
Eastern Virginia Medical School/ Old Dominion University	Yes	No	Social Marketing (1)	4 credits
Emory University	Yes	Yes	Epidemiology of Cancer (2) ; Build Environment & Public Health (2); Public Health Biology (2); Diet and Chronic Disease (2); Opportunities in Global Cancer Prevention & Control (1)	300
Florida A & M University	Yes	Yes	Epidemiology of Chronic Diseases (3); Topics in Public Health (3); Cancer Epidemiology (3)	100
Florida State University	Yes	No	Chronic Disease Epidemiology (3)	400
George Mason University	Yes	No	Chronic Disease (3)	200
George Washington University	Yes	Yes	Cancer Epidemiology (2); Epidemiology Surveillance in Public Health (2); Epidemiology of Infectious Agents Associated with Human Cancer (1); Exercise in Selected Chronic Diseases (3)	120
Georgia Southern University	Yes	Yes	Epidemiology of Chronic Disease (3)	300
Georgia State University	Yes	Yes	Cancer and Society (3); Public Health & Reproductive Health (3); Urban Health (3)	3 credits
Harvard University	Yes	Yes	Epidemiology of Cancer; Cancer Prevention; Use of Biomarkers in Epidemiologic Research; Applied Biomarkers in Cancer Epidemiology; Molecular Biology for Epidemiologists; Infections & Cancer; Advanced Seminar in Cancer Epidemiology; Screening; Translational Research Methods; Pathology of for Epidemiologists; Society & Health; Health Promotion through Mass Media; Approaches to International Tobacco Control; Nutritional Epidemiology of Cancer; Advanced Topics in Nutrition and Cancer	128–320
Hunter College-City University of New York	Yes	Yes	Reproductive & Perinatal Epidemiology	210–300
Indiana University, Indianapolis	Yes	Yes	Cancer Epidemiology (3); Chronic Disease Epidemiology (3)	Unknown
Jackson State University	Yes	Yes	Chronic & Infectious Diseases Epidemiology (3)	400

(continued)

TABLE 13.1 (Continued)

INSTITUTION	DEGREE		COURSE TITLE (CREDIT HOURS) COURSES-CONTAINING CANCER TOPICS	FIELD TRAINING HOURS OR CREDITS
	MPH	PHD		
John Hopkins University	Yes	Yes	Special Studies-Current Topics in Biochemistry & Molecular Biology (1); Stem Cells & the Biology of Aging & Disease (3); Molecular Endocrinology (4); Genome Integrity & Cancer (3); MHS Thesis in Reproductive & Cancer Biology (5); Statistical Machine Learning: Methods, Theory, & Applications (4); Fundamentals of Clinical Oncology for Public Health Practitioners (3); Toxicology: The Molecular Basis (4); Molecular Epidemiology & Biomarkers in Public Health (4); Immunology of Environmental Disease (3); Epidemiology & Natural History of Human Viral Infections (6); Methodologic Issues in Cancer Epidemiology (3); Etiology, Prevention, & Control of Cancer (4); Epidemiology in Evidence-Based Policy (2); Problem Solving in Public Health (4); Introduction to Genetic Counseling (2); Introduction to Human Genetics I (2); Introduction to Human Genetics II (2); Current Topics in Molecular Genetics I (1); Current Topics in Molecular Genetics II (1); Introduction to Medical Genetics (2); Cancer Genetics: Managing the Risks Through Testing & Counseling (2); Early Detection in Cancer: Recent Developments & Challenges (3); Principles of Human Nutrition (4); Advanced Nutrient Metabolism (3); Biologic Basis of Vaccine Development (3); Principles of Human Nutrition (4); Clinical Immunology (3); Clinical Aspects of Reproductive Health (3); Reproductive & Perinatal Epidemiology (4)	60–100
Loma Linda University	Yes	Yes	Epidemiology of Cancer (3)	240
Louisiana State University	Yes	Yes	Cancer Epidemiology (3); Chronic Disease Epidemiology (3)	200
Missouri State University	Yes	No	Chronic Disease Epidemiology (3)	200
Montclair State University	Yes	No	Human Diseases (3)	180
Mount Sinai School of Medicine	Yes	No	Disease Prevention & Health Promotion for Non-Health Professionals (2)	150
New Mexico State University	Yes	No	Many courses on the Aged	Unknown

Institution			Course	
New York Medical College	Yes	Yes	Topics in Cancer Epidemiology	140
New York University	Yes	Yes	Advanced Seminar: Cancer (1); Epidemiology of Cancer (4); Nutritional Epidemiology (3); Health Psychology (3)	180
Northeastern University	Yes	No	Exercise in Health & Disease	Unknown
Northern Illinois University	Yes	No	If want courses on cancer would have to take nursing courses	300
Northwest Ohio Consortium (Bowling Green State University & University of Toledo)	Yes	No	Cancer Epidemiology (3)	275
Northwestern University	Yes	No	Cancer Epidemiology	200
Ohio State University	Yes	Yes	Chronic Disease Epidemiology; Cancer Epidemiology; Molecular Epidemiology of Cancer	120
Oregon MPH Program (Oregon Health & Science University, Oregon State University, & Portland State University)	Yes	No	Chronic Disease Epidemiology (3)	200
Saint Louis University	Yes	Yes	Cancer Epidemiology	360
San Diego State University	Yes	Yes	Epidemiology Chronic Diseases (3)	180
Simon Fraser University	Yes	Yes	Perspectives on Cancer, Cardiovascular & Metabolic Diseases; Cancer, Cardiovascular Disease	440
St. George's University	Yes	No	Chronic Disease Epidemiology (3)	240
Stony Brook University-State University of New York	Yes	Yes	Epidemiology for Public Health (3)	varies
Texas A&M	Yes	Yes	Cancer Epidemiology (3); Environmental Carcinogenesis (3)	200
The State University of New York Downstate Medical Center	Yes	Yes	Chronic Disease Epidemiology (3); Cancer Epidemiology(3)	200
Thomas Jefferson University	Yes	Yes	Geographic Information System (GIS) Mapping (2)	Unknown

(continued)

TABLE 13.1 (Continued)

INSTITUTION	DEGREE		COURSE TITLE (CREDIT HOURS) COURSES-CONTAINING CANCER TOPICS	FIELD TRAINING HOURS OR CREDITS
	MPH	PHD		
Tulane University	Yes	Yes	Cancer Epidemiology (3); Molecular Epidemiology (3); Human Molecular Genetics (3); Epidemiologic Perspectives on Nutrition & Chronic Disease (3)	200
Uniformed Services University of Health Sciences	Yes	Yes	Molecular Epidemiology (2) Fundamentals of Human Physiology for Public Health (2)	Unknown
Université de Montréal	Yes	Yes	Chronic Disease	Unknown
University at Albany The State University of New York	Yes	Yes	Cancer Epidemiology (3)	720
University at Buffalo The State University of New York	Yes	Yes	Cancer Epidemiology (3); Advanced Cancer Epidemiology & Prevention (3); Cancer Control & Prevention (3); Oncology for Scientists (4); The Public Health Practice of Tobacco Control (3); Cancer Pathology (3)	240
University of Alabama at Birmingham	Yes	Yes	Cancer Epidemiology & Control (2) Epidemiology of Chronic Diseases (3); Molecular & Genetic Basis of Obesity (3)	240
University of Alaska-Anchorage	Yes	No	Circumpolar Health Issues	225
University of Arizona	Yes	Yes	Cancer Epidemiology & Prevention (3)	Unknown
University of Arkansas	Yes	Yes	Interdisciplinary Perspectives on Cancer Control; Principles of Toxicology in Public Health; Cancer Epidemiology	135
University of California, Berkeley	Yes	Yes	Epidemiology of Neoplastic Diseases (3); Viruses & Human Cancer (2–3)	480
University of California, Davis	Yes	No	Cancer Epidemiology (3)	300
University of California, Irvine	Yes	Yes	Cancer Epidemiology (4)	240
University of California, Los Angeles	Yes	Yes	Cancer Epidemiology (4); Molecular Epidemiology of Cancer (4); Research Methods in Cancer Epidemiology (2) Epidemiology of Infections & Cancer (2) Seminar: Environmental & Occupational Cancer Epidemiology (2) Seminar: Epidemiology-Cancer (2) Topics in Population Genetics and Nutrition (2)	400

Institution			Courses	Credits
University of Connecticut	Yes	Yes	Occupational & Environmental Health Policy (3); Toxicology & Risk Assessment (3); Intermediate Epidemiology (3)	3 credits
University of Florida	Yes	Yes	Epidemiology & Prevention Of Chronic Diseases; Public Health Biology; Human Health Risk Assessment (4)	240–384
University of Georgia	Yes	Yes	Cancer Epidemiology (3); Special Topics in Health Promotion & Behavior: Cancer Prevention & communication (1-3); Chronic Disease Prevention	300
University of Illinois at Chicago	Yes	Yes	Survey of Cancer Epidemiology (3); Advanced Cancer Epidemiology (2) ; Genetics in Epidemiology (2) Occupational & Environmental Epidemiology (2) Special Topics: Social Epidemiology (3); Special Topics: Surveillance Epidemiology (3); Nutritional Epidemiology (3); Evaluation of Nutritional Status (3); Cancer Epidemiology (3); Epidemiology of Non-Infectious Diseases (3)	320
University of Iowa	Yes	Yes	Cancer Registration Internship; Cancer Epidemiology & Control; Cancer Molecular Epidemiology Seminar	200
University of Kansas	Yes	No	Cancer Epidemiology (3); Tobacco in Public Health (3)	400
University of Louisville	Yes	Yes	Epidemiology of Cancer (2) Research in Cancer (1); Disease Surveillance & Health Statistics (3); Epidemiology of Chronic Disease (3)	6 credits
University of Maryland	Yes	Yes	Chronic Disease Epidemiology (3)	240
University of Maryland at Baltimore	Yes	Yes	Environmental & Occupational Health (3); Molecular Biology in Public Health Research (1); Critical Issues in Global Health (3); Complex Disorders Seminar (2)	240
University of Medicine & Dentistry of New Jersey	Yes	Yes	Epidemiology of Chronic Diseases	400
University of Memphis	Yes	Yes	Cancer Epidemiology (3); Infections Disease Epidemiology (3)	240
University of Miami	Yes	Yes	Cancer Epidemiology (3); Chronic Disease Epidemiology (3)	300
University of Michigan	Yes	Yes	Biostatistics in Cancer Seminar (1); Principles of Environmental Health Sciences (3); Genes& the Environment (2); Radiation Biology 3; Epidemiology of Chronic Diseases (3); Cancer Epidemiology (3); Principles & Practice of Preventive Medicine (2); Sex, Gender & Vulnerability (3); Aging & Health Behavior (3)	318–636

(continued)

TABLE 13.1 (Continued)

INSTITUTION	DEGREE		COURSE TITLE (CREDIT HOURS) COURSES-CONTAINING CANCER TOPICS	FIELD TRAINING HOURS OR CREDITS
	MPH	PHD		
University of Minnesota	Yes	Yes	Cancer Epidemiology (2) Pathophysiology of Human Disease (4)	120–300
University of Nebraska	Yes	No	Chronic Disease Prevention & Control: Research Concepts & Methodology (3) Cancer Epidemiology in Special Populations (1); Topics in Cancer Prevention I (1); Topics in Cancer Prevention II (1); Principles and Methodologies in Cancer Research (3).	12 credits
University of Nevada, Las Vegas	Yes	Yes	Chronic Disease Epidemiology	150
University of Nevada, Reno	Yes	Yes	Epidemiology of Chronic Disease; Cancer Epidemiology	250
University of New Mexico	Yes	No	Cancer Epidemiology (2) Chronic Disease Epidemiology & Surveillance (2)	160
University of North Carolina at Chapel Hill	Yes	Yes	Cancer Epidemiology & Pathogenesis (3); Cancer Epidemiology Methods (3); Cancer Prevention & Control Seminar (3); Advanced Cancer Epidemiology: Classic & Contemporary Controversies in Cancer Causation (2) Diet & Cancer (3); Seminar in Oral Epidemiology (1)	200–400
University of North Florida	Yes	No	Chronic Disease Epidemiology (3)	3 credits
University of North Texas	Yes	Yes	Cancer Epidemiology (3)	3 credits
University of Oklahoma	Yes	Yes	Cancer Epidemiology & Prevention 3; Survival Data Analysis (3)	160
University of Pennsylvania	Yes	No	Behavioral & Social Sciences in Public Health (1); Anthropology & Public Health; Anthropology & Risk	108
University of Pittsburgh	Yes	Yes	Cancer Epidemiology (2) Advance Topic Cancer Epidemiology Prevention (2) Epidemiology & Health Services (2) Biomarkers & Molecular Epidemiology (2)	200
University of Rochester	Yes	Yes	Cancer Biology (4)	3 credits
University of Saskatchewan	Yes	Yes	Chronic Disease Epidemiology	480
University of South Carolina	Yes	Yes	Investigative Epidemiology: Cancer (3)	250

University			Course(s)	
University of South Florida	Yes	Yes	Cancer Epidemiology (3)	135
University of Southern Mississippi	Yes	No	Chronic Disease Epidemiology	400
University of Texas	Yes	Yes	Molecular & Cellular Approaches in Human Genetics (3); Genetic Epidemiology of Chronic Diseases (2) Pediatric Epidemiology (3); Epidemiology Seminar (1); Occupational Epidemiology (3)	3 credits
University of Utah	Yes	Yes	Cancer Epidemiology (3)	180
University of Washington	Yes	Yes	Epidemiologic Studies of Cancer Etiology & Prevention (3–4); Introduction to Cancer Biology (3); Cancer Prevention Research Laboratory (3)	120
University of Wisconsin-Madison	Yes	No	Cancer Epidemiology (2)	400
Virginia Commonwealth University	Yes	Yes	Cancer Epidemiology (3)	180
Washington University in St. Louis	Yes	No	Cancer Epidemiology (3)	360
Wayne State University	Yes	No	Health, Disease, and Aging (3)	3 credits
Western Kentucky University	Yes	No	Health Problems of the Aged (3)	480
Yale University	Yes	Yes	Epidemiology of Cancer; Introduction to Environmental Genetics; Environmental Hormones and Human Health; Health of Women and Children; Nutrition & Chronic Disease; Molecular Epidemiology of Chronic Disease; Directive Reading: Exercise and Cancer; Directive Reading: Environmental Cancer Epidemiology; Vaccines: Concepts in Biology; Health Disparities by Race & Sex: Epidemiology & Intervention; Preventive Interventions: Theory, Methods, & Evaluation	400

Topics of these courses are centered around introductory cancer epidemiology, cancer etiology and causation, infection and cancer, viral carcinogenesis, cancer biology, genetics and cancer, molecular cancer epidemiology, environmental carcinogenesis, biomarkers in cancer epidemiology, behavioral and social epidemiology of cancer, screening, cancer prevention and control, genetic counseling, oncology in public health practice, and global cancer. The most common course is the introductory or comprehensive cancer epidemiology. Students take this course to fulfill requirements of academic programs or training grants or because of the students' personal interest in learning about the subject. The topic of cancer is appealing to a wide variety of students because of the frequent discussion of the topic in the media and because of its relevance to many personal lives.

Teaching of an introductory cancer epidemiology course is not easy because of the different backgrounds of students who usually take the course and the wide range of topics that are usually covered in it. However, to make this course appealing to students, the course should be multidisciplinary in terms of the topics covered to engage students from different backgrounds.

Some of the students who take this introductory course on cancer epidemiology may have strong backgrounds in molecular biology, which has become an integral part of understanding cancer etiology. These students may find parts of this course too easy for them and may even have more advanced knowledge of molecular biology than a mid-career or senior faculty who teach the course and whose knowledge in molecular biology may not match the molecular biology level of fresh undergraduates.[2] To make this course appealing to a wide variety of students from different backgrounds, the course should progress from the basic nomenclature of cancer vocabulary to basic molecular pathways of cancer, cancer incidence and mortality, cancer registration, social epidemiology, genetic, molecular, and gene-environment interactions. For example, students from strong biology background would benefit from learning about study design, methods of assessment of and environmental and genetic factors in epidemiologic studies, cancer registration, and application of cancer epidemiology to cancer prevention and controls. On the other hand, students with behavioral and social sciences backgrounds need to learn about molecular biology related to cancer, study design, and cancer prevention and control. After students learn the basic cancer epidemiology concepts of design, implementation of studies and analysis, students from different backgrounds could be divided into team projects to formulate a hypothetical research grant on a cancer epidemiology topic of specific cancer sites. The research project exercise allows the students to apply the foundations of cancer epidemiology, find the gaps in the literature, and explore setting and methods to apply the theoretical knowledge into applied and practical skills for cancer epidemiology research.

Other learning opportunities include the summer courses offered by the National Cancer Institute (NCI), the International Agency for Research on Cancer (IARC) or the International Epidemiology Institute in Italy (Please see Chapter 15 of this section). Major universities in the United States have also summer epidemiology courses that address the introduction to cancer epidemiology, molecular and genetic epidemiology, and translation of epidemiology to cancer prevention and control. The University of Michigan offers two of its summer courses in developing countries. These courses are attended by clinicians, epidemiologists, and cancer prevention researchers from developing countries, and the contents of the courses are centered around on cancer epidemiology and translation to cancer prevention and controls.

CULTURE OF SCHOOLS OF PUBLIC HEALTH IN RELATION TO CANCER EPIDEMIOLOGY EDUCATION

In the United States

The effectiveness of schools of public health in cancer epidemiology education and training relies on the structure and culture of the schools, curriculum, and students. These factors may be categorized into two groups of factors

School and Faculty Factors

A matrix of factors helps influence the degree to which cancer epidemiology education and training will have a presence in the school's curriculum. These factors include the following:

- organizational set-up of the school with respect to number and specialization of departments or programs, number of faculty and whether cancer is their primary focus
- other expertise in departments of epidemiology (e.g., infectious, social, or environmental epidemiology)
- level of funding available for cancer training from training or educational grants, networks and collaboration with the surrounding communities
- whether the programs include minority populations
- interest and activities of the school, department, and faculty in global health
- tenure and promotion criteria
- protected time for faculty for travel time needed for global cancer research.

Students and Curricular Factors

There are generally two types of students who may be involved in cancer epidemiology education and research training, doctoral and master students. Doctoral students may receive different levels of educational and research training experience depending on the availability of faculty members who specialize in cancer epidemiology and their sub-specialties in the field, available courses, and available research and training grants for them. In most schools, doctoral students can engage more in cancer epidemiology because (1) they chose to come to this field, (2) they intend to pursue future careers in the field, (3) they have some flexibility in the required period to earn the degree, (4) they have previous work and possibly research experience that provide more maturing and in-depth thinking than master students, (5) and if they are required to have a multidisciplinary advisory committee of faculty with cognates from departments other than epidemiology.

Master students who wish to learn about cancer epidemiology do not have the educational and learning opportunities available to doctoral students. First, master students have a busy curriculum and must take core course that may not be related to cancer epidemiology. Second, the main focus of most MPH programs is not completely focused on research but more on practice. Third, there are very limited funds available to train master students in cancer epidemiology, but more opportunities for training in infectious disease epidemiology. Fourth, the job market provides more opportunities for a general public health task force rather than specialized researchers who are graduates of MPH programs. However, master students in most schools are required to have a practicum or internship with a wide range of variances in terms of levels of requirements of format, duration, and expected outcomes of the practicum or internship. The more developed models for practicum/internship format include preparation of a proposal before the internship, duration of 8–14 weeks in field research, and analysis and write-up of the outcome of the internship. (Examples of field internship programs are described later in this chapter and in Chapter 14.)

Public Health Programs in Countries Other than the United States

In other countries, the main program at the entry level of professional public health education is a master of science in public health (MSc).

These programs exist in Canada, the United Kingdom, Ireland, Belgium, Iceland, Sweden, Spain, The Netherlands, and several other European countries. Programs are also offered in many countries in Africa, Asia, Latin America, and Australia and New Zeeland. For complete list of the schools and programs, the following websites can be of help: http://mph-selection.org.uk, www.fphm.org.uk; http://spuweb.siu.edu.ar/studyinargentina/pages/study1603.php; http://www.degreesoverseas.com/all-degrees/degree-programs-in-australia/public-health-degree-programs/ The websites of the Latin American Global Health Alliance, Asia Pacific Academic Consortium for Public Health, Association of Schools of Public Health in Africa, and Association of Schools of Public Health in the European Region are also useful.

The Association of Schools of Public Health in the European Region (ASPHER) is the major body of European organizations focused on strengthening the importance of public health by enhancing education and training of public health professionals for both practice and research. The association was established in 1966 and includes 80 members located in different parts of the member states of the European Union (EU), Council of Europe (CE), and European affiliates of the World Health Organization.[3]

The MSc programs are geared toward research while the MPH program is more of a multidisciplinary practice. The MSc program requires a thesis and data collection process, but there are several opportunities for the MPH program type practicum. The format of the practicum/internship vary from field training, use of data for analysis, hands-on experience in a field setting, and may be writing of a report or a mini thesis.

Like the United States, no separate departments of cancer epidemiology exist at universities outside the United States.[4] However, in most countries, graduate students who are interested in cancer epidemiology usually earn their degrees and write their dissertations on cancer epidemiology topics from departments of epidemiology.[4]

■ CURRENT STATUS OF CURRICULA AND PROGRAMS FOR TRAINING IN CANCER EPIDEMIOLOGY IN MEDICAL SCHOOLS: THE EXPERIENCE OF MEDICAL SCHOOLS

In the United States

Population health is not a major part of the curriculum in medical schools in the United States. Apart from a required, brief introduction to population health, epidemiology, and biostatistics in the beginning of medical school education, usually in the first year, only limited training is provided in population health or epidemiology in US medical school curricula. The required course on population health, epidemiology, and biostatistics enables students to understand and critically evaluate presentations, analysis, and interpretation of data in the biomedical publications and literature. This course also makes students aware of fundamentals of hypothesis generation and testing, study design, and statistical inference. Students enrolled in such a course may also acquire skills in internal and external validity of research studies and evaluating the study designs for appropriateness of testing specific questions and reaching the possible study outcomes.

Based on this description of medical school training in epidemiology, it follows that cancer epidemiology is not touched upon in medical school education. However, medical students have 2 opportunities to learn about cancer epidemiology. First, with the growing interest and increasing number of students in global health, they have increased opportunities for global health training and education. Global health field training may involve cancer internships and possibly cancer epidemiology field training. Although this is not a systematic way of training, some medical students involved in field training may encounter opportunities for orientation about cancer and possibly cancer epidemiology. These opportunities increase if the medical school and or its university have an infrastructure for field training of students in international settings (see Chapter 3).

Second, there is an increasing trend of US medical schools to provide MPH programs either in between medical school years of education or combined with the medical school education. The programs usually offer one year of the MPH education through condensed courses with little or no field training. The programs include education about population heath, and cancer may be one of the elective courses in the curriculum. The MD-MPH program does not aim to create population scientists out of medical students, but rather seeks to make them think about populations at large and special populations or underserved minorities and international medicine in addition to their practice on individual patients. Because of the short one-year program and the limited opportunities for practical work, field training in cancer is rarely included. Some medical schools with departments of epidemiology or public health may also offer joint MSc or MPH degrees.

Other Countries

Medical students in countries outside the United States have more opportunities to learn about cancer because departments of public health or community medicine are frequently parts of medical schools in other countries. In developing countries, especially those following the British system of education, chronic disease epidemiology, including cancer, is part of the curriculum. However, the extent of inclusion of cancer epidemiology is limited. In HI and LMI countries, there are no masters or doctoral degrees in cancer epidemiology.[4] Nonetheless, students' master theses and dissertations may be focused on cancer epidemiology based on the interest of the mentoring faculty members, and available cancer epidemiology resources in terms of hospital, cancer center, or patient population.

▨ SUMMARY

Cancer epidemiology education is not a core part of the master-level curricula in the United States or other countries. There are no master's or doctoral degrees in cancer epidemiology in the United States or other countries. When cancer epidemiology courses exist in the curriculum of schools or programs of public health, they are usually offered as electives and their extent and varieties depend on the existing cancer epidemiology research programs and faculty on campus. In the United States, presence of a comprehensive cancer center on campus increases the opportunities for cancer epidemiology education and training of students because of the population science faculty and research resources required for the comprehensive status.

▪ REFERENCES

1. Association of Schools of Public Health. Annual data report, 2010. Washington DC: ASPH, 2010.
2. Trichopoulos D, Lagiou P. Are epidemiologists becoming victims of the success of their discipline? *Soz Praventivmed.* 2001;46(6):347–348.
3. ASPHER. The association of schools of public health in the European region. www.old.aspher.org. Updated 03/11/2011. Accessed 03/06, 2012.
4. Mosavi-Jarrahi A, Azargashb E, Mousavi-Jarrahi Y, Mohagheghi MA. The state of cancer epidemiology curricula in postgraduate schools worldwide. *J Cancer Educ.* 2011;26(3):566–571.

CHAPTER 14

UNIVERSITY RESOURCES FOR ACADEMIC AND FIELD RESEARCH TRAINING IN CANCER EPIDEMIOLOGY

AMR S. SOLIMAN AND ROBERT M. CHAMBERLAIN

This chapter delineates the existing educational and training programs in the United States that fund programs for training students and trainees in the fields of cancer epidemiology, cancer research, and cancer prevention. The chapter also provides descriptions of the global health programs available at top-tier schools of public health in the United States and their field training resources, including cancer epidemiology research training. Finally, the chapter provides an example of a field training program in cancer epidemiology in low- and middle-income (LMI) countries from the University of Nebraska College of Public Health.

EXISTING PROGRAMS FOR GRADUATE STUDENTS AND POSTDOCTORAL FELLOWS

In 1982, the National Cancer Institute (NCI) issued a new grant mechanism for cancer education. Grants funded through this mechanism were mainly available to medical schools for developing curricula and providing medical students with experience in cancer practice and possibly research. Approximately a decade later, the first program announcement (PA) was issued by NCI seeking applications for grants on cancer education, research training, and cancer prevention and control. In the mid-1990s, NCI divided the PA into 2 grant mechanisms: an educational grant mechanism (R25E) and a training grant mechanism (R25T). The two programs focus on cancer education and training from different angles.

The R25E mechanism is for "cancer education" grants. The grants target a wide range of audiences, including students and researchers in health and biomedical sciences with a primary focus on cancer and education of students, communities, and practitioners in all aspects of cancer research and cancer prevention. Grants aimed at educating students, cancer scientists, cancer care professionals, clinicians, or community health providers are usually awarded for developing and using curriculum-based short-term educational experiences. The curriculum content of these programs may range from cancer biology and genetics to cancer prevention, control, and palliative care. This section of R25E grants is the one mainly dealing with education and research training of students. It is important to note that nonstudent groups and projects may be eligible for funding through this mechanism. Examples of grants not focused on students include those to community health care providers or community settings to facilitate the diffusion of evidence-based findings within a relatively short time. "Research dissemination" projects that target public health workers, community organizations, and clinicians for cancer prevention and control programs are also eligible for grants. Disseminating findings into patient and lay communities through this mechanism is also eligible for grant applications. Further details about this mechanism are available under

http://grants.nih.gov/grants/guide/pa-files/PAR-12–049.html

Table 14.1 provides a complete list of grants that are funded through this mechanism, which can be found at the website of the NCI Funded Research Portfolio and the following link:

http://fundedresearch.cancer.gov/search/ResultManager?fy=PUB2011&mech=R25 &pd=Erica+Rosemond

The Cancer Education and Career Development Program (R25T) mechanism funds the development and implementation of curriculum-dependent programs to train predoctoral and postdoctoral candidates in cancer research settings that are highly interdisciplinary and collaborative. This program is particularly applicable to cancer prevention and control, epidemiology, nutrition, and the behavioral and population sciences. Details of the Program Announcement Reviewed by NIH Institute (PAR) are available through the following website: http://grants.nih.gov/grants/guide/pa-files/PAR-10–165.html

Table 14.2 provides a complete list of grants that are funded through this mechanism, which can be found at the website of the NCI Funded Research Portfolio and the following link:

http://fundedresearch.cancer.gov/search/ResultManager?fy=PUB2010&mech=R25 &pd=Dorkina+Myrick

A third grant mechanism for training is the Ruth L. Kirschstein National Research Service Award (NRSA) (T32). This award supports institutional training grants that develop or enhance research training opportunities for early-stage investigators committed to cancer research. Details of the PAR can be found under the following link:

http://www.cancer.gov/researchandfunding/cancertraining/outsidenci/T32

Table 14.3 provides a complete list of grants that are funded through this mechanism, which can be found at the website of the NCI Funded Research Portfolio and the following link:

http://fundedresearch.cancer.gov/search/ResultManager?fy=PUB2010&mech=T32

■ EXISTING FIELD TRAINING IN LOW- AND MIDDLE-INCOME COUNTRIES FOR GRADUATE STUDENTS IN THEUNITED STATES

Over the past decade, many schools of public health in the United States have created or expanded global health programs. Although in past decades a limited number of international epidemiology programs existed at top schools, global health programs, concentrations, and certificates in increasing numbers of public health programs in the United States

TABLE 14.1 R25E Programs funded by NCI focused on Cancer Epidemiology

PROGRAM NAME	PRINCIPAL INVESTIGATOR	INSTITUTION	PROGRAM OUTLINE
PROGRAMS WITH FULL FOCUS ON CANCER EPIDEMIOLOGY			
Cancer Epidemiology Education in Special Populations	Soliman, Amr	University of Nebraska Medical Center, College of Public Health	**Description:** Four-month summer curriculum-based and summer research field experiences in special populations (minority and international settings). **Aim:** To motivate public health students to pursue future careers in cancer in special populations **Participants:** students from the University of Michigan School of Public Health. Predominately MPH students with some slots for PhD students
PROGRAMS WITH PARTIAL FOCUS ON CANCER EPIDEMIOLOGY			
Cancer Prevention Education: Student Research Experiences	Chang, Shine	University of Texas MD Anderson Cancer Center	**Description:** Three to six month curriculum-based, short-term research experiences in cancer prevention research and education **Aim:** To motivate students to pursue careers in cancer prevention research. **Participants:** Graduate students and minority undergraduates from the basic biomedical sciences, biostatistics, epidemiology, genetics, behavioral and social sciences, nursing, medicine, and related public health disciplines
Short-Term Training on Epidemiologic Methods	Lyon, Joseph	Society of Epidemiologic Research, Utah	**Description:** One-week educational program to enhance the education of doctoral students in cancer research. **Aim:** To provide a forum for doctoral-level students to interact with their peers and senior epidemiologists. **Participants:** Doctoral-level students working on theses on cancer at any U.S. institution.

are now providing ample opportunities for students to learn about field epidemiology in LMI countries. These programs are funded through training grants, such as the grants listed previously, foundation training resources, the National Institutes of Health Fogarty Training Programs, school funding, or other mechanisms.

The field training opportunities for public health students in epidemiology are provided through internships or practicum experience through different levels of structures, requirements, and outcomes or through participation in faculty research projects in LMI countries.

TABLE 14.2 R25T Programs funded by NCI focused on Cancer Epidemiology (1990 to 2013, discontinued 2013)

PROGRAM NAME	PRINCIPAL INVESTIGATOR	INSTITUTION	PROGRAM OUTLINE
PROGRAMS WITH FULL FOCUS ON CANCER EPIDEMIOLOGY			
Interdisciplinary Training in Cancer Epidemiology at UB	Freudenheim, Jo	State University of New York at Buffalo, New York	**Description:** Training for pre-doctoral fellows in Cancer Epidemiology and Control. **Aim:** To train scientists prepared for the rapidly changing field of cancer epidemiology, increase skills epidemiologic methods, with an integrated understanding of the biology of cancer. **Participants:** Pre-doctoral students in epidemiology
Mayo Cancer Genetic Epidemiology Training Program	Petersen, Gloria	Mayo Clinic. Minnesota	**Description:** Interdisciplinary training to prepare post-doctoral fellows to meet the challenges of bridging the laboratory-translational interface, and to stimulate improvements in cancer detection, prevention, and treatment. **Aim:** To produce investigators capable of developing an independent academic career in the evolving arena of cancer research that transects the disciplines of genetics, epidemiology, bioinformatics, and biostatistics. **Participants:** Post-doctoral fellows
Moffitt Post-doctoral Training Program in Molecular & Genetic Epidemiology	Egan, Kathleen	H. Lee Moffitt Cancer Center & Research Institute, Florida	**Description:** A specialized curriculum to prepare future academic researchers to integrate the latest technologies and full spectrum of outcomes (from risk to survival) in observational molecular and genetic epidemiology **Aim:** Provide multidisciplinary training in cancer prevention **Participants:** Post-doctoral fellows from epidemiology, biostatistics, medicine, or other related fields
Nutritional Epidemiology of Cancer Education and Career Development Program	Stampfer, Meir	Harvard University (School of Public Health), Massachusetts	**Description:** To train researchers in nutritional epidemiology of cancer **Aim:** To discover new ways in which changes in diet can reduce the risk and burden of cancer **Participants:** Post-doctoral fellows with research in nutritional epidemiology of cancer

(continued)

TABLE 14.2 (Continued)

PROGRAM NAME	PRINCIPAL INVESTIGATOR	INSTITUTION	PROGRAM OUTLINE
Training in Computational Genomic Epidemiology of Cancer	Elston, Robert	Case Western Reserve University, Ohio	**Description:** Developing expertise in innovative cancer research by training scientists. Researchers with interdisciplinary training across these fields of genetic epidemiology **Aim:** To define a novel, transdisciplinary area of training at the intersection of cancer research, epidemiology, biostatistics, genetics, and computer science **Participants:** Postdocotoral fellows with a mixture of backgrounds, including molecular biology, oncology, medicine, epidemiology, biostatistics, genomics/genetics, and computer science
Training in Molecular & Genetic Epidemiology of Cancer	Witte, John	University of California, San Francisco	**Description:** Train scientists in multidisciplinary molecular, genetic, and biostatistical epidemiology **Aim:** To develop independent researchers in the interdisciplinary field of genetic and molecular epidemiology of cancer **Participants:** Post-doctoral fellows with training in genetic and molecular epidemiology of cancer (GMEC)
Training Program in Cancer-Related Population Sciences	Neugut, Alfred	Columbia University Health Sciences, New York	**Description:** Curriculum-based multi-disciplinary training in Epidemiology, biostatistics, and environmental health sciences **Aim:** To develop a multi-disciplinary training program for graduate students and fellows **Participants:** Pre- and post-doctoral fellows

PROGRAMS WITH A PARTIAL FOCUS ON CANCER EPIDEMIOLOGY

PROGRAM NAME	PRINCIPAL INVESTIGATOR	INSTITUTION	PROGRAM OUTLINE
Cancer Control Education Program	Earp, Jo Anne	University of North Carolina, Chapel Hill	**Description**: Cancer training and education program **Aim:** Cancer prevention and control research **Participants:** Pre- and post-doctoral fellows
Cancer Prevention & Control Training Program	Nagy, Timothy	University of Alabama at Birmingham, Alabama	**Description**: Cancer training and education program **Aim:** Cancer prevention and control research **Participants:** Pre- and post-doctoral fellows

(continued)

TABLE 14.2 (Continued)

PROGRAM NAME	PRINCIPAL INVESTIGATOR	INSTITUTION	PROGRAM OUTLINE
Cancer Prevention & Control: Multidisciplinary Training	Redd, William	Mount Sinai School of Medicine, New York	**Description:** Cancer training and education Program **Aim:** Cancer prevention and control research **Participants:** Post-doctoral fellows
Cancer Prevention and Control Translational Research	Alberts, David	University of Arizona, Tucson, Arizona	**Description**: Didactic and research experiences needed for a collaborative post-graduate career in cancer prevention and control **Aim:** Cancer prevention and control research **Participants:** Post-doctoral fellows
Cancer Prevention Training in Nutrition, Exercise & Genetics	White, Emily	University of Washington, Seattle	**Description:** Emphasizes the interrelationship of human nutrition, exercise, genetics and metabolic pathways in cancer susceptibility and prevention. **Aim:** To gain didactic and research experience to become knowledgeable investigators on multidisciplinary cancer prevention research projects **Participants:** Pre- and post-doctoral fellows
Education Program in Cancer Prevention	Weissfeld, Joel	University of Pittsburgh at Pittsburgh	**Description**: Multidisciplinary training in cancer epidemiology, prevention, and control **Aim:** Cancer epidemiology and prevention **Participants:** Pre-doctoral candidates
Epidemiologic and Basic Science in Cancer Prevention	Marshall, James	Roswell Park Cancer Institute Corporation, New York	**Description**: To develop the ability for interdisciplinary collaboration in cancer prevention research based on the "bench to sidewalk" model **Aim:** Study and treat malignant disease **Participants:** Post-doctoral fellows
Harvard Education Program in Cancer Prevention Control	Sorensen, Glorian	Harvard University (School of Public Health), Massachusetts	**Description:** Cancer prevention and control **Aim:** Create a cadre of researchers in cancer prevention and control **Participants:** Pre- and post-doctoral fellows

(*continued*)

TABLE 14.2 (Continued)

PROGRAM NAME	PRINCIPAL INVESTIGATOR	INSTITUTION	PROGRAM OUTLINE
Integrating Population and Basic Science in Cancer Research	Schildkraut, Joellen	Duke University, North Carolina	**Description**: Interdisciplinary cancer training program **Aim:** Training in population science including epidemiology, survival analysis, genetics, pharmacogenomics, & statistical modeling **Participants:** Junior and more experienced basic scientists
M.D. Anderson Education Program in Cancer Prevention	Chang, Shine	University of Texas M.D. Anderson Cancer Center	**Description**: Cancer Prevention, control research, and practice **Aim:** Multi-disciplinary research in cancer prevention and control **Participants:** Pre- and post-doctoral trainees
Nutritional & Behavioral Cancer Prevention in a Multiethnic Population	Maskarinec, Gertraud	University of Hawaii at Manoa, Hawaii	**Description**: Prepare young scientists to elucidate the causes of cancer and develop strategies to reduce cancer incidence and mortality **Aim:** Nutritional epidemiology and behavioral cancer prevention in a multiethnic population **Participants:** Post-doctoral fellows
Prevention Research Educational Post-doctoral (PREP) Training Program	Rose, Julia	Case Western Reserve University, Ohio	**Description**: Focuses on research on behavioral aspects of cancer prevention, detection, and control **Aim:** Research on behavioral aspects of cancer prevention, detection, and control **Participants:** Post-doctoral fellows
Training Program for Quantitative Population Sciences in Cancer	Moore, Jason	Dartmouth College, Hanover, New Hampshire	**Description**: Combines specialized research knowledge and methodologies in bioinformatics, biostatistics and epidemiology. **Aim:** To accelerate cancer research by enhancing the existing pool of cancer researchers with the skills needed to meet the present and future needs in translational cancer research in the population sciences. **Participants:** Post-doctoral fellows
UCLA Career Development Program in Cancer Prevention and Control Research	Bastani, Roshan	University of California Los Angeles	**Description**: Transdisciplinary research **Aim:** To train transdisciplinary scientists to conduct cancer prevention and control research to reduce the population burden of cancer **Participants:** Pre- and post-doctoral fellows

TABLE 14.3 T32 Programs funded by NCI focused on Cancer Epidemiology

PROGRAM NAME	PI	INSTITUTION	ABSTRACT
PROGRAMS WITH FULL FOCUS ON CANCER EPIDEMIOLOGY			
Cancer Clinical Epidemiology Training Grant	Strom, Brian	University of Pennsylvania, Philadelphia,	**Description**: To prepare clinicians and researchers in independent careers as clinical investigators capable of using the range of approaches in public health, including etiology, prognosis, prevention and early detection, treatment, clinical economics, quality of patient care. **Participants**: Most trainees matriculate in the Master of Science in Clinical Epidemiology (MSCE) degree program. Only individuals who have completed training in a relevant medical specialty or hold a PhD in epidemiology or a related field are eligible **Main Focus**: To provide in-depth knowledge of research techniques appropriate for clinical cancer research and supervised research experiences with mentors in clinical epidemiology and cancer research.
Cancer Epidemiology and Biostatistics Training	Vaughan, Thomas	University of Washington, Seattle,	**Description**: Interdisciplinary training program in cancer epidemiology and biostatistics **Participants**: Pre- and post-doctoral trainees **Main Focus**: To provide skills in epidemiology and biostatistics that enable the trainee to address this problem through the conduct of high quality cancer research
Cancer Epidemiology Training Center	Zhang, Zuo-Feng	University of California Los Angeles	**Description**: Interdisciplinary program of cancer molecular and genetic epidemiology **Participants**: Pre- and post-doctoral trainees **Main Focus**: To implement innovative, multidisciplinary, and collaborative research training in cancer epidemiology in an interdisciplinary program of cancer molecular and genetic epidemiology
Cancer Epidemiology, Biostatistics and Environmental Sciences	Neugut, Alfred	Columbia University Health Sciences, New York	**Description**: A program in cancer epidemiology, biostatistics, and environmental health premised on the belief that high-quality investigators in these areas require a broad-based, multidisciplinary perspective. **Participants**: Pre- and Post-doctoral fellows **Main Focus**: Cancer epidemiology, biostatistics, environmental health, molecular genetics, clinical oncology, toxicology, and behavioral science

(continued)

TABLE 14.3 (Continued)

PROGRAM NAME	PI	INSTITUTION	ABSTRACT
PROGRAMS WITH PARTIAL FOCUS ON CANCER EPIDEMIOLOGY			
Cancer Etiology, Prevention, Detection and Diagnosis	Giaccia, Amato	Stanford University, California	**Description**: Interdisciplinary program in cancer biology **Participants**: Pre- and post-doctoral fellows **Main Focus**: To provide students with education and training that enable them to make significant contributions to cancer biology
Cancer Health Disparities Training Program	Campbell, Marci	University of North Carolina, Chapel Hill	**Description**: To address and understand cross-cutting health disparity issues in cancer across the cancer continuum from etiology and primary prevention to survivorship **Participants**: Post-doctoral fellows **Main Focus**: Educational and research knowledge necessary for the cancer health disparities research, survivorship, and critical thinking and synthesis

The epidemic of HIV/AIDS has resulted in increased clinical and epidemiologic research. The research funding that has supported this effort has enabled academic institutions from HI countries to establish semipermanent field research stations in LMI countries in Africa. The stations have provided a base for student research projects in a variety of fields, including cancer. The model has helped in capacity building and joint collaborations with physicians and scientists in these countries. These long-term collaborations can be valuable in providing infrastructure and mentoring for epidemiology students to carry out research in LMI countries. Similar long-term collaborations in certain LMI countries have been a feature of cancer epidemiology field training, as illustrated in the University of Nebraska program described in the next section.

Table 14.4 provides a list of the top 10 schools of public health, based on the *U.S. News and World Report* ranking of 2011 along with examples of countries and diseases or fields of experience that are provided for students in field epidemiology in LMI countries. The list of schools can be found under the following link:

http://grad-schools.usnews.rankingsandreviews.com/best-graduate-schools/
    top-health-schools/public-health-rankings

▦ AN EXAMPLE OF A FIELD TRAINING PROGRAM IN CANCER EPIDEMIOLOGY IN LMI COUNTRIES, THE UNIVERSITY OF NEBRASKA COLLEGE OF PUBLIC HEALTH

While cancer epidemiology training may be provided through student participation in faculty research projects on cancer in LMI countries or through occasional and unplanned global health opportunities, the University of Nebraska sponsors a program that combines funding in an educational research training grant through NCI (from an R25E mechanism),

TABLE 14.4 List of top 10 U.S. Schools of Public Health and examples of countries of field training and diseases or fields of research and training

SCHOOL	OFF-CAMPUS COUNTRIES	DISEASES OR FIELD OF RESEARCH AND/OR TRAINING
Johns Hopkins University	Ethiopia, Chad, Ghana, Malawi, Nigeria, Uganda, Congo, South Africa, Tanzania, Botswana, Namibia, Madagascar, Mauritania, Mali, Niger, Zambia, Egypt, Bangladesh, China, Panama, Philippine, Peru, Colombia, Brazil, Bolivia, Venezuela, Mongolia, Afghanistan, Turkey, Iraq, Iran, United Arab Emirates, Pakistan India, Ukraine, France, Norway, Sweden, Finland, and Italy.	Diarrheal diseases, HIV/AIDS, HPV, malaria, hepatitis, cardiovascular diseases, diabetes, obesity, cancer, bioinformatics, reproductive health, women's health, childhood diseases, vaccination, injuries, environmental exposures, and health systems
http://www.hopkinsglobalhealth.org/		
University of North Carolina	South Africa, Egypt, Angola, Cote d'Ivoire, Congo, Ethiopia, Ghana, Guinea, Kenya, Liberia, Madagascar, Mali, Mozambique, Namibia, Nigeria, Rwanda, Senegal, Sudan, Swaziland, Tanzania, Togo, Uganda, Zambia, Zimbabwe, Bangladesh, Burma, China, Laos, Thailand, Vietnam, Brazil, Dominican Republic, El Salvador, Guatemala, Guyana, Haiti, Honduras, Jamaica, Mexico, Nicaragua, Panama, Paraguay, and Peru.	HIV/AIDS, health systems, bioethics, infectious diseases, malaria, HIV/AIDS, child health, nutrition, aging environmental exposures, and capacity building.
http://www.sph.unc.edu/globalhealth/		
Harvard University	China, Taiwan, Bangladesh, Scandinavian countries, Italy, central America, Africa, and the Middle East.	Maternal and child health, health systems, ethical issues, human rights, aging, health inequalities, exposure to chemicals, infectious diseases, cardiovascular diseases, and cancer.
http://www.hsph.harvard.edu/departments/global-health-and-population/ http://www.hsph.harvard.edu/departments/epidemiology/		
University of Michigan	Iraq, Ghana, Kenya, Ethiopia, Malawi, Zimbabwe, South Africa, Zambia, Nigeria, Mexico, Argentina, Brazil, Colombia, Peru, Ecuador, Dominican Republic, Haiti, India, Pakistan, Nepal, Bangladesh, China, Taiwan,	Environmental exposures, environmental justice, heavy metals, climate changes, infectious diseases, HIV/AIDS, hepatitis, vaccines, maternal and child health, nutrition, social determinants of health, human rights, and health economics,
http://www.sph.umich.edu/global/ http://www.globalhealth.umich.edu/		

(continued)

TABLE 14.4 (Continued)

SCHOOL	OFF-CAMPUS COUNTRIES	DISEASES OR FIELD OF RESEARCH AND/OR TRAINING
Columbia University	Kenya, Mozambique, Rwanda, South Africa, Uganda, Zambia, Jordan, Thailand,	HIV/AIDS and infectious diseases,

http://www.mailman.columbia.edu/academic-departments/select-programs/global-health-initiative

Emory University	Ethiopia, Kenya, Ghana, Tanzania, Nigeria, Rwanda, Madagascar, Mali, South Africa, Peru, Bolivia, Ecuador, Honduras, Mexico, Dominican Republic, Haiti, Bangladesh, Cambodia, India, and China.	Vaccination, water and sanitation, hygiene, food production, primary health care, climate change, maternal and child health, environmental exposures, HIV/AIDS, and health systems.

http://www.sph.emory.edu/cms/departments_centers/gh/index.html

University of Washington	China, Cambodia, Pakistan, India, Timor, Nepal, Sudan, Botswana, Ethiopia, Kenya, Malawi, Mozambique, Namibia, South Africa, Senegal, Uganda, Caribbean, Honduras	HIV/AIDS, HHV-8, HPV, cervical cancer, field epidemiology, malaria, maternal and child health, heart disease, stroke, operations research, health systems, and trauma

http://globalhealth.washington.edu/

University of California-Berkeley	Kenya, Tanzania, Ghana, Japan, Haiti, Chile, Guatemala, Argentina, India, and Bangladesh	Radiation, water, smoke exposure, pneumonia, cognitive impacts, Schistosomiasis, arsenic exposure, and early childhood exposures.

http://sph.berkeley.edu/students/degrees/areas/gh.php

University of Minnesota	Uganda, India, Uruguay, Europe, Thailand	Zoonotic disease, infectious diseases, disease surveillance, food safety, animal health, nutrition, mental health, and alcohol,

http://www.sph.umn.edu/outreach/engagement/fe.asp
http://www.sph.umn.edu/outreach/go/gouganda.asp

University of California-Los Angeles	Kenya, Ghana, Uganda, Ethiopia, Angola, South Africa, Congo, Cameroon, Madagascar, South Africa, Egypt, Iran, Lebanon, India, Thailand, China, Philippine, Paraguay, Cuba, Costa Rica, Mexico, Chile, Puerto Rico.	Nutrition, maternal and child health, medical anthropology, aging, environmental health, disaster response, HIV/AIDS, STDs, health services, and metal health.

http://www.ph.ucla.edu/globalhealth/global_health_faculty.php

as listed in Table 14.1. The program, the called Cancer Epidemiology Education in Special Populations (CEESP) Program, started at the University of Michigan in 2006, then moved to the University of Nebraska in 2012. It builds upon the university's existing global health infrastructure in international settings, as well as adding educational and curricular opportunities through the funding from the NCI training grant. After successfully securing grant funding from NCI, the program was initiated in 2006 and renewed in 2011.

The rest of this chapter highlights the lessons learned from establishing, implementing, and continuing such field training programs in cancer epidemiology in LMI countries. This experience can be used by faculty in high-income countries (HI) to develop similar programs and also by mentors in LMI countries for training students from HI countries.

The objective of the program has been to develop and implement an educational program to prepare public health students in the field of cancer epidemiology research in special populations (international and minority settings in the United States). The program has developed a curriculum, including 3 new courses and a research-training infrastructure, and has trained 10 students per year. A new feature was added to the program in 2011 with the addition of up to 2 of the 10 positions for doctoral students.

The aims of the program are to:

1. Recruit and select first-year MPH and PhD students to fill 10 positions during each year.
2. Develop and maintain a core curriculum to prepare students for summer field research experiences in cancer epidemiology in special populations. A follow-up component of the curriculum occurs after the summer field research experience. A new educational innovation that was introduced to the program after the first 5 years included the development of 3 new educational modules related to data capturing, epidemiology subspecialties, and measurements in cancer epidemiology.
3. Maintain and increase the pool of the University of Nebraska faculty mentors and off-campus field site research mentors.
4. Maintain and enhance review and oversight functions of a cancer epidemiology educational advisory committee, consisting of both internal and external experts in cancer education and epidemiology.
5. Maintain and enhance the process and outcome evaluation, long-term tracking, and dissemination of the program to other educational institutions in the United States.

This program defines cancer epidemiology in special populations as a future career discipline for students in the field of public health and provides a source of trained professionals needed to carry out large projects in cancer epidemiology in special populations.

Topics of Research: Topics of research are focused on descriptive, molecular, environmental, and social epidemiology of colorectal, breast, pancreatic, liver, and thyroid cancers in international settings and migrant and minority populations in the United States. Other topics include knowledge about attitudes about cancer, cancer registration among ethnic and minority populations, and risk factors of cancer.

Field Sites: All students' projects built upon the existing research infrastructure of the University of Michigan faculty mentors' research. In international settings, the projects were located in Morocco, Tunisia, Egypt, Jordan, Israel, Uganda, Malawi, Ghana, and Tanzania. While the program primarily focuses on Africa and the Middle East, additional projects have been conducted in Mexico and India. Domestic internships in migrant and minority populations have been located in communities with large numbers of Arab Americans, migrant farm workers, Native Americans, and African Americans.

Course Development: The program has created a new course on cancer epidemiology in special populations, a seminar on cancer epidemiology, and a seminar on the translation of cancer epidemiology to cancer control and prevention. All courses have attracted double the number of students enrolled in the cancer education program. For the existing core course on cancer epidemiology, the number of students enrolled every year since the beginning of the program accounts for 3 times the number of enrolled students each year prior to the program. In other words, the program has motivated nonprogram students to learn about cancer epidemiology and to pursue summer internships in cancer epidemiology. The favorable evaluations students gave to all these courses meant that these courses were among the most highly rated courses at University of Michigan School of Public Health. Another indication of the quality and perception of the value of the new courses is that the school adopted them as permanent courses.

SELECTION OF STUDENT APPLICANTS

Selection of student applicants to the program is the responsibility of the advisory committee. Applications are accepted on an annual basis, with committee members receiving complete application packets on December 15 of each year before the annual meeting of the committee. All committee members score every applicant by ballot on a scale of 1.0 to 10.0, similar to the National Institutes of Health scoring system. Most successful applicants are anticipated to achieve scores in the range of 2.0–3.0. A completed application includes a proposal for admission to the program, in which students outline their suggested list of courses and how these courses can help their internship projects and future career. The proposal also includes the following information about the 4-month research experience:

1. Description and time line of the 4-month research project
2. Description of the research resources, mentor's research program, lab resources, data availability, etc.
3. The student's existing skills that make the project feasible
4. Student's learning objectives for the 4-month period, including new skills that the student acquires during the short-term research experience
5. PhD students are also expected to include in their plan a discussion of dissertation possibilities growing out of the 4-month summer research experience

ESTABLISHING EACH STUDENT'S EDUCATIONAL OBJECTIVES

During the application process, student candidates meet with faculty members of the program to discuss the educational opportunities of various projects and to clarify mutual expectations. From this meeting, an educational plan is developed that describes the skills and/or knowledge that the students are expected to learn in courses and field experiences, their obligations to the project in terms of calendar and schedule, and the form of the students' final report. Acceptance of the students' application is primarily influenced by the overall educational benefit and feasibility of the research plan along with evidence of satisfactory academic performance in their respective programs. Past experience indicates that students frequently overestimate what can be accomplished. Adequate faculty counseling at the beginning of the students' program usually results in appropriate course selection and a realistic research plan. Experience has shown that careful preparation of learning objectives, methods, and time line planning helps ensure a successful research experience and subsequent career plans.

▧ OVERSIGHT OF STUDENT PROGRESS

Oversight and evaluation of the student's work in this program is primarily the responsibility of the faculty mentor. The mentor is asked to file a brief report each month on the student's progress according to the previously established time line. As demonstrated by the existing research infrastructure in international and ethnically diverse populations, the program faculty have the interest and ability to mentor the students during their traineeship period.[1] In addition, a member of the leadership team of the program carries out annual site visits to international and domestic minority populations involved in the program that are not visited by other faculty mentors. Also, the monthly reports are sent to the members of the advisory committee for their review.

▧ MAINTAINING AND INCREASING THE POOL OF MENTORS

The program began with a core group of faculty mentors who represent a variety of cancer disciplines. The group is maintained to provide active academic support for the students before, during, and after the summer internship program. New mentoring materials are developed and provided to new faculty and special courses offered on mentoring skills, advising and mentoring trainees, and developing educational objectives. To help recruit new faculty members to the mentoring team, advisory committee members conduct routine direct interpersonal contact and communications with new faculty recruited by the College of Public Health and the Cancer Center.

▧ ADVISORY COMMITTEE RECOMMENDATIONS

The 7-member advisory committee consists of internal university faculty and external cancer educators. This mix has been found to be extremely valuable. The committee evaluates all components of the program, including recruitment, selection, curriculum, evaluation, and dissemination. The following section summarizes action items and judgment of the committee.

In the first year evaluation, the committee concluded that the program had accomplished its aims. The committee judged the epidemiology curriculum as crowded in the first year, so they recommended increasing flexibility for the program's students by allowing some streamlining of coursework, reducing the total number of courses for students, thus providing them more time for the required core courses of the program. The committee approved the policy of accepting students with a grade point average of at least 6.0 (representing the top 60% of students on the school's 1.0–9.0 grade point range) at the end of their first term at the University of Michigan School of Public Health.

In the second year evaluation, the committee confirmed that the Department of Epidemiology had streamlined the first year curriculum for students, as recommended by the committee in the earlier report. The advisory committee reviewed the program's dissemination efforts, including a presentation at national conferences, which was designed to increase the interest of other Schools of Public Health in adopting the program. Dissemination efforts had also included sponsored workshops on cancer in Africa hosted by the University of Michigan. The advisory committee reviewed the workshop's impact on increasing student and faculty awareness of the program and the productive interactions between students and on-site and off-site mentors. To enhance the program's impact, the committee recommended focusing on selected geographical regions in the United States and abroad for field sites with existing research infrastructure and ongoing projects of University of Michigan faculty in place. The committee also recommended that students focus on field research projects with limited, attainable objectives that could be accomplished in four months.

In the third year evaluation, the committee cited the program's accomplishments, particularly the student publication rate (70%) in comparison to < 5% among other MPH students at the University of Michigan. They also noted the evidence of program success as indicated by the students seeking advanced degrees in cancer epidemiology and special population research. The committee recommended maintaining the core curriculum developed in the past three years that prepared students for summer field research experiences in cancer epidemiology in special populations. They also recommended maintaining the follow-up component of the curriculum in which students participate after the summer field research experience. However, in the committee's annual review of students' presentations and site mentors' evaluations, they identified a few gaps in special areas of knowledge and skills relevant to specific research projects. They sought to avoid adding to the students' already demanding curriculum and therefore recommended focused short courses with a range from 5 to 10 contact hours to cover the following aspects: data capturing, epidemiologic subspecialties (molecular, social, and environmental epidemiology), and measurements in cancer epidemiology. Planning and implementation of the modular courses was included after the initial 5 years of the program.

▦ ESTABLISHED MANAGERIAL POLICIES FOR SUMMER INTERNSHIPS

Based upon the experience and from the advice of the advisory committee, a standard policy for all aspects of the summer research experiences both in the United States and abroad was established. These policies are compiled in a binder, made accessible to faculty and students, and updated regularly. For example, it was essential that students have a continuous work period and schedule holidays for tourism before or after, not during, the summer research. A second example was based on feedback from students who lived in cities away from their research sites. Students were advised to live near their research site to reduce time lost to commuting.

▦ PROGRAM EVALUATION AND TRACKING SYSTEM FOR LONG-TERM IMPACT

The evaluation strategy of the program includes a number of distinct components designed to ensure ongoing assessment of the program and rapid corrective actions where indicated, as in the current cycle. The program evaluation measures are used to guide midstream corrective actions by the advisory committee. The evaluation is focused on the aims of the program as follows:

Evaluating Recruitment and Selection of Applicants

Based on the experience of the program, it is anticipated that the program will receives at least 20 qualified student applications each year from which the 10 most suitable applicants will be selected. The validity and adequacy of the selection criteria based on the performance of the students and their project productivity are periodically evaluated.

Evaluating, Maintaining, and Enhancing the Existing Core Curriculum of the Program and Modules

The evaluation of the curriculum includes faculty ratings of students' research proposals and adherence to guidelines for conducting, analyzing, and presenting research. Evaluation of the curriculum also includes mentors' review of student performance in courses and summary of strengths and limitations of previous field research experiences. The advisory committee reviews the evaluation results on an annual basis.

Evaluating, Maintaining, and Increasing the Pool of Potential Mentors

The program monitors the number of faculty who potentially can serve as mentors from different schools and centers on campus. Research-site and university mentors are continuously evaluated by the program students.

Evaluating, Maintaining, and Enhancing the Process and Outcome Evaluation, Long-Term Tracking, and Dissemination of the Program to Other Educational Institutions in the United States

The success of the program is evaluated by the short- and long-term gains. Short-term gains include achieving educational and research training aims and satisfactory rating by the advisory committee. Long-term success is evaluated by the benchmark of at least 50% of participating MPH and PhD students' continuing careers in cancer-related fields. With students' consent, students' contact information is retained to track their future careers and update their CV file annually. For each student, the evaluation methods include: (1) student trainee evaluation questionnaire, (2) mentor's progress reports, (3) checklist of field skills completed by each student trainee, (4) form for student's evaluation of off-site and on-site mentors, (5) the program director's exit interview, and (6) the students' formal presentation. All questionnaires and forms are in the appendix of this chapter.

■ DISSEMINATION PLAN

The program dissemination focuses on US institutions that have some form of existing field research internships, as well as other institutions that do not yet have such experience. First, the program established a special interactive website (http://unmc.edu/publichealth/ceesp). The program website is open for browsing and registration for students and institutions free of charge. This helps establish website interaction with faculty who are interested in adopting all or parts of the program. The website includes a description of the program curriculum, courses, students' field projects and results, publications, and feedback of students, mentors, and advisory committees' evaluations. Second, the program works with professional associations, such as the American College of Epidemiology, the American Public Health Association, and the American Association for Cancer Education to distribute CDs of the program activities to public health, medical, and nursing schools with an interest in initiating similar programs. Third, program students and faculty present the results of their educational and research training programs at national and international scientific conferences. In addition, the program provides extensive mentoring that has assisted 70% of our students to publish in peer-review journals.

■ SUMMARY

This chapter has reviewed the US funding mechanisms and active programs available for cancer education, cancer research, and cancer prevention. Because of the increasing student interest in global health, many schools of public health run programs for field research and training in LMI countries. These programs may include cancer as a topic of research and training of students. The University of Nebraska CEESP program is an illustration of a specialized cancer education and cancer research training program in LMI countries and minority populations in the United States. Lessons learned from this program have a wide applicability to other universities for initiating or developing cancer training in similar settings.

▪ REFERENCE

1. Soliman AS, Mullan PB, Chamberlain RM. Research training of students in minority and international settings: Lessons learned from cancer epidemiology education in special populations. *J Cancer Educ.* 2010;25(2):263–269.

■ SUPPLEMENTAL MATERIALS

Outcome Tools (Questionnaires and Forms) for Evaluation

Trainee Feedback Questionnaire
Trainee Evaluation of the Faculty Mentor
Faculty Evaluation of Trainee
Faculty Checklist of Trainee Skills

Cancer Epidemiology Education in Special Populations Program
Trainee Feedback Form

Name of trainee: _____ **Date:** _____
Current Degree: _____ **in** _____ **field/specialty. Date earned** _____
Future degree: _____ **in** _____ **field/specialty. Date expected** _____

1. How satisfied were you with:

A. Your laboratory or other field setting (overall)

0 _____|_____100

Comments:

B. Knowledge you acquired (overall)

0 _____|_____100

Comments:

C. The amount of time your faculty mentor spent with you

0 _____|_____100

Comments:

D. The amount of time other faculty and research assistants spent with you

0 _____|_____100

Comments:

E. The lab equipment and lab supplies available   ____Check here if NOT APPLICABLE

0 _____|_____100

Comments:

F. The computers provided for your use   _____Check here if NOT APPLICABLE

0 _____|_____100

Comments:

G. The desk and space provided for your work   _____Check here if NOT APPLICABLE

0 _____|_____100

Comments:

H. Laboratory bench space provided for you   Check here if NOT APPLICABLE

0 _____|_____100

Comments:

I. Library facilities made available to you   Check here if NOT APPLICABLE

0 _____|_____100

Comments:

J. The stipend paid to you   Check here if NOT APPLICABLE

0 _____|_____100

Comments:

K. The help from the program coordinator in administrative matters

0 _____|_____100

Comments:

2. If you could make your decision again, would you choose the Multidisciplinary Cancer Epidemiology Traineeship, or another alternative?

_____ I would make the same choice _____ I would select another alternative

3. If a very good friend was considering a traineeship would you recommend this program?

_____ I would recommend it strongly
_____ I would recommend it moderately
_____ I would not recommend it

Comments:

4. Do you believe that there might be a future for you in multidisciplinary cancer epidemiology research?

_____ Yes, definitely.
_____ Yes, maybe
_____ No, unlikely
_____ No, very unlikely

Comments:

5. Please tell us anything that you believe would make our program better.

Date:_____

Cancer Epidemiology Education in Special Populations Program
Trainee Evaluation of the Faculty Mentors

Name of Student: _____   _____,
LAST   FIRST

Name of Faculty Mentor: _____   _____,
LAST   FIRST

University Faculty Mentors

1. The amount of time your faculty mentor spent with you.

   0_____|_____100 DK/NA

   Comments:

2. The amount of interest your faculty mentor had in your intellectual development.

   0_____|_____100 DK/NA

   Comments:

3. The amount of interest your faculty mentor had in career advising and career opportunities.

   0_____|_____100 DK/NA

   Comments:

4. The amount of interest your faculty mentor had in you as a person.

   0_____|_____100 DK/NA

   Comments:

5. When seeking a job, would you ask your faculty mentor for a recommendation?

   ____Very Likely   ____Somewhat Likely   ____Neutral
   ____Somewhat Unlikely   ____Very Unlikely

   Comments:

Off-site Faculty Mentors

6. The number of visits your faculty mentor made to the local offsite.

   0_____|_____100 DK/NA

   Comments:

7. The amount of time your family mentor spent with you during local offsite visits.

   0_____|_____100 DK/NA

   Comments:

Date:_____

Cancer Epidemiology Education in Special Populations Program
Faculty Evaluation of Trainee

Name of Trainee: _____   _____,
                              LAST   FIRST

1. Please rate how well prepared your trainee was to perform the work she or he was assigned.

    0_____|_____100 DK/NA

2. Rate your trainee's self-discipline in relation to his or her work.

    0_____|_____100 DK/NA

3. Rate your trainee's intellectual inquisitiveness as it relates to his or her work.

    0_____|_____100 DK/NA

4. Rate your trainee's:

    a. Personal integrity   0_____|_____100 DK/NA
    b. Laboratory skills   0_____|_____100 DK/NA
    c. Judgment and maturity   0_____|_____100 DK/NA
    d. Poise and tactfulness   0_____|_____100 DK/NA
    e. Ability to work with others   0_____|_____100 DK/NA

5. Rate your trainee on his or her reliability and work habits.

    0_____|_____100 DK/NA

6. Rate your trainee on his or her communication skills.

    0_____|_____100 DK/NA

7. If your trainee were to ask for your recommendation, how strongly would you support him or her for a research position?

    0_____|_____100 DK/NA

8. Rate your trainee's potential as:

    a. A field researcher   0_____|_____100 DK/NA
    b. A cancer researcher   0_____|_____100 DK/NA

9. Rate your trainee's skill as:

    a. A lab or research technician 0_____|_____100 DK/NA
    b. An analyst of data   0_____|_____100 DK/NA
    c. A writer of research reports 0_____|_____100 DK/NA
    d. A writer of articles   0_____|_____100 DK/NA
    e. An oral presenter   0_____|_____100 DK/NA
    f. A literature searcher   0_____|_____100 DK/NA

10. Rate your trainee's overall performance.

    0_____|_____100 DK/NA

Date:_____

Cancer Epidemiology Education in Special Populations Program
Checklist of Skills Learned During Training

SKILL	YES	NO	NOT APPLICABLE	ALREADY KNOWN	EXAMPLES
Study design					
Sampling					
Questionnaire development					
Questionnaire testing					
Data collection					
Data coding					
Data entry					
Handling cultural traditions					
Abstraction of data from records					
Interviewing					
Field supervision					
Work with foreign researchers					
Obtaining biological specimens					
Separate serum from blood					
Isolate DNA					
Laser Capture Microdissection					
Immunohistochemistry					
Sequencing					
Using statistical genetics software					

NON-UNIVERSITY TRAINING PROGRAMS IN CANCER EPIDEMIOLOGY, EMPHASIZING PARTICIPATION FROM LOW- AND MIDDLE-INCOME COUNTRIES

JESSICA M. FAUPEL-BADGER

This chapter includes examples of focused, non-university based programs in cancer epidemiology and prevention that emphasize training individuals from low- and middle-income countries (LMICs) (Table 15.1). Opportunities offered on-site by various agencies at their facilities vary in length from short courses (e.g. one to several weeks) to long-term postdoctoral training. These on-site courses are highlighted in the beginning of the chapter followed by examples of funding mechanisms from the Union for International Cancer Control (UICC) and Fogarty International Center (FIC) designed to support additional training in the fields of cancer epidemiology and prevention for individuals from LMICs. The chapter concludes with a description of a recent program aimed at providing US-trained individuals with the opportunity to conduct research in LMICs and be mentored by a senior scientist in that country. Formal degree-granting programs at US Schools of Public Health and other academic institutions are not included here as these are presented in a prior chapter. This chapter is not meant to be all-inclusive of organizations providing training in cancer epidemiology for individuals from LMICs but rather to highlight a few well-established examples where one can obtain training and may also serve as models for developing new training programs.

Structured, comprehensive, and up to date training in cancer epidemiology and prevention is necessary to develop a workforce capable of addressing the global cancer burden. Cancer is the leading cause of death worldwide, with approximately 12.7 million cases and 7.6 million deaths in 2008[1]. This number is projected to increase to 26 million cases by 2030, with LMICs experiencing the greatest rise in cancer burden.[1] Over 60% of cancer cases will be in LMICs by 2030.[2]

Recognizing the "health tsunami" of not only cancer but other chronic diseases as well, the United Nations General Assembly scheduled a Non-Communicable Disease (NCDs) Summit for September 2011.[3,4] Multiple international health groups advocated for this

TABLE 15.1 Examples of focused training opportunities in cancer epidemiology offered by international funding agencies and institutions

	SOME TRAINING AS INFORMAL PART OF ONGOING STUDY IN REGION	SHORT-TERM (<12 MONTHS) STRUCTURED TRAINING/ FORMAL COURSE	LONG-TERM (≥12 MONTHS) STRUCTURED TRAINING	APPLICANT'S CAREER STAGE
ON-SITE AND/OR STRUCTURED TRAINING FOR INDIVIDUALS FROM LMIC:				
National Cancer Institute (US)	X[a]	X[b]	X[a]	Postdoctoral
International Agency for Research on Cancer	X	X[c]	X	Postdoctoral
Centers for Disease Control and Prevention			X[d]	Postdoctoral
FUNDING FOR TRAINING EXPERIENCES/PROJECTS FROM LMIC APPLICANTS:				
Union for International Cancer Control[e]		X	X	Postdoctoral
Fogarty International Center	X	X	X[f]	Graduate/ Medical Student, Postdoctoral
OPPORTUNITIES FOR US-TRAINED INDIVIDUALS TO CONDUCT RESEARCH IN LMICS:				
Fogarty International Center			X[g]	Graduate/ Medical Student, Postdoctoral

[a] Division of Cancer Epidemiology & Genetics.

[b] Cancer Prevention Fellowship Program—cancer prevention short-course.

[c] Short-courses on cancer epidemiology and cancer registries.

[d] US Centers for Disease Control and Prevention Field Epidemiology Training Program.

[e] Various funding opportunities (both cancer prevention and epidemiology training).

[f] D43 funding mechanisms for non-communicable disease and global infectious disease (can include cancer epidemiology training).

[g] International Clinical Research Scholars & Fellows (includes cancer epidemiology training).

summit and prepared documents to help guide the summit. The NCD Alliance is comprised of the International Diabetes, Federation, International Union against Tuberculosis and Lung Disease, the World Heart Federation, and the Union for International Cancer Control (UICC). All four of these organizations agree prevention must be at the forefront of efforts to address the NCDs with the greatest impact on public health (cancer, cardiovascular disease, chronic respiratory disease, and diabetes). These diseases have shared risk factors—obesity, physical activity, poor diet, and tobacco use—and suggested approaches to curb these risk factors are highlighted in a proposed outcomes document from The NCD Alliance.[5]

Similarly, the UICC released an outcomes document focused exclusively on cancer. This document contains laudable but aggressive goals related to leadership, prevention, and early-detection (http://www.uicc.org/advocacy/cancer-outcomes-statement-un-summit-ncds). The UICC document calls for initiating or strengthening population-based cancer registries in all countries by 2015 and implementing national comprehensive (i.e. prevention to palliative care) cancer control plans by 2018. Other goals include developing population-based screening and early detection programs for cervical and breast cancer, and increasing human papilloma virus (HPV) and hepatitis B virus (HBV) vaccination coverage to 80% of high-risk individuals. There also is a call to "strengthen the evidence base to support innovative strategies for cancer prevention, early detection, and treatment."

Achieving the goals of the documents from the UICC or The NCD Alliance requires a workforce of health care providers, policy makers, and scientists who understand the principles of cancer epidemiology and prevention. Individuals who are already in the workforce must be trained to tackle the growing cancer burden evident now and to make progress towards the goals in the UICC document. Many LMICs do not have sufficient cancer epidemiology expertise and capacity to accomplish the goals in the UICC document. Training in cancer epidemiology is scattered and individuals eager to learn more about this area must seek out the few experts available in-country.

Training the current workforce and building the future one is necessary to have the expertise and capacity to launch national cancer registries. The data from these registries can then be used to develop targeted, measurable goals in cancer control plans and also develop (and test) more sophisticated hypotheses about cancer etiology. Finally, there are prevention messages that can be delivered now and policies that could be developed to decrease exposure to risk factors for cancer. These combined efforts require training individuals in a wide array of health disciplines (epidemiology, clinical, social and behavioral science and laboratory) and also educating those with positions in governments in the principles of cancer epidemiology and prevention.

EXAMPLES OF ON-SITE AND STRUCTURED TRAINING FOR INDIVIDUALS FROM LMIC: NCI SUMMER CURRICULUM IN CANCER PREVENTION

The National Cancer Institute's (NCI) Cancer Prevention Fellowship Program (CPFP) is a postdoctoral training program bringing individuals from a multitude of health-related disciplines together to focus their talents on cancer prevention research with a public health perspective[6,7]. Each year, the CPFP hosts a summer course in cancer prevention research and epidemiology methods designed for incoming fellows as well as both US and international attendees who are beginning careers in this area.

This cancer prevention training is entitled, "NCI Summer Curriculum in Cancer Prevention," and is divided into two courses offered July through mid-August of each year. A four-week course entitled, "The Principles and Practice of Cancer Prevention and Control" (hereafter referred to as "Principles") covers the full spectrum of cancer prevention research (e.g. epidemiology, clinical, social and behavioral research).[8] Within this session, there are a few select talks that also emphasize basic science/laboratory research findings that have advanced cancer prevention research. However, an additional one-week course entitled, "Molecular Prevention," immediately follows the Principles course and focuses solely on the molecular underpinnings of cancer biology and prevention. These two sessions can be taken concurrently or independently.

The central focus of the curriculum is cancer prevention, which sets this particular training apart from other short courses emphasizing cancer epidemiology and/or cancer registry training. The Principles and Molecular Prevention courses are largely taught in a lecture format with three lectures given daily. The lectures are structured to be approximately 60 minutes followed by a 30 minute discussion. Two-thirds of the faculty for the courses is comprised of scientists from the NCI, with the remainder being scientists from US academic and medical research centers.

The Principles course is organized into nine thematic modules and two special presentations (Table 15.2). The first module is designed to provide an introduction to epidemiology methods, including considerations when interpreting results from a given study and the level of evidence needed to make inferences about causation. This module is strategically placed so that all course participants start off with a shared understanding of epidemiology research as most subsequent presentations refer back to the methods and core principles necessary to conduct these studies. Week two focuses on lifestyle factors related to cancer incidence and screening. Week three is a variety of lectures focused on specific primary cancer sites (e.g. breast, lung, colon, and prostate). Topics for this week are cancers that have high incidence and/or high mortality and for which there are known preventive measures. The course finishes with exploring current topics in behavioral and social research, including an emphasis on special populations and health disparities. Final talks address policy implications for cancer prevention research and disseminating information from research studies. Translating information to the community is an area of interest for many course participants and high-priority for NCI leadership.

The special sessions in the course include International Day, held at the end of the first week, and the keynote "Annual Advances in Cancer Prevention" lecture. On International Day, course participants, typically representing 30–35 countries, present an overview of cancer prevention efforts in each of their home countries. Cancer control and prevention activities are as varied as the countries the participants represent. The exchange of information

TABLE 15.2 2011 Principles and practice of cancer prevention and control course modules

MODULE	TITLE
Module 1:	Introduction to the Cancer Problem
International Day:	Cancer Prevention: An International Perspective
Module 2:	Health Disparities and Cancer Prevention in Diverse Populations
Module 3:	Diet, Physical Activity, and Cancer Prevention
Module 4:	Applications of Cancer Prevention
Module 5:	Epidemiology, Prevention, and Control of Site-Specific Tumors
Special Lecture:	Annual Advances in Cancer Prevention
Module 6:	Behavioral Science and Community Interventions
Module 7:	Occupational and Environmental Exposures in Cancer
Module 8:	Cancer Prevention Research: Multiple Perspectives
Module 9:	Disseminating Scientific Knowledge

and design of the day presents an opportunity for course participants to network with each other early in the four-week curriculum. The "Annual Advances in Cancer Prevention" lecture, held in the latter half of the course, is a comprehensive view of cancer prevention by an internationally-recognized scientist in the fields of cancer prevention and control. Topics have included chemoprevention, survivorship, molecular targets, and care of high-risk individuals.

While selected talks in the Principles course do address current advances in laboratory research, an additional one-week course focuses solely on the molecular underpinnings of cancer biology and prevention. This is entitled, "Molecular Prevention," and incorporates the concepts and methods, issues, and applications of molecular biology in cancer prevention efforts and genetics of cancer. Participants gain a broad-based perspective of basic laboratory methodology and theory of how molecular techniques are applied to molecular epidemiology, bionutrition, chemoprevention, biomarkers, and translational research. The overall objective is to provide participants with knowledge that will facilitate critical appraisal of the molecular approaches, methodologies, and theory used in the field of cancer prevention.

Current attendance is approximately 90 individuals for the Principles and 70 for the Molecular Prevention course, with half of the attendees being international participants, mostly from LMICs (Table 15.3). The remaining 50% of the class is divided between US participants (35% of total) and the NCI Cancer Prevention Fellows (15% of total).

TABLE 15.3 Number of participants in NCI Summer Course[a] 1998–2011

YEAR	NCI CPFP FELLOWS	LMIC PARTICIPANTS	OTHERS	TOTAL[b]
1998	7	9	95	111
1999	11	16	92	119
2000	12	9	109	130
2001	14	27	33	74
2002	13	22	43	78
2003	15	23	44	82
2004	19	28	34	81
2005	12	20	47	79
2006	15	36	46	97
2007	7	43	19	69
2008	6	40	28	74
2009	10	40	26	76
2010	11	41	34	86
2011	14	39	37	90
Totals	152	354	650	1156

[a]Summer Course includes the "Principles and Practice of Cancer Prevention and Control" Course (2000–2010), and formerly the Cancer Prevention and Control Academic Course (1998–2000).

[b]Countries represented by 2011 Course Attendees: Albania, Brazil, Canada, Chile, Egypt, Ghana, India, Indonesia, Northern Ireland, Republic of Ireland, Israel, Jordan, Republic of Korea, Malaysia, Mauritania, Mexico, Montenegro, Morocco, Namibia, Nepal, Nigeria, Senegal, Serbia, Singapore, Sri Lanka, United Kingdom, United States, Viet Nam, Zambia, Zimbabwe.

The CPFP, in partnership with the NCI Office of International Affairs (OIA), began accepting applications from international participants in 1998. The NCI OIA has placed an emphasis on recruiting individuals from LMICs to attend the NCI Summer Curriculum in Cancer Prevention due to the dramatically increasing cancer burden in these countries and corresponding shortage of individuals trained in cancer prevention and control. OIA provides financial support to offset living expenses and accommodations for the duration of the training. Many attendees of the summer curriculum are self-nominated and apply directly through the CPFP website[9] for this opportunity. These applications are reviewed both by OIA and CPFP staff for acceptance into the course.

Additional international applications are accepted through the International Atomic Energy Association's (IAEA) Programme of Action for Cancer Therapy (PACT). In 2007, the NCI partnered with the IAEA-PACT to expand cancer treatment and prevention efforts in low and middle income countries. As part of this partnership, the NCI Summer Curriculum in Cancer Prevention was opened to applicants from low and middle-income countries nominated via IAEA-PACT. The IAEA-PACT nomination process begins with the IAEA conferring with either IAEA or World Health Organization (WHO) representatives located in member states to solicit names of potential nominees. IAEA-PACT participants are nominated from across all IAEA member states (151 as of November 2010.[10] The addition of IAEA-PACT nominees increased the international presence in the NCI Summer Curriculum in Cancer Prevention, reflected in Table 15.3, and changed the distribution of participants by geographic region, with increased attendance from individuals from Sub-Sahara Africa and Latin America.

Application materials for both courses include a curriculum vitae and letter of nomination from a supervisor. International applicants must also submit a statement of English proficiency. Each year, there are more applicants than can be accommodated in the course. Acceptance is determined by CPFP leadership and selection is based on who is in the best position to put the course information received into practice. Preference is given to individuals with MD, PhD, and/or MPH level training. The prerequisites of having education or experience in epidemiology, biostatistics, and/or cancer biology also are recommended.

Recently, NCI's OIA conducted follow-up evaluations of participants from LMICs supported by this office to attend the NCI summer curriculum in cancer prevention from 1998–2009 and presented these findings at the 2010 UICC meeting in China.[11] Out of 269 individuals who participated in the training, 123 returned the survey. The geographic representation of the respondents included 27% from Asia, 24% from Sub-Saharan Africa, 20% from North Africa/Middle East, 16% from Europe, and 13% from Latin America/Caribbean, which is similar to the distribution of all LMIC participants from 1998–2009. The majority (59%) of respondents had a medical degree, 18% had a doctoral degree, 10% held both medical and doctoral degrees, and 13% marked "other."

Approximately 43% of the respondents indicated having grant funding currently or in the past, with half of these individuals having funding focused on cancer prevention. After taking the NCI summer curriculum in cancer prevention, 65% indicated they presented or published information on cancer prevention based on the knowledge gained during the NCI training and 97% marked that the course addressed specific needs and helped achieve research goals, prepared them for effective contributions to home country activities, and/or enhanced their cancer prevention knowledge and skills.

Important for all participants of the NCI Summer Curriculum in Cancer Prevention, there is no registration fee, and individuals attending 80% or more of the sessions receive a certificate of completion. In addition to the comprehensive introduction to cancer prevention research, participants have the opportunity to benefit from a number of different networking opportunities. Participants may chose to use the time at NCI to meet with NCI Staff regarding mutual research interests, establishing long-distance collaborations. In a few cases, Principles course participants have returned to the NCI in Visiting Fellow positions to work with research groups on-site. Many Principles course participants also maintain contact with each other and have developed an international network of colleagues interested in cancer prevention.

▩ NCI DIVISION OF CANCER EPIDEMIOLOGY AND GENETICS VISITING FELLOWS AND SCIENTISTS

Long-term training opportunities in cancer epidemiology exist within the NCI Division of Cancer Epidemiology and Genetics (DCEG) intramural research program. Applicants from both the US and abroad can apply to be postdoctoral fellows and train with scientists in DCEG. Each year a few early-career scientists from LMICs are accepted into these positions.

NCI's DCEG also conducts cancer epidemiology research abroad, with recent locales including China, Iran, Costa Rica, and Africa. As part of these studies, DCEG investigators collaborate with local health care workers and scientists and provide training as it relates to the goals of the study. These international studies often result in scientists from abroad travelling to the NCI for additional short-term training or to collaborate on specific, focused projects that are part of the larger study.

▩ IARC SUMMER SCHOOL PROGRAM

The International Agency for Research on Cancer (IARC) in Lyon, France is an autonomous international research and training institution that is part of the World Health Organization (WHO). IARC supports a multidisciplinary research and training portfolio that emphasizes epidemiology, laboratory, and biostatistical methods and furthers the IARC mission, "Cancer Research for Cancer Prevention." Education and training is highlighted as one of five core principles for the IARC mission and have been consistent activities since the agency's beginning in 1966[12]. IARC's education and training program is centered on two key objectives: international collaboration and training. The program is aimed at junior researchers, with special emphasis on those from LMICs, particularly in the areas of cancer epidemiology and cancer registration. A summer school with courses devoted to these two topics has been offered annually in Lyon since 1996.

The current summer school format consists of two modules (Table 15.4). "Cancer Registration: Principles and Methods" is the first module and is one-week in duration, typically offered at the end of June. The second module "Introduction to Cancer Epidemiology" immediately follows and runs over two weeks. The first module covers collection and recording of data for cancer registries using IARC and international standards. The second module emphasizes methods that can be implemented to analyze data from epidemiological studies or cancer registries. The main purpose of these courses is to enhance capacity for developing cancer registries and cancer epidemiology studies in LMICs. Without credible cancer registries to provide information on the scope of the cancer problem, it is difficult to establish meaningful national cancer control plans.

These two modules include homework and small group projects, in addition to lectures. The course attendees are assigned to groups that are balanced across gender and geographic region. Course participants provide a suggestion for the group project based on a real question or problem they would like to address. Each group may select only one project to focus on throughout the course. The group work demonstrates the course participants' ability to

TABLE 15.4 2011 IARC Summer School Program Offered in Lyon, France

MODULE	2011 DATES	TOPICS
Cancer Registration	20–24 June	* Sources of information, case-finding and methods of data abstraction; * Classification of tumors and coding according to ICD and ICD-O; * Quality control, measures of comparability, standard definitions according to IACR * Data analysis and reporting
Introduction to Cancer Epidemiology	27 June–8 July	* Introduction to biostatistics * Measures of occurrence and association * Descriptive epidemiological studies in cancer surveillance and research * Standardization * Cross-sectional, cohort and case-control studies * Bias and confounding * Interaction * Topics in cancer epidemiology * Cancer prevention

work independently and collaboratively, while providing a glimpse into the issues that arise when conducting international projects. IARC summer school attendees often are interested in becoming IARC Fellows and/or initiating collaborations with IARC scientists. In addition to providing a real project for the participants to finish, the group work provides insight into whether the course participants would be capable collaborators with IARC staff in the future.

The summer school program attracts approximately 250 applicants each year, of which approximately 40 are admitted to each module. There is overlap in participants between the two modules as some individuals are admitted for the entire three-week session. The most important selection criteria when reviewing applicants is determining if the individual will be able to put the coursework into practice back in their home country. This includes both reviewing the applicant's qualifications as well as understanding how they will use the knowledge and skills gained during the course after returning home. Many summer school attendees use their knowledge from the IARC courses to train colleagues and students once returning home. This "train-the-trainer" effect extends the reach of the summer school beyond those attending the courses.

■ IARC INTERNATIONAL SHORT COURSES

In addition to the summer school program in Lyon, IARC offers between 5–10 international short courses per year, ranging from one day to several weeks in duration (Table 15.5). These short courses have been offered by IARC since the start of the agency. Each course is reviewed and approved by the IARC Advisory Committee on Education and Training, and the location and topics of the courses depend on science being conducted at IARC and the needs of the research program sponsoring the course. The Section of Cancer Information and the Screening Group within the Section of Early Detection and Prevention predominantly sponsor these courses.

TABLE 15.5 Examples of IARC short courses taught in country in fall 2010/spring 2011

DATES	TITLE	LOCATION	ATTENDANCE
15–17 September 2010	Workshop on Cancer Registration	South Africa	54
12–15 October 2010	CanReg5	Japan	17
6–10 November 2010	Cervical Cancer Prevention	India	200
28 February-4 March 2011	Cancer Registration and Descriptive Epidemiology: Principles and Methods	India	29
10–11 February 2011	Basic Epidemiology Course	Belgium and Luxembourg	26
5–9 March 2011	VIA, colposcopy and treatment of cervical neoplasia	India	30

Both the international short courses and the summer school program in Lyon are evaluated by the participants each year and changes are made based on the feedback. Over time, for example, the courses on cancer registration have shifted to focus not only on developing cancer registries but also on how to conduct research studies with registry data. More recent changes have included incorporating communications into the curriculum (i.e. annual reports, national cancer control plans).

▦ IARC FELLOWSHIPS PROGRAM

There are longer-term postdoctoral training opportunities sponsored by IARC. The IARC Fellowships Program provides postdoctoral training to junior scientists from all over the world who are committed to pursuing a career in cancer research and who have little or no prior postdoctoral experience[12]. The program admits between six and eight new Fellows each year for one year of training, renewable for a second year subject to satisfactory appraisal. The fellowships are tenable in any research Group at the Agency in Lyon, France. It is anticipated that with widened experience gained from working at the Agency, the Fellows will return to their home institute, able to make an increasing contribution to cancer research. In addition to the postdoctoral fellowships, the IARC offers an "Expertise Transfer Fellowship" to enable an established scientist to transfer his knowledge and expertise to a host institute in a low- and medium-income country. This focus on developing countries is a unique feature of the IARC program, facilitating global collaboration and playing a particularly important role in the transfer of knowledge and skills to individuals in countries with limited cancer research and control programs.

Between 1966–2010, 562 scientists were IARC Fellows and approximately 40% were from developing countries (E. Seleiro, personal communication and).[12] Most of the IARC Fellows have focused their research training on molecular aspects of carcinogenesis including: cell biology, genetics, biochemistry, molecular biology, and viral or chemical carcinogenesis. Epidemiology training also is prominent in the IARC Fellowships Program, with approximately 23% (n=127) of the fellowship awardees during this time period focused on epidemiology and biostatistics. Approximately 54% of the fellowships in epidemiology/biostatistics were awarded to individuals from LMICs.

Additional research opportunities at IARC in Lyon include the Senior Visiting Scientist Award program. Senior Visiting Scientists are qualified and experienced senior investigators who bring innovative research to IARC, ideally of benefit to several research Groups, and can be from any country. Senior scientists from LMICs have been invited to conduct research with the IARC Groups through this official program.

Nearly 50 years after its start, the education and training program of IARC remains one of the key elements of its mission. By focusing on the development of local expertise in countries where resources for the control of cancer, and chronic diseases in general, are limited, and by strengthening local research institutions through international collaborations, IARC and its education and training program aims to provide the opportunity to form a new generation of cancer researchers with the motivation and skills to tackle the global cancer burden.

■ FIELD EPIDEMIOLOGY TRAINING PROGRAMS SPONSORED BY NATIONAL AND INTERNATIONAL AGENCIES

Like the NCI and IARC, the US Centers for Disease Control and Prevention (CDC) devotes significant resources to training in areas that support the CDC mission of, "collaborating to create the expertise, information, and tools that people and communities need to protect their health—through health promotion, prevention of disease, injury and disability, and preparedness for new health threats." This mission extends not only to the US but across the world as the CDC seeks to improve global health.

The Epidemic Intelligence Service (EIS) is the flagship training program at the CDC and serves the CDC mission by providing a cadre of individuals with training in epidemiology methods and application. This two-year postdoctoral training program, originated in 1951, combines formal coursework with "on the job" practical experience.[13–15] EIS officers are expected to demonstrate competency in several areas, including experience with field studies, familiarity with public health data and public health surveillance systems, and writing and submitting papers.[15]

Initially developed to tackle infectious diseases and bioterrorism threats, the program expanded to include other topics, such as noncommunicable disease, as the focus of the CDC grew. Current areas of interest for the EIS program include infectious disease, injury prevention, violence, environmental health, occupational safety, maternal and child health, and chronic disease including cancer. Approximately 70–90 individuals are selected to be EIS officers each year and serve at the CDC or in state and local health departments. Many EIS officers continue in public health careers, some in senior and influential posts in the US government.[14]

Given the success of the EIS program in contributing to the public health workforce in the US, the CDC developed the Foreign Epidemiology Training Program (FETP). The CDC works with Ministries of Health and other partner organizations to develop these programs in-country. The long-term goal is for each country to take ownership of the FETP but the CDC provides substantial support to initiate and launch the program, including an in-country resident advisor for the first 4–6 years. There are multiple steps required for the establishment of an FETP sponsored by the CDC and this framework can be found on the website (http://www.cdc.gov/globalhealth/fetp/pdf/FE(L)TP_development_process.pdf). Since 1980, the CDC has helped establish 35 programs that have transitioned to being operated by the respective country, with 15 of these currently supported by CDC resident advisors. An additional 10 programs are in various stages of development (Table 15.6).

The structure of the CDC-FETP closely follows that of the EIS program. The FETP also is a two-year training program combining coursework with field epidemiology experience.

TABLE 15.6   Geographic regions of US CDC-supported FETPs 1980–2009*

OWNERSHIP OF PROGRAM	GEOGRAPHIC REGIONS
US CDC-supported but now self-sustaining	Thailand, Indonesia, Mexico, Taiwan, Saudi Arabia, Philippines, Peru, Australia, Columbia, Italy, Zimbabwe, Spain, Uganda, Germany, Vietnam, Japan, Jordan, Brazil, Indian (Chennai)
Currently US CDC-supported	Central American Regional, China, Central Asian Republic, Kenya Regional, South Africa, Pakistan, India, Ghana, Nigeria, Tanzania, South Caucasus Regional, Ethiopia, Iraq, Rawanda, West Africa
Under development with US CDC	Afghanistan, Angola, Bangladesh, Belize, Central Africa, Morocco, Mozambique, Panama, Paraguay

*Adapted from tables found at http://www.cdc.gov/globalhealth/FETP/pdf/factoid_poster.pdf, Accessed 8/4/2011.

The particular training can be adapted to the priority health needs of a given country. The FETP officer and supervisor, with input from others involved in the program, select a project, define the analyses and plan studies. The projects can vary substantially between programs since each has a different disease emphasis or focus. FETP officers could design a project focused on cancer outcomes, if this fit within the goals of the particular program. It is important to note, however, that projects focused on non-communicable diseases are relatively new within the FETP and it may be challenging to find appropriate subject matter experts who could advise a cancer-related project.

National Field Epidemiology Training Programs or Applied Epidemiology Training Programs similar to those of the CDC-FETP are present in other regions, including in LMICs.[16–18] With an increasing number of these programs being developed, interest has grown in creating a standardized format and developing shared competencies graduates from these programs should achieve.[18,19] In 1997, the Training Programs in Epidemiology and Public Health Interventions Network (TEPHINET) was formed to help achieve cohesiveness across the programs.[20] TEPHINET provides shared resources for best practices and standard curriculum, in addition to other services, to the FETPs.[18] In 2005, the African Field Epidemiology Network (AFENET) formed to support FETPs and applied epidemiology in African countries.[21] In Europe, the European Programme for Intervention Epidemiology Training (EPIET) is an FETP program sponsored by the European Centre for Disease Prevention and Control that involves institutes across many European Union Member States.[22] In addition, EPIET can provide logistical assistance for other national FETPs in Europe.[16]

Almost all of the FETPs outlined here, including those in high-income countries or sponsored by the US CDC, focus on infectious disease and acute health threats.[16–19] Infectious diseases are a top health priority for many countries; however, it is important to pay attention to shifting demographics and trends in disease, including the aging populations and increasing cancer burden in LMICs.[1] Administrators and leaders of FETPs could incorporate cancer-related projects as either a main or secondary focus within the program. A starting point for other programs could be to build on existing expertise in infectious disease training to incorporate projects focused on cancers with known viral (e.g. cervical and liver cancer) or bacterial (e.g. stomach cancer) etiology. Some programs may already be moving in this direction. Publications documenting the incorporation of cancer-related projects into FETPs would help inform others in the community who may have an interest in this area. With the strong central support from ministries of health and defined training structure, FETPs seem uniquely situated to bring additional expertise in cancer prevention and control to LMICs. Further, using existing FETP structure would be an expeditious way to build capacity and bring cancer expertise to the existing public health workforce facing the growing burden of cancer in their countries.

■ UNION FOR INTERNATIONAL CANCER CONTROL FUNDING OPPORTUNITIES FOSTERING TRAINING IN CANCER EPIDEMIOLOGY FOR LMIC APPLICANTS

The Union for International Cancer Control brings together 463 member organizations (governmental and non-governmental) focused on cancer control and ministries of health[23] that together represent 123 countries. The UICC provides members with an opportunity to share resources and to have one voice in the international political arena, such as the recently drafted UICC Cancer Outcomes Statement for the United Nations Summit on Non-Communicable Diseases mentioned in the introduction to this chapter. Among the UICC activities is a fellowships program that includes mechanisms for funding individuals from LMICs who would like to conduct cancer epidemiology and prevention research. These funding opportunities are supported by the UICC membership and applications are reviewed by a scientific panel comprised of representatives from UICC member organizations. Similar to the IARC program, the UICC fellowships provide training to individuals from LMICs who will return to their home countries to transfer the knowledge gained during the fellowship to other members of the local workforce. In fact, return to the home country is a requirement of the UICC funding to individual investigators. Current funding mechanisms supporting cancer epidemiology and prevention studies include beginning investigator, technology transfer, and study grants to individuals and support for training workshops (Table 15.7).

The American Cancer Society international fellowships for beginning investigators (ASCBI) funds scientists early in their independent (i.e. no longer in a mentored/training setting) research careers to conduct research with a mentor at a not-for-profit institution in another country. The investigator must make a commitment to return to his or her home country to contribute to cancer control efforts following the fellowship. The ASCBI are exclusively for individuals from LMICs and epidemiology projects are strongly encouraged. In 2010, ASCBI grants supported four individuals from Nigeria, Malaysia, Slovenia, and China. The individual from Malaysia elected to work with a mentor in the United Kingdom, the other three grantees were at various institutes in the United States.

The Yamagiwa-Yoshida (YY) Memorial international study grants fund three-month training experiences in a country different from the applicant's home country. These grants are designed to promote international collaboration and prevention projects are highly desired. There are no geographic restrictions as to who can apply for the award or where the training must take place. In 2010, there were 10 YY awardees, one of whom was from a LMIC.

The international cancer technology transfer fellowship (ICRETT) mechanism has provided funding to over 2500 recipients from 110 different countries. The primary focus of this mechanism is to provide funding for one month technical training that develops immediate new skills in research technologies and methods. These fellowships support individuals across a multitude of disciplines important to cancer research. There is no geographic requirement for either the applicant or the training site.

TABLE 15.7 UICC fellowships providing training in epidemiology to individuals from low- and middle-income countries[a]

FELLOWSHIP	DURATION OF AWARD[b]	NUMBER OF AWARDS PER YEAR	NUMBER OF AWARDS SINCE INCEPTION	NUMBER OF COUNTRIES REPRESENTED BY AWARDEES	SPECIAL EMPHASIS GEOGRAPHICALLY	SPECIAL EMPHASIS IN DISCIPLINE
American Cancer Society Beginning Investigator (ACSBI)	12 months	6–8	450	63	Low- and middle-income countries	Encourages epidemiology applications
Yamagiwa-Yoshida Memorial International Study Grants (YY)	3 months	14–16	330	40	No	Encourages prevention projects, includes epidemiologists
International Cancer Technology Transfer (ICRETT)	1 month	120–150	2500	110	No	Encourages prevention projects, includes public health professionals

[a]Information compiled from www.uicc.org/fellowships.

[b]For all UICC Fellowships, an additional extension period equal to the length of the duration of the award can be requested, pending funding from other sources and at no cost to UICC.

More details on the individual awards outlined above can be found at the UICC fellowships website and in Table 15.7. All of these mechanisms support epidemiology and prevention-focused projects. In addition, the UICC provides funding for training workshops. The goal of the workshop funding is to bring a small (up to 3 people), knowledgeable faculty to LMICs to provide training on-site for up to 50 individuals engaged in cancer research or care. Topics for these workshops could include cancer epidemiology and prevention. Since 2005, the UICC has funded 55 workshops in LMICs.

■ FOGARTY INTERNATIONAL CENTER FUNDING FOR CANCER EPIDEMIOLOGY TRAINING IN LMICS

The Fogarty International Center (FIC), one of the 27 Institutes and Centers of the National Institutes of Health in the United States, funds research conducted in LMICs. The FIC funding portfolio includes mechanisms (known as "D43" grants) that support training of individuals in LMICs in global infectious disease and in NCDs across the lifespan. These grants are designed to partner US institutions with institutions in LMICs to build the local workforce capacity necessary to sustain research efforts. Research projects are combined with training efforts that can span the spectrum of short courses to long-term degree granting programs or postdoctoral research. The training efforts need not be focused only on doctoral level individuals but rather should educate a varied workforce (e.g. nurses, study managers, etc.) capable of facilitating research. Cancer epidemiology projects could fit within the scope of the NCD training program but would need to focus on cancers with an infectious disease etiology to be appropriate for the global infectious disease training program. FIC also recently launched the Medical Education Partnership Initiative (MEPI) to provide funding to Sub-Saharan African countries to strengthen medical education and increase the health care workforce. The countries eligible for this program also receive support from the President's Emergency Plan for AIDS Relief (PEPFAR); therefore, the currently funded education programs focus predominantly on infectious disease. These curricula could be expanded over time to incorporate NCDs, including cancer prevention and control, where appropriate.

▦ EXAMPLE OF AN OPPORTUNITY FOR US-TRAINED INDIVIDUALS TO CONDUCT RESEARCH ON-SITE WITH SENIOR SCIENTISTS IN LMICS

Fogarty International Clinical Research Scholars and Fellows Program

FIC also supports a unique one-year mentored training program known as the Fogarty International Clinical Research Scholars and Fellows Program. This program focuses on clinical research in LMICs and is designed for US students and postdoctoral fellows engaged in the health sciences. FIC defines "clinical research" broadly to cover research focused on "patient oriented health conducted with human subjects, or research on the causes and consequences of disease in human populations involving material of human origin (such as tissue specimens and cognitive phenomena) for which an investigator or colleague directly interacts with human subjects in an outpatient or inpatient setting to clarify a problem in human physiology, pathophysiology or disease, or epidemiologic or behavioral studies, outcomes research or health services research, or developing new technologies, therapeutic interventions, or clinical trials." The ultimate goal of the Fogarty International Clinical Research Scholars and Fellows programs is to inspire early-career scientists to pursue careers in global health-related research. These programs provide an opportunity for senior scientists in LMICs to directly mentor US students in clinical research in low-resource settings. Mentors also receive funding to support their efforts on these projects.

The FIC Clinical Research Scholars (FICRS) program is for students pursuing a doctoral degree (MD or PhD) in the US. Each Scholar is paired with a mentor in the LMICs. This program began in 2004 and, since that time, approximately 200 US Scholars and an equal number of mentors from LMICs have participated in the program. FIC has designated approved training sites for this opportunity to ensure a strong environment for health-related clinical research. A requirement for each approved site is funding support from both FIC and an NIH clinical research grant, appropriate policies in place for protection of research subjects, adequate infrastructure, and a proven track-record in mentoring students. The National Cancer Institute participates in this FIC initiative and funds scholars who propose cancer-related research.

The FICRS program was expanded to include scientists still in training at the postdoctoral level (MD and PhD). This initiative started in 2008 and is known as the Fellows Program (or ICRF for International Clinical Research Fellows) to distinguish it from the Scholars program for students in graduate or medical school. Applications to the Fellows program must include a research plan and identify the site where the study would be conducted, in addition to demonstrating a record of scholarly achievement and potential. In contrast to the Scholars program with approved sites for study, Fellows may elect to complete their project at an approved site or may identify a site that is not currently approved but meets the requirements of having US Government funding related to the research program, continued research support, and commitment to mentorship activities. Representatives from FIC review these proposals and determine if the research is feasible and of interest to FIC. The overseas sight and mentor are as important as the research proposal. Approximately 45 US Fellows and 43 International Mentors have participated in the program since 2008. The NCI provided support to nine US Fellows, between 2008–2010, who focused on cancer-related projects including early phase clinical trials and epidemiologic studies.

■ SUMMARY

This chapter focused on two broad types of cancer epidemiology training efforts for individuals from LMICs. These include on-site programs ranging from short courses to long-term training and funding mechanisms that support either individuals to obtain additional training or training programs. Some of these examples had cancer as a core focus while others could incorporate cancer epidemiology as a new emphasis within the existing structure. As stated in the beginning of the chapter, this section was not meant to be all-inclusive but to highlight some of the programs available that could also serve as models for other organizations interested in supporting cancer epidemiology training. Indeed, there are organizations besides those mentioned here that have developed cancer epidemiology curricula based on either the IARC cancer registries course or the NCI CPFP Cancer Prevention Summer Curriculum.

Cancer epidemiology training outside of formal degree granting programs can vary dramatically. The US CDC FETP provides field training experience, the IARC summer school focuses on establishing cancer registries, and the NCI CPFP provides training in cancer prevention. Each of these programs fulfills a distinct need within the cancer workforce.

There are gaps in the current cancer epidemiology training programs featured here. Most of the examples in this chapter are aimed at individuals who have achieved a doctoral degree. The cancer epidemiology and prevention workforce requires individuals across the career spectrum, with doctoral-level individuals being only a small percentage of the total number of people working in these fields. New and existing training opportunities should consider content appropriate for the different careers represented in the field. A well-trained study team is as important to the success of the project as the study designer. Some of the courses mentioned here are adapted to be offered abroad to intact work groups. Other methods for reaching a broader audience include developing distance learning curricula to provide access to the course content remotely. While there are advantages to training an intact work unit together on-site, there is still a place for attending international courses offered at research institutions abroad. These courses provide the opportunity to cultivate new relationships and learn about experiences in other countries from fellow course participants.

Another gap among most of the current programs is a lack of outcomes evaluation after the training. Each program has records of who has enrolled in a course or received funding; therefore, the number of people receiving training is known but the number acting on the training and the ways the training is incorporated remain largely unknown. An exception is the UICC, which requires follow-up reports from all individuals who received funding. The NCI OIA recently conducted a follow-up survey of past participants of the Summer Curriculum in Cancer Prevention. The majority of respondents indicated preparing presentations, publications, and grant applications based on material presented in the curriculum. More detailed information on the types of presentations, examples of publications and success of grant applications would provide a greater assessment of the impact of the program. For example, are the presentations following a "train-the-trainer" model where individuals who participated in the training are presenting the information to others or are these presentations to policy makers who can influence how health care funds are spent? For grant applications, what aspect of cancer prevention was the focus of the application and how will the funding be utilized? For programs that have been successful in evaluating outcomes of the participants, these results should be communicated so that others have models to follow to assess the successes and potential gaps in their programs.

Much of the current cancer epidemiology training in LMICs focuses on describing the cancer problem. This is an appropriate place to be for beginning cancer prevention and control programs. As capacity grows in LMICs, there should be a second level of training that builds on this foundation. This next level of training could address designing interventions tailored to the available resources and culture, identifying high-risk or especially vulnerable populations, and contributing to molecular epidemiology and etiology studies.

There is expertise in health care and research in LMICs that could be capitalized on now to help address rising global cancer incidence. For much of this workforce, considering NCDs such as cancer is a new area, however, the existing workforce could apply their experience with the infrastructure and resources for addressing infectious disease issues to new found skills in cancer epidemiology. Short-courses and structured training offered by the organizations highlighted here are providing these skills, especially when many individuals involved in health care do not have the time or means available to pursue formal degrees in cancer epidemiology. In most LMICs, there also would not be the expertise to launch formal degree-granting programs in these areas. Beyond addressing the immediate public health burden of cancer, it is critical that the current workforce be trained in cancer epidemiology and prevention methods to provide mentors for students considering addressing cancer in the future. This will build capacity and sustain research efforts over the long-term as cancer becomes a greater focus of national health and research agendas.

■ REFERENCES

1. Ferlay J, Shin H, Bray F, Forman D, Mathers C, Parkin DM. Estimates of worldwide burden of cancer in 2008: GLOBOCAN 2008. *International Journal of Cancer*. 2010;127(12):2893–2917.

2. Thun MJ, DeLancey JO, Center MM, Jemal A, Ward EM. The global burden of cancer: Priorities for prevention. *Carcinogenesis*. 2010;31(1):100–110.

3. Morris K. UN raises priority of non-communicable diseases. *Lancet*. 2010;375(9729):1859.

4. Beaglehole R, Bonita R, Alleyne G, et al. UN high-level meeting on non-communicable diseases: Addressing four questions. *Lancet*. 2011;378(9789):449–455.

5. NCD Alliance. Proposed outcomes document for the United Nations high-level summit on non-communicable diseases. Accessed at: http://www.ncdalliance.org/node/3317; last accessed 02/03/2013. 2011.

6. Husten CG, Weed DL, Kaluzny AD. Training researchers in cancer prevention and control: A description and evaluation of NCI's cancer prevention fellowship program. *J Cancer Educ*. 1993; 8(4):281–290.

7. Chang S, Hursting SD, Perkins SN, Dores GM, Weed DL. Adapting postdoctoral training to interdisciplinary science in the 21st century: The cancer prevention fellowship program at the national cancer institute. *Acad Med*. 2005;80(3):261–265.

8. Faupel-Badger JM, van Bemmel DM, Wiest JS, Nelson DE. Expanding cancer prevention education to national and international audiences: The national cancer institute's principles and practice of cancer prevention and control annual summer course. *J Cancer Educ*. 2011;26(4):619–625.

9. US National Cancer Institute (NCI). NCI summer curriculum in cancer prevention. Cancer Prevention Fellowship Program (CPFP) Web site. https://cpfp.cancer.gov/summer/summer.php. Updated 2012.

10. International Atomic Energy Agency (IAEA). Member states of the IAEA. http://www.iaea.org/About/Policy/MemberStates/index.html. Updated 2010. Accessed November, 2010.

11. Williams MK, Harford JB, Otero IV, eds. *Evaluation of the NCI summer curriculum in cancer prevention's impact on international participants from low- and middle-income countries.* Shenzhen, China: Union for International Cancer Control 2010 World Cancer Congress; 2010.

12. Montesano R, Akroud EE. International agency for research on cancer fellowships programme-over 30 years of experience. *Carcinogenesis.* 1999;20(11):2041–2044.

13. Buffington J, Lyerla RL, Thacker SB. Nonmedical doctoral-level scientists in the centers for disease control and prevention's epidemic intelligence service, 1964–1997. *Am J Prev Med.* 1999;16(4): 341–346.

14. Koo D, Thacker SB. In snow's footsteps: Commentary on shoe-leather and applied epidemiology. *Am J Epidemiol.* 2010;172(6):737–739.

15. Thacker SB, Dannenberg AL, Hamilton DH. Epidemic intelligence service of the centers for disease control and prevention: 50 years of training and service in applied epidemiology. *Am J Epidemiol.* 2001;154(11):985–992.

16. Krause G, Aavitsland P, Alpers K, et al. Differences and commonalities of national field epidemiology training programmes in Europe. *Euro Surveill.* 2009;14(43):19378.

17. López A, Cáceres VM. Central America field epidemiology training program (CA FETP): A pathway to sustainable public health capacity development. *Human resources for health.* 2008;6(1):27.

18. White ME, McDonnell SM, Werker DH, Cardenas VM, Thacker SB. Partnerships in international applied epidemiology training and service, 1975–2001. *Am J Epidemiol.* 2001;154(11):993–999.

19. Traicoff DA, Walke HT, Jones DS, Gogstad EK, Imtiaz R, White ME. Replicating success: Developing a standard FETP curriculum. *Public Health Rep.* 2008;123 Suppl 1:28–34.

20. Training Programs in Epidemiology and Public Health Interventions Network (TEPHINET). http://www.tephinet.org/. Updated 2012.

21. African Field Epidemiology Network (AFENET). http://www.afenet.net/. Updated 2012.

22. European Centre for Disease Prevention and Control (ECDC). The European programme for intervention epidemiology training (EPIET). http://ecdc.europa.eu/en/epiet/Pages/HomeEpiet.aspx. Updated 2012.

23. Union International Cancer Control. Global cancer control. http://www.uicc.org/. Updated 2012.

Helpful Websites

US National Cancer Institute (NCI) Cancer Prevention Fellowship Program (CPFP) Summer Curriculum in Cancer Prevention—https://cpfp.cancer.gov/summer/summer.php

NCI Office of International Affairs (OIA)—http://oia.cancer.gov/

NCI Division of Cancer Epidemiology and Genetics (Training)—http://dceg.cancer.gov/fellowships

International Agency for Research on Cancer (IARC) Education and Training (Fellowships)—http://www.iarc.fr/en/education-training/index.php

IARC Education and Training (Summer School in Cancer Epidemiology)—http://www.iarc.fr/en/education-training/training-courses.php

US Centers for Disease Control and Prevention (CDC) Field Epidemiology Training Program (FETP)—http://www.cdc.gov/globalhealth/FETP/

Training Programs in Epidemiology and Public Health Interventions Network (TEPHINET)—http://www.tephinet.org/

African Field Epidemiology Network (AFENET)—http://www.afenet.net/english/index.php

European Programme for Intervention Epidemiology Training (EPIET)—http://ecdc.europa.eu/en/epiet/Pages/HomeEpiet.aspx

Union International Cancer Control Fellowships—http://www.uicc.org/fellowships

Fogarty International Center Research Scholars and Fellows (FICRS-F)—http://www.fogartyscholars.org/

Fogarty International Center D43 funding mechanism for Chronic, Non-Communicable Diseases and Disorders Across the Lifespan: Fogarty International Research Training Award (NCD-LIFESPAN)—http://grants.nih.gov/grants/guide/pa-files/PAR-10-257.html

Fogarty International Center D43 funding mechanism for Global Infectious Disease Research Training Program—http://grants.nih.gov/grants/guide/pa-files/PAR-10-260.html

Fogarty International Center Medical Education Partnership Initiative—http://www.fic.nih.gov/programs/pages/medical-education-africa.aspx

NEEDS AND OPPORTUNITIES FOR EPIDEMIOLOGIC TRAINING OF EARLY-CAREER CLINICIANS AND SCIENTISTS SEEKING TO CONDUCT CANCER RESEARCH IN LOW- AND MIDDLE-INCOME COUNTRIES

AMR S. SOLIMAN AND
ROBERT M. CHAMBERLAIN

Recognizing the multidisciplinary nature of cancer prevention research, the National Cancer Institute (NCI) and other cancer-focused agencies have developed extramural award mechanisms for early career cancer researchers.[1] These awards usually provide individual training and research funds to junior faculty who are focusing their careers on cancer research. An example is the K07 mechanism, which specifies certain research topics and relevant disciplines as high priorities for early career development grants.[2] These disciplines include human genetics, genetic predisposition to cancer, detection of precursor lesions, patient-oriented research on cancer prevention, behavioral research and interventions, molecular and genetic cancer epidemiology, biostatistics, survivorship, health policy, and decision analysis. Each of these disciplines and sub-disciplines can be effectively utilized in studies of special populations.

The significance of this type of research is enforced by the availability of the NCI, Department of Defense (DoD), and American Cancer Society (ACS) cancer education and training awards to junior faculty. Most "K" grant award mechanisms focus on career development for new scientists. In contrast, the R25 mechanism of the NCI provides grant awards to academic institutions for the development of cancer curricula and training. In 1992, the DoD inaugurated various programs supporting cancer research education and training with an emphasis on innovative approaches by researchers at the beginning of their careers through mentoring, formal educational plans, and research projects. These educational methods have become a model for developing the careers of junior scientists as independent researchers.

In keeping with the theme of this section of the book, this chapter will focus on methods for providing education and training for early-career scientists in cancer epidemiologic research in LMI countries and special populations in HI countries. In the United States, most of these scientists are located in research-based universities, medical schools, schools of public health, and academic cancer centers. The faculties of these institutions have the expertise to provide high-quality mentoring in a variety of areas, but are frequently lacking in mentoring expertise and/or research collaborations in LMI countries and in special population research. Without this mentoring expertise, early-career scientists will not know about or be able to pursue research experience in LMI countries or special populations in the United States or abroad. One solution might be to bring early-career scientists together for a short period at a major university where there is a critical mass of faculty expertise in LMI country and special population research. Such a training center could be a magnet for junior scientists seeking this experience. Early-career scientists who are already located in such universities would not have a need for such a program, and in fact their university could potentially develop a "magnet training program" for their region. With regard to feasibility, certain points should be considered: (1) minimizing the off-campus time required for participation in a magnet program; (2) maintaining close contact with home-institution mentors of the participants to provide continuity; and (3) scheduling any domestic or foreign field experience to meet the scheduling requirements of the participants at their home institutions. Clearly, a curriculum component would need to be compressed into modules, of no more than a week or two. These modules could be done virtually or at the magnet campus.

▪ ASSESSMENT OF TRAINING NEEDS

To estimate the demand for an early-career training program, the authors of this chapter conducted a national survey in 2010, to explore the interest of junior faculty and senior postdoctoral fellows in acquiring the skills required for cancer prevention research in LMI countries and/or in special populations.[3] The purpose of the survey was to determine, from the perspective of both cancer research trainees and R25T program directors, the level of interest among trainees in careers in cancer research in LMI countries and/or special populations. The electronic surveys were e-mailed to trainees with active career development awards for the period 2005–2010 in the NCI K01, K07, and K08 programs, as well as the DoD Breast and Prostate Control Programs. In addition, PIs of NCI R25 training programs were included, as were key individuals in NCI-designated Comprehensive Cancer Centers, to elicit their perspective on their trainees' career development needs and preferences. The brief five-question survey consisted of four structured questions, with Likert-scale response options ranging from "Strongly Disagree" to "Strongly Agree," and one open-ended question. The survey inquired about career plans, perceived training content needs, and preferred duration of a proposed magnet training program at a major university. The open-ended question elicited reflections on other skills, program features, or barriers the trainees might wish the proposed program to address.[3] Response rates from all but one of the trainee groups exceeded 65%; the K08 trainees had a lower response rate (49%). Table 16.1 shows the results of the survey based on direct report from trainees (i.e., K01, K07, K08 and DoD training participants), followed by the R25 and Comprehensive Cancer Center Principal Investigators' characterization of trainees' needs and interests (Table 16.2).

▪ NEEDS ASSESSMENT SURVEY RESULTS OF TRAINEES

As expected, almost all (94–100%) respondents from each trainee group affirmed their intention of preparing for a career in cancer research. About 70% of respondents from all but the K08 trainee group identified an interest in research in US minority populations. A substantial

TABLE 16.1 Distribution of survey responses from career development award junior faculty aggregated over all (K01, K07, K08, and DoD) NIH-training programs (response options ranged from Strongly Agree "SA" to Strongly Disagree "SD")

QUESTION	SA	A	D	SD
1. I am planning a career that will include:				
Cancer research	177 (85.1%)	24 (11.6%)	0	6 (2.9%)
Cancer research in US minority groups and populations	49 (32.9%)	57 (38.2%)	31 (20.8%)	12 (8.0%)
Cancer research in international populations	37 (26.0%)	50 (35.2%)	35 (24.6%)	21 (14.7%)
2. Please indicate your interest in a brief (1–4-week) extramural focused training program that includes:				
Grant writing and budgeting	73 (35.1%)	101 (45.6%)	24 (11.5%)	10 (4.8%)
Presentation skills in various formats, such as podium presentations and PowerPoint	39 (18.9%)	87 (42.2%)	62 (30.1%)	18 (8.8%)
Manuscript writing	65 (31.4%)	76 (36.7%)	52 (25.1%)	14 (6.8%)
Conducting collaborative research	71 (34.1%)	94 (55.2%)	35 (16.8%)	8 (3.9%)
Modular courses on specific prevention & control topics	46 (22.3%)	104 (50.5%)	48 (23.3%)	11 (5.3%)
Mentoring and being mentored	56 (26.8%)	101 (48.3%)	41 (23.3%)	8 (3.9%)
Career planning	78 (37.3%)	94 (45.0%)	32 (15.3%)	5 (2.4%)
3. Thinking back to the time when you were preparing your career development (e.g. K01, K07, DoD, ACS etc) application, a brief training program like the one we are planning would have complemented and augmented the required career development of your application if it included:				
Structured education and experiential training in US minority group and populations research	41 (23.7%)	57 (32.9%)	58 (33.5%)	17 (9.8%)
Structured education and experiential training in international cancer research	28 (16.0%)	62 (35.4%)	65 (37.1%)	20 (11.4%)
Financial support participants	80 (42.8%)	76 (40.6%)	25 (13.4%)	6 (3.3%)
4. Considering your training plan, it would have been feasible for you to be away from your home institution to participate in our brief proposed program for:				
One week	96 (47.8%)	90 (44.8%)	9 (4.5%)	6 (3.0%)
Two weeks	26 (13.7%)	74 (38.9%)	57 (30.0%)	33 (17.4%)
Three weeks	7 (3.7%)	28 (14.8%)	87 (46.0%)	67 (35.4%)
Four weeks	10 (5.2%)	14 (7.3%)	75 (39.3%)	92 (48.2%)

TABLE 16.2 Distribution of survey responses from directors of cancer training programs aggregated over NIH-R25T (n=24) and NCI-designated Comprehensive Cancer Centers (n=17)

QUESTION	TOTAL	AVERAGE	SA	A	D	SD
1. Please indicate the number of trainees who, in an average year, would be interested in a career that includes:						
Cancer Research	271	7.1				
Cancer research in US minority groups and populations	145	3.6				
Cancer research in international populations	48	1.3				
2. As a program director, you would permit your trainees to participate in a brief extramural training program if it included:						
Financial support for participants			16 (40.0%)	21 (52.5%)	2 (5.0%)	1 (2.5%)
Structured education and experiential training in US minority groups and population cancer research			9 (23.1%)	26 (66.7%)	4 (10.2%)	0
Structured education and experiential training in international cancer research			6 (15.0%)	24 (60.0%)	10 (25.0%)	0
3. Considering your program, it would be feasible for your trainees to be away from your home institution to participate in our brief proposed program for:						
One week			22 (57.9%)	16 (42.1%)	0	0
Two week			12 (30.8%)	22 (56.4%)	5 (12.8%)	0
Three weeks			4 (10.8%)	8 (21.6%)	20 (54.1%)	5 (13.5%)
Four weeks			4 (10.5%)	6 (15.8%)	17 (44.7%)	11 (29.0%)
4. The following topics are being considered in our program planning. Your trainees would be interested in:						
Grant writing and budgeting			17 (42.5%)	16 (40%)	5 (12.5%)	2 (5.0%)
Presentation skills in various formats, such as podium presentations and PowerPoint presentations			11 (27.5%)	20 (50.0%)	6 (15.0%)	3 (7.5%)
Manuscript writing			15 (37.5%)	12 (30.0%)	10 (25.0%)	14 (6.8%)
Conducting collaborative research			71 (34.1%)	94 (55.2%)	10 (25.9%)	3 (7.5%)
Modular courses on specific cancer prevention and control topics			8 (20.0%)	25 (62.5%)	6 (15.0%)	1 (2.5%)
Mentoring and being mentored			10 (25.0%)	21 (52.5%)	7 (17.5%)	2 (5.0%)
Career planning			15 (38.5%)	17 (43.6%)	6 (15.4%)	1 (2.5%)

percent of trainees in all but the K08 group indicated that their plans also include cancer research in international settings. The full distribution of responses from the aggregated set of trainees (i.e., combined across DoD, K01, K07, and K08 programs), across all item response categories, is summarized in Table 16.1. Based on the responses, K08 awardees appear to be an unlikely group for cancer prevention training in international settings.

Table 16.1 also lists the skills trainees identified as important for a brief (one-to-four-week) extramural focused training program. In terms of trainee perceptions of the amount of time available for participating in an extramural training program, the majority reported that a two-week program would represent a feasible time away from their home institution.

The survey's fifth and final question was open-ended, asking respondents to identify other career development skills, program features, and barriers that the trainees wished the program could address. The categories into which all responses could be included were as follow: preferences for additional knowledge and skills training; mentors; preferences for additional program activities; constraints to participation; challenges to program need; and affirmation for the need and features of the proposed extramural program.[3]

■ NEEDS ASSESSMENT SURVEY RESULTS OF R25T PROGRAM DIRECTORS AND DIRECTORS OF PREVENTION AT NCI-DESIGNATED COMPREHENSIVE CANCER CENTERS

The distribution of responses from the aggregated set of directors (i.e., combining the R25 and Comprehensive Cancer Center Directors of Prevention Programs) across all item-response categories is summarized in Table 16.2. Overall, program directors identified more of their trainees as potentially interested in careers in US minority groups and populations than in international populations. They also responded to our questions about the financial and educational aspects of our proposed program and its educational components (Table 16.2).

Most comments from the R25 program directors (40%) affirmed the importance of the proposed program's components, but characterized these as similar to components already featured in their own local programs. Exceptions cited by the program directors were the unique contributions that the proposed program could offer, including the structured education and field experience in international research. Reinforcing trainees' comments, the R25 program directors also identified the need for financial support to trainees, particularly for housing during the one to two weeks of training at the magnet university campus. Program directors also cited the proposed program as a potential source for trainees for special population research. One program director explained "one other thing they've [trainees] asked for … is how to prepare a research portfolio—demonstrating the outcomes of work other than through a CV. Something that helps them establish appropriate lifelong goals in cancer research." Another program director suggested clarifying whether the program would target behavioral or clinical researchers, noting: "I am not sure if the fellows you're targeting are behavioral or clinical researchers. I think all the experiences could have potential benefit, depending on the fellow up."

■ POTENTIAL APPLICANT POOL AND POSSIBLE RECRUITMENT PROCEDURES

Applicants to this kind of program are anticipated to be senior postdoctoral fellows and junior faculty members, with or without career development awards. Recruitment material for websites and brochures are critical. There are likely four general recruitment targets: (1) potential and current awardees of NCI K awards, DoD and ACS career development grants, and directors of NCI R25 T programs; (2) junior faculty members and senior postdoctoral fellows in biomedical sciences in US universities and cancer centers, regardless of whether they currently have external career development funding or not; (3) senior cancer researchers, such as K05 awardees, who are likely to be mentoring potential participants in the program; and (4) a network of referral partners who are senior cancer prevention and control scientists.

Intensive Brief Modular Courses: The Program faculty would be required to create intensive high-level curricula focused on anticipated specific needs of junior faculty participants. In doing so, they could use resources from existing semester-long courses and content from other faculty. Specifically, four areas of course content are believed to be important: field research, data capturing, early detection/down-staging, and career development. Each of these areas would be uniquely focused on research in special populations.

▪ EXAMPLE: AN EDUCATIONAL PLAN AND MODULAR COURSES FOR THE CORE CURRICULUM

The table below illustrates a possible time line of general activities.

EDUCATIONAL PLAN OF A TYPICAL POSTDOCTORAL FELLOW OR JUNIOR FACULTY

Year 1

Application, interview and selection	Conference calls and video conference with mentoring team →	1-Week summer residential education program →	1-Week field site visit either immediately following a residential period or later in Yr 1 →

Year 2

Home Institution Activities: Communication with the magnet campus faculty and home institution faculty and field-site mentors for research, publication, and grant writing on special populations every 3 months →	Video report & presentations to the magnet campus team & participant's home institution faculty →	Final video report presentations to the magnet campus team and participant's home institution key faculty →

▪ THE PROPOSED MODULAR CORE CURRICULUM

During the residential educational summer program, all participants would be at the magnet campus during the same one-to-two-week period. During this time, they would meet with their magnet campus mentoring team and complete new modules specifically designed for the program. These modules should focus on the following 4 areas: (1) field research; (2) data capturing; (3) early detection/down-staging; and (4) career development. More details of a proposed core curriculum are described in Figure 16.1 and Table 16.3.

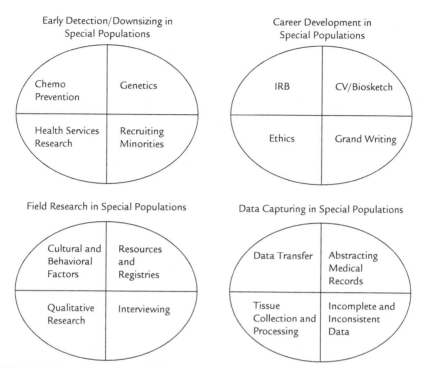

FIGURE 16.1 Examples of possible modular courses for trainees.

▪ ONE-TO-TWO-WEEK FIELD RESEARCH SITE VISIT WITH MAGNET CAMPUS MENTOR (EITHER IMMEDIATELY FOLLOWING BRIEF SUMMER RESIDENTIAL PROGRAM PERIOD OR LATER IN YEAR 1)

Field experiences are based on the magnet campus mentoring team's special population field research. For example, if the mentor is conducting a special population study on cancer in Native Americans, the field experience would include opportunities for applied skills in defining ethnic background, cultural believes and practices of special populations, biological differences between ethnic groups, and management of cancer based on ethnic background and local resources. Another example could be related to cancer survivorship. For example, if the mentor has a study on cancer survivorship of a minority or international population, the participant would learn about setting up the survivorship registries; understanding cultural barriers to follow up; and evaluating clinical outcomes for survivors, secondary cancers, and developmental complications of treatment in these special populations. A third example would be a mentor conducting a study on health services research within a special population, where the participant would learn about lower access and utilization of screening facilities among African Americans at higher risk for prostate and breast cancer incidence and/or mortality.

The overall objective of the program would not be to conduct research, but rather focus on training and early career development. The outcomes of this education could be in several directions: participants would (1) utilize the ongoing projects, research data, and/or specimens from ongoing collaborative studies in special populations in the US or in LMI countries, (2) utilize the field research site to develop new research projects in collaboration

TABLE 16.3 Examples of new educational modular topics and competencies

NEW EDUCATIONAL MODULES	TOPICS AND FOCUS FOR COMPETENCIES
Module 1: Field Research in Special Populations	**Competency to be evaluated**: Recognize and interact with field site collaborations and populations from different cultural backgrounds. Identify & access research data from minority & international settings.
a. Resources and registries	**Focus:** State/SEER registries resources for minorities, Int'l. Registries, migrants & seasonal farm workers, NCI rare cancer consortia, data & specimen repositories in minority & international settings.
b. Interviewing and IRB/ Ethics	**Focus:** Cultural sensitivity factors of interviewing minority and international populations, special Federal-Wide-Assurance requirements in minority and international settings, IRB & vulnerable groups in minority and international settings.
c. Qualitative research	**Focus:** Sampling procedures, self-reporting, social norms, local beliefs and their role in reporting in behavioral and cancer prevention research in minority and international settings.
d. Cultural and behavioral factors	**Focus:** Cancer stigma, barriers to prevention, "hot-cold balance," herbal medicine, traditional healers and fatalism for early detection and behavioral interventions in minority and international settings.
Module 2: Data Capturing in Special Population Research	**Competency to be evaluated**: Being able to abstract, manage, and access data and develop strategies for dealing with incomplete and inconsistent data from minority and international settings
a. Abstracting medical records	**Focus:** Accessing medical records, filing systems, confidentiality of information, multiple records for the same patients, multiple names of patients, and lack of electronic systems in developing countries.
b. Data management	**Focus:** Variability of data abstraction procedures from pathology reports, medical records, tumor registries & population-based registries of minority & international settings.
c. Data transfer	**Focus:** Data quality verification, permits for accessing & transporting data, website entry from remote sites, variability of standard softwares in minority & international settings.
d. Incomplete and Inconsistent data	**Focus:** Model-based data inference, using models for missing-data mechanism, and using likelihood-based inferential techniques.
Module 3: Early Detection/ Down-staging in Special Population Research	**Competency to be evaluated**: To be able to formulate strategies for risk assessment of sub-populations and tailor appropriate cancer prevention and control interventions
a. Genetic susceptibility and tailored prevention	**Focus:** Consanguinity, founder mutations, GWAS, tailored prevention, risk assessment in minority & international settings.
b. Recruiting minorities in clinical and prevention trials	**Focus:** Composition of the target population, recruitment strategies in minority and international settings.

TABLE 16.3 (Continued)

NEW EDUCATIONAL MODULES	TOPICS AND FOCUS FOR COMPETENCIES
c. Health services research	**Focus:** Racial/ethnic factors in health disparities, socioeconomic factors in cancer risk, social barriers in screening/prevention, outcome research in minorities and international settings.
d. Chemoprevention and epigenomic research	**Focus:** Polymorphism and nutrient metabolism, preexisting conditions and utilization of chemoprevention, dietary supplementation, high-risk groups in cancer prevention
Module 4: Career Development in Special Population Research	**Competency to be evaluated**: To be able to formulate short- and long-term career plans. Therefore, each participant will have unique benchmarks to be evaluated.
a. CV/Biosketch development	**Focus:** Cover letter, executive summary, formatting, highlighting and important achievements
b. Publications	**Focus:** Scientific technical writing, writing styles, authorship rules, editorial procedures, and response to reviewers
c. Grant writing	**Focus:** Proposal development, generating preliminary data, locating funding sources, peer-review and resubmission
d. Research careers	**Focus:** Networking, research cultures, interview preparation, switching careers, leadership skills & time management

with the field site mentor, and/or (3) learn from this experience and apply their knowledge to a different special population research site.

▓ PROPOSED CAREER DEVELOPMENT ACTIVITIES AT THE PARTICIPANT'S HOME ACADEMIC INSTITUTION

After the summer modular training and subsequent field training experiences, participants will return to their home academic institutions, but continue to communicate with the magnet campus mentoring team. This can happen through video conference and/or simultaneous document sharing through Adobe Connect or Google or other software. Communicating at least every three months allows participants to continue to receive guidance from the magnet campus mentoring team, as well as the field site researchers. The majority of this communication would relate to drafting manuscripts about the research and new grant application drafts. Plans for these manuscripts and applications would be a part of the educational plan of each participant.

▓ PRELIMINARY VIDEO REPORT PRESENTATIONS TO THE MAGNET CAMPUS MENTORS AND TO THE PARTICIPANT'S HOME INSTITUTION MENTORS AND FIELD SITE MENTORS

Magnet campus mentors would assist and coach the participants in developing their presentations. In the first six months of Year 2, each participant could be scheduled to make at least one presentation via video from their home institutions. The topics of these presentations should be focused on research grant development, manuscripts in progress, and research progress and results for special population research.

▨ FINAL VIDEO CONFERENCE

Two months before the end of Year 2, participants could be scheduled to present their entire progress and future plans to the magnet campus team and home institution mentors. This video conference could include a final presentation of research grant development, finalized and/or submitted manuscripts, and any additional research results for their special population research.

▨ SUMMARY

The chapter helps define LMI country and special population research training as an important focus in cancer prevention and control. The survey results included in this chapter indicate that training programs in cancer epidemiology would be likely to attract early-career researchers from universities and cancer centers in high-income countries and could help them launch their professional careers. The development and implementation of such a program should have widespread applicability to enhance career development of cancer researchers and research in cancer prevention and control.

▨ REFERENCES

1. National Cancer Institute (U.S.). The center for cancer training. National Cancer Institute Web site. www.cancer.gov/CCT. Updated 2012.
2. National Cancer Institute (U.S.), National Institute of Health. Cancer prevention, control, behavioral, and population sciences career development award (K07). . 2011. http://grants.nih.gov/grants/guide/pa-files/PAR-09-078.html.
3. Soliman AS, Mullan PB, O'Brien KS, Thaivalappil S, Chamberlain RM. Career development needs assessment in cancer prevention and control: Focus on research in minority and international settings. J Cancer Educ. 2011;26(3):409–419.

4

Illustrative Examples of Collaborative Field Studies

CHAPTER 17

HEPATITIS B VIRUS, AFLATOXIN, AND PRIMARY LIVER CANCER

W. THOMAS LONDON, TIMOTHY M. BLOCK, KATHERINE A. MCGLYNN

THE DISCOVERY OF HEPATITIS B VIRUS

The method of discovery of the hepatitis B virus (HBV), the search for serum protein polymorphisms by the late Baruch Blumberg, both identified the virus and simultaneously revealed the wide distribution of chronic infection with the virus around the world.[1]

In the late 1950s, while a doctoral student in the laboratory of Professor A.G. Ogston at Oxford University, Blumberg became interested in the role of evolution and natural selection in medical science. A.C. Allison working in the department of biochemistry in Oxford introduced Blumberg to the concept of polymorphism. As defined by E.B. Ford, it was "the occurrence together in the same habitat of two or more inherited discontinuous forms of a species in such proportions, that the rarest of them cannot be maintained merely by recurrent mutation."[2] Polymorphisms of the red blood cell groups were already known, as was the role of sickle cell heterozygosity (Hb^s/Hb^A) in resistance to the most severe form of malaria, Falciparum malaria.[3] That is, sickle cell homozygotes died of severe anemia usually before reproductive life thereby removing two Hb^s genes from the population, but because of the advantage given by malaria resistance, heterozygotes persisted in the population at levels well above that accounted for by recurrent mutation.

Allison and Blumberg then began a collaboration to examine whether serum protein polymorphisms could provide new insights into the biology of human diseases. To further their research, they collected blood samples from several geographically disparate populations and used them to study the distribution of several known polymorphic traits.[4,5] To identify new polymorphisms they used the immunodiffusion in agar gel method introduced by Ouchterlony to react serum samples from multiply transfused patients with "normal" sera from members of different populations. They soon discovered an immunoprecipitin between one such multiply transfused individual and many serum samples from individuals in several geographic locations. The antibody in the transfused patient reacted against inherited antigenic specificities on low density lipoproteins. They called the antigenic determinants the Ag system.[6]

Having been successful in identifying one new polymorphic system, Blumberg, now collaborating with Harvey Alter at the National Institutes of Health (NIH), Bethesda,

MD, used the same methodology to search for additional ones. Within a short time, they observed a precipitin band between a serum from a multiply transfused boy with hemophilia in New York City and a member of the aboriginal population of Australia (Figure 17.1). This was the first demonstration of the Australia antigen (Au). It was quite distinct from the Ag precipitin both antigenically and in staining strongly for protein and only weakly for lipid.[7,8]

They began the investigation of Au by determining its distribution in serum samples from normal and clinical populations. Au was rare in the United States among healthy people, but relatively common in several foreign populations. Particularly striking were prevalences of 20% among a tribe of Cashinahua Indians from Peru, 9% among Ghanaians, 13% among Chinese in Taiwan, 5 to 6% among Filipinos, and 2 to 7% among Pacific Islanders. In persons from whom samples were collected over several years, those who were positive, initially, remained positive; those who were Au negative remained negative. Because both Alter and Blumberg were working at the NIH they tested samples from patients being treated at the NIH Clinical Center. To their surprise, they observed that 11% of children with acute leukemia were positive for Au.[7]

Blumberg hypothesized that Au might be a marker of susceptibility to leukemia. To test this notion, he studied children with Down's syndrome who were known to have an increased risk of leukemia. This study yielded a key observation; about 30% of boys with Down's living in an institution in New Jersey were positive.[9] Working with Sutnick, Gerstley

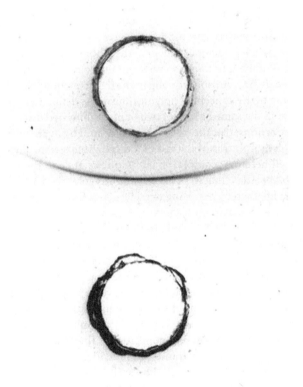

FIGURE 17.1 Double diffusion Ouchterlony experiment showing formation of precipitin line between serum from a leukemia patient and serum from a hemophilia patient. Originally published, 1965.

and London at the Institute for Cancer Research (now the Fox Chase Cancer Center) in Philadelphia, Blumberg did studies comparing boys with Down's syndrome who were Au positive with boys who were Au negative. One of these boys was negative when first tested, but positive on a second test. Studies of this individual showed that he had mildly elevated liver enzymes. A liver biopsy revealed that he had a mild hepatitis. Comparisons of ALT (alanine aminotransferase) levels of Down's syndrome patients with and without Australia antigen showed that ALT was significantly higher among the positive individuals.[9,10]

Subsequent tests of patients with clinical acute hepatitis determined that about 20% were Au positive.[11] When tested over time, such patients were positive only transiently. Electron microscopic studies of isolated Au showed that that the antigen was a particle compatible with a virus.[12] Studies by many investigators then showed that Au was the surface antigen of a virus that caused one form of hepatitis, hepatitis B. Subsequent studies of patients with chronic hepatitis and cirrhosis showed high frequencies of individuals who were positive.[13]

Because HBV was discovered by searching for serum protein polymorphisms in diverse populations, a rough approximation of the global distribution of chronic infection with the virus was available shortly after its identification.

HEPATITIS B VIRUS INFECTION

Chronic hepatitis B is defined as persistence of HBsAg (hepatitis B surface antigen) in serum for at least six months following initial infection.[14,15] In epidemiologic surveys of populations, a single sample testing positive is usually accepted as the presence of a chronic infection, because newly acquired infections would be relatively rare in a population except during an epidemic.

Risk of chronic HBV infection is inversely related to age at infection: approximately 90% of infants infected in the perinatal period and 30% of children infected before 5 years of age become chronically infected, compared with 2%–6% of adults.[16] Among adults, about half of newly acquired infections are symptomatic, whereas infections of infants and children are usually silent (asymptomatic). Although HBV can be transmitted by injection of illicit drugs, by blood transfusion and through sexual contact, in areas of the world where chronic HBV infection is endemic, most infections are acquired perinatally or in early childhood.[15,17] Perinatal transmission is thought to result from exposure of a newborn to the blood of a chronically infected mother during or shortly after birth. In utero transmission has been documented,[18] but accounts for a very small fraction of perinatally acquired infections. The mechanism of horizontal transmission in childhood remains an enigma. Premastication of food, contact with open sores, bites, and contact with contaminated toys or other objects in the environment have been proposed as routes of transmission, but not proven.[19]

Chronic HBV infection usually proceeds through 3 or 4 sequential phases.[15,20] Phase 1 is an immune tolerance period that invariably follows perinatal infection. It may last 15 to 45 years. During this phase, viral replication and viral load are high and hepatitis B e antigen (HBeAg) is detectable in serum.[21] Phase 2, is an immune reactive period in which the immune system attempts to clear the virus infection. During this phase, HBeAg usually becomes undetectable in serum and viral load falls. Often there are repeated bouts of liver inflammation (hepatitis). Fibrosis of the liver and cirrhosis often occur and progress during this time.[22] Chronic HBV infections in adults usually have a brief or undetected tolerant phase and proceed quickly to the immuno-reactivity phase. Phase 3 is a period of low viral replication and, consequently, low viral load. Liver disease becomes inactive. In some individuals there is a fourth phase in which viral reactivation occurs, viral titers rise and liver damage resumes.

In summary, in populations around the world in which HBV infection is endemic, most infections are acquired in infancy or early childhood. When adults in these populations are studied for risks of chronic liver disease and hepatocellular carcinoma (HCC), it can be assumed individuals who are HBsAg positive have been chronically infected for the number of years they have lived, minus 0 to 5 years. At least half of these adults will be in the immuno-reactive phase of their disease and at risk of developing the deadly consequences of chronic HBV, cirrhosis, and HCC.

Global Distribution of HBV Infection

Chronic HBV infection rates around the world vary widely (Figure 17.2). The highest rates (≥8% of the population chronically infected) are found in eastern Asia and sub-Saharan Africa. Medium rate countries, with infection rates between 2% and 7%, are found in northern Africa, western and southern Asia, and eastern Europe. The lowest rates in the world (< 2% of the population chronically infected) are found in North America, western Europe, southern South America and Australia. Within each area, however, HBV rates tend to vary by race and ethnicity. For example, in the United States, HBV infection rates are notably higher among Asians/Pacific Islanders[23] and Native Americans[24] than they are among black and white persons.[25]

▪ HEPATOCELLULAR CARCINOMA

Hepatocellular carcinoma (HCC) is the most common histology of primary liver cancer in almost all countries, thus liver cancer rates are a close approximation of HCC rates around the world. An exception is northeast Thailand, where intrahepatic cholangiocarcinoma, a

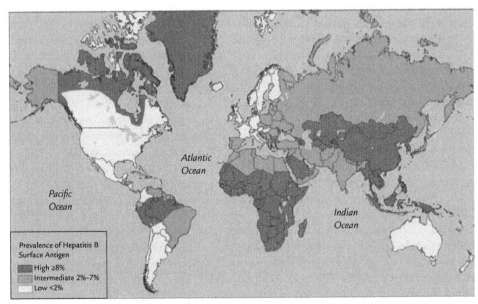

FIGURE 17.2 Global prevalence of chronic infection with hepatitis B virus, 2006. Centers for Disease Control and Prevention: http://wwwnc.cdc.gov/travel/yellowbook/2010/chapter-5/hepatitis-c.aspx.

cancer arising in the cells lining the intrahepatic bile duct, is the dominant histologic type of primary liver cancer.[26]

Global Incidence of HCC

Globally, there is a notable concurrence between HBV chronic infection rates and liver cancer incidence rates. Overall, liver cancer incidence rates are two and a half times higher in the less developed regions of the world (13.1/100,000) than in the developed regions (5.2/100,000).[27] The highest liver cancer incidence rates in the world occur in eastern Asia and sub-Saharan Africa (Figure 17.3).[27] Collectively, these areas account for approximately 85% of all liver cancers. Mongolia has the highest reported incidence in the world, by far, with an age-standardized rate of 94 per 100,000 persons. Other high-rate Asian countries, all with rates between 20 and 35/100,000 are Taiwan, Laos, Viet Nam, China, and South Korea. Mongolia's very high incidence rate is likely due to high rates of mono- and co-infections with HBV, HCV and hepatitis D virus (75% of persons infected with HBV are also infected with HDV).[28,29] In addition, it has been suggested that alcohol consumption is more widespread in Mongolia than in other Asian countries.[30] In contrast, the dominant HCC risk factor in other high rate Asian countries, with the exception of Japan, is HBV infection alone.

The African country with the highest reported incidence is The Gambia, with a rate of 36/100,000. Other high-rate African countries, with incidence rates between 15 and 20/100,000 are the Democratic Republic of Congo, Ghana, Guinea-Bissau, Senegal, Liberia, and Sierra Leone. Although the incidence in African countries appears to be somewhat lower than the incidence in Asian countries, the data from Africa may be less reliable

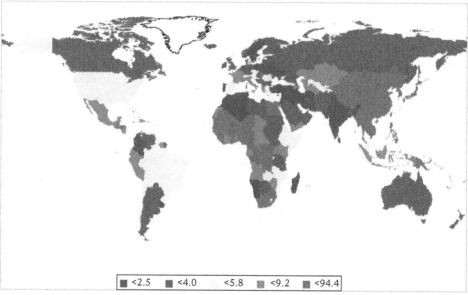

| ▩ <2.5 | ▩ <4.0 | <5.8 | ▩ <9.2 | ▩ <94.4 |

FIGURE 17.3 Global estimated age-standarized incidence rate of liver cancer per 100,000. Ferlay J, Shin HR, Bray F, Forman D, Mathers C and Parkin DM.GLOBOCAN 2008 v1.2, Cancer Incidence and Mortality Worldwide: IARC CancerBase No. 10 [Internet]. Lyon, France: International Agency for Research on Cancer; 2010. Available from: http://globocan.iarc.fr, accessed on 15/10/2011.

than the data from other areas, as in Africa there are few long-term cancer registries. The incidence in The Gambia, where a long-term HBV project has been underway for many years, may be more representative of the actual incidence in other sub-Saharan African countries.[31] The dominant risk factor for HCC in sub-Saharan Africa is HBV infection. In contrast, in northern African countries such as Egypt, HCV is the dominant risk factor.[32]

In contrast to Asia and Africa, countries in northern Europe and North America tend to be low-rate areas. For example, age-standardized incidence rates in the Nordic countries are between 1.5 and 3.1/100,000, while rates in Canada and the United States range from 3.3 to 4.5/100,000. Intermediate rate HCC areas, where the incidence rates are typically between 5 and 10/100,000, include central Europe (e.g., Italy, France, Switzerland, Greece) and Central America (Nicaragua, Mexico, El Salvador, Costa Rica).

Regardless of the magnitude of the incidence, in most areas, rates among males are two to three-fold higher than rates among females (Figure 17.4). The discrepancy, however, is not more pronounced in high-rate HCC areas. Overall, the largest male:female ratios occur in western (3.4) and southern Europe (3.1). In contrast, the lowest male:female ratios in the world occur in Central (1:0) and South America (1.4). In fact, in a number of Central and South American countries, incidence rates are slightly higher among females. For example, the male:female ratio is 0.8 in Bolivia, Ecuador, and Peru and between 0.7 and 0.9 in El Salvador and Nicaragua. The reasons that males have higher rates of liver cancer than females in most populations are not well understood, but may be explained, in part, by the sex-specific prevalence of risk factors. Males are more likely to be chronically infected with HBV and HCV, consume alcohol, smoke cigarettes, and have increased iron stores. Males have also been reported to have higher levels of serum aflatoxin B_1 (AFB_1) markers than do females.[33] There is also some evidence that androgen metabolism in males may be related to increased risk.[34–36]

In addition to variability by gender, HCC incidence rates in most areas also vary by race/ethnicity. In the United States, HCC incidence is highest among Asians/Pacific Islanders (11.7/100,000) and lowest among white persons (3.9/100,000).[37] Intermediate to these rates are those of Hispanics (8.0/100,000), black persons (7.0/100,000) and American Indians/Alaska Natives (6.6/100,000). Just as divergent as the rates among various ethnic groups residing in one area are the rates among members of a single ethnic group living in various locations. For example, incidence rates among Chinese populations are notably lower in the United States than they are in either China or in Singapore. As with gender differences, race/ethnic differences in risk are likely to be related, at least in part, to the prevalence of major risk factors in each group.

Liver cancer incidence rates increase with age in all populations, with the highest age-specific rates occurring among persons aged 75 years and older. The age-specific curves look slightly different in various areas of the world, but in no area do the rates decline among older persons (Figure 17.5a–b). In a low-rate area, such as northern Europe, rates are generally very low prior to age 40 years, then rise linearly with age throughout adulthood. In high rate areas of eastern Asia, rates become elevated in childhood, then continue to rise with age. In the extremely high rate country of Mongolia, rates increase dramatically until age 70 years, and then appear to stabilize. In contrast, in the high rate area of sub-Saharan Africa, rates increase until age 55 years, plateau until age 70, then rise again. The reasons for the slightly different patterns in Africa and Asia are not certain, but may be related to overall life-expectancy, competing causes of mortality, difference in mean ages at HBV infection, and/or differences in HBV viral replication patterns in the two areas. In regard to life expectancy, sub-Saharan Africa has the lowest life expectancy of any region in the world, with more than 20 countries having a life expectancy of less than 50 years.[38]

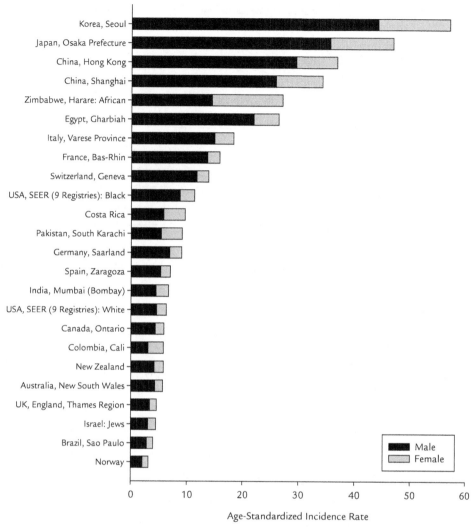

FIGURE 17.4 Age-adjusted incidence rates per 100,000 of liver cancer by gender, 1998–2002. *Cancer Incidence in 5 Continents*, Vol IX. Age adjusted to world standard.

Trends in Liver Cancer Incidence

During the interval between 1983–1987 and 1998–2002, liver cancer incidence increased in many areas of the world. Increases were seen in northern Europe, North and South America, Oceania, and in most countries of southern Europe, India and Israel (Figure 17.6).[39] In Spain and in most far east Asian countries, however, incidence rates declined. Although the reasons for the increase in incidence in most areas are not entirely clear, factors such as HCV infection, increasing rates of obesity and diabetes and improved survival from cirrhosis are likely to be related. The reasons for the declining rates in some far east Asian countries are likely to be several. In Japan, the cohort of individuals infected with HCV in the 1930s and 1940s is growing ever smaller and thus the rate of HCV-related HCC is declining.[40] The declining HCC rates in China and Singapore, areas where HBV

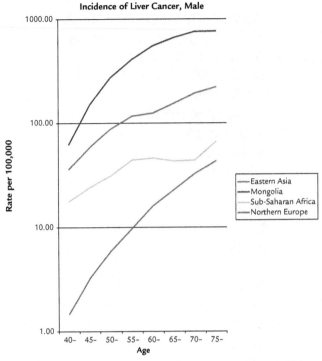

FIGURE 17.5A Age-specific incidence rates of liver cancer per 100,000 among males by region. *Cancer Incidence in 5 Continents,* Vol IX. Age adjusted to world standard.

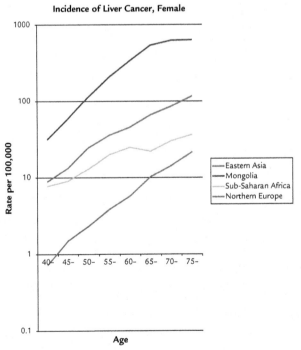

FIGURE 17.5B Age-specific incidence rates of liver cancer per 100,000 among females by region. *Cancer Incidence in 5 Continents,* Vol 9. Age adjusted to world standard.

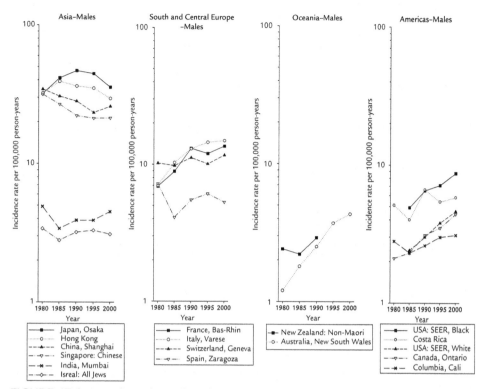

FIGURE 17.6 Age-adjusted trends in liver cancer incidence among men by region, 1978–1982 to 1998–2002. *Cancer Incidence in 5 Continents,* Vol 9. Age adjusted to world standard.

is the major risk factor, are more likely due to the elimination of other HCC co-factors. Although HBV vaccination began in these areas in the mid-1980s, the vaccine was initially only given to newborns. Thus, the vaccinated population is still too young to have a large influence on current HCC incidence rates.

Prognosis of HCC

The prognosis of liver cancer, even in developed countries, is poor. In the United States, one-year survival is less than 50%, and five-year survival only 18%.[37,41] Survival is even less favorable in developing countries. As a result, mortality rates in all locations are roughly equivalent to incidence rates.

Relationship between HBV and HCC

The first large prospective study of risk of HCC among persons chronically infected with HBV was reported in 1981. Beasley and colleagues followed a cohort of 22,707 adult male government workers in Taiwan. After 75,000 person years (py) of follow-up, there were 57 deaths from HCC or cirrhosis among 3454 HBV carriers compared with 3 deaths from HCC or cirrhosis among 19,253 noncarriers. The initial relative risk (RR) in this study was 223.[42] With longer follow-up, the RR for HCC among chronic HBV carriers decreased to 98.[43]

Although many prospective studies of persons with chronic HBV infection have been performed over the 30 years since Beasley's study, very few population-based, as opposed to clinic-based or hospital-based cohort studies, have been done in low- and middle-income countries. Two such studies were initiated in the early 1990s; one study by London and colleagues in Haimen City, Jiangsu Province, China[44] and one by Chen and colleagues in Taiwan.[45] In addition, there is a cohort of 2 million women in Taiwan enrolled at the time they were screened for HBV infection during pregnancy and followed for more than 11 years.[46] These three studies differ in design, advantages and limitations, but taken together they demonstrate the remarkable magnitude of risks of death, HCC and chronic liver disease imparted by chronic HBV infection.

In Haimen City, China, the cohort was assembled between February 1992 and December 1993. Study teams traveled to 1008 villages in each of the 35 townships of Haimen City to enroll 90,836 subjects between the ages of 25 and 64 years. At entry, each subject completed a brief questionnaire and donated a sample of blood. Questionnaire data collected included residence, date of birth, occupation, tobacco use, alcohol consumption, tea consumption, past pesticide exposure, drinking water source, staple food by decade from 1960s to 1990s (corn, rice, wheat), history of acute hepatitis, history of jaundice, history of cirrhosis, and family history of HCC. The male cohort included 58,545 men, 15.0% of whom were HBV carriers. The female cohort included 25,340 women, 10.7% of whom were HBV carriers.

After 8 years, 434,718 person-years of follow-up were accumulated, and 1092 deaths from HCC had occurred. The overwhelming risk factor for HCC mortality was chronic HBV infection; for men the relative risk (RR) of HCC was 18.8, and for women the relative risk was 33.5. Other risk factors that were significant but at much lower levels (RR between 1.5 and 2.5) were: family history of HCC, history of acute hepatitis, and occupation (peasant). Alcohol consumption, which was high among men and relatively uncommon among women, was not associated with risk of HCC. The risk of cigarette smoking varied by gender. Smoking was almost universal among men and was not associated with HCC risk. In contrast, smoking was less common and less frequent among women and was associated with risk (RR = 4.2 for more than 10 cigarettes smoked per day).[47]

In the REVEAL study, a community-based study conducted in Taiwan, C.J. Chen and colleagues enrolled a cohort of 23,820 men and women, age 30 to 65 years, from 7 townships in 1991–1992.[48] HBsAg positivity among men ranged from 26.7% at 30–34 years of age to 13.4% at 60–65 years. The prevalence of HBsAg positivity in women was 16.1% at 30–34 years and 12.1% at 60–65 years. There were 1814 deaths during 12.5 years (282,323.7 person-years of follow-up). Persons positive for HBsAg at study entry had significantly ($P < .01$) higher adjusted hazard ratios (HR) for all causes of mortality (1.7), liver cancer mortality (22.4), and chronic liver disease and cirrhosis mortality (5.4).[49]

In the nationwide study of women in Taiwan ascertained during pregnancy, 313,749 (15%) of the 2,087,994 women tested, were HBsAg(+).[46] The mean age at enrollment was 26.5 years, but ranged from less than 20 years to more than 36 years. After 11.4 years of follow-up, 14,524 of the women had died. The all cause mortality rate for the population was 60.9 per 10^5 person years, 58.9 for the HBsAg negative women and 72.0 for the HBsAg positive women yielding a HR of 1.24 for HBsAg positives vs. negatives. There were 356 deaths from liver cancer (not necessarily all HCC, cholangiocarcinomas and other liver tumors could have been included). Ninety-eight liver cancer deaths occurred among the HBsAg(–) women and 258 among the HBsAg(+) women yielding a HR of 15.5 for HBsAg(+) vs. HBsAg(–). Three hundred eighty-four women died from non-cancer liver diseases. The HR of liver disease death among HBsAg(+) women vs HBsAg(–) women was 3.1. The investigators also observed elevated HRs for extrahepatic bile duct and gall bladder cancers (HR = 2.0) and non-Hodgkin lymphoma (HR = 2.4).

Overall, this study demonstrates a remarkable increased risk of death among this cohort of young women from chronic HBV infection. HCC is less common among women than men and liver cancer incidence is usually low before the age of 40 years, peaking in the 5th or 6th decade. The likelihood is that with further years of follow-up the risks of HCC and chronic liver disease among HBV infected women will only increase unless ameliorated by anti-viral therapy.

The next topic addressed by the Haimen City and the REVEAL study was the identification of factors that increase or decrease the risk of HCC and death among persons chronically infected with HBV. In both the Haimen and Taiwan communities, viral load, the concentration of HBV DNA in serum, was assessed in conjunction with other risk variables. In Haimen, HBV viral load was assayed by real-time polymerase chain reaction (PCR) in stored samples from cohort entry (1992–1993) among 2763 HBsAg positive adults. Major end points were death from HCC or chronic liver disease (CLD). There were 447 deaths. Viral load was divided into three categories: undetectable (<1.6 10^3 copies/mL); low titer (<10^5 copies/mL); and high titer (10^5 copies/mL). There was a significant increase in HCC mortality across viral load categories ($p_{trend} < 0.001$). Compared to the HBV undetectable category, the RR for HCC mortality in the low viral load group was 1.7 and 11.2 in the high viral load group. For CLD mortality, the RRs were 1.5 and 15.2 respectively ($p_{trend} < 0.001$). The RR associated with high viral load did not change with increased follow-up time.[45]

In the REVEAL study after 11 years of follow-up of 3563 HBsAg(+) persons at study entry, the incidence of HCC increased with serum HBV DNA level (assayed by real-time PCR) in a dose-response relationship ranging from 108 per 10^5 person-years for an HBV DNA level of less than 300 copies/mL to 1152 per 10^5 person-years for an HBV DNA level of ≥10^6 copies/ml (RR about 10). After adjustment for sex, age, cigarette smoking, alcohol consumption, HBeAg serostatus, serum alanine aminotransferase level, and liver cirrhosis at study entry, the biological gradient of HCC by serum HBV DNA levels remained significant (P < .001). The incidence of cirrhosis increased in a similar manner with respect to HBV DNA level. Hazard ratios (HR) went from 1.0 for the referent category of HBV DNA undetectable to 9.8 for HBV DNA levels of ≥ 10^6 copies/ml.[48]

The REVEAL study also assessed the risk of HCC by HBV genotype. Genotype C had a modestly greater RR of 1.7 compared with genotype B. In contrast, the pre-core mutant (G1896A) compared with wild-type was associated with a lower HR of HCC (0.34). The double mutant of the basal core promoter (A1762T/G1764A) compared with wild-type had a slightly elevated HR of HCC (1.73).

Taken together these studies indicate that viral load, measured as concentration of HBV DNA in serum or plasma, is the major risk factor for HCC among persons infected with HBV.

■ AFLATOXIN

Aflatoxins are mycotoxins produced by the fungi *Aspergillis flavus* and *Aspergillis parasiticus*. While the fungi can grow on a wide variety of agricultural products both preharvest and postharvest, *A. flavus*, has a particular affinity for peanuts, maize, cottonseed and groundnuts, while *A. parasiticus* rarely contaminates maize.[50] Although most human exposure to aflatoxins is via food consumption, occupational exposure via airborne dust also occurs.[51,52] The aflatoxins were first identified in the United Kingdom in 1960 when an epizootic of mycotoxicosis killed 100,000 turkey poults.[53,54] The ensuing investigation found that the turkeys' feed had been contaminated by four toxic metabolites of *A. flavus*, which were designated as aflatoxin B_1, aflatoxin B_2, aflatoxin G_1, and aflatoxin G_2, depending on whether they fluoresced blue or green under ultraviolet light. Subsequent research determined that aflatoxin B_1 (AFB_1) was both the most abundant and most potent of the four naturally occurring aflatoxins.[55] Aflatoxins M_1 and M_2 are metabolites of aflatoxin B_1 and B2, and can contaminate the milk of animals ingesting aflatoxin-contaminated feed.

Aflatoxin-exposure has been demonstrated to cause liver tumors in a wide variety of animal species including rainbow trout,[56] rats,[57] mice,[58] ducks,[59] fish,[60] marmosets,[61] tree shrews,[62] and monkeys.[63] Based on the accumulated animal data, in 1987, the International Agency for Research on Cancer (IARC) determined there was sufficient evidence to classify aflatoxins as carcinogenic.[55]

While the animal data on the carcinogenicity of the aflatoxins became convincing by the mid-1980s, the human evidence lagged behind. Early epidemiologic studies were hampered by the lack of biomarkers to determine aflatoxin exposure, the paucity of long-term, high-quality cancer registries in high-rate HCC areas, and the failure of studies to account for major risk factors such as HBV infection. Many epidemiologic studies conducted in the 1970s and 1980s were either ecologic studies or cross-sectional studies that correlated the incidence of HCC in a location with the amount of AFB_1 found in foodstuffs. Studies reporting a positive correlation were conducted in a number of high-rate HCC areas in sub-Saharan Africa and Asia.[64–76] In contrast to the positive studies, several ecologic studies found little association between AFB_1 levels in sample foods and HCC rates.[74,75,77]

Even the positive ecologic studies however, could only correlate AFB_1 and HCC in a population, not in a person. Attempts to circumvent this problem by studying the relationship at the individual level led to the conduct of several dietary case-control studies.[78–80] These studies reported inconsistent findings, which is not unexpected in that they relied on self-reported intake of foods likely to be contaminated with aflatoxins. As there is seasonal variability in aflatoxin contamination, great variability in contamination across a single food product and imprecision in the recall of dietary intake, the dietary studies could only estimate, very roughly, whether the individual had been exposed.

The development of aflatoxin biomarkers for human specimens, beginning in the 1980s, was critical to gaining a better understanding of the AFB_1-HCC relationship. Biomarker development was made possible by the appreciation that AFB_1's hepatocarcinogenic effect is mediated not by AFB_1 itself, but by its metabolites. AFB_1 is metabolized primarily in the liver by p450 enzymes (CYP3A4, 3A5, 3A7, 1A2) to create AFB_1-8, 9-*exo*-epoxide and AFB_1 8,9-*endo*-epoxide.[81,82] AFB_1 8,9-*exo*-epoxide binds to DNA to form the 8,9-dihydro-8-(N7-guanyl)-9-hydroxy AFB_1 adduct that is used as major urinary biomarker.[81] Detoxification of both epoxides is accomplished via glutathione S-transferase conjugation[83] or via hydrolysis to AFB_1 8,9-dihydrodiol. The glutathione-conjugate epoxide can be metabolized to aflatoxin-mercapturic acid, which is used as another urinary biomarker. A third urinary biomarker, aflatoxin M_1, is an oxidative metabolite of AFB_1. The urinary biomarkers reflect AFB_1 exposure over the past several days while a serum biomarker, aflatoxin-albumin adducts, reflects exposure over the past several weeks. In addition, a specific mutation in the *TP53* tumor suppressor gene, a G to T transversion in the third nucleotide of codon 249,[84] has been used as an AFB_1 biomarker. The association of the codon 249 mutation with AFB_1 exposure was first reported in 1991 by studies conducted in Qidong, China[85] and in South Africa.[86] Fifty percent of the HCCs from Qidong, and 40% of the HCCs from South Africa carried the codon 249 mutation. Subsequent research reported high rates of the mutation in tumors from AFB_1 endemic areas,[87,88] and low rates among tumors from non-AFB_1 endemic areas.[89–91] The codon 249 mutation has also been detected in serum of persons with HCC, making it useful as a serum biomarker in epidemiologic studies.[92,93]

Identification of AFB_1 biomarkers permitted the conduct of more rigorous epidemiologic studies. Several early case-control studies which incorporated biomarkers found conflicting results, however. While Olubuyide et al found a signification association between AFB_1 and HCC in Nigeria,[94] neither Srivatanakul et al. in Thailand[77] nor Mandishona et al in South Africa[95] detected associations. Some of the inconsistency may have been due to the relatively small size of the studies, the unrepresentativeness of the control groups and/or to the determination of AFB_1 levels among persons who already had liver cancer. Case-control studies also had the disadvantage that they were studying a cancer that had been initiated many years in the past, so the relevance of a biomarker determined at the present time was questionable.

Many of the limitations of ecologic, cross-sectional or case-control studies were overcome by the use of prospective study designs which examined AFB_1 biomarkers among persons prior to the development of cancer. In a seminal cohort study conducted in Shanghai, China, the investigators demonstrated that men positive for any biomarker of aflatoxin exposure were at significantly greater risk of developing HCC (RR = 5.0) than were men negative for any AFB_1 biomarker.[95–97] Furthermore, the study found that men positive for both AFB_1 and HBsAg had a synergistically higher risk of HCC (RR = 59.0) than men negative for both exposures. Though the synergism had been suggested by earlier studies,[71,98] the Shanghai cohort study was the first to demonstrate the magnitude of the dual effect. A subsequent report from a cohort in Taiwan, confirmed the findings of the Shanghai study.[99] In the Taiwan cohort, the relative risk associated with AFB_1 was 3.8, while the relative risk associated with AFB_1 and HBsAg together was 112, confirming that AFB_1 and HBV infection together conferred a much higher risk of HCC than did either exposure alone. Whether AFB_1 also amplifies the risk associated with HCV infection is not as clear, although there is some evidence that synergism does exist.[100–102] A combined effect of AFB_1 and HCV on HCC risk, however, is less important from a public health perspective, as AFB_1 and HCV co-occur much less frequently than do AFB_1 and HBV.

Although the *Aspergilli* fungi are fairly ubiquitous, AFB_1 exposure is most common in warm, humid environments. A 2006 report estimated that more than 55 billion people in the world, primarily in Africa and Asia, were chronically exposed to AFB_1.[103] The number of cases of HCC that might be prevented if AFB_1 exposure were reduced or eliminated has been estimated by several groups,[104,105] and most recently by Liu and Wu.[106] The authors estimated that of the 550,000 to 600,000 incident cases of HCC that arise each year, anywhere from 4.6% to 28.2% could be attributable to AFB_1. Thus, if the upper estimate of attributable risk is accurate, eradication of AFB_1 could have a major effect on reducing the incidence of HCC.

Intervention strategies to control AFB_1 include both primary and secondary approaches. Primary intervention methods include preventing mold growth, preharvest and postharvest, or adding trapping agents, such as sodium calcium aluminosilicate, to the diet to prevent uptake of aflatoxin.[107] Secondary prevention strategies, aimed at enhancing the internal elimination of the toxic metabolites of AFB_1, have focused on agents such as chlorophyllin, Oltipraz, sulforaphane, and green tea polyphenols.[108] While all of these approaches show promise, the synergistic effect of AFB_1 and HBV on HCC risk in many high-rate areas indicates that universal HBV vaccination might go a long way to ameliorating aflatoxin's effect on HCC risk.

▪ PREVENTION OF HCC

Primary Prevention via Vaccination

Chronic HBV infection is 90% preventable with proper use of the hepatitis B vaccine.[109] The vaccine, originally derived from hepatitis B surface antigen particles in plasma and approved in the United States in 1982, has remarkably few adverse effects. In 1986, a recombinant vaccine was introduced and has largely replaced the plasma derived vaccine.

Studies from Taiwan, where universal immunization of newborns was introduced in 1984, showed a significant reduction in the incidence of HCC among 6- to 14-year-old children 15 years after vaccination was introduced.[110,111] More recently, the investigators provided a 20 year follow-up of this population. Comparing HCC rates in vaccinated children aged 6–19 years with HCC rates among children of earlier birth cohorts, the authors found that HCC risk was remarkably reduced: 64 HCCs occurred among vaccinees during 37,709,304 person-years (py) of follow-up vs. 444 HCCs among unvaccinated children during 78,496,406 py. The age- and sex-adjusted relative risk of HCC was 0.31 for persons vaccinated at birth.[112] As the vaccinated population moves into their early 20s, it will be important to see whether this magnitude of protection is maintained or possibly increased.

The investigators also ascertained whether children who were diagnosed with HCC after the initiation of the vaccine program had HBsAg-positive and HBeAg-positive mothers. Among children whose mothers were HBsAg positive, 44 of 729,420 children in the vaccinated population developed HCC compared with 8 of 3,656,182 vaccinated children of HBsAg(−) mothers (OR = 29.50). Among 35 children with HCC whose mothers were HBsAg(+), 27 had HBeAg(+) mothers and should have received HBIG (hepatitis immune globulin) at birth, in addition to 3 or more doses of HBV vaccine. In fact, 19 of these 27 children received HBIG at birth and at least 3 doses of HBV vaccine. These properly treated children, however, still had a higher rate of HCC than children of HBsAg(+)/HBeAg(−) mothers (OR = 5.13). The remaining eight of the 27 high-risk children did not receive HBIG at birth, leading to an even higher rate of HCC (OR = 9.43) compared to children of HBsAg(+)/HBeAg(−) mothers. Therefore, some babies born to HBeAg(+) mothers were not fully protected by HBV vaccination and HBIG and, as a result, had an increased risk of developing HCC later in life.

Finally, the investigators determined whether those individuals who developed HCC after universal vaccination was initiated, had been properly dosed and immunized. Among those children who received fewer than 3 doses of HBV vaccine, 14 of 395,976 persons developed HCCs compared with 42 of 5,128,459 persons who were fully vaccinated (OR = 4.32). That is, children who were incompletely vaccinated had a higher risk of developing HCC than children who were fully vaccinated.

The challenge now is to expand hepatitis B vaccination coverage to the populations at greatest risk of HBV infection and HCC. In 1992, the World Health Organization (WHO) set a goal for all countries to integrate HBV vaccination into their universal childhood vaccination programs by 1997. That goal was not achieved, but significant progress is being made. By 2009, 178 (92%) of the 193 WHO member states had universal infant or childhood HBV vaccination programs.[17] Globally, 70% of infants had received 3 doses of the vaccine. Through the efforts of the Global Alliance for Vaccines and Immunization (GAVI), the cost of vaccine has been reduced from $100 to $1.00 per pediatric dose for very low income countries. This support has allowed GAVI and the WHO to set a goal of universal 3-dose vaccination, including a birth dose, with the intention of having 90% coverage in all countries. From studies done in several high-risk countries, we can predict that vaccination programs will reduce the prevalence of chronic HBV infection from between 8 and 20% to less than 1%[17] and this should lead to major decreases in the incidence of HCC in the coming decades.

Secondary Prevention of HCC

Surveillance of high-risk groups with ultrasonography and serum AFP determination is recommended by the European Association for the Study of the Liver,[113] the American Association for the Study of Liver Diseases,[114] and the Japan Society of Hepatology.[115] In practice however, the evidence that surveillance can decrease the HCC death rate, even in developed countries, is not persuasive. Randomized, controlled trials of HCC surveillance in low and middle income countries have reported inconsistent results. Surveillance of HBV carriers in Qidong, China, a very high-risk HCC area, found little benefit.[116] In contrast, a surveillance trial in Shanghai, China reported a sizable reduction in HCC mortality,[117] but this study had a follow-up rate below 20%. A major consideration in screening high risk groups in low-income countries, however, is whether individuals in whom early stage HCCs are detected, can be offered potentially curative therapies such as liver resection or transplantation. Without access to effective therapies, screening can have no effect on HCC mortality.

Clinicians in developed countries commonly screen patients chronically infected with HBV or HCV, with or without cirrhosis, with annual or semiannual determinations of serum alpha-fetoprotein (AFP) levels and ultrasonography (US) to detect small, incident HCCs. Whether such screening confers a survival advantage is still uncertain. Randomized clinical trials are difficult to justify ethically and those that have been done have either not shown a mortality benefit or have had methodological problems. There are several components to screening for HCC that limit its value including: (1) the sensitivity and specificity of AFP, (2) the quality and maintenance level of the US equipment, particularly in developing countries, (3) the skill of the US operator in identifying small tumors, (4) the availability of high quality surgery, and (5) cost.[15,118]

AFP has been used clinically since it was first reported as a serum marker of HCC in 1968.[119] As with all tests, the sensitivity of AFP can be increased to 100% if the cut-off level is set low enough, but only at the cost of loss of specificity. The most commonly used cut-off level for HBV carriers is 20 ng/ml, which yields sensitivities between 50 and 75% and a specificity of 90%.[15] The sensitivity of US to detect HCCs less than 3 cm in diameter among HBV infected individuals has ranged from 68 to 87%, but the specificity has been 80% or less.[118]

The results of surgery for HCC are highly dependent on the experience and skill of the surgeon and the quality of surgical facilities. Even in the best of hands, however, the recurrence rate and the development of new tumors are high. Orthotopic liver transplantation (OLT) has been used successfully to treat patients with small solitary HCCs and decompensated cirrhosis caused by HBV or HCV.[120] One year survival is about 80% and 5-year survival 65 to 70%.[121–124] The demand and need for an OLT is far higher than the supply of donor organs, even in high income countries. Presently, in the United States about 18,000 patients are on waiting lists, but only 5000 patients are transplanted each year.[122] Furthermore, the first year cost of an OLT is $80,000 to $200,000. Therefore, OLT is not an option in low income countries and most middle income countries. Recently, ablative methods, particularly radiofrequency ablation (RFA), have been used to treat small HCCs with good benefit. Such methods may be appropriate in middle income countries and possibly in low income countries.[125–127]

Biomarkers of HCC

Even though periodic screening with AFP and US is of limited value, it is the best currently available means for secondary prevention. Because of the limitations, however, there have been many efforts to discover new serum markers for the early detection of HCC.[128] These potential biomarkers include des-gamma-carboxyprothrombin (DCP), glypican, serum glycan, protein fragments, and several other biomarkers. However, none of these candidate markers has proven superior to AFP in multicenter, large blinded studies.

To discover new biomarkers of HCC, genome-wide array studies are being used to analyze HCCs to identify specific "signatures."[129] Such signatures may eventually be adapted to serum-based tests, but none have been reported yet. Using HCCs occurring in woodchucks infected with the woodchuck hepatitis virus (WHV, a close relative of human HBV), Marrero and colleagues[130] identified a glycoprotein in the Golgi organelle, Golgi protein 73 (GP73), which had previously been reported by Kladney et al in human serum.[131] In several studies in humans, GP73 was associated with HCC with better sensitivity and specificity than AFP.[132,133] Changes in glycosylation, particularly fucosylation, have also been associated with the development of HCC. Levels of fucosylated kininogen (Fc-Kin) and fucosylated alpha-1-antitrypsin were analyzed individually and in combination with AFP and GP73, for the ability to distinguish between a diagnosis of cirrhosis and HCC. Serum samples from 113 patients with cirrhosis without HCC and 164 samples from patients with cirrhosis and HCC were analyzed. The levels of Fc-Kin and fucosylated alpha-1-antitrypsin were significantly higher in persons with HCC than persons with cirrhosis ($P < 0.0001$). Greatest performance was achieved through the combination of Fc-Kin, AFP, and GP73, giving an optimal sensitivity of 95%, a specificity of 70%, and an area under the receiver operating curve of 0.94.[134] Therefore, glycosylated serum proteins can act as potential biomarkers of HCC when used independently or, especially, in combination with other markers of HCC.

There is reason to be optimistic that in the next few years more sensitive and specific serum biomarkers of HCC will be identified. In the future one or more of these tests may be used alone or in combination to screen populations for HCC in low and middle income countries where chronic HBV infection is endemic. Ultimately such biomarkers could be used in epidemiologic studies to estimate, more accurately, the incidence and prevalence of HCC, as well as to identify HCCs at an earlier, treatable stage.

Tertiary Prevention of HBV Associated HCC

There are about 350 to 400 million people in the world who are chronically infected with HBV. There is good evidence that treatment of these individuals, at least those who meet current treatment guidelines,[135] will reduce or, more likely, delay the risk of developing HCC.[136] In a placebo controlled clinical trial, lamivudine, the first anti-viral approved for treatment of chronic HBV infection, reduced the incidence of HCC in the treated group to 3.9% in contrast to 7.85% in the placebo group (HR = 0.49).[137] Lamivudine is the least effective of the currently approved antiviral therapies. Therefore, it is assumed although not demonstrated, that the newer drugs would have an even more profound effect on reducing the risk of HCC.[138]

■ SUMMARY

Blumberg considered eradication of HBV infection from the human population the ultimate goal of the public health approach to prevention of HCC.[139] He foresaw this happening as a combination of universal vaccination of all newborns to prevent new HBV infections and treatment of persons chronically infected with HBV to reduce or eliminate their risk of developing HCC. Currently anti-viral therapies are very expensive, thus limiting their use in low and middle income countries, but they are not as costly as combination therapies used to treat HIV infections. In the future, governmental and nongovernmental bodies could provide the resources to reach Baruch Blumberg's goal of the universal eradication of HBV.

■ REFERENCES

1. Blumberg BS. Australia antigen and the biology of hepatitis B. In: Lindsten L, eds. *Nobel lectures, physiology or medicine, 1971–1980*. Singapore; River Edge, N.J.: World Scientific; 1992:275–296.
2. Ford EB. *Genetics for medical students*. London: Methuen; 1956:202 p.
3. ALLISON AC. Protection afforded by sickle-cell trait against subtertian malareal infection. *Br Med J*. 1954;1(4857):290–294.
4. BLUMBERG BS, ALLISON AC, ALBERDI-LOPEZ-ALEN F. Contribution of blood groups to the study of the anthropology of the Basques. *Rev Clin Esp*. 1957;67(1):27–31.
5. BLUMBERG BS, ALLISON AC, GARRY B. The haptoglobins and haemoglobins of Alaskan Eskimos and Indians. *Ann Hum Genet*. 1959;23:349–356.
6. ALLISON AC, BLUMBERG BS. An isoprecipitation reaction distinguishing human serum-protein types. *Lancet*. 1961;1(7178):634–637.
7. BLUMBERG BS, ALTER HJ, VISNICH S. A "new" antigen in leukemia sera. *JAMA*. 1965;191:541–546.
8. Alter HJ, Blumberg BS. Further studies on a "new" human isoprecipitin system (Australia antigen). *Blood*. 1966;27(3):297–309.
9. Blumberg BS, Gerstley BJ, Hungerford DA, London WT, Sutnick AI. A serum antigen (Australia antigen) in Down's syndrome, leukemia, and hepatitis. *Ann Intern Med*. 1967;66(5):924–931.
10. Blumberg BS, Gerstley BJS, Sutnick AI, Millman I, London WT. Australia antigen, hepatitis virus and Down's syndrome. *Ann N Y Acad Sci*. 1970;171(2):486–499.
11. London WT, Sutnick AI, Blumberg BS. Australia antigen and acute viral hepatitis. *Ann Intern Med*. 1969;70(1):55–59.
12. Bayer ME, Blumberg BS, Werner B. Particles associated with Australia antigen in the sera of patients with leukaemia, Down's syndrome and hepatitis. *Nature*. 1968;218(5146):1057–1059.
13. Gitnick GL, Gleich GJ, Schoenfield LJ, et al. Australia antigen in chronic active liver disease with cirrhosis. *Lancet*. 1969;2(7615):285–288.
14. London WT, Drew JS, Lustbader ED, Werner BG, Blumberg BS. Host responses to hepatitis B infection in patients in a chronic hemodialysis unit. *Kidney Int*. 1977;12(1):51–58.
15. Lok AS, McMahon BJ, Practice Guidelines Committee, American Association for the Study of Liver Diseases. Chronic hepatitis B. *Hepatology*. 2001;34(6):1225–1241.
16. Centers for Disease Control and Prevention (CDC). Hepatitis B information for health professionals. http://www.cdc.gov/hepatitis/HBV/hbvfaq.htm#treatment. Updated 2011. Accessed 10/01, 2011.
17. World Health Organization (WHO). Hepatitis B. Immunizations, vaccine and biologicals Web site. http://www.who.int/immunization/topics/hepatitis_b/en/index.html. Updated 20102010.
18. Ohto H, Lin HH, Kawana T, Etoh T, Tohyama H. Intrauterine transmission of hepatitis B virus is closely related to placental leakage. *J Med Virol*. 1987;21(1):1–6.
19. Davis LG, Weber DJ, Lemon SM. Horizontal transmission of hepatitis B virus. *Lancet*. 1989;1(8643): 889–893.
20. Yim HJ, Lok AS. Natural history of chronic hepatitis B virus infection: What we knew in 1981 and what we know in 2005. *Hepatology*. 2006;43(2 Suppl 1):S173–S181.
21. Chang MH, Hwang LY, Hsu HC, Lee CY, Beasley RP. Prospective study of asymptomatic HBsAg carrier children infected in the perinatal period: Clinical and liver histologic studies. *Hepatology*. 1988;8(2):374–377.

22. Chen DS. Natural history of chronic hepatitis B virus infection: New light on an old story. *J Gastroenterol Hepatol.* 1993;8(5):470–475.

23. Centers for Disease Control and Prevention (CDC). Screening for chronic hepatitis B among Asian/Pacific islander populations—New York City, 2005. *MMWR Morb Mortal Wkly Rep.* 2006;55(18):505–509.

24. McMahon BJ, Holck P, Bulkow L, Snowball M. Serologic and clinical outcomes of 1536 Alaska natives chronically infected with hepatitis B virus. *Ann Intern Med.* 2001;135(9):759–768.

25. Wasley A, Kruszon-Moran D, Kuhnert W, et al. The prevalence of hepatitis B virus infection in the United States in the era of vaccination. *J Infect Dis.* 2010;202(2):192–201.

26. Ferlay J, Parkin DM, Curado MP, et al. *Cancer incidence in five continents,* volumes 1 to 9: IARC Cancer Base no.9. Geneva: World Health Organization; 2010.

27. Ferlay J, Shin HR, Bray F, Forman D, Mathers C, Parkin DM. GLOBOCAN 2008 v1.2, cancer incidence and mortality worldwide: IARC Cancer Base no. 10 [internet]. 2010. Accessed 07/02/2012.

28. Oyunsuren T, Kurbanov F, Tanaka Y, et al. High frequency of hepatocellular carcinoma in Mongolia; association with mono-, or co-infection with hepatitis C, B, and delta viruses. *J Med Virol.* 2006;78(12): 1688–1695.

29. Dondog B, Lise M, Dondov O, Baldandorj B, Franceschi S. Hepatitis B and C virus infections in hepatocellular carcinoma and cirrhosis in Mongolia. *Eur J Cancer Prev.* 2011;20(1):33–39.

30. Alcorn T. Mongolia's struggle with liver cancer. *Lancet.* 2011;377(9772):1139–1140.

31. The Gambia hepatitis intervention study. The Gambia hepatitis study group. *Cancer Res.* 1987;47(21): 5782–5787.

32. Darwish MA, Issa SA, Aziz AM, Darwish NM, Soliman AH. Hepatitis C and B viruses, and their association with hepatocellular carcinoma in Egypt. *J Egypt Public Health Assoc.* 1993;68(1–2):1–9.

33. Sun CA, Wu DM, Wang LY, Chen CJ, You SL, Santella RM. Determinants of formation of aflatoxin-albumin adducts: A seven-township study in Taiwan. *Br J Cancer.* 2002;87(9):966–970.

34. Tanaka K, Sakai H, Hashizume M, Hirohata T. Serum testosterone: Estradiol ratio and the development of hepatocellular carcinoma among male cirrhotic patients. *Cancer Res.* 2000;60(18):5106–5110.

35. Yu MW, Yang YC, Yang SY, et al. Hormonal markers and hepatitis B virus-related hepatocellular carcinoma risk: A nested case-control study among men. *J Natl Cancer Inst.* 2001;93(21):1644–1651.

36. Yuan JM, Ross RK, Stanczyk FZ, et al. A cohort study of serum testosterone and hepatocellular carcinoma in Shanghai, China. *Int J Cancer.* 1995;63(4):491–493.

37. Altekruse SF, McGlynn KA, Reichman ME. Hepatocellular carcinoma incidence, mortality, and survival trends in the United States from 1975 to 2005. *J Clin Oncol.* 2009;27(9):1485–1491.

38. United Nations, Department of Economic and Social Affairs, Population Division. *World population prospects: 2006 revision.* New York: United Nations; 2007.

39. McGlynn KA, London WT. The global epidemiology of hepatocellular carcinoma: Present and future. *Clin Liver Dis.* 2011;15(2):223–243, vii–x.

40. Tanaka H, Imai Y, Hiramatsu N, et al. Declining incidence of hepatocellular carcinoma in Osaka, Japan, from 1990 to 2003. *Ann Intern Med.* 2008;148(11):820–826.

41. Altekruse SF, McGlynn KA, Dickie LA, Kleiner DE. Hepatocellular carcinoma confirmation, treatment, and survival in surveillance, epidemiology, and end results registries, 1992–2008. *Hepatology.* 2012;55(2):476–482.

42. Beasley RP, Hwang LY, Lin CC, Chien CS. Hepatocellular carcinoma and hepatitis B virus. A prospective study of 22 707 men in Taiwan. *Lancet.* 1981;2(8256):1129.

43. Beasley RP. Hepatitis B virus. the major etiology of hepatocellular carcinoma. *Cancer.* 1988;61(10): 1942–1956.

44. London WT, Evans AA, McGlynn K, et al. Viral, host and environmental risk factors for hepatocellular carcinoma: A prospective study in Haimen city, China. *Intervirology.* 1995;38(3–4):155–161.

45. Chen G, Lin W, Shen F, Iloeje UH, London WT, Evans AA. Past HBV viral load as predictor of mortality and morbidity from HCC and chronic liver disease in a prospective study. *Am J Gastroenterol.* 2006;101(8):1797–1803.

46. Fwu CW, Chien YC, Nelson KE, et al. Mortality after chronic hepatitis B virus infection: A linkage study involving 2 million parous women from Taiwan. *J Infect Dis*. 2010;201(7):1016–1023.

47. Evans AA, Chen G, Ross EA, Shen FM, Lin WY, London WT. Eight-year follow-up of the 90,000-person Haimen city cohort: I. hepatocellular carcinoma mortality, risk factors, and gender differences. *Cancer Epidemiol Biomarkers Prev*. 2002;11(4):369–376.

48. Chen CJ, Yang HI, Su J, et al. Risk of hepatocellular carcinoma across a biological gradient of serum hepatitis B virus DNA level. *JAMA*. 2006;295(1):65–73.

49. Huang YT, Jen CL, Yang HI, et al. Lifetime risk and sex difference of hepatocellular carcinoma among patients with chronic hepatitis B and C. *J Clin Oncol*. 2011;29(27):3643–3650.

50. IARC Working Group on the Evaluation of Carcinogenic Risks to Humans. Some traditional herbal medicines, some mycotoxins, naphthalene and styrene. *IARC Monogr Eval Carcinog Risks Hum*. 2002;82:1–556.

51. Hayes RB, van Nieuwenhuize JP, Raatgever JW, ten Kate FJ. Aflatoxin exposures in the industrial setting: An epidemiological study of mortality. *Food Chem Toxicol*. 1984;22(1):39–43.

52. Olsen JH, Dragsted L, Autrup H. Cancer risk and occupational exposure to aflatoxins in Denmark. *Br J Cancer*. 1988;58(3):392–396.

53. Blount W. Turkey "X" disease. *Turkeys*. 1961;9:55–58.

54. Asplin F, Carnaghan R. The toxicity of certain groundnut meals for poultry with special references to their effect on duckling and chickens. *Vet Rec*. 1961;73:1215–1219.

55. Hopkins J. IARC monographs on the evaluation of carcinogenic risks to humans overall evaluations of carcinogenicity: An updating of IARC monographs volumes 1 to 42. supplement 7. IARC, Lyon, 1987. pp. 440. sw.fr 65.00. ISBN 92-833-1411-0. *Food and Chemical Toxicology*. 1989;27(8):549.

56. Halver JE. Aflatoxicosis and trout hepatoma. *Bull Off Int Epizoot*. 1968;69(7):1249–1278.

57. Butler WH, Hempsall V. Histochemical studies of hepatocellular carcinomas in the rat induced by aflatoxin. *J Pathol*. 1981;134(2):157–170.

58. Vesselinovitch SD, Mihailovich N, Wogan GN, Lombard LS, Rao KV. Aflatoxin B 1, a hepatocarcinogen in the infant mouse. *Cancer Res*. 1972;32(11):2289–2291.

59. CARNAGHAN RB. Some biological effects of aflatoxin. *Proc R Soc Med*. 1964;57:414–416.

60. Sinnhuber RO, Lee DJ, Wales JH, Ayres JL. Dietary factors and hepatoma in rainbow trout (*salmo gairdneri*). II. cocarcinogenes by cyclopropenoid fatty acids and the effect of gossypol and altered lipids on aflatoxin-induced liver cancer. *J Natl Cancer Inst*. 1968;41(6):1293–1301.

61. Lin JJ, Liu C, Svoboda DJ. Long term effects of aflatoxin B1 and viral hepatitis on marmoset liver. A preliminary report. *Lab Invest*. 1974;30(3):267–278.

62. Reddy JK, Svoboda DJ, Rao MS. Induction of liver tumors by aflatoxin B1 in the tree shrew (*tupaia glis*), a nonhuman primate. *Cancer Res*. 1976;36(1):151–160.

63. Adamson RH, Correa P, Dalgard DW. Occurrence of a primary liver carcinoma in a rhesus monkey fed aflatoxin B 1. *J Natl Cancer Inst*. 1973;50(2):549–553.

64. Alpert ME, Hutt MS, Wogan GN, Davidson CS. Association between aflatoxin content of food and hepatoma frequency in Uganda. *Cancer*. 1971;28(1):253–260.

65. Keen P, Martin P. Is aflatoxin carcinogenic in man? the evidence in Swaziland. *Trop Geogr Med*. 1971;23(1):44–53.

66. Purchase IF. Aflatoxin residues in food of animal origin. *Food Cosmet Toxicol*. 1972;10(4):531–544.

67. Shank RC, Bhamarapravati N, Gordon JE, Wogan GN. Dietary aflatoxins and human liver cancer. IV. incidence of primary liver cancer in two municipal populations of Thailand. *Food Cosmet Toxicol*. 1972;10(2):171–179.

68. Peers FG, Linsell CA. Dietary aflatoxins and liver cancer—a population based study in Kenya. *Br J Cancer*. 1973;27(6):473–484.

69. Peers F, Bosch X, Kaldor J, Linsell A, Pluijmen M. Aflatoxin exposure, hepatitis B virus infection and liver cancer in Swaziland. *Int J Cancer*. 1987;39(5):545–553.

70. Armstrong B. The epidemiology of cancer in the People's Republic of China. *Int J Epidemiol*. 1980;9(4):305–315.

71. Yeh FS, Mo CC, Yen RC. Risk factors for hepatocellular carcinoma in Guangxi, People's Republic of China. *Natl Cancer Inst Monogr.* 1985;69:47–48.
72. Wang YB, Lan LZ, Ye BF, Xu YC, Liu YY, Li WG. Relation between geographical distribution of liver cancer and climate-aflatoxin B1 in China. *Sci Sin B.* 1983;26(11):1166–1175.
73. Van Rensburg SJ, Cook-Mozaffari P, Van Schalkwyk DJ, Van der Watt JJ, Vincent TJ, Purchase IF. Hepatocellular carcinoma and dietary aflatoxin in Mozambique and Transkei. *Br J Cancer.* 1985;51(5):713–726.
74. Autrup H, Seremet T, Wakhisi J, Wasunna A. Aflatoxin exposure measured by urinary excretion of aflatoxin B1-guanine adduct and hepatitis B virus infection in areas with different liver cancer incidence in Kenya. *Cancer Res.* 1987;47(13):3430–3433.
75. Campbell TC, Chen JS, Liu CB, Li JY, Parpia B. Nonassociation of aflatoxin with primary liver cancer in a cross-sectional ecological survey in the People's Republic of China. *Cancer Res.* 1990;50(21):6882–6893.
76. van Rensburg SJ, van Schalkwyk GC, van Schalkwyk DJ. Primary liver cancer and aflatoxin intake in Transkei. *J Environ Pathol Toxicol Oncol.* 1990;10(1–2):11–16.
77. Srivatanakul P, Parkin DM, Khlat M, et al. Liver cancer in Thailand. II. A case-control study of hepatocellular carcinoma. *Int J Cancer.* 1991;48(3):329–332.
78. Bulatao-Jayme J, Almero EM, Castro MC, Jardeleza MT, Salamat LA. A case-control dietary study of primary liver cancer risk from aflatoxin exposure. *Int J Epidemiol.* 1982;11(2):112–119.
79. Lam KC, Yu MC, Leung JW, Henderson BE. Hepatitis B virus and cigarette smoking: Risk factors for hepatocellular carcinoma in Hong Kong. *Cancer Res.* 1982;42(12):5246–5248.
80. Omer RE, Verhoef L, Van't Veer P, et al. Peanut butter intake, GSTM1 genotype and hepatocellular carcinoma: A case-control study in Sudan. *Cancer Causes Control.* 2001;12(1):23–32.
81. Wild CP, Turner PC. The toxicology of aflatoxins as a basis for public health decisions. *Mutagenesis.* 2002;17(6):471–481.
82. Kamdem LK, Meineke I, Godtel-Armbrust U, Brockmoller J, Wojnowski L. Dominant contribution of P450 3A4 to the hepatic carcinogenic activation of aflatoxin B1. *Chem Res Toxicol.* 2006;19(4):577–586.
83. Guengerich FP, Johnson WW, Shimada T, Ueng YF, Yamazaki H, Langouet S. Activation and detoxication of aflatoxin B1. *Mutat Res.* 1998;402(1–2):121–128.
84. Foster PL, Eisenstadt E, Miller JH. Base substitution mutations induced by metabolically activated aflatoxin B1. *Proc Natl Acad Sci U S A.* 1983;80(9):2695–2698.
85. Hsu IC, Metcalf RA, Sun T, Welsh JA, Wang NJ, Harris CC. Mutational hotspot in the p53 gene in human hepatocellular carcinomas. *Nature.* 1991;350(6317):427–428.
86. Bressac B, Kew M, Wands J, Ozturk M. Selective G to T mutations of p53 gene in hepatocellular carcinoma from southern Africa. *Nature.* 1991;350(6317):429–431.
87. Ozturk M. P53 mutation in hepatocellular carcinoma after aflatoxin exposure. *Lancet.* 1991;338(8779):1356–1359.
88. Scorsone KA, Zhou YZ, Butel JS, Slagle BL. p53 mutations cluster at codon 249 in hepatitis B virus-positive hepatocellular carcinomas from China. *Cancer Res.* 1992;52(6):1635–1638.
89. Hayward NK, Walker GJ, Graham W, Cooksley E. Hepatocellular carcinoma mutation. *Nature.* 1991;352(6338):764.
90. Murakami Y, Hayashi K, Hirohashi S, Sekiya T. Aberrations of the tumor suppressor p53 and retinoblastoma genes in human hepatocellular carcinomas. *Cancer Res.* 1991;51(20):5520–5525.
91. Sheu JC, Huang GT, Lee PH, et al. Mutation of p53 gene in hepatocellular carcinoma in Taiwan. *Cancer Res.* 1992;52(21):6098–6100.
92. Jackson PE, Qian GS, Friesen MD, et al. Specific p53 mutations detected in plasma and tumors of hepatocellular carcinoma patients by electrospray ionization mass spectrometry. *Cancer Res.* 2001;61(1):33–35.
93. Kirk GD, Lesi OA, Mendy M, et al. 249(ser) TP53 mutation in plasma DNA, hepatitis B viral infection, and risk of hepatocellular carcinoma. *Oncogene.* 2005;24(38):5858–5867.

94. Olubuyide IO, Maxwell SM, Hood H, Neal GE, Hendrickse RG. HBsAg, aflatoxins and primary hepatocellular carcinoma. *Afr J Med Med Sci.* 1993;22(3):89–91.

95. Mandishona E, MacPhail AP, Gordeuk VR, et al. Dietary iron overload as a risk factor for hepatocellular carcinoma in black Africans. *Hepatology.* 1998;27(6):1563–1566.

96. Ross RK, Yuan JM, Yu MC, et al. Urinary aflatoxin biomarkers and risk of hepatocellular carcinoma. *Lancet.* 1992;339(8799):943–946.

97. Qian GS, Ross RK, Yu MC, et al. A follow-up study of urinary markers of aflatoxin exposure and liver cancer risk in shanghai, People's Republic of China. *Cancer Epidemiol Biomarkers Prev.* 1994;3(1):3–10.

98. Yeh FS, Yu MC, Mo CC, Luo S, Tong MJ, Henderson BE. Hepatitis B virus, aflatoxins, and hepatocellular carcinoma in southern Guangxi, China. *Cancer Res.* 1989;49(9):2506–2509.

99. Wang LY, Hatch M, Chen CJ, et al. Aflatoxin exposure and risk of hepatocellular carcinoma in Taiwan. *Int J Cancer.* 1996;67(5):620–625.

100. Kuang SY, Lekawanvijit S, Maneekarn N, et al. Hepatitis B 1762T/1764A mutations, hepatitis C infection, and codon 249 p53 mutations in hepatocellular carcinomas from Thailand. *Cancer Epidemiol Biomarkers Prev.* 2005;14(2):380–384.

101. Kirk GD, Bah E, Montesano R. Molecular epidemiology of human liver cancer: Insights into etiology, pathogenesis and prevention from the Gambia, West Africa. *Carcinogenesis.* 2006;27(10): 2070–2082.

102. Wild CP, Montesano R. A model of interaction: Aflatoxins and hepatitis viruses in liver cancer aetiology and prevention. *Cancer Lett.* 2009;286(1):22–28.

103. Strosnider H, Azziz-Baumgartner E, Banziger M, et al. Workgroup report: Public health strategies for reducing aflatoxin exposure in developing countries. *Environ Health Perspect.* 2006;114(12):1898–1903.

104. Henry SH, Bosch FX, Troxell TC, Bolger PM. Policy forum: Public health. Reducing liver cancer—global control of aflatoxin. *Science.* 1999;286(5449):2453–2454.

105. Shephard GS. Risk assessment of aflatoxins in food in Africa. *Food Addit Contam Part A Chem Anal Control Expo Risk Assess.* 2008;25(10):1246–1256.

106. Liu Y, Wu F. Global burden of aflatoxin-induced hepatocellular carcinoma: A risk assessment. *Environ Health Perspect.* 2010;118(6):818–824.

107. Wang JS, Luo H, Billam M, et al. Short-term safety evaluation of processed calcium montmorillonite clay (NovaSil) in humans. *Food Addit Contam.* 2005;22(3):270–279.

108. Kensler TW, Roebuck BD, Wogan GN, Groopman JD. Aflatoxin: A 50-year odyssey of mechanistic and translational toxicology. *Toxicol Sci.* 2011;120 Suppl 1:S28–S48.

109. Kane MA, Brooks A. New immunization initiatives and progress toward the global control of hepatitis B. *Curr Opin Infect Dis.* 2002;15(5):465–469.

110. Chang MH, Chen CJ, Lai MS, et al. Universal hepatitis B vaccination in Taiwan and the incidence of hepatocellular carcinoma in children. Taiwan childhood hepatoma study group. *N Engl J Med.* 1997;336(26):1855–1859.

111. Lee CL, Ko YC. Hepatitis B vaccination and hepatocellular carcinoma in Taiwan. *Pediatrics.* 1997; 99(3):351–353.

112. Chang MH, You SL, Chen CJ, et al. Decreased incidence of hepatocellular carcinoma in hepatitis B vaccinees: A 20-year follow-up study. *J Natl Cancer Inst.* 2009;101(19):1348–1355.

113. Bruix J, Sherman M, Llovet JM, et al. Clinical management of hepatocellular carcinoma. Conclusions of the Barcelona-2000 EASL conference. European association for the study of the liver. *J Hepatol.* 2001;35(3):421–430.

114. Bruix J, Sherman M, American Association for the Study of Liver Diseases. Management of hepatocellular carcinoma: An update. *Hepatology.* 2011;53(3):1020–1022.

115. Kudo M, Izumi N, Kokudo N, et al. Management of hepatocellular carcinoma in Japan: Consensus-based clinical practice guidelines proposed by the Japan society of hepatology (JSH) 2010 updated version. *Dig Dis.* 2011;29(3):339–364.

116. Chen JG, Parkin DM, Chen QG, et al. Screening for liver cancer: Results of a randomised controlled trial in Gidong, China. *J Med Screen.* 2003;10(4):204–209.

117. Zhang B, Yang B, Tang Z. Randomized controlled trial of screening for hepatocellular carcinoma. *J Cancer Res Clin Oncol.* 2004;130(7):417.

118. Gebo KA, Chander G, Jenckes MW, et al. Screening tests for hepatocellular carcinoma in patients with chronic hepatitis C: A systematic review. *Hepatology.* 2002;36(5 Suppl 1):S84–S92.

119. Alpert ME, Uriel J, de Nechaud B. Alpha-1 fetoglobulin in the diagnosis of human hepatoma. *N Engl J Med.* 1968;278(18):984–986.

120. Figueras J, Jaurrieta E, Valls C, et al. Survival after liver transplantation in cirrhotic patients with and without hepatocellular carcinoma: A comparative study. *Hepatology.* 1997;25(6):1485–1489.

121. Mazzaferro V, Regalia E, Doci R, et al. Liver transplantation for the treatment of small hepatocellular carcinomas in patients with cirrhosis. *N Engl J Med.* 1996;334(11):693–699.

122. Wright TL. Treatment of patients with hepatitis C and cirrhosis. *Hepatology.* 2002;36(5 Suppl 1):S185.

123. Busuttil RW, Farmer DG, Yersiz H, et al. Analysis of long-term outcomes of 3200 liver transplantations over two decades: A single-center experience. *Ann Surg.* 2005;241(6):905–916; discussion 916-8.

124. Saab S, Wang V, Ibrahim AB, et al. MELD score predicts 1-year patient survival post-orthotopic liver transplantation. *Liver Transpl.* 2003;9(5):473–476.

125. Rossi S, Di Stasi M, Buscarini E, et al. Percutaneous radiofrequency interstitial thermal ablation in the treatment of small hepatocellular carcinoma. *Cancer J Sci Am.* 1995;1(1):73–81.

126. Shiina S, Teratani T, Obi S, et al. A randomized controlled trial of radiofrequency ablation with ethanol injection for small hepatocellular carcinoma. *Gastroenterology.* 2005;129(1):122–130.

127. Nguyen KT, Geller DA. Radiofrequency abiation of hepatocellular carcinoma. In: Carr BI, ed. *Hepatocellular carcinoma diagnosis and treatment.* New York: Humana Press; 2010:421–452.

128. Block TM, Marrero J, Gish RG, et al. The degree of readiness of selected biomarkers for the early detection of hepatocellular carcinoma: Notes from a recent workshop. *Cancer Biomark.* 2008;4(1):19–33.

129. Llovet JM, Chen Y, Wurmbach E, et al. A molecular signature to discriminate dysplastic nodules from early hepatocellular carcinoma in HCV cirrhosis. *Gastroenterology.* 2006;131(6):1758–1767.

130. Marrero JA, Romano PR, Nikolaeva O, et al. GP73, a resident golgi glycoprotein, is a novel serum marker for hepatocellular carcinoma. *J Hepatol.* 2005;43(6):1007–1012.

131. Kladney RD, Cui X, Bulla GA, Brunt EM, Fimmel CJ. Expression of GP73, a resident golgi membrane protein, in viral and nonviral liver disease. *Hepatology.* 2002;35(6):1431–1440.

132. Gu Y, Chen W, Zhao Y, Chen L, Peng T. Quantitative analysis of elevated serum golgi protein-73 expression in patients with liver diseases. *Ann Clin Biochem.* 2009;46(Pt 1):38–43.

133. Tian L, Wang Y, Xu D, et al. Serological AFP/ golgi protein 73 could be a new diagnostic parameter of hepatic diseases. *Int J Cancer.* 2010;129(8):1923–1931.

134. Wang M, Long RE, Comunale MA, et al. Novel fucosylated biomarkers for the early detection of hepatocellular carcinoma. *Cancer Epidemiol Biomarkers Prev.* 2009;18(6):1914–1921.

135. Lok AS, McMahon BJ. Chronic hepatitis B: Update 2009. *Hepatology.* 2009;50(3):661–662.

136. Blumberg BS, London WT. Hepatitis B virus and the prevention of primary hepatocellular carcinoma. *N Engl J Med.* 1981;304(13):782–784.

137. Liaw YF, Sung JJ, Chow WC, et al. Lamivudine for patients with chronic hepatitis B and advanced liver disease. *N Engl J Med.* 2004;351(15):1521–1531.

138. Lai CL, Yuen MF. Chronic hepatitis B—new goals, new treatment. *N Engl J Med.* 2008;359(23): 2488–2491.

139. Blumberg BS. Viruses and Cancer: A historical perspective—HBV and prevention of a cancer. In: Robertson ES, ed. *Cancer associated viruses.* Boston, MA: Springer US; 2012:25–43.

CHAPTER 18

NATIONAL CANCER INSTITUTE– COSTA RICA STUDIES ON HUMAN PAPILLOMA VIRUS AND CERVICAL CANCER

ROLANDO HERRERO

INTRODUCTION

Cervical cancer is a leading cause of cancer incidence and mortality. The most recent estimates from Globocan[1] indicate that cervical cancer is the third leading cancer among women in the world, with 530,000 new cases in 2008. In some developing countries, it remains the leading malignancy (eastern Africa, south-central Asia, and Melanesia). More than 85% of cervical cancers occur in developing countries. The mortality incidence ratio is close to 50%, with about 275,000 deaths a year. Some developed countries have succeeded at reducing incidence and mortality thanks to extensive and costly screening programs based on cervical cytology. However, control of the disease has been difficult in developing countries, in many of which there are no screening efforts in place while in others, despite serious attempts, limited impact has been obtained. In most places in Latin America, incidence rates are very high, and there are important regional variations both between and within countries, with the less developed areas typically presenting the highest rates. The age of occurrence of cervical cancer is typically younger than for most tumors, and it is much more common among poor women, who are often the main support of their numerous families, making the social consequences of this problem even more severe. Moreover, cervical cancer is a disease with detectable and curable precursors that precede the disease for many years. In this context, the occurrence of invasive cancer is a sign of negligence and a serious failure of the health system, and society in general, to control a preventable condition of poor women.

Demographic changes characterized by population aging will produce an important increase in the burden of disease in the next decades. It has been estimated that for Latin America[2] even if current incidence rates remain unchanged, the number of cases will increase by nearly 75% in the next 20 years solely as a consequence of those demographic changes.

The association of cervical cancer with sexual behavior has been noted for more than 150 years, but only in the last 20 years it has been possible to identify its etiologic agents, the human papillomaviruses (HPVs), a growing family of more than 120 viral types, of which nearly 20 have clearly identified oncogenic properties in the genital tract and other epithelia.[3]

In the 1980s there was limited knowledge of the etiology and natural history of cervical cancer. Around 1985, the US National Cancer Institute launched an initiative to investigate risk factors for cervical cancer in Latin America, which generated a series of research studies spanning almost three decades, particularly in Guanacaste, Costa Rica, that have produced dozens of publications and contributed extensively to the knowledge of cervical cancer etiology and the development of preventive methods against the disease.[4] The studies have also transferred state-of-the-art research technology to Costa Rica, where a large research center named the Proyecto Epidemiológico Guanacaste (PEG), almost entirely dedicated to the study of this disease, is in operation. In this chapter we present the major characteristics of the studies conducted to date and discuss their methodology, organization, main scientific findings and public health implications as an example of successful collaborative research between two nations each offering its own advantages.

▦ THE LATIN AMERICAN CASE-CONTROL STUDY

The Latin American case-control study of cervical cancer originated from an initiative of the Environmental Epidemiology Branch, Division of Cancer Epidemiology and Genetics of the United States National Cancer Institute (NCI), which issued a request for proposals to conduct a multicentric case-control study of invasive cervical cancer in the region. The contract was awarded to the Gorgas Memorial Laboratory in Panama. Local investigators and participating centers were identified in Colombia, Costa Rica, Mexico and Panama, and detailed protocols and study manuals prepared.

The design was a case-control study with recruitment of women under the age of 70 years diagnosed with incident, histologically confirmed invasive cervical cancer in the participating areas, with an attempt to recruit into the study a comprehensive sample of all cases diagnosed during the study period from defined geographical areas between January 1986 and June 1987.[5] Hospital (all centers) and community controls (two centers), frequency-matched on age to the age distribution of cervical cancer cases in the community in previous periods were selected with a 1:2 case-control ratio. In order to prevent selection bias associated with the use of hospital controls, the diagnoses of control women eligible to be included in the study were restricted to those not associated with the exposures under study as suspected cervical cancer risk factors (neoplastic, endocrinologic, nutritional, psychiatric, circulatory, gynecologic or smoking-related diagnoses). Potential community controls were selected by randomly selecting several women from the censal segments where the cases came from. They were visited at home and invited to participate, and those with a history of cancer were replaced. However, eligible hospital and community controls who refused to participate were not replaced. Both cases and controls had to be residents in the study areas for at least 6 months before recruitment to be considered eligible for the study.

Cases and controls had an extensive personal interview on potential cervical cancer risk factors, including demographic characteristics, sexual, reproductive, smoking, medical and socioeconomic data, in addition to employment history, dietary, contraceptive and hygienic practices. In order to determine the presence of HPV DNA, a swab of the tumor was collected from each case and an endocervical swab was obtained from controls. In addition, blood was obtained for immunologic and nutritional tests, and was processed and separated into its components (plasma, buffy coats) in the evening of collection at local laboratories.

To investigate the role of the male factor in cervical cancer etiology isolated from women's sexual behavior, the husbands or partners of case and control women reporting only one lifetime sexual partner (40% of the cancer patients and 52.8% of the controls) were also invited to participate and recruited. The interviewers, most of them male physicians, conducted an interview with each male participant to obtain information on sociodemographic factors, sexual and medical history, genital hygiene and family history of cancer, after which they performed a physical examination with emphasis on the genital area in order to assess hygiene, circumcision and signs of venereal diseases. To investigate the presence of HPV, a cotton tip applicator was used to obtain a smear of the coronal sulcus and another from the distal urethra. All samples for HPV testing were stored in phosphate-buffered saline (PBS), frozen as soon as possible and stored at –20 degrees Celsius until tested.

Detailed procedures and field manuals were elaborated and the field work strictly supervised. The staff was extensively trained on all study procedures and the necessary resources to conduct the study were provided through agreements with the local governments, including study materials, equipment, vehicles and salaries for the staff. Specimens were shipped periodically to the Gorgas Laboratory in Panama. The study was supervised by the NCI and local IRBs and all participants signed informed consent.

Participation rates were near complete for all study components (Figure 18.1). Thus, of 766 eligible cases, 759 were included in the study (99%), and of 1532 eligible controls, 1467 were interviewed (95.8%). Similarly, 99.6% of cases and 95.4% of controls agreed to the collection of biological specimens. In the case of male partners of monogamous women, after excluding women whose only lifetime partner had died, interviews were conducted with 204 partners of patients (corresponding to 78.5% of the living subjects) and 485 were

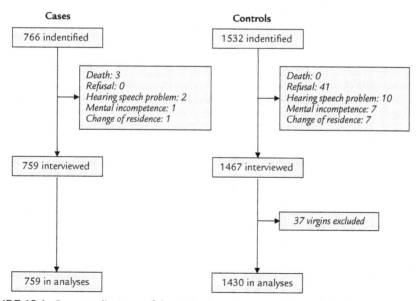

FIGURE 18.1 Consort diagram of the Latin American Case Control Study.

conducted with partners of controls (71.1% of living subjects). Of the husbands of cases, 97.5% agreed to donate biological specimens vs. 95.2% of the control husbands.

Multivariate models were developed including behavioral and biological markers of exposure (Table 18.1). In such models, the study confirmed the clear association of sexual behavior of women and risk of invasive cervical cancer.[6] Both age at first sexual intercourse and the number of lifetime sexual partners were associated with risk of cervical cancer. The number of steady sexual partners (relationships of more than 3 months) was the main determinant of this association, while the number of casual partners did not increase risk. A history of anal sexual intercourse was also associated with increased risk.

Another important determinant of risk in the multivariate models was the number of live births, which showed a strong trend of increasing risk. Women with 12 or more live births had an almost 4-fold increase in risk, while cesarean sections were associated with a borderline statistically significant reduction in risk.[7]

This was the first epidemiological study that included molecular testing for HPV using an early detection method (filter in situ hybridization, FISH) and demonstrated an association between HPV and cervical cancer.[8] As shown in Table 18.1, 47% of the cases and 18% of the controls had detectable HPV 16 or 18, with an associated OR of 5.2 (95% CI = 4.1–6.6). These results contrast with recent data using more sensitive and specific tests showing that the fraction of cancers associated with these two viral types is around 70%, and the ORs are one order of magnitude higher. Moreover, HPV testing was relatively high in controls and HPV infection did not show the expected correlations with age and sexual behavior.

This finding was the subject of intensive debate and theoretical speculation and lead to the search of more precise measurement of HPV infection. The debate between basic scientists and epidemiologists ensued, because epidemiologist demanded strong population evidence before accepting the causal association proposed by molecular biologists.[9,10]

In this population where smoking is relatively rare (only about 5% of controls reported smoking 20 or more cigarettes per day), a weak association was observed with smoking large amounts of cigarettes in the unadjusted models, but given the correlation of smoking with sexual behavior, the association was not present in the multivariate models.[11]

We also took the opportunity of having collected data on screening histories of cases and controls to evaluate the impact of screening behavior on risk of cervical cancer.[12] Several important methodologic aspects needed to be taken into consideration, including the fact that the diagnosis of cervical cancer is strongly linked to screening activity, and this can produce the false impression that screening is ineffective. To circumvent this limitation, the analyses were restricted to tests conducted at least one year before diagnosis. As shown in Table 18.1, women who reported never having had a Pap test had a 3-fold increase in risk compared to those with a test in the previous 2 years.

As mentioned above, in addition to women with cancer and their corresponding controls, the husbands of women reporting lifetime monogamy were also recruited and specimens collected.[13] In this analysis, the behavior of the partner also increased risk of invasive cervical cancer (Table 18.2), with a trend of increasing risk associated with increasing number of sexual partners of the men. There was also an inverse association with education of the partners, but not with a history of visits to prostitutes, circumcision or the presence of smegma on physical exam.

Other hormonal factors investigated were oral[14] and injectable contraceptives,[15] with detection of moderately increased risk for long-term users.

Another contribution of this study was the assessment of the association of diet and nutritional status with cervical cancer using both dietary and serologic measurements. Subjects were interviewed about their adult consumption of 58 food items, including the

TABLE 18.1 Relative risks of invasive cervical cancer associated with selected cervical cancer risk factors

	CASES	CONTROLS	RR[1]	RR[2]	95% CI
Age at first sexual contact:					
≥ 20	170	521	1.0	1.0	
18–19	139	284	1.5	1.2	0.9–1.7
16–17	189	303	1.9	1.3	1.0–1.8
14–15	217	233	2.9	1.8	1.3–2.4
<14	42	84	1.5	1.1	0.7–1.7
p for trend			<0.0001	0.0007	
Total number of sex partners:					
1	303	783	1.0	1.0	
2–3	340	489	1.8	1.6	1.3–2.0
4–5	65	92	1.8	1.4	1.0–2.1
≥6	51	64	2.1	1.7	1.1–2.5
p for trend			<0.0001	0.0009	
Number of steady sex partners:[3]					
0–1	416	1,015	1.0	1.0[4]	
2	203	270	1.8	1.5	1.2–2.0
3	90	93	2.3	2.0	1.4–2.9
4	30	27	2.7	1.8	1.0–3.3
>4	19	19	2.4	2.0	1.0–4.3
p for trend			<0.0001	<0.0001	
Number of nonsteady sex partners:					
0	561	1,068	1.0	1.0[5]	
1	101	181	1.1	1.1	0.8–1.5
2	35	71	0.9	1.0	0.6–1.6
3–4	26	57	0.9	0.9	0.5–1.5
≥5	35	47	1.4	1.1	0.7–1.9
p for trend			0.45	0.85	
Frequency of anal sexual relations:[6]					
Never	631	1,248	1.0	1.0	
Once	35	44	1.6	1.5	0.9–2.6
More than once	88	103	1.7	1.9	1.3–2.6
p for trend			0.0002	0.0003	

(*continued*)

TABLE 18.1 (Continued)

	CASES	CONTROLS	RR[1]	RR[2]	95% CI
Number of live births:					
0–1	39	146	1.0	1.0[7]	
2–3	152	387	1.5	1.8	1.2–2.8
4–5	180	334	2.1	2.2	1.4–3.5
6–7	148	211	2.9	2.8	1.8–4.5
8–9	99	145	3.0	2.6	1.6–4.4
10–11	70	101	3.2	2.2	1.3–3.8
≥12	57	53	5.0	3.7	2.0–6.7
p for trend			<0.0001	0.0001	
History of cesarean section:					
No	668	1,164	1.0	1.0[8]	
Yes	74	197	0.6	0.7	0.5–1.0
HPV types 16/18:					
Negative	273	833	1.0	1.0	
+/–	109	173	1.9	2.2	1.6–2.9
Positive	339	219	4.8	5.2	4.1–6.6
HPV types 6/11:					
Negative	595	1,143	1.0	1.0	
+/–	77	59	2.5	2.1	1.5–3.1
Positive	49	23	4.1	4.2	2.4–7.2
Cigarettes per day:					
Nonsmoker	523	1,028	1.0	1.0	
<20	183	329	1.1	1.1	0.8–1.3
≥20	53	73	1.4	1.1	0.7–1.7
p for trend			0.06	0.55	
Length of oral contraceptive use:[9]					
Non	568	1,072	1.0	1.0	
<5 years	101	204	0.9	1.1	0.8–1.5
5–9 years	61	101	1.1	1.4	1.0–2.1
≥10 years	27	51	1.0	1.3	0.8–2.3
p for trend			0.76	0.50	
Time elapsed since last Pap smear:[10]					
<2 years	123	384	1.0	1.0	
2–3 years	109	345	1.0	0.9	0.7–1.3
4–5 years	45	84	1.7	1.6	1.0–2.5

(continued)

TABLE 18.1 (Continued)

	CASES	CONTROLS	RR[1]	RR[2]	95% CI
≥6 years	66	139	1.6	1.5	1.0–2.2
Never done	372	409	3.0	3.0	2.3–4.0
Not known	44	69			

[1] Adjusted for age, unknowns excluded.

[2] Adjusted for age, number of sexual partners, age at first sexual contact, presence of HPV DNA, time elapsed since last Pap smear, number of pregnancies, and socioeconomic status.

[3] In relationships lasting 3 months or more.

[4] RR[2] also adjusted for number of nonsteady sex partners.

[5] RR[2] also adjusted for number of steady sex partners.

[6] Including only women with at least one stead sex partner.

[7] Also adjusted for number of stillbirths, spontaneous abortions, and induced abortions.

[8] Also adjusted for number of pregnancies.

[9] Excluding cases and controls for whom the duration of use was unknown.

[10] Excluding cytology done in the year immediately preceding the diagnosis or interview.

major sources of putative protective agents (vitamin A, carotenoids, vitamin C, and folacin).[16] In multivariate models, a slightly lower risk was observed for the highest quartiles of consumption of fruit and fruit juices, while no reductions in risk were associated with vegetables, foods of animal origin, complex carbohydrates, legumes, or folacin-rich foods. When nutrient indices were derived, significant trends of decreasing risk were observed for vitamin C (adjusted odds ratio (OR) = 0.69 for the highest vs. the lowest quartile; p for trend = 0.003), beta-carotene (OR = 0.68; p = 0.02), and other carotenoids (OR = 0.61; p = 0.003). However, the associations were driven by associations restricted to two of the study sites and among women of higher socioeconomic status. Furthermore, adjustment for HPV infection was not possible given the limitations of the assay employed, leaving open the possibility of selection bias, effects of unidentified aspects of dietary patterns or residual confounding by HPV.

In a subgroup of 387 cases and 670 controls we evaluated the association with risk of eight micronutrients.[17] The serologic analyses were restricted to a sample of subjects with stage I and II disease to minimize effects of the disease on the serologic markers. Blood samples were analyzed for carotenoids, retinol, and tocopherols by high-pressure liquid chromatography. Cases did not differ significantly from controls in mean serum levels of retinol, cryptoxanthin, lycopene, alpha-carotene, lutein, or alpha-tocopherol. The mean level of beta-carotene was lower and the mean level of gamma-tocopherol was higher among cases as compared with controls. In multivariate models, a trend of decreasing risk was associated with higher levels of beta-carotene (p for trend = 0.05), with the adjusted odds ratio decreasing to 0.72 for the highest versus the lowest quartile. Beta-carotene results were similar by stage of disease, arguing against an effect of disease progression on nutrient values. Unexpectedly, increasing risks were observed as the level of gamma-tocopherol increased (odds ratio = 2.09; p for trend = 0.03); however, levels were higher among stage II cases as compared with stage I cases, suggesting a metabolic alteration resulting from the disease process. The concordance in the strength and direction of the blood and dietary results was

TABLE 18.2 Relative risks of invasive cervical cancer associated with monogamous women's male partners—in terms of the male partners' education, sexual behavior, and physical examination results.

	PARTNERS OF PATIENTS	PARTNERS OF CONTROLS	RR	95% CI
Education:				
≥ 10 years	26	92	1.0[1]	
7–9 years	27	53	1.8	0.9–3.4
4–6 years	76	182	1.6	0.9–2.7
1–3 years	56	118	2.0	1.1–3.6
None	19	40	2.2	1.0–4.8
Number of sex partners:				
1–5	39	128	1.0[2]	
6–10	53	128	1.4	0.9–2.3
11–25	54	125	1.5	0.9–2.5
≥26	58	104	2.0	1.2–3.4
p for trend			0.005	
Age at first sexual contact:				
≥18	57	151	1.0[3]	
16–17	50	137	0.8	0.5–1.3
14–15	69	133	1.1	0.7–1.7
<4	28	64	0.9	0.5–1.5
Number of visits to prostitutes:				
None	63	156	1.0	
<50	50	97	1.3	0.8–2.0
50–249	23	67	0.7	0.4–1.3
≥250	55	128	0.8	0.5–1.3
Unknown	13	37	1.0	0.5–2.0
Circumcised (data from physical examination):				
No	157	362	1.0	
Yes	47	123	0.9	0.6–1.3
Presence of smegma:				
No	150	381	1.0	
Yes	48	79	1.5	1.0–2.3
Unknown	6	25	0.6	0.2–1.6

[1] Adjusted for age (mean age of patients' partners = 49.2 years and controls' partners = 49.6 years) and number of sex partners.

[2] Adjusted for age and years of education.

[3] Adjusted for age, years of education, and number of sex partners.

considered supportive of a role for beta-carotene or foods rich in beta-carotene in the etiology of cervical cancer. The study also indicated that simultaneous analysis using serologic and dietary nutrient indicators allows better discrimination of the association.

Similarly, specimens were analyzed for folate concentrations by radioassay.[18] Cases did not differ significantly from controls in mean levels of folate (5.00 and 4.90 ng/ml, respectively). No associations were observed between quartiles of serum folate and risk of cervical cancer after adjustment for other risk factors, and no interactions with established risk factors were observed; thus findings did not support a role for serum folate in the etiology of invasive cervical cancer.

The fact that we recruited community controls that were matched on age and geographical region to the cases allowed an ecologic analysis of risk factors to explore the explanation of the vast differences in incidence of cervical cancer in Costa Rica.[19] The coastal areas have traditionally much higher incidence than the central, more developed areas, according to data gathered by the Costa Rica National Tumor Registry. We used the prevalence of specific risk factors, including HPV, using our FISH assay to compare between regions at high and low risk of cervical cancer. This ecological analysis, based on a survey of data from individuals, established that the main explanation was a difference in screening practices and not a difference in sexual behavior (number of sexual partners or age at first intercourse) or HPV detection. This lack of association with HPV could be related to the limited sensitivity and specificity of the testing assay.

An article describing epidemiological considerations for conducting case-control studies in 4 developing countries was also produced, emphasizing advantages and disadvantages of case-control studies.[20] Among the advantages we discussed the high participation rate of these populations that have limited access to medical care and see in their participation an opportunity to receive high quality care. Among the disadvantages we discussed the lack of experienced staff for this kind of studies and the limited expertise for handling contractual issues, in addition to the difficulties of communication and transportation, which can be overcome with appropriate training and supervision. The positive experience with this study set the stage for the continued collaboration of the Costa Rican and NCI investigators.

THE HPV NATURAL HISTORY STUDY (GUANACASTE PROJECT)

This study originated in discussions between the Costa Rican and US investigators after the success of the Latin American case-control study and was designed with the purpose of investigating the natural history of HPV infection and cervical neoplasia, in addition to evaluating a series of new screening techniques. The initial plan was to include two high incidence areas of Costa Rica, namely the Limon Province on the Caribbean area, and Guanacaste, an area in the northwest of the country. However, a major earthquake that seriously disrupted communications and demographics in the former made us decide to conduct it only in Guanacaste, a rural area with perennially high rates of invasive cervical cancer (around 30 per 100,000 women in the 1980s). From the beginning, the study received enthusiastic support from the local authorities, who facilitated the use of tens of clinics spread around the Province, provided office space and made the study part of medical care in the area.

The design was a prospective cohort study and a detailed publication of methods has been published.[21] We recruited approximately 20% of the entire female adult population of the Province, identified by a census conducted with the collaboration of the vast network of outreach workers from the Ministry of Health of Costa Rica. After proper training by our demographer and census supervisors, they visited every house in 20% of randomly selected censal segments in the Province and developed a list of women older than 18 years of age, including their address and other contact details. A total of 11742 women constituted the target for the population-based cohort (Figure 18.2).

Women in the sample were invited via a personal letter, and for those who accepted to participate, a private standardized interview on demographic, socioeconomic, sexual, medical, reproductive, and smoking history was administered and collection of blood and specimens for HPV testing was carried out. Nurses with special training conducted a pelvic exam on all women reporting previous sexual intercourse, including a physical exam and referral to colposcopy in case of obvious abnormalities suggestive of cancer. In addition, pH measurement and cervical cells for conventional and liquid-based cytology and HPV testing were obtained. After collection of cells, the cervix was rinsed with 5% acetic acid and two photographic images of the cervix were taken (Cervigrams). The film was sent periodically to National testing Laboratories in the United States for developing, processing, and evaluation. Finally, each participant was asked to donate blood that was centrifuged the same day and aliquotted into plasma, buffy coats and red blood cells. Several cytology readings were available from each woman, conventional cytology read in Costa Rica, liquid based cytology read in the United States and automated cytology read in the United States (same slides as conventional). Women with abnormalities in cytology or in the Cervigram were referred to colposcopy, biopsies and treatment as needed. After pathology and cytology review in the United States, a final baseline diagnosis was established for each woman.

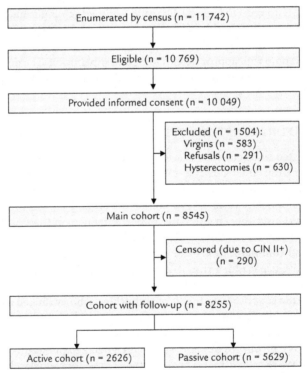

FIGURE 18.2 Consort diagram of the natural history study. *(Adapted from Castle et al., BMJ 2009;339:b2569) CIN: cervical intraepithelial neoplasia.*

A total of 10,049 women were recruited with a participation rate of 94% for all components of the study (Figure 18.2). Detailed procedures and field manuals were elaborated and the field work strictly supervised. This extremely high participation rate was the result of (1) the use of multiple local clinics spread all over the Province that allowed relatively easy access of women, (2) the deployment of extensive resources for invitation of women and their transportation, (3) the recruitment of only female nurses to conduct the examinations, (4) the difficulties often experienced by the women to obtain preventive care within the health system in Guanacaste, (5) the natural good will and interest of the community, (6) the extensive support of the local health authorities, (7) the extraordinary dedication of the staff, and (8) our conviction that in this population, being part of the study was a definitive benefit for women and prevention of cervical cancer.

Despite the relatively large number of participants, the number of prevalent cervical cancers was expected to be low. Therefore, to increase the numbers of this outcome, we also recruited all cases diagnosed in the province during the period when the main cohort was enrolled, and obtained from them as much information and specimens as possible (using the same protocol as for all women in the cohort). For the analyses including these cases, the entire population-based cohort was a totally appropriate control group as it represents the population from which cases originated.

Based on the final diagnosis given to each woman at the end of the enrollment phase, active follow-up of several subcohorts was carried out. All women with suspected CIN2 or worse were censored from the study regardless of whether CIN2 was confirmed. Detailed description of the followup design and procedures has been published.[22] Women considered to be at higher risk of developing CIN2+ were followed actively, including those with 5 or more sexual partners, abnormal enrollment cytology, HPV infection as determined by an early Hybrid Capture assay, and a random group of the rest of the cohort. Procedures and specimen collection during follow up were similar to recruitment procedures. Retention in the study during follow up was high, with more than 90% continued participation.

The main test used for HPV DNA testing was the MY09/M11 L1 degenerate primer polymerase chain reaction (PCR) method. Dot blot hybridization of PCR products for HPV genotype specific detection was conducted for low and high risk HPV types.

This epidemiological study has generated ample information on multiple aspects of the natural history of HPV infection. Based on recruitment data alone, several publications analyzed the epidemiology of HPV infection and disease using interview data and diverse biomarkers, in addition to the performance of multiple screening methods.

Overall HPV prevalence was 26.5%, with 13.7% of oncogenic types and 17.5% of non oncogenic types.[23] Prevalence of HPV had a peculiar U-shape with a peak of 36.9% among women <25 years, declining to about 20% in middle ages and increasing again to 31.4% after age 65 (Figure 18.3).[24] The second peak was more pronounced for the nononcogenic HPV types. The most common oncogenic HPV type in the general population was HPV 16 (prevalence of 3.6%), followed by HPV 58 (prevalence of 2.0%).

Risk factors for HPV infection were mainly those related to sexual behavior both of the women and, in the case of monogamous women, the behavior of their sexual partners as reported by the women. Risk factors were similar for oncogenic and nononcogenic HPV types. Multiple infections were very common, particularly in young women among whom almost 30% had more than one HPV type detected.

An interesting finding had to do with the HPV type distribution among women who did not have an intact uterus.[25] They tended to have a similar overall prevalence of HPV as women with an intact uterus, but in women after hysterectomy, there was an increased

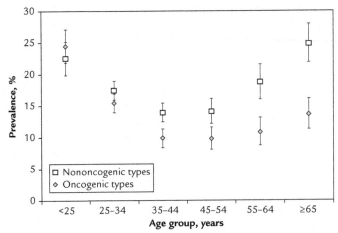

FIGURE 18.3 Prevalences of oncogenic human papillomavirus (HPV) types (16, 18, 26, 31, 33, 35, 39, 45, 51, 52, 56, 58, 59, 66, 68, 73, and AE2 [82 subtype]) and nononcogenic HPV types (2, 6, 11, 13, 26, 32, 34, 40, 42–44, 53–55, 57, 61, 62, 64, 67–72, 74, AE10 [74 variant], 81–85, 89, and AE9), by age group. Bars indicate binomial exact 95% confidence intervals. (Herrero et al., IJD 2005;191:1796–807).

detection of nononcogenic types, suggesting that nononcogenic types may have a specific tropism for the vaginal epithelium.[26]

HPV serology for types 16, 18, 31 and 45 was also investigated using an early ELISA method.[27] Seropositivity for these HPV types was between 10% and 15%, and only between 28% and 51% of women infected with HPV DNA at the cervix was positive for antibodies against the corresponding HPV type. The prevalence of antibodies against HPV 16, 18, 31 and 45 by age had an inverted u shape, being lowest among women under 25 and maximum in middle age, with a subsequent decline after age 50 (Figure 18.4). The determinants of serologic conversion and seropersistence of antibodies against HPV 16 were also investigated prospectively.[28] Overall, 55% of women who were seropositive at enrollment remained seropositive after 5–7 years of follow up. Seropersistence tended to be similar by age, but seroconversion was much more common among younger than among older women.

We also investigated if natural antibodies conferred protection against reinfection with the same HPV type[29] We tested for the presence of antibodies against HPV16, 18, and 31 using an ELISA method and calculated ORs for detection of same-type HPV infection during follow up. In this analysis, there was no clear evidence of protection against any of the viruses. However, as will be described later, with the more recent testing methods the results are different.[30]

In terms of associations of HPV with disease, we confirmed the presence of HPV in 97% of women with cancers and precursor lesions as compared to 22% of normal women.[23] HPV type distribution was similar by age group. Multiple infections were very common and analyses to investigate possible interactions between the different types indicated that infections with different HPV types are independent of each other,[31] a finding consistent with a similar analysis in the vaccine trial cohort.[32]

In the context of this study, we were able to investigate cofactors of HPV with adjustment for the presence of the virus. This was accomplished by restricting the analyses to cases and controls that were HPV positive. As mentioned before, we detected similar cofactors

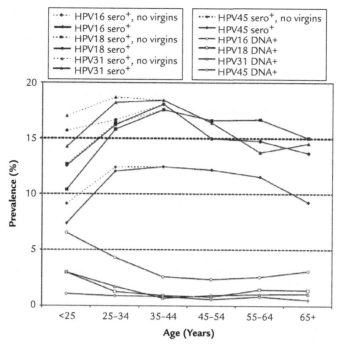

FIGURE 18.4 Age distribution of HPV-16, -18, -31, and -45 seroprevalence* and DNA-prevalence** in Guanacaste, Costa Rica women. *Populationbased HPV-16, -18, -31, and -45 serology prevalence is shown in black lines and includes study virgins. Black dotted lines denote seroprevalence excluding study virgins. **HPV DNA prevalence does not include study virgins. (Wang et al., British Journal of Cancer 2003;89:1248–1254). HPV: Human papillomavirus.

when adjusting for HPV in this manner as we had found in the case-control study without adjustment. Smoking, oral contraceptives (among women reporting fewer than 3 children), and increasing number of children were the main cofactors identified in the enrollment phase of the cohort study.[33] In addition, we investigated the possible role of inflammation as a cofactor by comparing cases of high grade lesions with controls that were HPV positive among women under 50 years of age.[34] Inflammation was assessed by counting the number of neutrophils in cervical cytology slides (Nugent score), and those with high numbers of neutrophils were categorized as having cervicitis, which was associated with a 2-fold increase in risk of CIN2+, suggesting the importance of inflammation as a cofactor.

Within the same HPV type, variants have been described when they present genomic differences with the prototype of less than 10%. We investigated risk associated with non-European variants of HPV 16 and detected a 3-fold higher risk of high-grade squamous intraepithelial lesion (HSIL) and an 11-fold higher risk of cancer when compared to the European variants.[35]

Another important area of our research has been the role of host genetics on risk of cervical precursors and cancer, in particular those related to immune mechanisms that may determine the ability of the host to deal with HPV infections (e.g., HLAs). Compared with women who were HPV negative, women with HLA-RRB1*1301 were associated with a 60% reduction in risk for cancer /HSIL and for LSIL/HPV. On the contrary, women with both HLA-B07 and HLA-DQB1*0302 had an 8-fold increase in risk of cancer and a 5-fold increase in risk of LSIL/HPV, indicating that multiple alleles may be needed to increase risk of cancer but a single allele may be enough for protection.[36]

Prospectively, we have conducted several analyses to investigate the fate of HPV infections. For example, we investigated outcomes of 800 carcinogenic HPV infections detected in 599 study participants. For individual infections, we calculated cumulative proportions of three outcomes (viral clearance, persistence without progression to CIN2+, and persistence with a newly diagnosed CIN2+) at successive 6-month time points for the first 30 months of follow-up.[37] Infections typically cleared rapidly, with 67% (95%CI = 63–70%) clearing by 12 months (Figure 18.5). However, among infections that persisted at least 6 months, the risk of CIN2+ diagnosis by 30 months was 21% (95% CI = 15–28%). The risk of CIN2+ was highest for women under 30 years of age with HPV 16 infections that persisted for more than 12 months (Figure 18.6).

We also evaluated the risk of subsequent disease associated with short- term persistence of HPV by calculating the 3-year and 5-year cumulative incidence of CIN2+ (n = 70) among 2282 women actively followed after enrollment.[38] Those who tested positive for a carcinogenic HPV at enrollment and after about one year (9–21 months) (positive/positive) had a 3-year cumulative incidence of CIN2+ of 17% (95% CI = 12.1–22.0%). Those who tested negative/positive (3.4%, 0.1–6.8), positive/negative (1.2%, –0.2–2.5%) and negative / negative (0.5%, 0.1–0.9) were at significantly lower risk. There was little difference in the cumulative incidence of CIN2+ between testing positive twice for any carcinogenic HPV type (same genotype or different genotypes) vs testing positive twice for the same carcinogenic HPV type (17.3% vs 21.0%, respectively). Short term persistence of HPV 16 strongly predicted CIN2+, with a 3-year cumulative incidence of 40.8% (26.4 to 55.1). Similar patterns were observed for the 5-year cumulative incidence of CIN2+ and CIN3+.

A group of 410 virgins under 26 years of age at enrollment provided an opportunity to investigate the acquisition and early natural history of HPV infections. They were followed every 6 months and the first time they reported sexual activity they had a pelvic exam and specimens were collected. Kaplan Meier curves of acquisition of infection were generated using standard methods. During the 5 year observation period, a 40% cumulative incidence was observed (Figure 18.7).[39]

As part of the investigation of the natural history, we investigated a group of long- term persistent infections that did not progress to cancer precursor lesions. We studied a group of 810 initially HPV positive women with at least 3 years of active follow-up, at least 3 screening visits and no evidence of cervical neoplasia.[40] Seventy-two prevalent infections in 58 women persisted until the end of the follow-up period (median follow-up of 7 years) without evidence of cervical precancer. At enrollment, women with long term persistence were more likely to have multiple prevalently detected HPV infections (p<0.001) than women who cleared their infections during follow-up. They were also more likely to have another newly detected HPV infection.

The risks of persistence and neoplastic progression to cancer and CIN3, differ markedly by HPV type. To study type-specific HPV natural history, we wished to separate viral persistence from neoplastic progression.[41] We observed a strong concordance of newly revised HPV evolutionary groupings with the separate risks of persistence and progression to CIN3/cancer. HPV16 was uniquely likely both to persist and to cause neoplastic progression when it persisted, underscoring its strong carcinogenic potential. Specifically, 19.9% of HPV16-infected women were diagnosed with CIN3/cancer at enrollment or during the five-year follow-up. Other carcinogenic types, many related to HPV16, were not particularly persistent but could cause neoplastic progression, at lower rates than HPV16, if they did persist. Some low-risk types were persistent but, nevertheless, virtually never

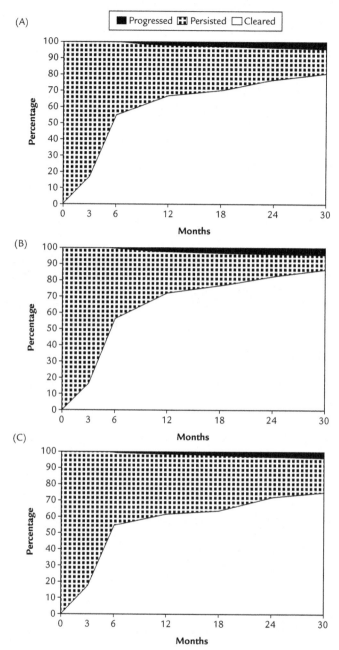

FIGURE 18.5 Clearance of carcinogenic human papillomavirus (HPV) infections during 30 months of follow-up. (A) All ages combined (n = 800 infections). (B) Women younger than 30 years (n = 393 infections). (C) Women aged 30 years or older (n = 407 infections). Carcinogenic types include HPV types 16, 18, 26, 31, 33, 35, 39, 45, 51, 52, 56, 58, 59, 66, 68, 73, 82, 82v. The x-axes represent months of follow-up, and the y-axes represent the percentage of infections that cleared (unshaded), persisted without evidence of cervical intraepithelial neoplasia grade 2 or worse (CIN2+; stippled), or persisted with evidence of CIN2+ (solid shading). The 3-month data represent nonrandom samples (36% for A, 38% for B, and 34% for C). (Rodriguez et al, J Natl Cancer Inst 2008;100: 513–517)

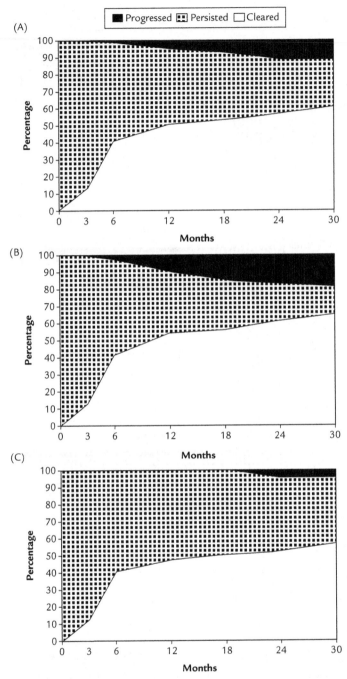

FIGURE 18.6 Clearance of human papillomavirus type 16 infections during 30 months of follow-up. (A) All ages combined (n = 115 infections). (B) Women younger than 30 years (n = 55 infections). (C) Women aged 30 years or older (n = 60 infections). The x-axes represent months of follow-up, and the y-axes represent the percentage of infections that cleared (**unshaded**), persisted without evidence of cervical intraepithelial neoplasia grade 2 or worse (CIN2+) (**stippled**), or persisted with evidence of CIN2+ (**solid shading**). The 3-month data represent nonrandom samples (38% for **A**, 44% for **B**, and 33% for **C**). *(Rodriguez et al, J Natl Cancer Inst 2008;100: 513–517)*

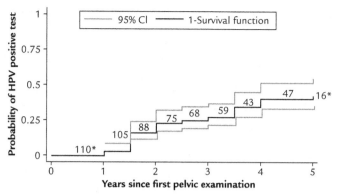

FIGURE 18.7 Human papillomavirus (HPV) infection acquisition among women who were HPV-negative at the time of the first pelvic examination after recent sexual debut. *Number of women at risk at the time period. Kaplan-Meier estimate. *(Rodriguez et al., Sexually Transmitted Diseases 2007;34(7):494–502)*

caused CIN3. Therefore, carcinogenicity is not strictly a function of persistence. Separately, we noted that the carcinogenic HPV types code for an E5 protein, whereas most low-risk types either lack a definable homologous E5 ORF and/or a translation start codon for E5. These results presented several clear clues and research directions to understand HPV carcinogenesis.

We also studied HPV variants prospectively,[42] exploring whether, on average, the oldest evolutionary branches within each carcinogenic type predicted different risks of ≥2-year viral persistence and/or precancer and cancer (CIN3+), using a nested case-control design. Infections were assigned to a variant lineage determined by phylogenetic parsimony methods based on URR/E6 sequences. We used the Fisher's combination test to evaluate significance of the risk associations, cumulating evidence across types. Globally, for HPV types including HPV16, the p-value was 0.01 for persistence and 0.07 for CIN3+. Excluding HPV16, the p-values were 0.04 and 0.37, respectively. For HPV16, non-European viral variants were significantly more likely than European variants to cause persistence (OR = 2.6, p = 0.01) and CIN3+ (OR = 2.4, p = 0.004). HPV35 and HPV51 variant lineages also predicted CIN3+. Our conclusion was that HPV variants generally differ in risk of persistence. For some HPV types, especially HPV16, variant lineages differ in risk of CIN3+. The findings indicate that continued evolution of HPV types has led to even finer genetic discrimination linked to HPV natural history and cervical cancer risk and that larger viral genomic studies are warranted, especially to identify the genetic basis for HPV16's unique carcinogenicity.

For the evaluation of screening methods used at enrollment, all women with abnormalities in any of the 3 cytologic modalities, visual inspection or cervigram, but not HPV positive women, were referred to colposcopy and final diagnosis. The final diagnosis was used as the gold standard to evaluate the performance of each screening method. Conventional cytology using atypical squamous cells of undetermined significance (ASCUS) as a cut point for referral resulted in 77.7% sensitivity and 94.2% specificity, with 6.9% of women referred to colposcopy.

For the Hybrid capture 2 method of HPV testing, the data permitted the evaluation of the ideal cut point for maximizing sensitivity and specificity of the assay using receiver operating characteristics analysis.[43] An analytic sensitivity of 1.0 pg/mL would have permitted detection of 89% of 138 high-grade lesions and cancers (all 12 cancers were HPV-positive), with colposcopic referral of 12.3% of women. The higher detection threshold of 10 pg/mL used with the original assay had a sensitivity of 74.8% and a specificity of 93.4%. Lower levels of detection with the second generation assay (<1 pg/mL) proved clinically nonspecific without gains in diagnostic sensitivity. This generated the conclusion that the cut point of 1.0 pg/mL permits sensitive detection of cervical high-grade lesions and cancer, yielding an apparently optimal trade-off between high sensitivity and reasonable specificity for this test.

For liquid-based cytology (ThinPrep),[44] there were significantly more women referred (12.7%) than with the conventional smear (6.7% in this analysis, P<0.001). Referral by ThinPrep slides detected 92.9% of cases with high grade squamous intraepithelial lesions (HSIL) and 100% of carcinoma cases. Conventional smears detected 77.8% of HSIL and 90.9% of carcinomas. Thus, liquid based cytology was significantly more sensitive in the detection of HSIL and cancer (McNemar test, P<0.001). Adjudication of cases in which the ThinPrep and smear diagnoses disagreed, using the final case diagnoses and the HPV DNA test results as reference standards, suggested that the ThinPrep method was detecting additional true SIL as opposed to false-positives. We concluded that liquid based cytology increased sensitivity at the expense of specificity. An important caveat of this analysis is that liquid based cytology was read by experts in the US while conventional cytology was read by the local pathologist.

The results of Cervigrams from 8460 women were also compared with the referent diagnosis and with the performance of conventional cytology.[45] Cervicography identified all 11 cancers, whereas cytologic testing missed 1. Cervicography yielded sensitivities for detecting high-grade squamous intraepithelial lesions or cancer of 49.3% overall (specificity, 95.0%), 54.6% in women younger than 50 years of age, and 26.9% in women 50 years of age and older. In contrast, sensitivity of cytology was 77.2% overall (specificity, 94. 2%), 75.5% in women younger than 50 years of age, and 84.6% in women 50 years of age and older. We concluded that cytology performed better than cervicography for the detection of high-grade squamous intraepithelial lesions and that cervicography should not be recommended for postmenopausal women.

We also assessed the screening performance of direct visual inspection with acetic acid and x2 magnification (VIAM) in our previously screened population, as performed by experienced gynecologic nurses with minimal training in VIAM.[46] Performance of VIAM was evaluated in 2080 women, 5 years after negative enrollment results of conventional and liquid-based cytologic analysis, cervigram, and human papillomavirus DNA by Hybrid Capture tube test. The VIAM results were compared with repeat conventional Pap smears, liquid-based cytologic examinations, and cervicography, with adjudication of differences by reference to MY09/MY11 L1 consensus primer PCR detection of oncogenic HPV DNA. Less than 5% of women were classified as having positive results using VIAM. The VIAM positivity was also very low among women with high-grade squamous intraepithelial lesion conventional Pap smear results (8.3%), high-grade squamous intraepithelial lesion liquid-based cytologic results (6.3%), or cervigrams suggesting cervical intraepithelial neoplasia 2–3 or cancer (30%). The VIAM positivity was not associated with human papillomavirus DNA positivity. We concluded that, as we practiced it, VIAM was not sensitive for detection of possibly serious incident cervical lesions in this previously screened population where cytologic screening is in place.

There are two articles describing the methodology employed in this study, emphasizing advantages and disadvantages of prospective studies.[21,22] Among the advantages are the highly cooperative population, relatively low costs, and direct applicability of the findings to a region where cervical cancer is common. Although Guanacaste is a relatively poor area of Costa Rica, the infrastructure was adequate for the logistics of a study like this one. In addition, local health authorities recognized the importance of this activity and offered full collaboration. Furthermore, it was possible to recruit educated and enthusiastic personnel, most of the roads were in good condition and there were excellent radio and telephone communication systems.

Among the disadvantages was the dearth of experienced investigators and adminis-trators, particularly with regard to contract negotiation and management, a situation that hampered the process of establishing the contract and initiating disbursement of funds. Another major difficulty was the preparation of equipments and materials, many of which were imported from the United States. The process of their importation and timely release from customs was a source of delays and additional cost. It was sometimes difficult to stan-dardize procedures, particularly laboratory methods that were unfamiliar to the staff. The tracking and shipment of thousands of biological specimens was a nearly overwhelming task, given the multiple requisites and permits established by the governments and airlines (and this was before September 11, 2011). Despite the difficulties, participation rates were almost 95%, not only for the interview component but for the exams and sample collec-tions. Also the existence of a census office and detailed political divisions made it possible to conduct a population-based census, which together with the almost complete participa-tion rates lend certainty to the claim that this is a true population-based cohort.

As has been demonstrated this collaboration produced a large number of high impact publications that have provided important knowledge on the natural history of HPV infec-tion and cervical neoplasia. The preparation and writing of manuscripts was done in col-laboration and under the leadership of both US and Costa Rica investigators, who have benefited largely from the learning experience. Currently we have plans to re-invite selected parts of the cohort for evaluation of the fate of HPV infections after 20 years of follow-up.

ANCILLARY STUDIES

After the cohort completed follow-up around the year 2000, we started preparations for an evaluation of the newly developed HPV vaccines, considering all the knowledge about HPV epidemiology and technical capacity developed in Guanacaste. However, there were important delays in the initiation of the vaccine trial and ,therefore, we designed additional studies among selected subcohorts of interest to address a series of hypotheses generated during the analysis of the natural history study. These studies were conducted after their individual approval by NCI and Costa Rican IRBs and all participants signed new informed consents for each of them.

The "Older Women Study"

This study was designed to further investigate the second peak in HPV prevalence observed among women older than 45 years of age in the natural history study. All women from the cohort in this age range, who were HPV positive at their 5–7 year visit and an equiva-lent number of HPV negative controls, frequency-matched to cases on age and time since enrollment, were asked to attend the study clinic (at their 7th to 9th anniversary of enroll-ment) for an additional study visit. At that visit, a questionnaire was given, cervical cells were collected for conventional and liquid-based cytology, additional cells were collected for PCR-based HPV DNA testing, and 40 mL of blood were collected in heparinized tubes from which peripheral blood mononuclear cells (PBMC) were isolated and cryopreserved. Cases (n = 324) and controls (n = 310) were selected for this study. Of these, 298 cases (92.0%) and 293 controls (94.5%) participated. Among these 591 participants, blood was successfully collected, cryopreserved, and tested for all but seven participants (5 cases and 2 controls). An additional nine cases with high-grade cervical disease were excluded, resulting in a final number of 284 cases and 291 controls for analysis. The median time between enrollment and the follow-up visit was 61 months for both cases and controls (57–98 months).

Proliferative responses to phytohemagglutinin (PHA), influenza virus (Flu), and HPV16 virus-like particles (VLP) were lower among women with persistent HPV infection [median counts per minute (cpm): 72,849 for PHA, 1241 for Flu, and 727 for VLP] than for the control group (median cpm: 107,049 for PHA, 2111 for Flu, and 2068 for VLP). The decreases were most profound in women with long-term persistence and were only observed for the oldest age group (≥65 years), indicating that an impairment in host immunologic responses was associated with persistent HPV infection. The fact that effects were evident for all studied proliferative responses was considered suggestive of a generalized effect.

Similarly, in order to characterize the phenotype of peripheral lymphocytes associated with persistent HPV infection,[47] we evaluated the expression of different cell surface markers in the PBMCs detected by immunological phenotyping via flow cytometry. Significant increases in risk of HPV persistence were observed for 3 marker subsets indicative of immune cell activation/differentiation. Relative risk estimates were 5.4 (95% CI = 2.2–13.3) for CD69(+)CD4(+), 2.6 (95% CI = 1.2–5.9) for HLADR(+)CD3(+)CD4(+) and 2.3 (95% CI = 1.1–4.7) for CD45RO(+)CD27(–)CD8(+). A significant decrease in HPV persistence was observed for a subset marker indicative of an immature, undifferentiated memory state CD45RO(+)CD27(+)CD4(+) (OR = 0.36; 95% CI = 0.17–0.76). Adjustment for these markers only partially explained the association between decreased lymphoproliferative responses and persistent HPV infection. We could not determine whether phenotypic alterations observed predispose to HPV persistence or result from it.

Detailed sexual behavior was also investigated.[48] Women with 2+ lifetime partners had 1.7-fold (95% CI = 1.1–2.7) higher risk than monogamous women, with similar findings if their partners had other partners. Women with 2+ partners after their last HPV-negative result had the highest risk (OR = 3.9; 95% CI = 1.2–12.4 compared with 0–1 partners). Among women with no sexual activity in the period before HPV appearance, reduced immune response to phytohemagglutinin was the only determinant (OR = 2.9; 95% CI = 0.94–8.8). We concluded that new infections among older women may result from sexual activity of women and/or their partners or reappearance of past (latent) infections possibly related to weakened immune response.

The "HSIL" Study

Risk of recurrent CIN2+ (including cervical intraepithelial neoplasia grade 2 [CIN2], CIN3, carcinoma and in situ, adenocarcinoma in situ or cancer) remains elevated for years following treatment. The HSIL study was designed to evaluate the role of long-term posttreatment HPV presence on subsequent risk of CIN2+ in the cohort. During enrollment and follow-up, 681 women were referred to colposcopy because of high-grade cytology, positive cervicography and/or suspicion of cancer based on visual assessment; 486 were judged to require treatment. After excluding women with <12 months of follow-up (N = 88), prior cancer or hysterectomy (n = 37) or other reasons (N = 14), 347 were included in the analysis. Infections were categorized as persistent if present at both pretreatment and post-treatment visits and new if detected only post-treatment. Median time between the treatment and post-treatment visits was 6.7 years (IQR 3.8 to 7.8). At the post-treatment visit, 8 (2.4%), 2 (0.6%), and 8 (2.4%) of the 347 treated women had persistent HPV16, HPV18, or other carcinogenic HPV, respectively. Two (0.8%), 3 (1.0%), and 14 (4.0%) had new HPV16, HPV18, and other carcinogenic HPV, respectively. Six CIN2+ cases were identified at the post-treatment visit, all with persistent infections (three HPV16, one HPV18, and two other carcinogenic HPV). No recurrent disease was observed among women with new HPV infections during the follow-up period. Thus, persistence of HPV infection a median of six years after treatment was uncommon but, when present, posed a substantial risk of subsequent CIN2+.[49]

The Genetic Susceptibility (GSS) Study

The GSS study was undertaken to investigate a series of host genetic factors potentially associated with risk of HPV persistent infection or cervical abnormalities. We selected (1) all women from the cohort with histologically confirmed prevalent or incident CIN3 or cancer ($n = 184$); (2) all women with evidence of HPV persistence, defined as women who tested positive for the same HPV type at 2 consecutive visits ($n = 432$; median duration of persistence, 25 months [range, 5–93 months]); and (3) a random selection of control subjects from the population based cohort ($n = 492$). We also identified additional individuals from Guanacaste who received a diagnosis of CIN3 or cancer during the period in which our cohort study was conducted (hereafter referred to as "supplemental case patients"). These supplemental case patients were initially identified from review of the Costa Rican National Tumor Registry and review of cytology listings from the National Cytology Laboratory in Costa Rica, followed by review of hospital and/or pathology records to verify that they had had histologically confirmed CIN3. Of 448 women identified as eligible, 331 (74%) of the women were included as supplemental case patients (median age, 42 years; range, 20–89 years). Twenty milliliters of peripheral blood were collected from the enrolled supplemental case patients, and DNA was extracted from one 10-mL tube.

From our initial analysis, we genotyped 92 single-nucleotide polymorphisms (SNPs) from 49 candidate immune response and DNA repair genes obtained from women with CIN3 or cancer, persistent HPV infections and random controls, calculating odds ratios and 95% confidence intervals (CIs) for the association of SNP and haplotypes.[50] A SNP in the Fanconi anemia complementation group A gene (FANCA) (G501S) was associated with increased risk of CIN3 or cancer. The AG and GG genotypes had a 1.3-fold (95% CI, 0.95–1.8-fold) and 1.7–fold (95% CI, 1.1–2.6-fold) increased risk for CIN3 or cancer, respectively (P(trend) = .008; referent, AA). The FANCA haplotype that included G501S also conferred increased risk of CIN3 or cancer, as did a different haplotype that included 2 other FANCA SNPs (G809A and T266A). A SNP in the innate immune gene IRF3 (S427T) was associated with increased risk for HPV persistence (P(trend) = .009). These results were considered to require replication but to support the role of FANCA variants in cervical cancer susceptibility and of IRF3 in HPV persistence.

Driven by findings that human papillomavirus (HPV)-induced degradation of p53 differs by a TP53 polymorphism at codon 72 (Pro72Arg), past studies of TP53 genetic variants and cervical cancer have focused on this nonsynonymous polymorphism, with mixed results,[51,52] we analyzed 11 common single nucleotide polymorphisms (SNP) across the TP53 locus in the GSS study.[53] We combined HPV persistence and CIN3+ into one case group because they did not differ in TP53 genotypic frequencies and calculated odds ratios and 95% confidence intervals (CI) for individual SNPs and inferred haplotypes. We observed that proline at codon 72 was associated with increased risk of CIN3+/persistence compared with population controls. Relative to GG (Arg), the CG (Pro/Arg) and CC (Pro) genotypes had a 1.3-fold (95% CI, 0.99–1.6) and 1.8-fold (95% CI, 1.2–2.7) increased risk, respectively (P(trend) < 0.01). rs12951053 and rs1642785 were also associated with CIN3+/persistence (P (trend), 0.05 and 0.04, respectively), as was a haplotype containing the codon 72 variant (rs1042522), rs12951053, rs1642785, and rs12947788 (odds ratio, 1.6; 95% CI, 1.1–2.3 versus the most common haplotype, which comprised the major alleles for all 11 SNPs). Although genetic variation in TP53 might affect the natural history of HPV and cervical cancer, further work was considered to be required to elucidate the possible mechanism.

Furthermore, we evaluated 7140 tag single nucleotide polymorphisms (SNPs) from 305 candidate genes hypothesized to be involved in DNA repair, viral infection and cell entry in the same population. We obtained pathway and gene-level summary of associations by computing the adaptive combination of p-values. Genes/regions statistically significantly associated with CIN3/cancer included the viral infection and cell entry genes 2′,5′ oligoadenylate synthetase gene 3 (OAS3), sulfatase 1 (SULF1), and interferon gamma (IFNG); the DNA repair genes deoxyuridine triphosphate (DUT), dosage suppressor of mck 1 homolog (DMC1), and general transcription factor IIH, polypeptide 3 (GTF2H4); and the EVER1 and EVER2 genes (p<0.01). From each region, the single most significant SNPs associated with CIN3/cancer were OAS3 rs12302655, SULF1 rs4737999, IFNG rs11177074, DUT rs3784621, DMC1 rs5757133, GTF2H4 rs2894054, EVER1/EVER2 rs9893818 (p-trends</=0.001). SNPs for OAS3, SULF1, DUT, and GTF2H4 were associated with HPV persistence whereas IFNG and EVER1/EVER2 SNPs were associated with progression to CIN3/cancer. However, the associations observed were less than two-fold. We identified variations in DNA repair, viral binding and cell entry genes associated with CIN3/cancer. Our results require replication but suggested that different genes may be responsible for modulating risk in the two critical transition steps important for cervical carcinogenesis: HPV persistence and disease progression.

The "Immunologic Study"

The objective of this analysis was to describe patterns and determinants of cervical immunoglobulin A (IgA) and G (IgG) levels during the menstrual cycle.[54] A total of 154 women who attended 3 visits coinciding with the follicular, periovulatory, and luteal phases of their menstrual cycle were studied. Cervical secretions were collected at each visit for determination of total IgA and IgG levels. Questionnaires administered at each visit inquired about demographic characteristics and behavioral practices. Total IgA and IgG levels were higher among oral contraceptive (OC) users than among naturally cycling women (hereafter, "non-OC users"). IgA and IgG levels decreased at midcycle, particularly among non-OC users (Figure 18.8). After adjustment for phase of the current cycle, specimen weight, and detection of blood in the sample, report of a recent illness was associated with lower IgA and IgG levels and increased age with higher IgA and IgG levels among OC users and non-OC users. Increased lifetime number of pregnancies was associated with a higher IgA level among non-OC users and a higher IgG level among OC users. Change in immunoglobulin levels between visits was associated with sample weight and the presence of blood for both OC users and non-OC users. Phase of the current menstrual cycle and OC use were significant determinants of cervical IgA and IgG levels. We considered that the impacts of endogenous and exogenous hormones on cervical immunoglobulin levels should be further investigated.

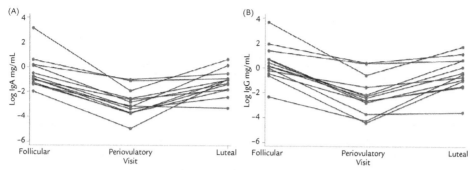

FIGURE 18.8 Patterns of log-transformed IgA levels (A) and IgG levels (B) among 13 women with a natural menstrual cycle in whom a surge in the luteinizing hormone level occurred on the day of the periovulatory visit. Median IgA levels were 0.39, 0.04, and 0.36 mg/mL during the follicular, periovulatory, and luteal visits, and median IgG levels were 1.14, 0.09, and 0.62 mg/mL, respectively. *(Safaeian et al., IJD 2009;199:445–63)*

▪ THE COSTA RICA HPV VACCINE TRIAL

The knowledge derived from these and many other studies clearly establishing the causal role of HPV in cervical cancer generated the expectation that a vaccine against HPV could be a useful tool to prevent this neoplasia. Investigators from the National Cancer Institute developed the virus-like particles (VLPs), composed of the main capsid protein of HPV (L1), which were tested in phase I and II studies demonstrating high antigenicity and acceptable safety.[55] Two prophylactic vaccines have been developed to date based on VLPs, the Merck vaccine (Gardasil®), which is a quadrivalent product against HPV types 6, 11, 16, and 18, adjuvanted with alum, and the GSK vaccine (Cervarix®), a bivalent product against HPV types 16 and 18 with a special adjuvant called ASO4 which is supposed to enhance the immune response. Both vaccine companies conducted large multicentric phase 3 trials that have now been completed and the two vaccines are licensed and broadly used worldwide, particularly in developed countries.

The Costa Rica Vaccine Trial (CVT) is a large, randomized double blind clinical trial to evaluate the efficacy of the bivalent vaccine. The study is an independent investigation started before licensure of the vaccine, funded by NCI and conducted under a clinical trials agreement with GSK. The planning and realization of such a study represented an important challenge for our study group given all the regulatory requisites associated with studies evaluating new products under an FDA IND (application for investigational new drug).

The study had ample support from the Ministry of Health of Costa Rica as well as from local health authorities and was conducted by the team of investigators of the Proyecto Epidemiologico Guanacaste (PEG). Some of the staff employed in the vaccine trial have been working continuously in our research projects for over 20 years.

The study was designed as a community-based clinical trial in which all women ages 18–25 in selected areas were invited to participate. Methodologic details have been published.[56] Prior to initiation of the study, a complete census of women 12–22 residing in the Province was conducted by the study staff in the year 2000. They visited all households in the province of Guanacaste and later on in selected areas of nearby Puntarenas, generating a target population in the age range of 18–25 at the time of recruitment of nearly 25,000 women (Figure 18.9).

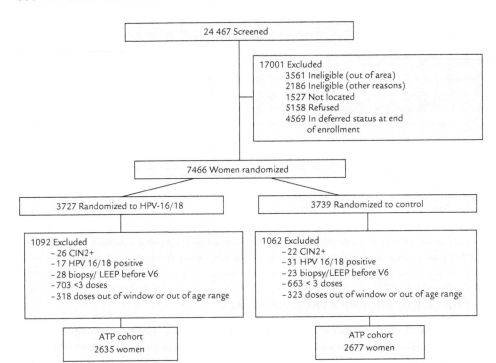

FIGURE 18.9 Consort diagram of the Costa Rica HPV vaccine trial. *HPV: Human papillomavirus; CIN: cervical intraepithelial neoplasia; LEEP: Loop electrical excision procedure; ATP: according to protocol.*

Potential participants were invited (June 2004–December 2005) to one of seven study clinics. After signing informed consent, an interview, medical history, physical exam and pregnancy test were conducted. For eligibility, women had to be healthy, not pregnant, not breastfeeding and using contraception during the vaccination period. Main exclusion criteria were chronic diseases, history of reactions to vaccines, and history of hepatitis A or vaccination against it. Women were recruited and randomized regardless of past sexual behavior, HPV status or cytology.

A pelvic exam was performed on sexually experienced women, collecting exfoliated cells in PreservCyt medium for cytology and HPV DNA testing. Blood was collected from all participants.

Participants were randomized with equal chance to Cervarix® or Hepatitis A vaccine. Each dose of the HPV16/18 vaccine contained HPV16 and HPV18 L1 virus-like-particle (20 μg of each) adjuvanted with 50 μg 3-O-desacyl-4′-monophosphoryl lipid A and 0.5 mg aluminum hydroxide. Each dose of the control hepatitis A vaccine contained 720 ELISA units (EU) of inactivated hepatitis A antigen and 0.5 mg aluminum hydroxide. Both were formulated in 0.5 ml doses with identical packaging and appearance to assure blinding. Vaccination schedule consisted of 3 doses at 0, 1 and 6 months. Desirable windows for vaccination defined periods beyond which the corresponding dose was not administered. At 6 months, sexually active women self-collected vaginal cells for HPV testing, with results comparable to clinician-collected specimens.

Each participant was scheduled for 4 annual follow-up examinations. Cytology was classified using the Bethesda system. Women with LSIL or HPV positive ASC-US were followed semi-annually for safety until obtaining 3 normal results. A repeat LSIL, HPV positive ASC-US, a single ASC-H, HSIL+ or glandular abnormalities prompted colposcopy and treatment as needed. Unsatisfactory cytology was managed as LSIL.

The study was approved and supervised by the IRBs of INCIENSA in Costa Rica and the NCI in the United States.

All participants were observed 30–60 minutes following vaccination. Adverse event and pregnancy information was actively collected during follow-up. An independent data and safety monitoring board (DSMB) met regularly during the study to examine unblinded adverse events and advise on trial continuation.

Broad spectrum PCR-based HPV DNA testing was performed at DDL Diagnostic Laboratory, based on amplification and probe hybridization using the SPF_{10} HPV DNA enzyme immunoassay (DEIA) system followed by typing using the $LiPA_{25}$ version 1 line detection system as described. To ensure that HPV16 and HPV18 infections were not missed, all specimens positive for HPV DNA using SPF_{10} DEIA but negative for HPV16 or HPV18 by $LiPA_{25}$ were also tested with type-specific primers/probes for the presence of HPV16 and HPV18 DNA.

ELISA was used for the detection and quantification of IgG antibodies against HPV16 and 18 separately by GSK as described.

A total of 7466 women participated in the study and have been followed for 4 years. In the main analysis,[57] evaluating efficacy against 1-year persistent infection (Median follow-up = 50.4 months), according-to-protocol (ATP) cohorts included compliant HPV-negative women. Intention-to-treat (ITT) cohorts included all randomized women. ATP vaccine efficacy (VE) was 90.9% (95%CI = 82.0, 95.9) against persistent HPV16/18 infections, 44.5% against HPV31/33/45 (95%CI = 17.5, 63.1) and 12.4% (95% CI = –3.5, 25.6) against any infection. ITT VE against HPV16/18 infections was 49.0% (95%CI = 38.1, 58.1). ATP efficacy was similar by age group, but ITT efficacy against HPV16/18 declined with age from 68.9% (95%CI = 53.1, 79.9) among 18–19 years old to 21.8% (95%CI = –16.9, 47.9) among 24–25 years old women. Similarly, ITT efficacy declined with time since first sexual intercourse and number of sexual partners (Figure 18.10). We concluded that vaccination is highly efficacious against HPV16/18 and affords partial protection against HPV31/33/45 among previously unexposed women, that efficacy among all women vaccinated decreases with age and sexual behavior with the implication that vaccination against HPV is most effective before initiation of sexual activity, which is important for vaccination programs and individual decisions.

Another important aspect we were particularly interested in is alternative delivery schedules for HPV vaccines, considering their high initial cost. Three-dose regimens for human papillomavirus (HPV) vaccines are expensive and difficult to complete, especially in low-resource environments where the need for cervical-cancer prevention is greatest. We evaluated vaccine efficacy (VE) of fewer than three doses.[58] For this purpose, after excluding women with no follow-up time or who were HPV16 and 18 DNA positive at enrollment, 5967 women received three vaccine doses (2957 HPV; 3010 Control), 802 women received two doses (422;380), and 384 women received one dose (196;188). Reasons for receiving fewer doses and other prerandomization and postrandomization characteristics were balanced within dose by arm. Within each dose group, the VE was calculated as one-minus the ratio of the attack rate (defined as number of events divided by number of women) for the HPV arm and the control arm. Attack rates of incident one-year persistent HPV16/18 infection in the control group were unrelated to number of doses received. VE was 80.9% for three doses (95%CI 71.1% to 87.7%; 25 and 133 events in the HPV and control arms, respectively), 84.1% for two doses (95%CI 50.2% to 96.3%; 3 and 17), and

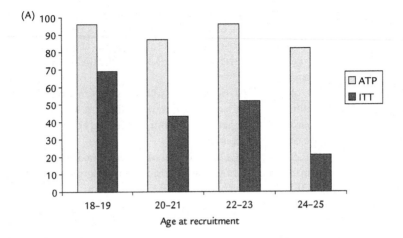

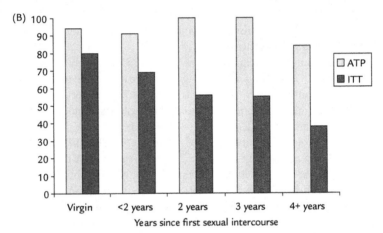

FIGURE 18.10 Efficacy of Human papillomavirus (HPV) 16/18 vaccine against 1-year persistent HPV injection in the Costa Rica vaccine trail by age group at vaccination (A) and by year since initiation of sexual life (B). *ATP: (according to protocol) cohort includes women who received all 3 doses within protocol—defined windows, complied with the protocol during the vaccination period did not have a biopsy or treatment (LEEP) prior to the 6-month visit and were HPV DNA negative (by PCR) for at least one of the HPV types in the endpoint at enrollment and at the 6-month visit. Women included all had at least one visit at least 12 months after the 6-month visit. ITT (intention to treat) analyses include all women randomized and vaccinated, regardless of prevalence of infection and follow-up visits.*

100% for one dose (95%CI 66.5% to 100%; 0 and 10). This was considered proof of principle that two, and maybe even one, dose(s) of the HPV16/18 vaccine are as protective as three doses against persistent HPV-16/18 infection in women without evidence of infection at vaccination, with important implications for implementation programs particularly in developing countries.

In this context, considering the possibility that levels of antibodies lower than those elicited by the vaccine could be protective, we followed up on the findings[29] in relation to the possible protection against reinfection by the usually low levels of antibodies elicited by natural HPV infection. At enrollment into the vaccine trial, 2813 control participants (not receiving the HPV vaccine) were negative for cervical HPV16 DNA and 2950 for

HPV18 DNA. Using Poisson regression, we compared rate ratios of newly detected cervical HPV16 or HPV18 infection among homologous HPV-seropositive and HPV-seronegative women, adjusting for age, education, marital status, lifetime number of sexual partners, and smoking. After controlling for risk factors associated with newly detected HPV infection, having high HPV16 antibody titer at enrollment was associated with a reduced risk of subsequent HPV16 infection (women in the highest tertile of HPV16 antibody titers, adjusted rate ratio = 0.50, 95% confidence interval = 0.26 to 0.86 vs HPV16-seronegative women). Similarly, having high HPV18 antibody titer at enrollment was associated with a reduced risk of subsequent HPV18 infection (women in the highest tertile of HPV18 antibody titers, adjusted rate ratio = 0.36, 95% confidence interval = 0.14 to 0.76 vs HPV18-seronegative women). We concluded that in this study population, having high antibody levels against HPV16 and HPV18 following natural infection was associated with reduced risk of subsequent HPV16 and HPV18 infections.[59]

HPV vaccines are considered prophylactic, as they were designed to prevent HPV infection and development of cervical precancers and cancer. However, women with oncogenic HPV infections might consider vaccination as therapy. To determine whether vaccination against HPV types 16 and 18 increases the rate of viral clearance in women already infected with HPV, we compared rates of type-specific viral clearance using generalized estimating equations methods at the 6-month visit (after 2 doses) and 12-month visit (after 3 doses) in 2189 women from the trial who were positive for HPV DNA at enrollment, had at least 6 months of follow-up, and had follow-up HPV DNA results (1088 from HPV vaccine arm and 1101 from the hepatitis arm). There was no evidence of increased viral clearance at 6 or 12 months in the group who received HPV vaccine compared with the control group. Clearance rates for HPV-16/18 infections at 6 months were 33.4% (82/248) in the HPV vaccine group and 31.6% (95/298) in the control group (vaccine efficacy for viral clearance, 2.5%; 95% confidence interval, –9.8% to 13.5%). Human papillomavirus 16/18 clearance rates at 12 months were 48.8% (86/177) in the HPV vaccine group and 49.8% (110/220) in the control group (vaccine efficacy for viral clearance, –2.0%; 95% confidence interval, –24.3% to 16.3%). There was no evidence of a therapeutic effect for other oncogenic or nononcogenic HPV categories, among women receiving all vaccine doses, among women with single infections, or among women stratified by the following entry variables: HPV-16/18 serology, cytologic results, HPV DNA viral load, time interval since sexual debut, Chlamydia trachomatis or Neisseria gonorrhoeae infection, hormonal contraceptive use, or smoking. We concluded that in women positive for HPV DNA, HPV-16/18 vaccination does not accelerate clearance of the virus and should not be used to treat prevalent infections.[59]

An additional study is also underway to investigate the efficacy of the vaccine against vulvar, oral and anal HPV infections, as well as the natural history of anal infections. Anal cancer remains rare (incidence of ~1.5 per 100,000 women annually) yet rates are increasing in many countries. Human papillomavirus-16 (HPV16) infection causes most cases. We evaluated vaccine efficacy (VE) of an ASO4-adjuvanted HPV16/18 vaccine against anal HPV16/18 infection.[60] In CVT, 4210 participants underwent anal specimen collection (4224 of 5968 = 70.8% of eligible women) at the final blinded study visit 4 years after vaccination to evaluate anal HPV16/18 VE. Cervical HPV16/18 VE among the same women at the same visit was calculated as a comparator. Analyses were conducted in a restricted cohort of women both cervical HPV16/18 DNA negative and HPV 16/18 seronegative prior at enrollment (N = 1989), and in the full cohort (all women with an anal specimen). In the restricted cohort, VE against prevalent HPV16/18 anal infection four-year post-vaccination was 83.6% (95%CI 66.7%

to 92.8%), which was comparable to cervical HPV16/18 VE (87.9%, 95%CI 77.4% to 94.0%). In the full cohort, HPV16/18 VE was statistically lower at the anus (62.0%, 95%CI 47.1% to 73.1%) compared to the cervix (76.4%, 95%CI 67.0% to 83.5%) (p for anatomic-site interaction =0.03). Significant and comparable estimates of vaccine efficacy against a composite endpoint of HPV31/33/45 cross-protection was observed at the anus and cervix. This was the first demonstration that the ASO4-adjuvanted vaccine affords strong protection against anal HPV in women, particularly among those more likely to be HPV naïve at vaccination.

One of the important aspects of this investigation is the evaluation of vaccine safety, particularly considering the age group of the subjects where reproductive outcomes are common. To assess whether vaccination against human papillomavirus (HPV) increases the risk of miscarriage,[61] we pooled data from this and another multicentre randomized controlled trial including 26 130 women aged 15–25 at enrolment; 3599 pregnancies eligible for analysis. The estimated rate of miscarriage was 11.5% in pregnancies in women in the HPV arm and 10.2% in the control arm. The one sided P value for the primary analysis was 0.16; thus, overall, there was no significant increase in miscarriage among women assigned to the HPV vaccine arm. In secondary descriptive analyses, miscarriage rates were 14.7% in the HPV vaccine arm and 9.1% in the control arm in pregnancies that began within three months after nearest vaccination. We concluded that there is no evidence overall for an association between HPV vaccination and risk of miscarriage.

The vaccine trial involved an important expansion of our study group and facilities, including the development of a quality control unit dealing with the proper documentation, training and conduct of all the study procedures under Good Clinical Practices, the establishment of a state-of-the-art specimen repository[62] and laboratories, and the handling of day-to-day external monitoring of all relevant procedures and audits. Recruitment started in 2004 with strong support from the Ministry of Health and enthusiasm in the community. However, after a few months, a series of criticisms were raised by several members of the media, politicians and religious authorities, some of which strongly opposed the study, concerned by the use of an investigational product in a large group of young women and the involvement of a commercial company and the US government. We required the assistance of professional public relations experts to convey the correct notion that all the necessary safeguards for human subject protection were in place and that the study was the only non-commercial, publicly funded trial of this vaccine that could provide invaluable independent data on its efficacy and safety, emphasizing the enormous disease burden and potential to prevent a large fraction of this serious public health problem. The negative coverage in the media slowed recruitment down and made it necessary to introduce corrective measures and recalculate sample size estimations. Our original target was to recruit at least 10,000 women, but the total recruitment was of only 7.466. A benefit back provision was part of the clinical trial agreement between NCI and GSK, indicating that in case the vaccine was proven effective, there would be some benefit for the communities involved, the amount to be negotiated directly with the Ministry of Health. In addition, participants were offered, if the vaccine was proven effective, to receive the vaccine they did not receive at recruitment at the end of the 4 years of follow up (crossover vaccination). This was accomplished with enthusiastic participation of the women.

Current plans include follow up of these subjects for up to 10 years to investigate the long term effect of vaccination. For this purpose, and considering that we are doing the crossover vaccination, we recently completed recruitment of an unvaccinated control group from the same age cohorts as the participants in the study. This group will replace the control group to evaluate long term efficacy and safety of the vaccine.

■ SUMMARY

The collaboration described in this chapter is an example of a highly successful collaborative effort between two countries of very different scientific development, each with its own strengths to make this happen. The United States provided epidemiological expertise, new technology and the necessary funds, while Costa Rica provided an enthusiastic group of collaborators eager to learn and a highly motivated community, in the context of its universal and highly developed health care system.

As shown in this vast scientific production, it is clear that the realization of state of the art scientific studies is highly feasible in developing countries, as long as there is sustained support, equal treatment of partners and personnel development. Professional staff from Costa Rica has always been actively engaged in the design, analysis, and publication of the studies, and have received extensive training in the United States and other places, an aspect that is crucial for the continuity of this kind of work.

The effort has involved more than 20,000 women from several generations in rural areas of Costa Rica who have generously maintained their strong support of the study and received the direct benefit of high quality cervical cancer prevention services. It has also involved several hundred collaborators in different capacities (field workers, interviewers, nurses, statisticians, laboratory staff, drivers, clerks, physicians, pharmacists, microbiologists, virologists, social workers, psychologists, quality experts etc.) who have worked together for the common goal of finding ways to control a major health problem of disadvantaged families. Both governments over the years have recognized the importance of this kind of work and provided ample support, and the awareness of the need for prevention in the community has increased. Cervical cancer mortality rates in the last 10 years have decreased in Costa Rica (Figure 18.11), and we consider that at least some of it is related to the vast technology transfer in this field that has happened as a consequence of our collaboration.

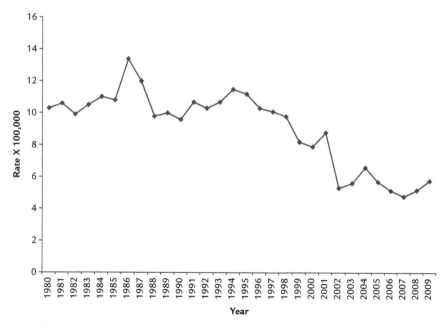

FIGURE 18.11 Age-adjusted cervical cancer mortality rates, Costa Rica (1980–2009).

There have been multiple challenges and difficulties but the common goal and trust between the groups have made it possible. Fortunately, the efforts have been very fruitful, and the accumulated knowledge generated by this and many other studies has lead to the discovery and availability of extremely powerful primary and secondary preventive tools. Our challenge is now to make the new tools available where they are needed.

Investigators (alphabetical order)

▨ **Latin America case-control study:**
María M. Brenes[a], Louise A. Brinton[b], Rosa C. de Britton[c], Eduardo Gaitán[d], Mariana García[a], Rolando Herrero[e], Francisco Tenorio[f], William E. Rawls[g], William C. Reeves[a].

▨ **HPV Natural history study (Guanacaste Project):**
Mario Alfaro[e], Concepción Bratti[h], Robert D. Burk[i], Philip E. Castle[b], Rolando Herrero[h], Allan Hildesheim[b], Jorge Morales[h], Ana C. Rodríguez[h], Mahboobeh Safaeian[b], Mark Schiffman[b], Mark E. Sherman[b], Sholom Wacholder[b].

▨ **Costa Rica HPV Vaccine Trial (CVT):**
Leen-Jan van Doorn[j], Paula González[h], Diego Guilleń[h], Rolando Herrero[h], Allan Hildesheim[b], Silvia Jimeńez[h], Hormuzd A Katki[b], Aimée R. Kreimer[b], Douglas R. Lowy[b], Jorge Morales[h], Carolina Porras[h], Wim Quint[j], Ana Cecilia Rodriguez[h], Mark Schiffman[b], John T. Schiller[b], Diane Solomon[b], Linda Struijk[j], Sholom Wacholder[b].

Affiliations (when the study was conducted)
[a] Gorgas Memorial Laboratory, Republic of Panama
[b] National Cancer Institute, NIH, USA
[c] Instituto Oncológico Nacional, República de Panamá
[d] Instituto Nacional de Cancerología, Colombia
[e] Caja Costaricense de Seguro Social, San Jose, Costa Rica
[f] Instituto Mexicano de Seguro Scial, México
[g] McMaster University, Canada
[h] Proyecto Epidemiológico Guanacaste, Fundación INCIENSA, Costa Rica
[i] Albert Einstein School of Medicine, USA
[j] DDL Diagnostic Laboratory, Voorburg, Netherlands

▨ REFERENCES

1. Arbyn M, Castellsague X, de Sanjose S, et al. Worldwide burden of cervical cancer in 2008. *Ann Oncol.* 2011;22(12):2675–2686.
2. Parkin DM, Almonte M, Bruni L, Clifford G, Curado MP, Pineros M. Burden and trends of type-specific human papillomavirus infections and related diseases in the Latin America and Caribbean region. *Vaccine.* 2008;26 Suppl 11:L1–L15.
3. Bouvard V, Baan R, Straif K, et al. A review of human carcinogens—part B: Biological agents. *Lancet Oncol.* 2009;10(4):321–322.
4. Robles SC, Periago MR. Guanacaste, Costa Rica: A landmark for cervical cancer prevention. *Rev Panam Salud Publica.* 2004;15(2):73–74.
5. Herrero R, Brinton LA, Reeves WC, et al. Risk factors for invasive carcinoma of the uterine cervix in Latin America. *Bull Pan Am Health Organ.* 1990;24(3):263–283.
6. Herrero R, Brinton LA, Reeves WC, et al. Sexual behavior, venereal diseases, hygiene practices, and invasive cervical cancer in a high-risk population. *Cancer.* 1990;65(2):380–386.

7. Brinton LA, Reeves WC, Brenes MM, et al. Parity as a risk factor for cervical cancer. *Am J Epidemiol.* 1989;130(3):486–496.

8. Reeves WC, Brinton LA, Garcia M, et al. Human papillomavirus infection and cervical cancer in Latin America. *N Engl J Med.* 1989;320(22):1437–1441.

9. Munoz N, Bosch X, Kaldor JM. Does human papillomavirus cause cervical cancer? the state of the epidemiological evidence. *Br J Cancer.* 1988;57(1):1–5.

10. Franco EL. The sexually transmitted disease model for cervical cancer: Incoherent epidemiologic findings and the role of misclassification of human papillomavirus infection. *Epidemiology.* 1991;2(2):98–106.

11. Herrero R, Brinton LA, Reeves WC, et al. Invasive cervical cancer and smoking in Latin America. *J Natl Cancer Inst.* 1989;81(3):205–211.

12. Herrero R, Brinton LA, Reeves WC, et al. Screening for cervical cancer in Latin Cmerica: A case-control study. *Int J Epidemiol.* 1992;21(6):1050–1056.

13. Brinton LA, Reeves WC, Brenes MM, et al. The male factor in the etiology of cervical cancer among sexually monogamous women. *Int J Cancer.* 1989;44(2):199–203.

14. Brinton LA, Reeves WC, Brenes MM, et al. Oral contraceptive use and risk of invasive cervical cancer. *Int J Epidemiol.* 1990;19(1):4–11.

15. Herrero R, Brinton LA, Reeves WC, et al. Injectable contraceptives and risk of invasive cervical cancer: Evidence of an association. *Int J Cancer.* 1990;46(1):5–7.

16. Herrero R, Potischman N, Brinton LA, et al. A case-control study of nutrient status and invasive cervical cancer. I. dietary indicators. *Am J Epidemiol.* 1991;134(11):1335–1346.

17. Potischman N, Herrero R, Brinton LA, et al. A case-control study of nutrient status and invasive cervical cancer. II. serologic indicators. *Am J Epidemiol.* 1991;134(11):1347–1355.

18. Potischman N, Brinton LA, Laiming VA, et al. A case-control study of serum folate levels and invasive cervical cancer. *Cancer Res.* 1991;51(18):4785–4789.

19. Herrero R, Brinton LA, Hartge P, et al. Determinants of the geographic variation of invasive cervical cancer in Costa Rica. *Bull Pan Am Health Organ.* 1993;27(1):15–25.

20. Brinton LA, Herrero R, Brenes M, et al. Considerations for conducting epidemiologic case-control studies of cancer in developing countries. *Bull Pan Am Health Organ.* 1991;25(1):1–15.

21. Herrero R, Schiffman MH, Bratti C, et al. Design and methods of a population-based natural history study of cervical neoplasia in a rural province of Costa Rica: The guanacaste project. *Rev Panam Salud Publica.* 1997;1(5):362–375.

22. Bratti MC, Rodriguez AC, Schiffman M, et al. Description of a seven-year prospective study of human papillomavirus infection and cervical neoplasia among 10000 women in Guanacaste, Costa Rica, *Rev Panam Salud Publica.* 2004;15(2):75–89.

23. Herrero R, Castle PE, Schiffman M, et al. Epidemiologic profile of type-specific human papillomavirus infection and cervical neoplasia in Guanacaste, Costa Rica. *J Infect Dis.* 2005;191(11):1796–1807.

24. Herrero R, Hildesheim A, Bratti C, et al. Population-based study of human papillomavirus infection and cervical neoplasia in rural Costa Rica. *J Natl Cancer Inst.* 2000;92(6):464–474.

25. Castle PE, Schiffman M, Bratti MC, et al. A population-based study of vaginal human papillomavirus infection in hysterectomized women. *J Infect Dis.* 2004;190(3):458–467.

26. Castle PE, Jeronimo J, Schiffman M, et al. Age-related changes of the cervix influence human papillomavirus type distribution. *Cancer Res.* 2006;66(2):1218–1224.

27. Wang SS, Schiffman M, Shields TS, et al. Seroprevalence of human papillomavirus-16, -18, -31, and -45 in a population-based cohort of 10000 women in Costa Rica. *Br J Cancer.* 2003;89(7):1248–1254.

28. Wang SS, Schiffman M, Herrero R, et al. Determinants of human papillomavirus 16 serological conversion and persistence in a population-based cohort of 10 000 women in Costa Rica. *Br J Cancer.* 2004;91(7):1269–1274.

29. Viscidi RP, Schiffman M, Hildesheim A, et al. Seroreactivity to human papillomavirus (HPV) types 16, 18, or 31 and risk of subsequent HPV infection: Results from a population-based study in Costa Rica. *Cancer Epidemiol Biomarkers Prev.* 2004;13(2):324–327.

30. Wentzensen N, Rodriguez AC, Viscidi R, et al. A competitive serological assay shows naturally acquired immunity to human papillomavirus infections in the guanacaste natural history study. *J Infect Dis.* 2011;204(1):94–102.

31. Vaccarella S, Franceschi S, Herrero R, et al. Clustering of multiple human papillomavirus infections in women from a population-based study in Guanacaste, Costa Rica. *J Infect Dis.* 2011;204(3):385–390.

32. Chaturvedi AK, Katki HA, Hildesheim A, et al. Human papillomavirus infection with multiple types: Pattern of coinfection and risk of cervical disease. *J Infect Dis.* 2011;203(7):910–920.

33. Hildesheim A, Herrero R, Castle PE, et al. HPV co-factors related to the development of cervical cancer: Results from a population-based study in Costa Rica. *Br J Cancer.* 2001;84(9):1219–1226.

34. Castle PE, Hillier SL, Rabe LK, et al. An association of cervical inflammation with high-grade cervical neoplasia in women infected with oncogenic human papillomavirus (HPV). *Cancer Epidemiol Biomarkers Prev.* 2001;10(10):1021–1027.

35. Hildesheim A, Schiffman M, Bromley C, et al. Human papillomavirus type 16 variants and risk of cervical cancer. *J Natl Cancer Inst.* 2001;93(4):315–318.

36. Wang SS, Wheeler CM, Hildesheim A, et al. Human leukocyte antigen class I and II alleles and risk of cervical neoplasia: Results from a population-based study in Costa Rica. *J Infect Dis.* 2001;184(10):1310–1314.

37. Rodriguez AC, Schiffman M, Herrero R, et al. Rapid clearance of human papillomavirus and implications for clinical focus on persistent infections. *J Natl Cancer Inst.* 2008;100(7):513–517.

38. Castle PE, Rodriguez AC, Burk RD, et al. Short term persistence of human papillomavirus and risk of cervical precancer and cancer: Population based cohort study. *BMJ.* 2009;339:b2569.

39. Rodriguez AC, Burk R, Herrero R, et al. The natural history of human papillomavirus infection and cervical intraepithelial neoplasia among young women in the Guanacaste cohort shortly after initiation of sexual life. *Sex Transm Dis.* 2007;34(7):494–502.

40. Castle PE, Rodriguez AC, Burk RD, et al. Long-term persistence of prevalently detected human papillomavirus infections in the absence of detectable cervical precancer and cancer. *J Infect Dis.* 2011;203(6):814–822.

41. Schiffman M, Herrero R, Desalle R, et al. The carcinogenicity of human papillomavirus types reflects viral evolution. *Virology.* 2005;337(1):76–84.

42. Schiffman M, Rodriguez AC, Chen Z, et al. A population-based prospective study of carcinogenic human papillomavirus variant lineages, viral persistence, and cervical neoplasia. *Cancer Res.* 2010;70(8):3159–3169.

43. Schiffman M, Herrero R, Hildesheim A, et al. HPV DNA testing in cervical cancer screening: Results from women in a high-risk province of Costa Rica. *JAMA.* 2000;283(1):87–93.

44. Hutchinson ML, Zahniser DJ, Sherman ME, et al. Utility of liquid-based cytology for cervical carcinoma screening: Results of a population-based study conducted in a region of Costa Rica with a high incidence of cervical carcinoma. *Cancer.* 1999;87(2):48–55.

45. Schneider DL, Herrero R, Bratti C, et al. Cervicography screening for cervical cancer among 8460 women in a high-risk population. *Am J Obstet Gynecol.* 1999;180(2 Pt 1):290–298.

46. Rodriguez AC, Morera LA, Bratti C, et al. Performance of direct visual inspection of the cervix with acetic acid and magnification in a previously screened population. *J Low Genit Tract Dis.* 2004;8(2):132–138.

47. Rodriguez AC, Garcia-Pineres AJ, Hildesheim A, et al. Alterations of T-cell surface markers in older women with persistent human papillomavirus infection. *Int J Cancer.* 2011;128(3):597–607.

48. Gonzalez P, Hildesheim A, Rodriguez AC, et al. Behavioral/lifestyle and immunologic factors associated with HPV infection among women older than 45 years. *Cancer Epidemiol Biomarkers Prev.* 2010;19(12):3044–3054.

49. Kreimer AR, Schiffman M, Herrero R, et al. Long-term risk of recurrent cervical human papillomavirus infection and precancer and cancer following excisional treatment. *Int J Cancer.* 2012;131(1):211–218.

50. Wang SS, Bratti MC, Rodriguez AC, et al. Common variants in immune and DNA repair genes and risk for human papillomavirus persistence and progression to cervical cancer. *J Infect Dis.* 2009;199(1):20–30.

51. Hildesheim A, Schiffman M, Brinton LA, et al. P53 polymorphism and risk of cervical cancer. *Nature.* 1998;396(6711):531–532.

52. Klug SJ, Ressing M, Koenig J, et al. TP53 codon 72 polymorphism and cervical cancer: A pooled analysis of individual data from 49 studies. *Lancet Oncol.* 2009;10(8):772–784.

53. Koshiol J, Hildesheim A, Gonzalez P, et al. Common genetic variation in TP53 and risk of human papillomavirus persistence and progression to CIN3/cancer revisited. *Cancer Epidemiol Biomarkers Prev.* 2009;18(5):1631–1637.

54. Safaeian M, Falk RT, Rodriguez AC, et al. Factors associated with fluctuations in IgA and IgG levels at the cervix during the menstrual cycle. *J Infect Dis.* 2009;199(3):455–463.

55. Schiller JT, Castellsague X, Villa LL, Hildesheim A. An update of prophylactic human papillomavirus L1 virus-like particle vaccine clinical trial results. *Vaccine.* 2008;26 Suppl 10:K53–K61.

56. Herrero R, Hildesheim A, Rodriguez AC, et al. Rationale and design of a community-based double-blind randomized clinical trial of an HPV 16 and 18 vaccine in Guanacaste, Costa Rica. *Vaccine.* 2008;26(37):4795–4808.

57. Herrero R, Wacholder S, Rodriguez AC, et al. Prevention of persistent human papillomavirus infection by an HPV16/18 vaccine: A community-based randomized clinical trial in Guanacaste, Costa Rica. *Cancer Discov.* 2011;1(5):408–419.

58. Kreimer AR, Rodriguez AC, Hildesheim A, et al. Proof-of-principle evaluation of the efficacy of fewer than three doses of a bivalent HPV16/18 vaccine. *J Natl Cancer Inst.* 2011;103(19):1444–1451.

59. Hildesheim A, Herrero R, Wacholder S, et al. Effect of human papillomavirus 16/18 L1 virus-like particle vaccine among young women with preexisting infection: A randomized trial. *JAMA.* 2007;298(7):743–753.

60. Kreimer AR, Gonzalez P, Katki HA, et al. Efficacy of a bivalent HPV 16/18 vaccine against anal HPV 16/18 infection among young women: A nested analysis within the Costa Rica vaccine trial. *Lancet Oncol.* 2011;12(9):862–870.

61. Wacholder S, Chen BE, Wilcox A, et al. Risk of miscarriage with bivalent vaccine against human papillomavirus (HPV) types 16 and 18: Pooled analysis of two randomised controlled trials. *BMJ.* 2010;340:c712.

62. Cortes B, Schiffman M, Herrero R, et al. Establishment and operation of a biorepository for molecular epidemiologic studies in Costa Rica. *Cancer Epidemiol Biomarkers Prev.* 2010;19(4):916–922.

CHAPTER 19

STUDIES OF TOBACCO SMOKING AND CONTROL

PRISCILLA REDDY, SHAMAGONAM JAMES,
NASHEEN NAIDOO, RONEL SEWPAUL,
KEN RESNICOW, ANTHONY MBEWU,
KOLA OKUYEMI

■ PREVALENCE IN DEVELOPING COUNTRIES

Accurate prevalence data of tobacco usage is important to assess the impact of tobacco control policies and interventions; and also to make projections of the future burden of disease that current tobacco usage is likely to cause. The Member States of the WHO collect four indicators of tobacco use to best represent tobacco use, i.e., current and daily prevalence rates of tobacco and cigarette smoking.[1]

More than 80% of the world's smokers live in low- or middle-income countries[2] and it is in these markets that tobacco usage and the associated burden of disease is growing most rapidly. Documenting tobacco use patterns in emerging economies is particularly important, as increased use is a common unintended consequence of economic growth and increasing disposable personal income. The subsequent tobacco-related morbidity and mortality, however, have significant negative effects on the economies of these countries due to days of work lost to tobacco-related illness; and the cost to their health systems of such morbidity.

In 2010, the Global Adult Tobacco Survey (GATS) was conducted in 14 lower and middle income countries representing 54% of the global population (Figure 19.1).[3] The highest rates were found in Bangladesh (43%) and the Russian Federation (39%), whilst the lowest was in Mexico (16%). These rates are driven predominantly by gender (male), urbanicity, lower education and lower income levels.

Approximately 30% of the world's cigarettes are consumed in China; and smoking prevalence remains high despite tobacco control interventions. The 2010 China Global Adult Smoking Survey (GATS) performed by the Chinese Centers for Disease Control reported that 53% of men and 2.4% of women aged 15 years and above were current smokers.[4] Current smoking among men was highest in the 25–44 year and 45–64 year age groups (59.3% and 63.0%, respectively), whereas current smoking rates for women rose with age from 0.7% among 15–24 year olds to 6.7% among those aged 65 years and older. Male smoking rates were higher in rural areas (56.1%) than in urban areas (49.2%).[5] In 1984

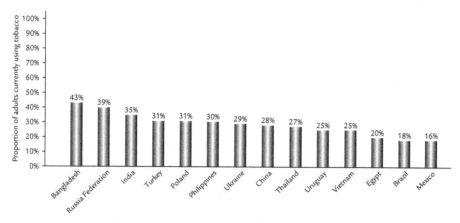

FIGURE 19.1 Tobacco use prevalence in 14 low- and middle-income countries, 2008–2010.[3]

there were approximately 250 million smokers in China (61% in men; 7% in women). This had increased to approximately 350 million by 2002.

Results from the Demographic and Health Surveys (DHS) conducted in 14 sub-Saharan African countries that had collected data on tobacco smoking reported that the prevalence of cigarette smoking among men ranged from 8.0% in Nigeria to 27.3% in the island nation of Madagascar.[6] In some countries, for example Nigeria, there were considerable geographical variations in smoking prevalence in the 2008 DHS ranging from 6.1% in the northeast to 12.4% in the southeast.[7] However, these results were not consistent with earlier (1998) data from the Nigerian Ministry of Health that reported smoking rates among adults to be 17.1% for males and 1.7% for females. The ministry also reported that total consumption of tobacco in Nigeria increased at an annual rate of 4.7% between 2001 and 2006.[8] In general, most smokers in Nigeria consume few cigarettes a day with two-thirds of smokers reporting smoking 1–5 cigarettes per day, and less than 20% reported smoking more than 10 cigarettes a day.[7]

Ethiopia (8.3%) and Ghana (8.8%) also had relatively low male cigarette smoking rates. The southern African nations of Mozambique, Lesotho, Zambia, Malawi, and Namibia ranked next with prevalence rates of between 14% and 18%. Higher male smoking prevalence rates were found in the eastern countries of Uganda (18.7%), Tanzania (21.0%), and Kenya (22.9%) as well as the southern African nation of Zimbabwe (22.1%). These rates are driven predominantly by male gender, urbanicity, lower education, lower work status and religion (Muslims (OR = 0.84) smoked more than Catholics (OR = 0.79) and then Protestants (OR = 0.51) compared to the referent groups of the others).[4,6]

Cigarette use among women in the counties surveyed was negligible with the exception of Namibia, where 5.9% of women smoked cigarettes. Smoking of other forms of tobacco was slightly higher than cigarette use among women. These differences may relate to cultural issues in Namibia where smoking by women is frowned upon, but chewing tobacco or snuff is acceptable. Furthermore in Namibia, as in South Africa, high rates of smoking among "colored" (mixed race) women is notable, driving up the figure for smoking prevalence in women in general.[9] Despite previous studies establishing that low socioeconomic status urban male residents are most at risk for cigarette use, this is less clearly defined for women due to the overall low levels of tobacco usage. Smoking of noncigarette tobacco among men was lower than cigarette use in most of the countries, though a few countries had more substantial rates of 11.9% in Mozambique, 17.7% in Madagascar, and 25.1% in Lesotho, while smoking of noncigarette tobacco by women, for example "snuff,"[10] is slightly more common than cigarette use.[6] Despite historically low rates of tobacco use in sub-Saharan Africa, annual cigarette consumption rates have been previously reported to be on the rise for both men and women in sub-Saharan Africa.[11]

As tobacco use is often initiated in adolescence, monitoring the levels of tobacco use among young people is therefore imperative in tobacco control efforts. As part of the WHO Global Tobacco Surveillance System (GTSS), youth and adolescent tobacco use is monitored through the Global Youth Tobacco Surveys (GYTS). The GYTS in Thailand in 2005 showed that 22.0% of males and 5.2% of females reported being current smokers. Current smoking according to the GYTS standards is defined as having smoked at least one cigarette in the 30 days preceding the survey.[12] Current smoking prevalence rates from the GYTS for school-going adolescents in Addis Ababa, Ethiopia were estimated at 4.5% for males and 1% for females, and is generally considered to be one of the lowest among adolescents in countries in Africa.[13]

Data from the Global Youth Tobacco Survey, 2006 in the Republic of Congo showed that 18% of in-school adolescents (n = 3034) reported using smokeless tobacco (chewing tobacco, "sniff" or "dip") in the last 30 days.[14]

National cross-sectional studies were also conducted among grade 8–10 learners in South African schools as a collaboration between WHO/CDC/MRC/National Departments of Health and Education—the GYTS in 1999, 2002, 2008 and 2011[15-17] and the Youth Risk Behavior Surveys in 2002 and 2008.[18,19] The South African GYTS in 2008 reported that 22.8% of boys and 10.5% of girls were current cigarette smokers.[17] The 2001 GYTS in Nigeria showed current smoking rates among adolescents 13–15 years old to be 7.7% for boys and 3.3% for girls.[20]

Results from GYTS surveys across all countries showed that an estimated 43% of 13–15 year olds were living in a home where others smoked. Globally, it is estimated that about one third of adults are regularly exposed to second-hand tobacco smoke (SHS).[20]

■ CORRELATES AND DETERMINANTS

Social diffusion theory[21] suggests that in countries in which social innovations such as cigarette smoking are introduced, the highly educated and affluent often experiment and accept the innovation first. It then diffuses to the lower socioeconomic groups where its adoption becomes fairly widespread and established. This theory has been used by some to explain the diffusion of cigarette smoking in developing countries and among women.[22,23] Tobacco use among these sub-populations would aggravate their already poor economic circumstances, leading to enormous social and health-related costs for the country.

Among adult men in sub-Saharan Africa, the highest cigarette use was found among urban men; those with lower education levels; and those working in service or manual jobs. Results for women showed much lower prevalence than men but similar social patterns of use.[6] Diffusion of smoking among women was shown to be more prominent among "colored" women (42%) than among black South African women (5%) in 2003.[24] Studies in Nigeria have also reported variation in smoking rates between various occupational groups such as 3.9%, 15.9%, and 13.9%, among physicians, soldiers, and (white collar) senior executives respectively.[25-27]

In China sociocultural factors contributing toward smoking behavior have also been identified. Smoking has been deeply integrated with Chinese social interactions through the acceptance of cigarettes as a traditional Chinese gesture of good will. The social changes and stresses caused by urban migration are associated with smoking initiation; and this is especially true among rural-urban migrant workers.[5] Second-hand smoking rates in China have also increased with cramped housing, poor ventilation and poor enforcement of smoke-free laws.[28] An estimated 50%–72% of Chinese nonsmokers (approximately 740 million) are regularly exposed to SHS.[3]

Many countries have conducted secondary analysis of data from their GYTS, to identify determinants and correlates of youth tobacco smoking. Data from the GYTS 2003 in Addis Ababa, Ethiopia reported that significant determinants of smoking among Ethiopian adolescents included being male, having one or both parents as smokers and having friends that smoke.[13] A four year cohort study of the predictors of smoking initiation among 441 nonsmoking school children in Tunisia showed that the predictors that were strongly associated with smoking initiation were previous experimentation with alcohol (OR = 11; 95%CI:5.82–20.9); having a smoking best friend (OR = 5.43; 95%CI:2.51–11.69); lack of school-based education about smoking (OR = 2.81; 95%CI:1.37–5.75); and believing that smoking makes one feel "cool" (OR = 2.41; 95%CI:1.04–5.57) and should not be forbidden in public places (OR = 2.81; 95%CI:1.54–5.13).[29]

The GYTS conducted in Punjab, India in 2003 (n = 2014) found that factors positively associated with current smoking in adolescents were receiving pocket money; having parents who smoked; and having chewed or applied tobacco. The following factors relating to perceptions about smoking were also positively associated with current smoking : adolescents who said that boys or girls who smoke or chew tobacco have more friends; adolescents who said that smoking or chewing tobacco makes boys look less attractive; adolescents who said that there is no difference in weight between smokers and nonsmokers; adolescents who said that smoking makes one gain weight; and adolescents who had most or all of their closest friends who smoked.[30] Analysis of cross-sectional data from the Thailand GYTS in 2005 (n = 18 368) found that determinants of adolescent smoking included being male (OR = 3.46; (95% CI:2.72–4.86); having parents who smoked (OR = 1.62; 95% CI:1.25–2.11); and friends who smoked (OR = 5.07; 95% CI:3.54–7.25) for "some friends smokers"; and OR = 26.71 (95% CI:18.26–39.06) for "most or all friends smokers" Older learners and learners who thought that smoking was harmful to health were less likely to report smoking.[12]

In Kurdistan, Iraq, where 15.3% of high school youth were current smokers, factors associated with adolescent current smoking included male gender; having parents who smoked; having close friends who smoked; having pocket money; and having perceptions that boys or girls who smoked were attractive.[30] Male gender, parents' smoking and close friends' smoking were also found to be determinants of current smoking among school-going adolescents in Lithuania[31] and Jamaica.[32]

Data from the World Health Survey in 48 low and middle income countries explored the impact of demographic and socioeconomic factors on the current smoking status of adult respondents. The data from these surveys provided information on 213,807 respondents aged 18 years or above. Results showed that individuals were more likely to smoke if they had little or no education. Wealth was inversely associated with smoking in the low-income countries but to a lesser extent, or not at all, in the middle-income countries.[2]

Overall, women in developing countries tend to have lower rates of smoking, initiate smoking later and consume fewer cigarettes daily than men. This can be attributed to sociocultural, religious, or economic factors. In some societies, it may be seen as "improper" or "indecent" for females to be seen smoking in public. This was apparent in a cross-sectional study among Kuwaiti Muslim adults, where the majority (85%) of female smokers preferred to smoke in the privacy of their homes.[33] In addition, there may also be religious arguments against smoking. Due to the negative sociocultural connotations of smoking, females in the study tended to underreport their smoking habits.[33]

The prevalence of tobacco use was shown to be low in Punjab, India where the main religion is Sikhism. Sikhism does not allow tobacco use as it was banned by a Sikh Guru in the 17th century.[34] Data from eight countries of the former Soviet Union showed that Muslims were less likely to smoke than non-Muslims. This pattern was most apparent in Kazakhstan and Kyrgyzstan, where the proportion of the population that is Muslim is higher. The age-adjusted odds ratios for smoking among Muslim respondents in these two countries were, respectively, 0.52 (99% CI:0.36–0.77) and 0.44 (99% CI:0.26–0.76) in males, and 0.33 (99% CI:0.17–0.64) and 0.07 (99% CI:0.03–0.18) in females.[35] Tobacco use among women in many countries in the Middle East, North Africa and South-East Asia with large proportions of Muslims, is much lower than among men, often <10%.[33] Studies from various settings suggest that religiousness in different faiths is associated with a lower prevalence of tobacco use.[36] Individuals of the same community seem to have similar patterns of tobacco use,[37] but it has been shown that where differences are present, it is unclear whether this is due to religion or to broader social differences, of which religion is only one.[38]

Studies suggest that cigarette prices are strong determinants of both smoking prevalence and cigarette consumption among current smokers, in low and middle income countries.[39–41] Kostova et al, using data on youth smoking from 17 low and middle income countries spread across the world (n = 315 353), showed that the total price elasticity of cigarette demand for the sample of youth was –2.11, implying that an increase in price of 10% would reduce youth cigarette consumption by 21.1% at the mean.[41] The new tax scheme implemented by Taiwan in 2002, after they joined the WTO, reduced annual cigarette consumption by 13.27 packs per person (10.5%). Male smokers who did not earn an income or who smoked light cigarettes were found to be more responsive to the changes in cigarette price.[39]

In summary, countries that have undertaken the GATS and despite intracountry differences, have shown similar determinants of tobacco use that is largely driven by gender (male), urbanicity, income (lower to middle), education (lower income), and religion (lower income).

POLICY IN DEVELOPING COUNTRIES

To date 174 countries, covering 87% of the world's population, have ratified the WHO Framework Convention on Tobacco Control (FCTC). The FCTC, introduced in 2005, is the world's first public health treaty. It sets international tobacco control standards in the areas of advertising, tax and price policy, product labeling, illicit trade, passive smoking, and others. To help countries fulfill the promise of the FCTC, WHO has established MPOWER, a package of cost-effective solutions that have been proven to reduce tobacco use. The six measures of the MPOWER package are (1) **monitor** tobacco use and prevention policies, (2) **protect** people from tobacco smoke, (3) **offer** help to quit tobacco use, (4) **warn** about the dangers of tobacco, (5) **enforce** bans on tobacco advertising, promotion and sponsorship and (6) **raise** taxes on tobacco.[42–44]

Since 2008, 16 additional countries have enacted national smoke-free laws covering all public places and workplaces. As a result, a total of 739 million people in 31 countries are now protected by comprehensive smoke-free laws. Among the low and middle income countries with complete smoke-free legislation in all public places (or at least 90% of the population covered by complete subnational smoke-free legislation), Thailand, Seychelles, Panama, Uruguay, Iran and Turkey stood out as having high levels of public compliance with their smoke-free laws.[42]

This report finds that more than one billion people in 19 countries are now protected by laws requiring graphic health warnings that cover 50% or more of tobacco packages.[1] However, the impact of warning labels depends upon many factors, including their size, comprehensiveness, visibility, and whether they are printed in the local language.[43]

WHO highlights that increasing the prices of tobacco products through higher taxes is the most effective intervention to reduce tobacco use and encourage smokers to quit.[42] Tax increases raise government revenues, which can be used for tobacco control and other public health program. Progress has recently been made by many countries in imposing revenue-generating tobacco taxes. Twenty-six countries and one territory have tobacco taxes that constitute the recommended minimum of 75% of retail price; although only eight of these are middle income countries and one a low income country. These include Madagascar, Argentina, Chile, Israel, Latvia, West Bank and the Gaza Strip, Estonia, Slovakia, and Turkey.[1] However governments often collect large tobacco tax revenues, but inadequately fund tobacco control activities, a deficit that is more marked in low- and middle-income countries.[1] Furthermore, taxes should be increased frequently to offset the effects of inflation and increased incomes. If tobacco prices do not increase faster than consumer purchasing power, tobacco becomes relatively more affordable and consumption rises.[44]

A review of empirical economic policy studies in support of raising tobacco taxes being progressive (affecting the higher socioeconomic groups more than the lower), are based on the premise that the poor are likely to be more sensitive to price changes and thus more likely to change their consumption by a greater proportion.[45] Research in Sri Lanka evaluated aggregate monthly data on cigarette consumption from 1999 to 2000 and concluded that a 10% increase in cigarette prices would reduce overall consumption by 2.3 to 9.1% and a 10% increase in income would increase overall cigarette consumption by 1.8 to 7.8%.[46] The 2002 estimates for China, based on economic models of addiction and using data from 1980 to 1996, concluded that a 10% increase in cigarette prices would decrease cigarette consumption by up to 5.4% in the short-run and by up to 6.6% in the long-run.[47]

Brazil has in recent years emerged as a global leader in tobacco control. Although it is the world's largest tobacco leaf exporter and one of the largest tobacco producers, Brazil has implemented stringent regulations that cover the full spectrum of tobacco control. It was the first country to create a body to regulate tobacco contents and emissions, and the first to ban the use of "light" and "mild" terms in describing tobacco products. It was also the second country (after Canada) to adopt graphic warnings on cigarette packages.[48] There are bans on the sale of cigarettes to minors (those under the age of 18), the distribution of free samples, Internet sales of tobacco, and the sale of tobacco in health centers and schools. Manufacturers must report on their product composition and on production and sales. Smoking bans are in place in public places and public transportation. However smoking is still permitted in some divided areas meeting specific ventilation criteria. Advertising tobacco products on television and radio is strictly prohibited, as are tobacco sponsorships. Point-of-sale advertisements are restricted and all tobacco packages must include health warnings. In 2002, Brazil began providing free support for smoking-cessation services, including both cognitive behavioral therapy and pharmaceutical products. Excise taxation is also implemented, and in 2001 cigarette taxes accounted for over 5% of the country's revenue. Health authorities have also considered legal action against the tobacco industry.[49]

A qualitative study including documentary analysis, key informant interview, focus group discussions, and key stakeholders analysis was conducted within the framework of the National Tobacco Control Policy (2000–2010) in Vietnam. Vietnam has a state-owned tobacco industry and is an important contributor to government revenue and GDP. This study concluded that tobacco control is not high in the priority policy agenda and is only likely to shift toward effective tobacco control if the economic framing is challenged.[50]

China signed the FCTC in 2003, which was ratified in 2005. Subsequently, health warnings occupying more than 30% of the cigarette packet surface have been in place since 2008. It is also illegal to promote tobacco on billboards or in magazines. The Ministry of Health has banned smoking in hospitals, schools and other places used by children, as well at the Olympic Games in Beijing in 2008 and at the Shanghai Expo in 2010.[5] Yet despite these legislative changes, China scored only 37.3 point out of 100 in a performance score measuring implementing the FCTC[51] and this is largely due to poor enforcement as evident by surveys showing tobacco advertising and public smoking is still prevalent.[52,53]

A number of developing countries, since ratifying the WHO FCTC, have had marginal success in adopting and enforcing tobacco control legislation. In Ecuador for example, the existing ban on smoking in public places was not fully maintained, as ventilated smoking zones continued to be allowed and voluntary compliance with smoking prohibitions was given to venues in the hospitality industry.[54] In Uganda, smoking in government buildings and advertising in certain media is restricted. Health warnings on cigarette packs are also required. However these measures fall short of the FCTC recommendations. Tobacco taxation accounts for 9% of total revenue.[55] In Liberia, smoking in educational and health facilities is prohibited, however, no other FCTC requirements are regulated.[55]

Kenya has comprehensive tobacco control legislation in the form of banning advertising in print and electronic media, on cigarette packs, and sporting and other events. Smoking is also banned in all public places and all cigarette packs are required to bear warnings and constituent information. Sales to minors are also prohibited. Tobacco taxation in Kenya accounts for 10% of total tax revenue. In Gambia, smoking is banned in public transport and is restricted in government buildings, worksites, and educational and health facilities. There is no legislation on the regulation of taxation, advertising, sponsorship and event promotion. Display of health warnings and constituents on tobacco packaging is not legally enforced, and there is no legal prohibition of sales to minors.[55] In 2011, Nigeria's national legislature passed a tobacco control legislation that requires health warnings on cigarette packages and bans cigarette smoking in public buildings;[56] the bill is awaiting the president's signature.

The South African tobacco control legislation experience has been previously well researched and documented. Tobacco control legislation in South Africa dates back to the 1970s when local governments banned smoking in cinemas, and during the 1980s with restrictions on smoking on domestic flights. In 1991 the Tobacco Action Group was formed, which raised public awareness of the harmful effects of tobacco use and the necessity for tobacco control. The group did not however reach the wider population, particularly the lower socioeconomic groups.[57]

The South African government passed the Tobacco Products Control Act of 1993, which had three main focus points: the regulation of smoking in public places, banning of sales to children under the age of 16, and the regulation of advertising of tobacco products in aspects such as labeling.[58] The Act did, however, have major limitations. It did not completely ban smoking in public places and its definition of public places was not specific, as uncertainty existed as to whether a workplace was a public place. The Act did not cover the licensing and placing of vending machines which provide minors with easy access to cigarettes. Furthermore the enforcement system of the Act was not adequately defined; especially regarding tobacco sales to minors, monitoring of smoking in public places and monitoring of health warning requirements. Tobacco advertising was also not completely prohibited in the 1993 Act despite persistent support for such a ban by individuals in the health sector. The advertising regulations excluded radio advertising. This was a large loophole, as at the time radio was the most significant communication medium, particularly among the poorest sectors of society. Instead the Act provided for health warnings. South Africa clearly needed a comprehensive tobacco control program, underpinned by supportive and enabling legislation. Research provided the evidence base for improving the country's tobacco control legislation. The democratic government, elected in 1994, embraced the health promotion approach and publicized the harmful effects of tobacco to the wider South African population. More groups began to join the movement for tobacco control and in 1995 President Nelson Mandela, together with the then Health Minister, Dr. Nkosazana Zuma, received the World Health Organization health medal for the country's efforts against tobacco.

The Tobacco Products Control Amendment Act No 12 of 1999[59] was developed with research support from the Medical Research Council, Health Promotion Office. The Act effectively addressed the flaws of the 1993 Act. Key features of the 1999 Act included:

- Prohibition of the direct advertising and promotion of tobacco products, as well as prohibition of advertising and promotion through sponsored events
- Prohibition of the free distribution of tobacco products and the receipt of gifts and cash prizes in contests, lotteries, or games
- Prescription of the maximum yields of tar, nicotine, and other constituents in tobacco products (as from December 2001: 15 mg per cigarette for tar; 1.5 mg for nicotine; as from June 1 2006: 12 mg and 1.2 mg, respectively)
- Ban on smoking of tobacco products in public places including work places and public transport
- No sales of tobacco products to children under 16
- Excise tax increases to 50% of the retail price

Increased efforts were also made to ensure stricter enforcements of the legislation, including increased fines for violation of laws.

South Africa played a significant role in developing the WHO FCTC and was one of the treaty's first signatories. The 1999 Act was further amended to address loopholes and to align South Africa's tobacco control activities with the requirements of the FCTC. The Tobacco Products Control Amendment Acts of 2007 and 2008 included stricter regulations on placement of vending machines and required prohibitions of tobacco sales to individuals under the age of 18.[60,61]

From the early 1990s research organizations, particularly the Medical Research Council of South Africa, conducted numerous research studies that provided the evidence underpinning the development of successful tobacco control legislation in South Africa. A monitoring and evaluation survey, the Health Warnings Evaluation (1996), was conducted to investigate adult South Africans' level of awareness of the health warnings and their ability to recall the health warning. Results from this study were used in support of the banning of tobacco advertising and also in assessing the status of health warnings on tobacco packages.[62]

▧ PREVENTION AND TREATMENT RESEARCH

During 2009 and 2010, 23 countries with a population of nearly two billion people aired strong mass media campaigns about the harmful effects of tobacco use.[1] Sustained anti-tobacco mass media communication programs in high-income countries, for example the "EX Plan" (http://www.becomeanex.org/) and the "TRUTH" campaign (http://www.protectthetruth.org/truthcampaign.htm), have shown success at changing smoking knowledge, attitudes, and behaviors.[63] Mullin et al cited case studies of mass media graphic campaigns and campaigns aimed at evoking negative emotions which were implemented successfully in three high-burden low and middle income countries: China, India, and Russia. The authors suggest that low and middle income country governments should consider resourcing and sustaining these interventions as key components of tobacco control strategies.[63]

Randomized controlled trials (RCTs) of intervention strategies from two school-based tobacco prevention programs (HRIDAY-CATCH and Project MYTRI) in India, were used by a local NGO to advocate for scaling up of the Government of India's national tobacco control program.[64] In South African schools Resnicow et al. conducted a three-armed trial testing two interventions: the "Harm Minimization" versus the "Life Skill" intervention among 5266 South African high school students involving interdisciplinary researchers across South Africa, United States, and Australia[65,66] and aimed to test the efficacy of the two contrasting interventions. Results from this trial showed a net change reduction of 6% in 30-day smoking from baseline to two-year follow-up in the control group compared to 3% in both the Harm Minimization and Life Skill interventions, the results of which were not statistically significant.[65] These interventions provide a basis from which to build more improved interventions that are targeted and tailored to young people, and which can be expanded to schools nationally. The intervention response was significantly moderated by both gender and race. The Harm Minimization intervention was more shown to be more effective for males, whereas the Life Skill intervention was more effective for females. The strongest effect was evident for black African students for the Harm Minimization intervention, whereas the strongest intervention effect for "colored" students was evident for the Life Skill intervention group.[65]

Meta-analyses evaluating tobacco cessation interventions recommend using a combination of behavioral interventions and pharmacotherapy. Pharmacotherapy has been shown to double or triple quit rates.[67,68] Nicotine replacement therapy (NRT), the most frequently used form of pharmacotherapy for tobacco cessation, has been associated with odds ratios of 1.5–1.8 for successful quitting.[69] NRT supplies patients with small amounts of nicotine to achieve constant levels of nicotine concentration and thereby alleviate cravings or withdrawal symptoms. NRT products include transdermal patches, nasal sprays inhalers and chewing gum. Varenicline and bupropion are also commonly used medications prescribed for tobacco cessation, and both have been shown to greatly improve quit rates. Most smoking cessation trials have been conducted in developed countries, and have yet to be conducted in low and middle income countries with vastly different educational cultural and economic factors to accurately assess the feasibility of these cessation strategies.

Success rates in quitting tobacco are generally low in India, as lack of awareness of harm, ingrained cultural attitudes, and lack of support for cessation maintains tobacco use. In 2002, tobacco cessation clinics were established in India to provide the first formal tobacco cessation intervention. Nineteen clinics were set up in oncology, cardiology, psychiatry, surgery and in NGO settings. Only behavioral interventions were used for 69% of the patients, and a combination of behavioral counseling and pharmacotherapy, typically bupropion and nicotine gums, were used for 31% of the patients. At 6 weeks, 14% had quit and 22% had reduced their tobacco use by at least half. Younger male patients and users of smokeless tobacco had relatively better outcomes at 3, 6, and 9 months.[69] Comparing the effect of behavioral counseling alone with counseling and medication (bupropion), the continuous tobacco abstinence rate in the counseling group at 1, 3, 6, and 12 months was 17%, 17%, 16%, and 15%, respectively, whereas in the medication group the rates were 60%, 58%, 54%, and 53%, respectively (P<0.001 for all comparisons).[70] The disadvantages of the cessation clinics were that they reached only a limited number of largely urban and educated tobacco users. Murthy and Saddichha (2010) suggest that tobacco cessation services in India need to be expanded at the primary, secondary, and tertiary care levels, so as to reach a wider population of users. In addition, increased availability and subsidies for NRT and other forms of pharmacotherapy can be introduced, wide-reaching cost-effective strategies, such as quit lines and group interventions should be developed and health professionals need to be trained in tobacco cessation.

Behavioral interventions have been shown to increase tobacco cessation rates in pregnant women.[71] There are few studies evaluating cessation interventions in low- and middle-income countries. In a cluster-randomized trial among pregnant women in the Lodz district of Poland, the intervention group (n = 205) received four midwife visits during pregnancy and one after delivery.[72] The control group (n = 181) received standard written information about the fetal health risks of prenatal smoking. Significantly higher smoking cessation rates were found in the intervention than in the control group (OR 2.5; 95%CI 1.8–3.7). A randomized controlled trial conducted in four Latin American cities (Rosario, Argentina; Pelotas, Brazil; Havana, Cuba and Mexico City, Mexico) studied the impact of a home-based health education and psychosocial support intervention targeting pregnant women (including education about prenatal smoking) on knowledge uptake, health behavior change, and perinatal outcomes.[73] Smoking cessation rates did not increase in the intervention group. Approximately one fifth of women in both the intervention and control groups smoked at study entry and at the end of pregnancy.

In South Africa, policy support was also provided by way of collating intersectoral data, for example health, economic and employment data, to create an impetus for decision makers and legislators.[74] National cross-sectional studies were conducted among adults (the National Adult Smoking Surveys—1993, 1994, 1996) to assess smoking behavior and compare trends over time. The surveys also provided key information during the legislative process.[62,75] Several qualitative and quantitative determinant studies of tobacco prevention[76] and smoking cessation[77,78] among school learners were also conducted.

Thus the formulation of tobacco control legislation in South Africa provides a singular case history of how health promotion and effective tobacco control strategies can radically change society, promote responsible health behaviors, and thus improve public health.

CLINICAL CAPACITY GAPS

Anti-tobacco warnings, campaigns, and cessation and prevention interventions should be evaluated to determine their effectiveness. In China, awareness of the health hazards related to tobacco smoking and second hand smoking was relatively poor considering the public education campaigns. A national survey showed that only 64.3% of the population were aware of serious diseases caused by SHS.[53]

Many countries in the developing world have a lack of nationally representative data on tobacco use. Published prevalence data in some African countries are nonexistent, e.g. Liberia, or are not standardized for inter-country comparison,[55] highlighting a major obstacle toward effective tobacco control in these countries. For sub-Saharan Africa, in particular, a weak knowledge base limits the targeting of strategies to combat the potential growth of tobacco use and its harmful effect on future mortality. Furthermore research on subgroups within a population is necessary, so as to identify high-risk populations and develop tailored interventions for these groups.

A lack of training and sensitization, as well as health professionals' misconceptions impacts on how effectively they can treat tobacco use behavior. One hospital-based study in Nigeria[79] found that 67% of the physicians reported being aware of smoking cessation therapy but only 30% had knowledge of specific treatments. The other study reported that 81% of physicians ever asked any patient about smoking status in the past 3 months.[80]

A study in Kerala showed that about one-third of doctors believed that smoking only becomes harmful when six or more cigarettes are smoked per day.[81] There is therefore a need to train health professionals in tobacco cessation counseling.

FUTURE RESEARCH AND NEEDS

In China, an emphasis on central leadership and multi-sector cooperation in tobacco control is needed, and this should be conveyed by relevant stakeholders to the central government.[5] Sustainable interventions including school-based anti-tobacco education, mass-media campaigns and community events are needed to raise public awareness of the health hazards of active smoking and second-hand smoking. Newer technologies such as Internet-based and telephone-based social networking systems, proven to be effective in randomized-controlled trials in younger western populations,[82] should be attempted on younger Chinese populations.[5]

The current cigarette pack warnings in China covering 30% of the front/back have been proven to be only marginally more effective than the previous warnings on the side of the pack,[83] suggesting that pictorial warnings may be required to improve the impact of health warnings.

In addition to collecting data on smoking prevalence and other measures of tobacco use, it is also necessary to monitor the activities of the tobacco industry. Many advocates foresee increasingly intense industry promotion and marketing as multinational tobacco companies focus on the potential customer base of the poorer countries of Africa, Asia, and Latin America.[49] Given the relatively low levels of tobacco use in Africa, the tobacco industry has in recent years greatly increased its presence in African countries and engaged in aggressive marketing campaigns, targeting youth in particular. In Nigeria for example, front groups were identified that were used by the tobacco industry to carry out its activities. Music concerts and other youth-centered events were sponsored by the industry, where cigarettes and tobacco-related merchandise were distributed freely.[20] Intensive efforts are thus required by the governments of these low- and middle-income countries to counteract the strategies of the tobacco industry.

Further research is needed into alternative sources of employment for workers in the tobacco industry (tobacco growing and product manufacturing). In the Philippines, efforts to promote alternative crops are hindered by the subsidies and incentives provided to growers by cigarette manufacturers.[49] Illicit trade and smuggling of tobacco products also hamper the effects of tobacco excise taxes. Thus, increased efforts are required by low- and middle-income countries to minimize these activities.

In terms of competing health priorities, countries in sub-Saharan Africa which are currently undergoing a rapid epidemiological transition, diseases such as HIV/AIDS have dominated health policy and practice both politically and financially. This has subsequently led to the unintended consequence of relegating chronic diseases to a disproportionately low priority status. As a result, these countries will likely not be adequately prepared for the coming wave of chronic diseases.

SUMMARY

Studies of Tobacco Smoking and Control

More than 80% of the world's smokers now live in low- or middle-income countries, and it is in these markets that tobacco usage and the associated burden of disease are growing most rapidly. The determinants of these high tobacco use rates are driven predominantly by gender (male), urbanicity, lower education, and lower income levels.

From a tobacco control policy perspective, there is substantial evidence to suggest that higher taxation on tobacco products is the most effective intervention to reduce tobacco use and encourage smokers to quit. The South African formulation of tobacco control policy is used as a singular case history of how health promotion and effective tobacco control strategies can influence responsible health behaviors.

Studies on the effectiveness of strong mass media campaigns, randomized controlled trials of intervention strategies from school-based tobacco prevention programs and meta-analyses evaluating tobacco cessation interventions using a combination of behavioral interventions and pharmacotherapy are further discussed. Major capacity gaps in effective tobacco control include a lack of nationally representative or nonstandardized data on tobacco use in many developing countries.

Future research needs include, in addition to collecting data on smoking prevalence and other measures of tobacco use, the necessity to monitor the activities of the tobacco industry. In countries currently undergoing a rapid epidemiological transition, diseases such as HIV/AIDS have dominated health policy and practice both politically and financially, thus relegating chronic diseases to a disproportionately low priority status leaving these countries inadequately prepared for the coming wave of chronic diseases.

REFERENCES

1. World Health Organization. WHO report on the global tobacco epidemic 2011. Warning about the dangers of tobacco. 2011. Geneva. (http://whqlibdoc.who.int/publications/2011/9789240687813_eng.pdf, accessed 27 January 2013).

2. Hosseinpoor AR, Parker LA, Tursan d'Espaignet E, Chatterji S. Social determinants of smoking in low- and middle-income countries: Results from the world health survey. *PLoS One*. 2011;6(5):e20331.

3. Centers for Disease Prevention and Control, Chinese Ministry of Health. Global Adult Tobacco Survey (GATS) China 2010 Country Report. 2010. Beijing. (http://who.int/tobacco/surveillance/survey/gats/en_gats_china_report.pdf, accessed 27 January 2013).

4. World Health Organization. Health situation analysis in the African region. Atlas of Health Statistics, 2011. 2011. Geneva. (http://www.afro.who.int/en/downloads/doc_download/7011-at-las-of-health-statistics-of-the-african-region-2011.html,, accessed 27 January 2013).

5. Zhang J, Ou JX, Bai CX. Tobacco smoking in China: Prevalence, disease burden, challenges and future strategies. *Respirology*. 2011;16(8):1165–1172.

6. Pampel F. Tobacco use in sub-Sahara Africa: Estimates from the demographic health surveys. *Soc Sci Med*. 2008;66(8):1772–1783.

7. National Population Commission (NPC) and ICF Macro. Nigeria Demographic and Health Survey 2008: Key Findings. 2009. Calverton, Maryland, USA: NPC and ICF Macro. (http://www.measuredhs.com/pubs/pdf/SR173/SR173.pdf, accessed 27 January 2013).

8. United Nations. Investment policy review: Nigeria. 2009. United Nations Conference on Trade and Development. Geneva. (http://unctad.org/en/docs/diaepcb20081_en.pdf, accessed 27 January 2013).

9. Steyn K, Jooste PL, Langenhoven ML, et al. Smoking patterns in the coloured population of the cape peninsula (CRISIC study). *S Afr Med J*. 1987;71(3):145–148.

10. Ayo-Yusuf OA, Reddy PS, van den Borne BW. Association of snuff use with chronic bronchitis among South African women: Implications for tobacco harm reduction. *Tob Control*. 2008;17(2):99–104.

11. Townsend L, Flisher AJ, Gilreath T, King G. A systematic literature review of tobacco use among adults 15 years and older in sub-Saharan Africa. *Drug Alcohol Depend*. 2006;84(1):14–27.

12. Rudatsikira E, Muula AS, Siziya S, Mataya RH. Correlates of cigarette smoking among school-going adolescents in Thailand: Findings from the Thai global youth tobacco survey 2005. *Int Arch Med*. 2008;1(1):8.

13. Rudatsikira E, Abdo A, Muula AS. Prevalence and determinants of adolescent tobacco smoking in Addis Ababa, Ethiopia. *BMC Public Health*. 2007;7:176.

14. Rudatsikira E, Muula AS, Siziya S. Current use of smokeless tobacco among adolescents in the republic of Congo. *BMC Public Health*. 2010;10:16.

15. Swart D, Reddy P, Pitt B, Panday S. The prevalence and determinants of tobacco-use among grade 8–10 learners in South Africa. The global youth tobacco school-based survey. 1999. South African Medical Research Council. Cape Town. (http://www.who.int/tobacco/surveillance/South%20Africa%201999.pdf, accessed 27 January 2013).

16. Swart D, Reddy P, Philip JL, Naidoo N, Ngobeni N. The 2002 global youth tobacco survey (GYTS): The 2nd GYTS in South Africa (SA)—A comparison between GYTS (SA) 1999 and GYTS (SA) 2002. 2004. South African Medical Research Council. Cape Town. (http://www.mrc.ac.za/healthpromotion/GYTS2002part1.pdf, accessed 27 January 2013).

17. Reddy SP, James S, Sewpaul R, Koopman F. The 2008 Global Youth Tobacco Survey: The 3rd GYTS in South Africa. 2010. South African Medical Research Council. Cape Town. (http://indicators.hst.org.za/indicators/Behaviour/GYTS_2008.pdf, accessed 27 January 2013).

18. Reddy SP, Panday S, Swart D, et al. Umthenthe Uhlaba Usamila – The South African Youth Risk Behaviour Survey 2002. South African Medical Research Council. Cape Town. (http://www.mrc.ac.za/healthpromotion/YRBSpart1.pdf, accessed 27 January 2013).

19. Reddy S, James S, Sewpaul R, et al. Umthente Uhlaba Usamila – The South African Youth Risk Behaviour Survey 2008. 2010. South African Medical Research Council. Cape Town. (http://www.mrc.ac.za/healthpromotion/yrbs_2008_final_report.pdf, accessed 27 January 2013).

20. Oberg M, Jaakkola MS, Woodward A, Peruga A, Pruss-Ustun A. Worldwide burden of disease from exposure to second-hand smoke: a retrospective analysis of data from 192 countries. *Lancet*. 2011;377(9760):139–146.

21. Rogers EM, Shoemaker FF. *Communication of innovations; a cross-cultural approach*. New York: Free Press; 1971:xix, 476 p.

22. Graham H. Smoking prevalence among women in the European community 1950–1990. *Soc Sci Med*. 1996;43(2):243–254.

23. King G, Grizeau D, Bendel R, Dressen C, Delaronde SR. Smoking behavior among French and American women. *Prev Med*. 1998;27(4):520–529.

24. Department of Health. South African Demographic and Health Survey (SADHS). 2003. Pretoria. South Africa. (http://www.info.gov.za/view/DownloadFileAction?id=90143, accessed 27 January 2013).

25. Harris-Eze AO. Smoking habits and chronic bronchitis in Nigerian soldiers. *East Afr Med J*. 1993;70(12):763–767.

26. Okojie OH, Isah EC, Okoro E. Assessment of health of senior executives in a developing country. *Public Health*. 2000;114(4):273–275.

27. Aina BA, Oyerinde OO, Joda AE, Dada OO. Cigarette smoking among healthcare professional students of University of Lagos and Lagos University teaching hospital (LUTH), Idi-Araba, Lagos, Nigeria. *Nig Q J Hosp Med*. 2009;19(1):42–46.

28. Wang CP, Ma SJ, Xu XF, Wang JF, Mei CZ, Yang GH. The prevalence of household second-hand smoke exposure and its correlated factors in six counties of China. *Tob Control*. 2009;18(2):121–126.

29. Harrabi I, Chahed H, Maatoug J, Gaha J, Essoussi S, Ghannem H. Predictors of smoking initiation among school children in Tunisia: A 4 years cohort study. *Afr Health Sci*. 2009;9(3):147–152.

30. Siziya S, Muula AS, Rudatsikira E. Correlates of current cigarette smoking among in-school adolescents in the Kurdistan region of Iraq. *Confl Health*. 2007;1:13.

31. Jamison B, Muula AS, Siziya S, Graham S, Rudatsikira E. Cigarette smoking among school-going adolescents in Lithuania: Results from the 2005 global youth tobacco survey. *BMC Res Notes*. 2010;3:130.

32. Muula AS, Siziya S, Rudatsikira E. Cigarette smoking and associated factors among in-school adolescents in Jamaica: Comparison of the global youth tobacco surveys 2000 and 2006. *BMC Res Notes*. 2008;1:55.

33. Memon A, Moody PM, Sugathan TN, et al. Epidemiology of smoking among Kuwaiti adults: Prevalence, characteristics, and attitudes. *Bull World Health Organ*. 2000;78(11):1306–1315.

34. Ministry of Health and Family Welfare, Government of India. Report on tobacco control in India. 2004. New Delhi. (http://www.who.int/fctc/reporting/Annex6_Report_on_Tobacco_Control_in_India_2004.pdf, accessed 27 January 2013).

35. Pomerleau J, Gilmore A, McKee M, Rose R, Haerpfer CW. Determinants of smoking in eight countries of the former Soviet Union: Results from the living conditions, lifestyles and health study. *Addiction*. 2004;99(12):1577–1585.

36. Jabbour S, Fouad FM. Religion-based tobacco control interventions: How should WHO proceed? *Bull World Health Organ*. 2004;82(12):923–927.

37. Gupta R, Gupta VP, Prakash H, Sarna M, Sharma AK. Hindu-Muslim differences in the prevalence of coronary heart disease and risk factors. *J Indian Med Assoc*. 2002;100(4):227–230.

38. Maziak W, Asfar T, Mzayek F. Socio-demographic determinants of smoking among low-income women in Aleppo, Syria. *Int J Tuberc Lung Dis*. 2001;5(4):307–312.

39. Lee JM, Hwang TC, Ye CY, Chen SH. The effect of cigarette price increase on the cigarette consumption in Taiwan: Evidence from the national health interview surveys on cigarette consumption. *BMC Public Health*. 2004;4:61.

40. Chung W, Lim S, Lee S, Choi S, Shin K, Cho K. The effect of cigarette price on smoking behavior in Korea. *J Prev Med Public Health*. 2007;40(5):371–380.

41. Kostova D, Ross H, Blecher E, Markowitz S. Is youth smoking responsive to cigarette prices? Evidence from low- and middle-income countries. *Tob Control*. 2011;20(6):419–424.

42. World Health Organization. WHO report on the global tobacco epidemic, 2009: Implementing smoke-free environments. 2009. Geneva. (http://whqlibdoc.who.int/publications/2009/9789241563918_eng_full.pdf, accessed 27 January 2013).

43. World Health Organization. WHO Report on the global tobacco epidemic, 2008: The MPOWER package. 2008. Geneva. (http://www.who.int/tobacco/mpower/mpower_report_full_2008.pdf, accessed 27 January 2013).

44. World Health Organization. MPOWER: A policy package to reverse the tobacco epidemic. 2008. Geneva. (http://www.who.int/tobacco/mpower/mpower_english.pdf, accessed 27 January 2013).

45. Ross H, Chaloupka FJ. Economic policies for tobacco control in developing countries. *Salud Publica Mex*. 2006;48 Suppl 1:S113–S120.

46. Ministry of Healthcare and Nutrition, Sri Lanka. World Health Organization Brief Profile on Tobacco Control in Sri Lanka. 2009. Sri Lanka. (http://209.61.208.233/LinkFiles/Tobacco_Free_Initiative_SEA-TFI-27.pdf, accessed 27 January 2013).

47. Hu TW, Mao Z. Effects of cigarette tax on cigarette consumption and the Chinese economy. *Tob Control*. 2002;11(2):105–108.

48. Lee K, Chagas LC, Novotny TE. Brazil and the framework convention on tobacco control: Global health diplomacy as soft power. *PLoS Med*. 2010;7(4):e1000232.

49. Douglas Blanks D and da Costa e Silva V. Tools for advancing tobacco control in the 21st century. Tobacco control legislation: an introductory guide. 2004. World Health Organization. Geneva. (http://www.who.int/tobacco/research/legislation/Tobacco%20Control%20Legislation.pdf, accessed 27 January 2013).

50. Higashi H, Khuong TA, Ngo AD, Hill PS. The development of tobacco harm prevention law in Vietnam: Stakeholder tensions over tobacco control legislation in a state owned industry. *Subst Abuse Treat Prev Policy*. 2011;6:24.

51. Li X, Li Q, Dong L, et al. Risk factors associated with smoking behaviour in recreational venues: Findings from the international tobacco control (ITC) China survey. *Tob Control*. 2010;19 Suppl 2:i30–i39.

52. Li L, Yong HH, Borland R, et al. Reported awareness of tobacco advertising and promotion in China compared to Thailand, Australia and the USA. *Tob Control*. 2009;18(3):222–227.

53. Yang Y, Wang JJ, Wang CX, Li Q, Yang GH. Awareness of tobacco-related health hazards among adults in China. *Biomed Environ Sci*. 2010;23(6):437–444.

54. Albuja S, Daynard RA. The framework convention on tobacco control (FCTC) and the adoption of domestic tobacco control policies: The Ecuadorian experience. *Tob Control*. 2009;18(1):18–21.

55. Nturibi EM, Akinsola AK, McCurdy SA. Smoking prevalence and tobacco control measures in Kenya, Uganda, the Gambia and Liberia: A review. *Int J Tuberc Lung Dis*. 2009;13(2):165–170.

56. National Assembly of the Federal Republic of Nigeria. National Tobacco Control Act 2008. 2008. (http://www.who.int/fctc/implementation/news/nig/en/index.html, accessed 27 January 2013).

57. Swart D and Reddy P. Strengthening Comprehensive Tobacco Control Policy Development in South Africa using Political Mapping. 1998. National Health Promotion Research and Development Office and The Chronic Diseases of Lifestyle Programme, South African Medical Research Council. Cape Town. (http://archive.idrc.ca/ritc/nhprdo.pdf, accessed 27 January 2013).

58. Department of Health, South Africa. Tobacco Products Control Act No 83 0f 1993. Government Gazette. July 1993. No 14916. Vol 512. (http://www.info.gov.za/view/DownloadFileAction?id=90146, accessed 27 January 2013).

59. Department of Health, South Africa. Tobacco Products Control Amendment Act No. 12 of 1999. Government Gazette. April 1999. No 19962.Vol 406. (http://www.doh.gov.za/show.php?id=1016, accessed 27 January 2013).

60. Department of Health, South Africa. Tobacco Products Control Amendment Act No. 63 of 2008. Government Gazette. January 2009. No. 31790. Vol. 523. (http://www.saflii.org/za/legis/num_act/tpcaa2008351.txt, accessed 27 January 2013).

61. Department of Health, South Africa. Tobacco Products Control Amendment Act No. 23 of 2007. Government Gazette February 2008. No. 30821. Vol. 512. (http://www.polity.org.za/article/tobacco-products-control-amendment-act-no-23-of-2007-2009-09-02, accessed 27 January 2013).

62. Reddy P, Meyer-Weitz A, Yach D. Smoking status, knowledge of health effects and attitudes toward tobacco control in South Africa. *South African Medical Journal*. 1996;86(11):1389–1393.

63. Mullin S, Prasad V, Kaur J, Turk T. Increasing evidence for the efficacy of tobacco control mass media communication programming in low- and middle-income countries. *J Health Commun*. 2011;16 Suppl 2:49–58.

64. Arora M, Stigler MH, Reddy KS. Effectiveness of health promotion in preventing tobacco use among adolescents in India: Research evidence informs the national tobacco control programme in India. *Glob Health Promot*. 2011;18(1):9–12.

65. Resnicow K, Reddy SP, James S, et al. Comparison of two school-based smoking prevention programs among South African high school students: Results of a randomized trial. *Ann Behav Med*. 2008;36(3):231–243.

66. Resnicow K, Zhang N, Vaughan RD, Reddy SP, James S, Murray DM. When intraclass correlation coefficients go awry: A case study from a school-based smoking prevention study in South Africa. *Am J Public Health*. 2010;100(9):1714–1718.

67. Rigotti N. Treatment of tobacco use and dependence. *N Engl J Med*. 2002;346:506–512.

68. Gorin SS, Heck JE. Meta-analysis of the efficacy of tobacco counseling by health care providers. *Cancer Epidemiol Biomarkers Prev*. 2004;13(12):2012–2022.

69. Murthy P, Saddichha S. Tobacco cessation services in India: Recent developments and the need for expansion. *Indian J Cancer*. 2010;47 Suppl 1:69–74.

70. Kumar R, Kushwah AS, Mahakud GC, Prakash S, Vijayan VK. Smoking cessation interventions and continuous abstinence rate at one year. *Indian J Chest Dis Allied Sci*. 2007;49(4):201–207.

71. Oncken CA, Dietz PM, Tong VT, et al. Prenatal tobacco prevention and cessation interventions for women in low- and middle-income countries. *Acta Obstet Gynecol Scand*. 2010;89(4):442–453.

72. Polanska K, Hanke W, Sobala W, Lowe JB. Efficacy and effectiveness of the smoking cessation program for pregnant women. *Int J Occup Med Environ Health*. 2004;17(3):369–377.

73. Belizan JM, Barros F, Langer A, Farnot U, Victora C, Villar J. Impact of health education during pregnancy on behavior and utilization of health resources. Latin American network for perinatal and reproductive research. *Am J Obstet Gynecol*. 1995;173(3 Pt 1):894–899.

74. Reddy P, Meyer-Weitz A, Abedian I, Steyn K, Swart D. Implementable strategies to strengthen comprehensive tobacco control in South Africa: Towards an optimal policy intervention mix. 1998. Policy Brief.

National Health Promotion and Development Office, South African Medical Research Council. Cape Town. (http://archive.idrc.ca/ritc/PolicyBrief2.htm, accessed 27 January 2013).

75. Reddy P, Meyer-Weitz A, Yach D. Smoking status, knowledge of health effects and attitudes towards tobacco control in South Africa. *S Afr Med J*. 1996;86(11):1389–93.

76. Swart D, Panday S, Reddy SP, Bergstrom E, de Vries H. Access point analysis: What do adolescents in South Africa say about tobacco control programmes? *Health Educ Res*. 2006;21(3):393–406.

77. Panday S, Reddy SP, Ruiter RA, Bergstrom E, de Vries H. Determinants of smoking cessation among adolescents in South Africa. *Health Educ Res*. 2005;20(5):586–599.

78. Panday S, Reddy SP, Ruiter RA, Bergstrom E, de Vries H. Determinants of smoking among adolescents in the southern Cape-Karoo region, South Africa. *Health Promot Int*. 2007;22(3):207–217.

79. Desalu OO, Adekoya AO, Elegbede AO, Dosunmu A, Kolawole TF, Nwogu KC. Knowledge of and practices related to smoking cessation among physicians in Nigeria. *J Bras Pneumol*. 2009;35(12):1198–1203.

80. Nollen N, Ahluwalia JS, Mayo MS, et al. A randomized trial of targeted educational materials for smoking cessation in African Americans using transdermal nicotine. *Health Educ Behav*. 2007;34(6):911–927.

81. Thankappan KR, Pradeepkumar AS, Nichter M. Doctors' behaviour & skills for tobacco cessation in Kerala. *Indian J Med Res*. 2009;129(3):249–255.

82. Grimshaw GM, Stanton A. Tobacco cessation interventions for young people. *Cochrane Database Syst Rev*. 2006;(4)(4):CD003289.

83. Fong GT, Hammond D, Jiang Y, et al. Perceptions of tobacco health warnings in China compared with picture and text-only health warnings from other countries: An experimental study. *Tob Control*. 2010;19 Suppl 2:i69–i77.

CHAPTER 20

HIV AND CANCER IN LESS DEVELOPED COUNTRIES

SAM M. MBULAITEYE

INTRODUCTION

Cases of Kaposi sarcoma (KS)[1,2] and aggressive B-cell non-Hodgkin lymphoma were reported in gay men in New York City in 1981,[3,4] and in Europe,[5] that marked the onset of the human immunodeficiency virus (HIV) pandemic. Shortly thereafter, dramatic increases in KS incidence were reported in sub-Saharan Africa, where the disease was known to occur endemically,[6,7] indicating deep penetration of the pandemic into sub-Saharan Africa.[8-10] KS, aggressive B cell NHL and opportunistic infections were reported to occur in persons suffering from severe depletion of cell-mediated immunity. The new pandemic was named acquired immunodeficiency syndrome" (AIDS). Studies conducted in the United States showed extraordinarily increased incidence rates for KS and NHL in people with HIV/AIDS. The high predictive value for AIDS in persons with these malignancies led to designating KS and aggressive B-cell NHLs as AIDS-defining cancers (ADCs)[11] to facilitate AIDS surveillance. Later, the incidence of cervical cancer was also noted to be increased in women with HIV and, although the increase was relatively modest (5–10 times), cervical cancer was declared an ADC to facilitate AIDS surveillance in women.[11] The close association between HIV/AIDS and risk for cancer noted at the outset of the HIV/AIDS pandemic triggered interest of many researchers who wanted to investigate and clarify the potential interactions of immunity, viruses, chemical and physical carcinogenic agents, and life style or geographical factors (Figure 20.1). The impact on other cancers was more modest and restricted to a handful of cancers, which were defined as non-AIDS-defining cancers (NADCs) that shared a viral or lifestyle etiology identified in patients with HIV/AIDS.[12] Information has accumulated about the impacts of HIV/AIDS on cancer in persons with HIV in different countries. Although, still incomplete, differences in the impact on cancers in different regions in developing countries are emerging (Figure 20.2). For example, although HIV/AIDS spread rapidly in countries in Asia, including India, KS has remained notably rare in the region's HIV infected persons.[13] Similarly, although Burkitt non-Hodgkin lymphoma risk is dramatically elevated in the West, it appears to be only slightly increased in Africa, where the disease predated the HIV/AIDS epidemic.[14-16]

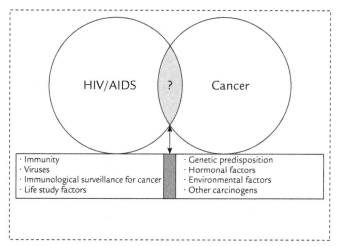

FIGURE 20.1 Understanding the overlap between HIV and cancer.

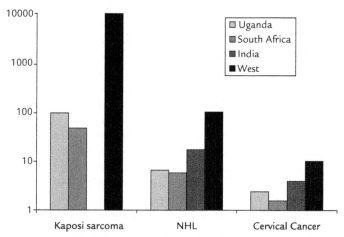

FIGURE 20.2 Estimates of association between AIDS-defining cancers (Kaposi sarcoma, Non-Hodgkin lymphoma, and cervical cancer) and HIV in representative studies conducted in different geographical regions.

In this chapter, we review current knowledge of the epidemiology of HIV/AIDS and cancers in less developed countries. Because our understanding of the epidemiologic patterns of cancers in persons with HIV has been shaped by studies conducted in developed countries, we briefly review these studies of specific ADCs and NADCs. This is followed by studies providing the best available evidence from developing countries to illustrate similarities and differences in the impact of HIV/AIDS on global cancer patterns. The chapter concludes by summarizing gaps in knowledge about the pathogenesis and spectrum of cancers in less developed countries and discussing opportunities to conduct studies that shed light on the general relationship between immunity and cancer.

▦ WHY QUANTIFY THE IMPACT OF HIV ON CANCER

First, an increase in cancer incidence due to HIV/AIDS, especially for cancers that are relatively common in the general population, would increase the overall cancer burden, potentially disrupting and further weakening the fragile economies and health infrastructure of the less developed countries. Thus, study of trends and patterns is useful for forecasting and planning and/or monitoring clinical and public health interventions. Second, epidemiologic studies may note novel patterns, which may suggest or provide clues to new infection-cancer associations and/or shed light on etiologic mechanisms. Finally, estimating the population attributable fraction (the proportion of cancer cases or deaths due to a specific cause), assists in assigning priorities in the use of scarce resources in cancer prevention and control programs.

Globally, the cancer burden has been increasing rapidly in many populations, in part, due to aging, urbanization, industrialization, and changing lifestyle practices.[17] This increase is notable in developing countries,[18] where a doubling of cancer cases has been observed over the past three decades.

Recent estimates from the UN Joint Program on AIDS (UNAIDS) indicate that 27.5–33.8 million people with HIV/AIDS (93% of the epidemic) live in less developed countries, including those in Africa (22.5 million or 67% of the epidemic),[19] in Asia, including India, and in Latin America, where 6.2 million people live with HIV/AIDS. However, less than 5% of studies on the link between HIV and cancer patterns have been conducted in Africa.[20] Although record-linkage studies have been essential in investigating the link between HIV and cancer in developed countries,[12,21–24] only one record-linkage study has been conducted in a developing country, namely Uganda.[16] This is due in part to a lower priority assigned to public health measures in cancer control in less developed countries, limited availability of pathologic confirmation of cancer cases, incomplete medical record files, and lack of cancer and HIV/AIDS registries. In addition, lack of unique personal identifying numbers, which can be used to track individuals from birth and through major life events, and regional cancer registries that record cancer incidence, or HIV/AIDS, detract from quality control of vital statistics. The few studies conducted in low- and middle-income countries described qualitative and quantitative differences in the pattern of cancers associated with HIV/AIDS. For example, KS, accounting for up to 10% of cancers in some countries in sub-Saharan Africa before the HIV/AIDS epidemic,[25] is the most common cancer in men, women, and children in Africa since the advent of the epidemic.[26,27] This change in incidence has been accompanied by a change in clinical progression, from an indolent disease with long survival to a more aggressive disease with a short median survival after diagnosis (approximately 15 months).[28] Conversely, KS was rare in Asia prior to the pandemic, and remains rare.[29] The reasons for this differential impact on KS in Africa and Asia are unclear, but may be related to low prevalence of Kaposi sarcoma-associated herpes virus (also called human herpes virus 8 or HHV8) in the general population and thus in patients with HIV/AIDS in Asia. Another example of differential impact is increased risk of squamous carcinoma of the conjunctiva in Africa, suggesting that this cancer is HIV-related in that region. However, whether this cancer is also increased in Asia or Latin America is unknown. Gradual increases in NHL incidence rates are being reported,[26,29,30] underscoring the potential impact of the HIV epidemic in less developed countries.[26] However, additional specific cancer sites that may be associated with HIV/AIDS, in low-and middle-income countries, such as uterine cervix, head and neck, and prostate, have not been adequately documented.[29,30]

AIDS-DEFINING CANCERS

Kaposi Sarcoma

Kaposi sarcoma was known to be endemic in Africa before the advent of the HIV/AIDS epidemic.[6,7] KS accounted for 5–18% of tumors in some areas, but its incidence showed marked geographic variation with the highest incidence noted in the Congo-Nile watershed area of Western Uganda, Eastern Congo, and south Kivu in Rwanda.[31] Onset of the HIV/AIDS epidemic was attended by a sudden increase in the number of KS cases recorded at hospitals in several African countries.[28,32] A careful analysis of cancer patterns from the Kampala Cancer Registry (KCR) for the period 1989–1991 by Wabinga et al.,[33] provided the first quantitative evidence of the population-level increase in KS incidence in Uganda, one of the first countries to be touched by the HIV epidemic. The KCR is one of the oldest continuously running cancer registries in Africa,[26] encompassing a population of about 1.2 million people residing in Kampala city and its suburbs. Routinely, cancer registrars visited local hospitals, histopathology laboratories, and Hospice centers to search for records of new cancer cases. Cases detected in the records were verified by reviewing hospital charts and abstracting data onto case report forms for keying into a computer using specialized software for cancer registration, or CANREG obtained from the International Agency for Research on Cancer (IARC).[34] Age-standardized KS incidence rates were calculated (cases per 100,000 person-years) for 1989–91, during the AIDS epidemic, and compared with 1954–1968, before the AIDS epidemic, to evaluate the impact of the HIV/AIDS epidemic on KS incidence in the local population. The proportional contribution of KS to all registered cancers, and to the incidence of KS, increased in both men and women during the AIDS epidemic (Figure 20.2). These initial results of population-level dynamics in KS incidence have been confirmed in later analyses using longer term data from 1960–1966 and 1995–1997 in Uganda.[26] KS incidence rates increased 12 times in men and 218 times in women during 1960–1966 and 1995–1997.[26] In Zimbabwe, KS incidence rates doubled both in men and women and KS now accounts for 31% of registered cancers and is the second most common malignancy in African women and children.[27,35]

Several case–control studies conducted in different countries have provided quantitative evidence suggesting that KS risk increased 22–95-fold with HIV (Table 20.1).[26,27,36] In Rwanda, the relative risk of KS was increased (approximately 35 times) with HIV, although the estimate was imprecise because of small sample size.[37] In South Africa, KS risk was elevated 22–47 times with HIV, based on two studies conducted in that country to date. In the first study, based on comparisons between 119 KS patients and 846 patients with other cancers or cardiovascular diseases enrolled at three tertiary hospitals in Johannesburg and Soweto from 1995 to 1999, the risk was 21.9 (95% CI=12.5–38.6).[38] In the second study including 5 more years of patient recruitment (1995–2004), the OR of KS was 47.1 (95% CI = 31.9–69.8), based on comparisons between 333 KS patients and 4399 patients with other cancers or cardiovascular diseases.[39] The impact of HIV on KS risk appears to be higher in children. The risk of KS with HIV was elevated 95 times (28.5–315.3) in a case–control study of children aged 15 years or younger in Uganda, but this estimate is imprecise due to limited sample size.[40]

The impact of HIV/AIDS on KS risk was evaluated among 12,607 HIV-infected persons attending a local AIDS organization called The AIDS Support Organization (TASO) in Kampala using record-linkage methods.[16] In this analysis, TASO, which was established in 1987 to provide social support to people with or affected by HIV, fulfilled the role of an HIV/AIDS registry. Cancer data were based on records from KCR. Individuals registered

TABLE 20.1 Association between AIDS-defining cancers with HIV in children and adults in studies conducted in sub-Saharan Africa

CANCER	COUNTRY	SUBJECTS	OR (95% CI)*	REFERENCES
Kaposi sarcoma	Uganda	Children	94.9 (28.5–315)	[40]
	Malawi	Children	93.5 (26.9–324)	[14]
	Uganda	Adults	6.4 (4.8–8.4)	[16]±
	Rwanda	Adults	35 (8.2–207)	[37]
	South Africa	Adults	22 (12.5–39)	[38]
	South Africa	Adults	47.1 (31.9–69.8)	[39]
Non-Hodgkin lymphoma				
Burkitt lymphoma	Uganda	Children	7.5 (2.8–20.1)	[40]
	Uganda	Children	2.2 (0.9–5.1)	[15]
	Malawi	Children	12.4 (1.3–116)	[59]
	Malawi	Children	2.2 (0.8–6.4)	[14]
	South Africa	Children	46.2 (16.4–130)	[60]
Non-Burkitt NHL	Malawi	Children	4.4 (1.1–17.9)	[14]
	South Africa	Children	5.0 (0.9–27.0)	[60]
	Uganda	Adults	6.2 (1.9–20)	[40]
	Uganda	Adults	6.7 (1.8–17)	[16]±
	South Africa	Adults	5.0 (2.7–9.5)	[38]
	South Africa	Adults	5.9 (4.3–8.1)	[39]
Cervical cancer	Uganda	Adults	1.6 (0.7–3.6)	[40]
	Uganda	Adults	2.4 (1.1–4.4)	[16]±
	South Africa	Adults	1.6 (1.1–2.3)	[38]
	South Africa	Adults	1.6 (1.3–2.0)	[39]

* OR Odds ratio; 95% CI 95% Confidence Interval; ± results are based on a record-linkage study and estimates represent standardized incidence ratios comparing risk of cancer in persons with HIV to the general population where cancers arose.

by TASO during 1988–2002 were linked to cancers registered with KCR during the same time period. To overcome lack of unique registry identifying numbers, the investigators used letters in individual names, age, and residence to create unique combinations of characters that could be linked to identify unique records in TASO and KCR using probabilistic matching algorithms. Cancers occurring in the period before registration with TASO were considered prevalent (Figure 20.3). For example, cancers occurring in the 0–3 month period were discounted because, being prevalent cancers, they were subject to detection bias associated with increased frequency of medical examination during assessments associated with registration at TASO. Cancers occurring from 3 months after registration with TASO to 5 years later were considered incident cancers.

The estimate of cancer risk in the early (3–27 months after registration) period is considered more accurate because competing mortality due to HIV is still low. However, estimates of cancer risk in the late (28–60 months) period may be less accurate because of biases

TABLE 20.2 Distribution of cancers observed in the Uganda HIV/AIDS Cancer Match Study*

CANCER TYPE	PERIOD OF ONSET AFTER REGISTRATION WITH TASO			
	PREVALENT	4–27 MONTHS	28–60 MONTHS	TOTAL
AIDS-defining cancers				
Kaposi sarcoma	107 (59%)	52 (54%)	53 (%)	212 (56%)
Non-Hodgkin lymphoma	3 (2%)	4 (4%)	1(1%)	8 (2%)
Cervix uteri	24 (13%)	10 (10%)	17 (17%)	41 (11%)
All AIDS defining cancers	134 (74%)	66 (69%)	71(70%)	261 (72%)
Non-AIDS defining cancers	47 (26%)	30 (31%)	30 (30%)	107 (28%)
Total	181 (48%)	96 (25%)	101 (27%)	378

*Based on the record-linkage study by Mbulaiteye et al.[16]

related to competing HIV-related mortality. Thus, standardized incidence ratios (SIRs) were calculated both for the early and late periods, as well as for both periods combined.

Overall, 378 cancers were linked (Table 20.2). Using the approach developed in western countries in classifying cancers (Figure 20.3), 48% of the linked cancers were prevalent; 25% occurred in the early AIDS period, and 28% in the late AIDS period. ADCs accounted for 72% and NADCs accounted for 28% of incident cancers. Among ADCs, the proportional contribution was 56% for KS, 11% for cervical cancer, and 2% for NHL. The SIR for KS was 6.4 (95% CI 4.8–8.4) during the 4–27 month period after registration (Figure 20.4). This increased risk was is less than that observed in case–control studies, as well as in studies conducted in western countries (SIR 3000–100,000).[22] The reasons for relatively modest increases in risk are unknown. One possible inference is that the risk of HIV-related KS in KS endemic regions may be lower in individuals in whom KSHV infection preceded HIV-related immunosuppression.[16] More likely, lower relative risks of KS in KS endemic regions may be due to competing mortality from opportunistic infections, to incomplete KS ascertainment, or confounded by the high background incidence of KS in the general population.[41] The SIRs were much higher when the investigators estimated SIRs using KS incidence rates in the 1960s before the AIDS epidemic. However, the interpretation of SIRs, when based on nonconcurrent incidence rates, may be confounded by period and cohort effects.

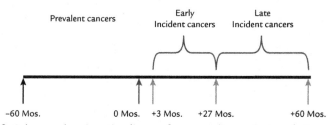

FIGURE 20.3 Schema showing timelines of cancer diagnosis in relation to time since registration with HIV/AIDS registry. The arrow at time "0" represents the time of registration with HIV/AIDS.

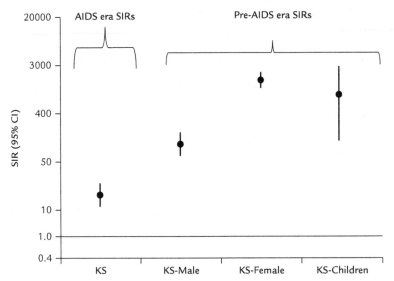

FIGURE 20.4 Standardized incidence ratios for Kaposi sarcoma (KS) for all subjects using KS rates calculated from during the AIDS era (1989–2002) and from the pre-AIDS era (1961–1971) for males, females, and children, based on data from the Uganda HIV/AIDS Cancer Match Study.

In contrast to the obvious impact of HIV on KS in Africa, the impact of HIV on KS in persons with HIV in Asia has not been convincingly shown.[29,42] KS was not observed in the largest study of the spectrum of cancers with HIV conducted by Dhir and colleagues[29] at Tata Memorial Hospital in Mumbai, India, during 2001–2005. Overall, 137 persons with cancers were found to be HIV positive; none of the cancers was KS. As TATA Memorial Hospital is the largest tertiary cancer referral medical center in India, the findings from this hospital are likely representative of the cancer patterns with HIV in India. The absence of KS despite a large HIV epidemic may be a clue to low prevalence of KSHV in the general population in India.

The study by Dhir et al.,[29] is also instructive from a methodological point of view. The investigators had access to hospital-based data, but they lacked precise information about the general population where cancers arose. Thus, the the impact of HIV on cancer was evaluated by calculating the age- and sex-adjusted proportional distribution of each cancer type in persons with HIV and dividing it by the corresponding proportional distribution of each cancer type registered in all patients with cancer seen at TATA Memorial Hospital in 2002. The resulting ratio is called a "proportional incidence ratio (PIR)" and may approximate the SIR. PIRs, similar to SIRs, provide a crude estimation of relative risk for cancers in persons with the exposure of interest. However, in contrast to SIRs, PIRs are sensitive to changes in the relative contribution of cancer types that may not be related to the etiologic co-factor under investigation. For example, an increase or decrease in the diagnosis of a given cancer in the study and/or reference group will influence the magnitude or direction of the ratio.

Elsewhere in Asia, in Thailand, where the AIDS epidemic has been documented for close to three decades, KS as in India, remains distinctly rare.[43] The picture is slightly different in Latin America, where KS is diagnosed frequently, but in homosexual men. For example, in Brazil, KS is an AIDS-defining condition in 25% of patients.[44] In these studies,

the diagnosis of KS is associated with homosexual contact and with being KSHV seropositive (Odds ratio 17–24).[45,46]

Taken together, studies conducted in developing countries indicate that the relative risk
of KS is elevated with HIV infection in sub-Saharan Africa, but the impact is comparatively
less than that observed in more developed countries. Conversely, KS risk is not elevated,
or only marginally elevated, in Asia.[13] The variations in the impact of HIV on KS may be
related to variations in KSHV prevalence,[47] in specific populations with HIV. As KSHV
viremia is linked to elevated KS risk,[48–50] one suggestion for differential impact in KS risk is
timing of KSHV infection relative to HIV infection. In developed countries, the incidence
of HIV-related KS has decreased following the introduction of combination antiretroviral therapies (cART).[51] Whether similar declines will be observed in less developed countries, where intervention treatment programs are expanding,[52] is possible and will require
documentation.

NON-HODGKIN LYMPHOMA

The background incidence of NHL in less developed countries is generally lower than
that in developed countries,[53] Burkitt lymphoma, which is an ADC, is endemic in certain
countries. However, the impact of HIV on NHL risk in less developed countries, including
those in Africa where Burkitt lymphoma is endemic, is still unclear. Available clinical and
epidemiologic evidence suggests that the cumulative probability of lymphoma with AIDS
is lower than in the West.[54]

A clinical report from Kenya, one of the countries impacted by the HIV epidemic, noted
that 19 of 26 NHL cases among persons aged 16 years or older diagnosed between 1992
and 1996 were HIV positive.[55] This number of NHLs in adults with HIV was higher than
would be expected, based on historical patterns before the HIV epidemic, and the median
age of the HIV positive cases with Burkitt lymphoma (35 years), which was higher than the
median age of 5–9 years typically observed in endemic Burkitt lymphoma. However, case
reports are limited because they do not allow risk to be estimated.

The best evidence we have of low impact of HIV on NHL risk comes from a systematic
case-series report of 247 persons aged 14 years or older who died of HIV-related disease and
underwent post-mortem diagnosis at a hospital in Abidjan Cote d'Ivoire.[56] The cumulative
risk of NHL was 2.8%, including 1.6% with visceral NHL and 1.2% with primary cerebral
lymphoma. This low risk contrasts with a cumulative risk of about 6% observed early in
the epidemic in the West.[57] This study included 78 HIV-positive children, but Burkitt lymphoma was not observed despite this region being endemic for the disease. The reasons
for this include competing mortality from HIV-related co-morbidity and, in many cases,
because of limited access to tumor specimens for pathologic classification of NHL.[30,58]

Data from population-based cancer registries in some African countries indicated that
population incidence of NHL may have increased during the AIDS epidemic. For example,
the incidence of NHL in Kampala in Uganda increased 3 times (2.3 to 6.6 per 100,000)
between 1961 and 1971 prior to the AIDS epidemic and in 1997 during the AIDS epidemic.[26] This increase was most marked for pediatric Burkitt lymphoma, which increased
4 times from 0.9 per 100,000 children before the AIDS epidemic to 3.8 during the AIDS
epidemic. While these data were suggestive, firm inferences could not be made because the
HIV status of individual cases was not known.

Results obtained from case–control studies have been inconsistent, with some studies
suggesting no association, while others describing associations of HIV and NHL as odds
ratios ranging from 2.2–46.2[14,15,40,59,60] (Table 20.1). Among adults, the association between

HIV and non-Burkitt lymphoma NHL ranged from 5.0–6.7 (Table 20.1). In the case–control study of adults in South Africa, Sitas et al. reported an OR of 5.0 (95% CI 2.7–9.5),[38] based on 105 histologically confirmed NHL cases and 844 hospital controls selected for cancers unrelated to HIV (in men) or vascular diseases (in women). These results were confirmed when final analyses were performed involving 154 adult NHL cases and 4399 controls.[39] In two case–control studies conducted in children, the OR for the association of non-Burkitt lymphoma with HIV was 4.4–5.0[14,60] (Table 20.1), but the result was statistically significant in only one study.[60] Significantly positive associations of HIV with Burkitt Lymphoma (OR 7.5–12.4) have been reported in two studies conducted in Uganda[40] and in Malawi,[59] based on cases diagnosed clinically or by histopathology. However, when the Ugandan data were re-analyzed using only cases confirmed by reviewed pathology, the association was no longer statistically significant (OR 2.1),[15] casting doubt on the validity of the previously reported significant associations. Recently, results from the HIV/AIDS-cancer record-linkage study in Uganda suggested that NHL incidence in HIV positive persons was increased nearly 7 times that of the incidence in the general population (SIR 6.7, 95% CI 1.8–17),[16] but independent histological verification of NHL was not done (Figure 20.5).

A recent study conducted in South Africa[60] reported an increased risk for the association of Burkitt lymphoma with HIV, based on 13/33 patients who were HIV positive. This contrasts with the experience in east and central Africa that patients with endemic Burkitt lymphoma are usually HIV negative.[61] Given that Burkitt lymphoma in South Africa is of the sporadic type, this result is reminiscent of the dramatically increased risk of HIV-related Burkitt lymphoma in developed countries,[62] and suggests a differential impact of HIV on endemic versus sporadic Burkitt lymphoma.

Limited data from Asia and Latin America suggest that NHL risk might be increased in persons with HIV from those regions. In India, the risk of NHL was increased in both men (PIR = 17) and women (PIR = 10), based on a study conducted at Tata Memorial

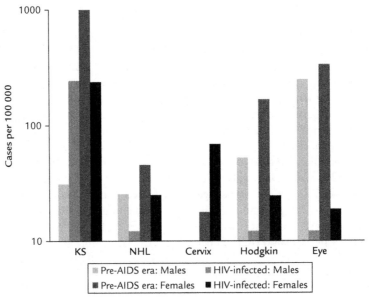

FIGURE 20.5 Incidence of selected cancers in persons with HIV/AIDS in The AIDS Support Organization, based on data from the Uganda HIV/AIDS Cancer Match Study.

Hospital. NHL was the most common type of cancer reported in this study, accounting for 38% of the cancers seen in males and 16% of all cancers in women. The lower PIR of NHL in women than in men may be confounded by the prominence of uterine cervical cancer. In Thailand, the population-based cancer registry data reported that the incidence of NHL had almost doubled from 2.7 per 100,000 during the early period in the AIDS epidemic in 1989–1991 to 4.8 per 100,000 in the later period in the AIDS epidemic in 1999–2001.[43] The incidence increased most steeply (11% per year, 95%CI, 8.6%–12.7%) for diffuse/high-grade lymphoma.[43] In one study in Hubei Province in China that measured the incidence of NHL in 3554 HIV-positive individuals from 2004 to 2007, the incidence of NHL was elevated 34 times (95% CI 11.7–89.9) when compared to the general population. Data from Brazil are scanty, but NHLs have been reported in persons with HIV and show a strong association with Epstein-Barr virus (EBV).[63] Taken together, results from less developed countries are consistent with the conclusion that NHL risk is increased with HIV, but the increase is less than that observed in developed countries. The lesser impact may be artifactual due to competing mortality from conditions that are prevalent in the region[56,64,65,66] Under-ascertainment and/or misclassification of cases remain in the diagnosis of lymphoma in less developed countries.[58] Final conclusions about the impact of HIV on NHL await results from studies using sound epidemiologic and laboratory design.

▪ CERVICAL CANCER

Cervical cancer is the first or second leading cause of cancer death in many developing countries,[67] where some of the world's highest incidence rates are observed.[53] Data from population-based cancer registries and case–control studies do not provide a clear picture of an impact of HIV on cervical cancer incidence. In Uganda, the incidence of cervical cancer in Kampala increased nearly three-fold from 17.7 per 100,000 during 1960–1966[26] to 52.4 during 1991–2006.[68] Whether this increase is due to HIV or temporal trends related to urbanization cannot be determined from cancer registry data. In Zimbabwe, another country severely impacted by HIV, the incidence of cervical cancer in Harare did not change between 1990–1992 and 1993–1995 and no change in the mean age at diagnosis was observed in cervical cancer cases diagnosed before and during the AIDS epidemic.[35]

Results from case–control studies conducted are compatible with a null or slight increase in risk for cervical cancer with HIV.[38–40] In Uganda, the association of cervical cancer with HIV was 1.6 (95% CI, 0.7–3.6), based on comparison of HIV prevalence in 65 women with cervical cancer vesus 112 women with other cancers or noncancerous conditions.[40] In South Africa, the corresponding OR was 1.6 (95% CI, 1.1–2.3), based on 1323 cases of cervical cancer and 556 women with non-HIV-related cancers or vascular disease.[38] This result has been replicated (OR 1.6, 95% CI 1.3–2.0) in the final analysis including 1586 cervical cancer cases and 2, 863 controls.[39] The risk of cervical cancer was increased 2.4 times with HIV in the record-linkage study in Uganda (SIR 2.4, 95% CI 1.1–4.4).[16] Taken together, studies conducted in sub-Saharan Africa using different epidemiological approaches are compatible with a weak, but potentially signficant increase in risk of cervical cancer with HIV. Although the impact of HIV on cervical cancer appears to be comparatively small, it may be important for public health because it could result in a large increase the number of cervical cancer cases and associated mortality from HIV-infected women in Africa.[53]

The impact of HIV on cervical cancer was slightly stronger in India (PIR = 4),[29] the country with the world's highest number of cervical cancer cases. The impact was even stronger in China (SIR 68.1, 95% CI 19.2–84.5), based on 14 cases observed among 1599 HIV infected women in Hubei Province in China during 2004 to 2008.[42] While these findings are based on only two studies and need to be confirmed, they are compatible with a potentially important public health impact of HIV in some regions.

NON AIDS-DEFINING CANCERS

Cancer patterns in the general population in low-and middle-income countries are different from those in the developed countries because of variations in socioeconomic, lifestyle, environmental and/or genetic factors. Thus, the impact of HIV on cancer is likely to vary from one population to another according to prevalence of local factors. Comparative studies of cancer patterns in HIV-infected populations in less developed versus more developed countries may help identify biologic agents associated with specific cancers. For example, KSHV and Merkel cell virus (MCV) were discovered after epidemiologic studies showed that risk for these cancers was dramatically increased in persons with AIDS.[47,69]

SQUAMOUS CELL CARCINOMA OF THE CONJUNCTIVA

Squamous cell carcinoma of the conjunctiva (SCCC) is a rare cancer whose incidence is inversely correlated with latitude, suggesting the etiologic role of exposure to ultraviolet light.[70,71] An impact of HIV on SCCC was suspected when analysis of population-based cancer data in Kampala in showed that the incidence of eye cancers increased 15 times from 0.2 per 100,000 in 1960–1966 before the AIDS epidemic to 3.0 in 1995–1997 during the AIDS epidemic.[26] The fraction of SCCC as a proportion of eye cancers increased from 23.5% to 71% in men and 0% to 85% in women in the respective periods.[26] A small case–control study conducted in Uganda showed that three quarters of 48 patients with SCCC were HIV positive compared to only 19% among 48 matched controls with non-malignant eye conditions.[72] These early findings have been confirmed in several case–control studies conducted in Uganda and elsewhere in tropical Africa,[70,73] but no positive associations were reported in South Africa.[39] Given that South Africa is quite distant from the equator, the negative findings may suggest that the impact of HIV on SCCC risk is mediated via interaction with ultraviolet light. The epidemiologic association of cutaneous squamous cell cancers with impaired immunity and ultraviolet radiation has been described in immunosuppressed organ transplant patients. Other preliminary studies of HIV and cutaneous and mucosal cancers have focused on associations with persistent human papillomavirus (HPV) infections.[70,71,74–76] The impact of HIV in India is unknown, although some cases have been reported suggesting SCCC occurs in HIV infected persons in that setting.[77] Firm conclusions must await analytic studies to provide quantitative estimates of risk.

HODGKIN LYMPHOMA

The risk of Hodgkin lymphoma is increased with HIV in developed countries,[22,24,78] but the evidence from low-and middle-income countries is less clear.[16,38,39] The evidence was equivocal in the preliminary analysis of the case–control study in South Africa (OR 1.4, 95% CI 0.7–2.8),[38] but subsequent analyses showed marginally significant results (OR 1.4, 95% CI 1.0–2.7).[39] The clearest evidence of elevated risk in less developed countries was noted in the Uganda HIV/AIDS record-linkage study (OR 5.7, 95% CI 1.2–17).[16] Although data from Asia are sparse, limited data from the TATA Memorial Hospital in India noted that the PIR was increased 200–400%, which was compatible with an associated risk with HIV.[29]

■ LIVER CANCER

Hepatocellular carcinoma (HCC) is one of the most common cancers in many less developed countries.[53] However, an association of HIV with HCC has not been demonstrated[16,39,40] However, recent studies have noted high frequency of co-infection between HIV and chronic hepatitis B and C infections in many countries in sub-Saharan Africa,[79,80] prompting concern that this might increase the risk of HCC. No association has been demonstrated between liver cancer and HIV in South Africa (OR 0.8, 95% CI 0.4–1.7)[39] or in Uganda (OR 1.2, 95% CI 0.3–4.2).[40] The reasons for lack of association are not known, but as liver cancer has a long induction period, it may be premature to come to conclusions about associations with HIV. Population-based rates of liver cancer have been stable among men in Uganda from 1960–1980 and 1991–2005,[81] consistent with lack of an impact from HIV. However, a slight increase in incidence was noted in women, which may be due to temporal trends unrelated to HIV. A recent study in China demonstrated an elevated risk (SIR 6.0, 95% CI 2.6–12.2),[42] but these results need to be confirmed. Studies in developed countries have revealed a slightly increased risk,[22] suggesting that co-infection with HBV and/or HCV, which is also prevalent in China,[82] may increase the risk of HCC in HIV patients.

■ CANCER SURVIVAL

Cancer is estimated to account for up to one-third of deaths in patients with HIV in western countries.[83,84] The relative increase in non-AIDS-defining cancers is, in part, due to increased survival and aging of HIV-infected populations in western countries. The unprecedented efforts to bring antiretroviral therapies to people with HIV/AIDS in sub-Saharan Africa is likely to change the importance of cancer in people with HIV in less developed countries.[19] Studies conducted thus far suggest that the pattern of cancer in less developed countries is similar to that observed in western countries,[20,85] but the impact appears to be quantitatively less, because proportionately more cancers in sub-Saharan Africa are linked to infectious etiology.[86] While proportionately more cancers in the western countries are linked to behavioral and environmental risk factors,[87] study of the link between HIV and cancer in these populations presents unique opportunities to acquire epidemiologic information about etiology and pathogenesis, and public health significance of cancer patterns in diverse settings.[20,85] Careful analysis of cancer risk patterns in persons with HIV/AIDS in low-and middle-income countries will provide extraordinary opportunities in planning of prevention and control programs in diverse racial and socio-cultural populations.[88]

■ SUMMARY

This chapter is an introduction to the epidemiology of human immunodeficiency virus (HIV)-associated cancers in less developed countries. The scientific and public health rationale for analyzing cancer patterns and trends in persons with HIV are reviewed. Specific studies that illustrate epidemiologic approaches to cancer patients with HIV/AIDS may serve to illuminate interactions between infectious agents, environmental and lifestyle factors, and impaired immunity in human carcinogenesis.

Briefly, the onset of the HIV epidemic, three decades ago, was heralded by Kaposi sarcoma (KS) and aggressive non-Hodgkin lymphomas (NHL). Concern that a cancer epidemic would follow in the wake of the HIV epidemic prompted studies to evaluate the impact of the HIV epidemic on cancer in developed countries, where reliable data were available. Three decades later, we recognized that a limited spectrum of cancers, mostly of infectious etiology, were increased. This knowledge was initially based on studies conducted in developed countries in which about 7% of the HIV epidemic was reported. Today, 93% of the estimated 27.5–33.8 million people living with the HIV infection reside in low-and middle-income countries (LMICs), including 67% in sub-Saharan Africa. Because proportionately more cancers in LMICs are linked to infections agents, namely more than 20% compared with less than 10% in developed countries, the evaluation of the impact of HIV on cancer in this setting has resulted in important insights about the interactions of innate and adaptive immune mechanisms.

■ REFERENCES

1. Friedman-Kien AE. Disseminated Kaposi's sarcoma syndrome in young homosexual men. *J Am Acad Dermatol.* 1981;5(4):468–471.
2. Hymes KB, Cheung T, Greene JB, et al. Kaposi's sarcoma in homosexual men-a report of eight cases. *Lancet.* 1981;2(8247):598–600.
3. Ziegler JL, Drew WL, Miner RC, et al. Outbreak of Burkitt's-like lymphoma in homosexual men. *Lancet.* 1982;2(8299):631–633.
4. Ziegler JL, Beckstead JA, Volberding PA, et al. Non-Hodgkin's lymphoma in 90 homosexual men. Relation to generalized lymphadenopathy and the acquired immunodeficiency syndrome. *N Engl J Med.* 1984;311(9):565–570.
5. Ebbesen P, Melbye M, Biggar RJ. Sex habits, recent disease, and drug use in two groups of Danish male homosexuals. *Arch Sex Behav.* 1984;13(4):291–300.
6. Taylor JF, Templeton AC, Vogel CL, Ziegler JL, Kyalwazi SK. Kaposi's sarcoma in Uganda: A clinico-pathological study. *Int J Cancer.* 1971;8(1):122–135.
7. Templeton AC, Hutt MS. Distribution of tumours in Uganda. *Recent Results Cancer Res.* 1973;41:1–22.
8. Downing RG, Eglin RP, Bayley AC. African Kaposi's sarcoma and AIDS. *Lancet.* 1984;1(8375):478–480.
9. Bayley AC. Occurrence, clinical behaviour and management of Kaposi's sarcoma in Zambia. *Cancer Surv.* 1991;10:53–71.
10. Ziegler JL, Katongole-Mbidde E. Kaposi's sarcoma in childhood: An analysis of 100 cases from Uganda and relationship to HIV infection. *Int J Cancer.* 1996;65(2):200–203.
11. Centers for Disease Control (CDC). Human immunodeficiency virus (HIV) infection codes. Official authorized addendum. ICD-9-CM (revision no. 1). Effective January 1, 1988. *MMWR Morb Mortal Wkly Rep.* 1987;36 Suppl 7:1S–20S.
12. Grulich AE. Cancer: The effects of HIV and antiretroviral therapy, and implications for early antiretroviral therapy initiation. *Curr Opin HIV AIDS.* 2009;4(3):183–187.
13. Biggar RJ, Chaturvedi AK, Bhatia K, Mbulaiteye SM. Cancer risk in persons with HIV/AIDS in India: A review and future directions for research. *Infect Agent Cancer.* 2009;4:4.
14. Mutalima N, Molyneux EM, Johnston WT, et al. Impact of infection with human immunodeficiency virus-1 (HIV) on the risk of cancer among children in Malawi—preliminary findings. *Infect Agent Cancer.* 2010;5:5.
15. Parkin DM, Garcia-Giannoli H, Raphael M, et al. Non-Hodgkin lymphoma in Uganda: A case-control study. *AIDS.* 2000;14(18):2929–2936.
16. Mbulaiteye SM, Katabira ET, Wabinga H, et al. Spectrum of cancers among HIV-infected persons in Africa: The Uganda AIDS-cancer registry match study. *Int J Cancer.* 2006;118(4):985–990.
17. Ferlay J, Shin HR, Bray F, Forman D, Mathers C, Parkin DM. GLOBOCAN 2008 v1.2, Cancer Incidence and Mortality Worldwide: IARC CancerBase no. 10 [internet]. 2010. Accessed 07/02/2012.
18. Lingwood RJ, Boyle P, Milburn A, et al. The challenge of cancer control in Africa. *Nat Rev Cancer.* 2008;8(5):398–403.
19. United Nations Programme on HIV/AIDS (UNAIDS), World Health Organization (WHO). AIDS Epidemic Update: November 2009. Geneva: WHO. 2009.

20. Sasco AJ, Jaquet A, Boidin E, et al. The challenge of AIDS-related malignancies in sub-Saharan Africa. *PLoS One.* 2010;5(1):e8621.

21. Cote TR, Biggar RJ, Rosenberg PS, et al. Non-Hodgkin's lymphoma among people with AIDS: Incidence, presentation and public health burden. AIDS/Cancer study group. *Int J Cancer.* 1997;73(5):645–650.

22. Goedert JJ, Cote TR, Virgo P, et al. Spectrum of AIDS-associated malignant disorders. *Lancet.* 1998;351(9119):1833–1839.

23. Dal Maso L, Braga C, Franceschi S. Methodology used for "software for automated linkage in Italy" (SALI). *J Biomed Inform.* 2001;34(6):387–395.

24. Grulich AE, Li Y, McDonald A, Correll PK, Law MG, Kaldor JM. Rates of non-AIDS-defining cancers in people with HIV infection before and after AIDS diagnosis. *AIDS.* 2002;16(8):1155–1161.

25. Hutt MS. Cancer in the black populations of East Africa. *Prog Clin Biol Res.* 1981;53:55–66.

26. Wabinga HR, Parkin DM, Wabwire-Mangen F, Nambooze S. Trends in cancer incidence in Kyadondo county, Uganda, 1960–1997. *Br J Cancer.* 2000;82(9):1585–1592.

27. Chokunonga E, Levy LM, Bassett MT, Mauchaza BG, Thomas DB, Parkin DM. Cancer incidence in the African population of Harare, Zimbabwe: Second results from the cancer registry 1993–1995. *Int J Cancer.* 2000;85(1):54–59.

28. Bayley AC. Aggressive Kaposi's sarcoma in Zambia, 1983. *Lancet.* 1984;1(8390):1318–1320.

29. Dhir AA, Sawant S, Dikshit RP, et al. Spectrum of HIV/AIDS related cancers in India. *Cancer Causes Control.* 2008;19(2):147–153.

30. Abayomi EA, Somers A, Grewal R, et al. Impact of the HIV epidemic and anti-retroviral treatment policy on lymphoma incidence and subtypes seen in the western cape of South Africa, 2002–2009: Preliminary findings of the Tygerberg lymphoma study group. *Transfus Apher Sci.* 2011;44(2):161–166.

31. Hutt MS. The epidemiology of Kaposi's sarcoma. *Antibiot Chemother.* 1981;29:3–11.

32. Serwadda D, Carswell W, Ayuko WO, Wamukota W, Madda P, Downing RG. Further experience with Kaposi's sarcoma in Uganda. *Br J Cancer.* 1986;53(4):497–500.

33. Wabinga HR, Parkin DM, Wabwire-Mangen F, Mugerwa JW. Cancer in Kampala, Uganda, in 1989–91: Changes in incidence in the era of AIDS. *Int J Cancer.* 1993;54(1):26–36.

34. Coleman MP, Bieber CA. CANREG: Cancer registration software for microcomputers. *IARC Sci Publ.* 1991;(95)(95):267–274.

35. Chokunonga E, Levy LM, Bassett MT, et al. Aids and cancer in Africa: The evolving epidemic in Zimbabwe. *AIDS.* 1999;13(18):2583–2588.

36. Banda LT, Parkin DM, Dzamalala CP, Liomba NG. Cancer incidence in Blantyre, Malawi 1994–1998. *Trop Med Int Health.* 2001;6(4):296–304.

37. Newton R, Grulich A, Beral V, et al. Cancer and HIV infection in Rwanda. *Lancet.* 1995;345(8961):1378–1379.

38. Sitas F, Pacella-Norman R, Carrara H, et al. The spectrum of HIV-1 related cancers in South Africa. *Int J Cancer.* 2000;88(3):489–492.

39. Stein L, Urban MI, O'Connell D, et al. The spectrum of human immunodeficiency virus-associated cancers in a South African black population: Results from a case-control study, 1995–2004. *Int J Cancer.* 2008;122(10):2260–2265.

40. Newton R, Ziegler J, Beral V, et al. A case-control study of human immunodeficiency virus infection and cancer in adults and children residing in Kampala, Uganda. *Int J Cancer.* 2001;92(5):622–627.

41. Chaturvedi AK, Mbulaiteye SM, Engels EA. Underestimation of relative risks by standardized incidence ratios for AIDS-related cancers. *Ann Epidemiol.* 2008;18(3):230–234.

42. Zhang YX, Gui XE, Zhong YH, Rong YP, Yan YJ. Cancer in cohort of HIV-infected population: Prevalence and clinical characteristics. *J Cancer Res Clin Oncol.* 2011;137(4):609–614.

43. Sriplung H, Parkin DM. Trends in the incidence of acquired immunodeficiency syndrome-related malignancies in Thailand. *Cancer.* 2004;101(11):2660–2666.

44. Yoshioka MC, Alchorne MM, Porro AM, Tomimori-Yamashita J. Epidemiology of Kaposi's sarcoma in patients with acquired immunodeficiency syndrome in Sao Paulo, Brazil. *Int J Dermatol.* 2004;43(9):643–647.

45. Keller R, Zago A, Viana MC, et al. HHV-8 infection in patients with AIDS-related Kaposi's sarcoma in brazil. *Braz J Med Biol Res.* 2001;34(7):879–886.

46. Zago A, Bourboulia D, Viana MC, et al. Seroprevalence of human herpesvirus 8 and its association with Kaposi sarcoma in Brazil. *Sex Transm Dis.* 2000;27(8):468–472.

47. Chang Y, Cesarman E, Pessin MS, et al. Identification of herpesvirus-like DNA sequences in AIDS-associated Kaposi's sarcoma. *Science.* 1994;266(5192):1865–1869.

48. Engels EA, Biggar RJ, Marshall VA, et al. Detection and quantification of Kaposi's sarcoma-associated herpesvirus to predict AIDS-associated Kaposi's sarcoma. *AIDS.* 2003;17(12):1847–1851.

49. Nsubuga MM, Biggar RJ, Combs S, et al. Human herpesvirus 8 load and progression of AIDS-related Kaposi sarcoma lesions. *Cancer Lett.* 2008;263(2):182–188.

50. Borok M, Fiorillo S, Gudza I, et al. Evaluation of plasma human herpesvirus 8 DNA as a marker of clinical outcomes during antiretroviral therapy for AIDS-related Kaposi sarcoma in Zimbabwe. *Clin Infect Dis.* 2010;51(3):342–349.

51. Engels EA, Pfeiffer RM, Goedert JJ, et al. Trends in cancer risk among people with AIDS in the united states 1980–2002. *AIDS.* 2006;20(12):1645–1654.

52. Mbulaiteye SM, Goedert JJ. Transmission of Kaposi sarcoma-associated herpesvirus in sub-Saharan Africa. *AIDS.* 2008;22(4):535–537.

53. Parkin DM, Sitas F, Chirenje M, Stein L, Abratt R, Wabinga H. Part I: Cancer in indigenous Africans—burden, distribution, and trends. *Lancet Oncol.* 2008;9(7):683–692.

54. Orem J, Otieno MW, Remick SC. AIDS-associated cancer in developing nations. *Curr Opin Oncol.* 2004;16(5):468–476.

55. Otieno MW, Remick SC, Whalen C. Adult Burkitt's lymphoma in patients with and without human immunodeficiency virus infection in Kenya. *Int J Cancer.* 2001;92(5):687–691.

56. Lucas SB, Diomande M, Hounnou A, et al. HIV-associated lymphoma in Africa: An autopsy study in Cote d'Ivoire. *Int J Cancer.* 1994;59(1):20–24.

57. Eltom MA, Jemal A, Mbulaiteye SM, Devesa SS, Biggar RJ. Trends in Kaposi's sarcoma and non-Hodgkin's lymphoma incidence in the United States from 1973 through 1998. *J Natl Cancer Inst.* 2002;94(16):1204–1210.

58. Ogwang MD, Zhao W, Ayers LW, Mbulaiteye SM. Accuracy of Burkitt lymphoma diagnosis in constrained pathology settings: Importance to epidemiology. *Arch Pathol Lab Med.* 2011;135(4):445–450.

59. Mutalima N, Molyneux E, Jaffe H, et al. Associations between Burkitt lymphoma among children in Malawi and infection with HIV, EBV and malaria: Results from a case-control study. *PLoS One.* 2008;3(6):e2505.

60. Stefan DC, Wessels G, Poole J, et al. Infection with human immunodeficiency virus-1 (HIV) among children with cancer in South Africa. *Pediatr Blood Cancer.* 2011;56(1):77–79.

61. Molyneux EM, Rochford R, Griffin B, et al. Burkitt's lymphoma. *Lancet.* 2012;379(9822):1234–1244.

62. Mbulaiteye SM, Parkin DM, Rabkin CS. Epidemiology of AIDS-related malignancies an international perspective. *Hematol Oncol Clin North Am.* 2003;17(3):673–696, v.

63. Sampaio J, Brites C, Araujo I, et al. AIDS related malignancies in Brazil. *Curr Opin Oncol.* 2007;19(5):476–478.

64. Boerma JT, Nunn AJ, Whitworth JA. Mortality impact of the AIDS epidemic: Evidence from community studies in less developed countries. *AIDS.* 1998;12 Suppl 1:S3–S14.

65. Morgan D, Mahe C, Mayanja B, Whitworth JA. Progression to symptomatic disease in people infected with HIV-1 in rural Uganda: Prospective cohort study. *BMJ.* 2002;324(7331):193–196.

66. Morgan D, Mahe C, Mayanja B, Okongo JM, Lubega R, Whitworth JA. HIV-1 infection in rural Africa: Is there a difference in median time to AIDS and survival compared with that in industrialized countries? *AIDS.* 2002;16(4):597–603.

67. Sylla BS, Wild CP. A million Africans a year dying from cancer by 2030: What can cancer research and control offer to the continent? *Int J Cancer.* 2012;130(2):245–250.

68. Parkin DM, Nambooze S, Wabwire-Mangen F, Wabinga HR. Changing cancer incidence in Kampala, Uganda, 1991–2006. *Int J Cancer.* 2010;126(5):1187–1195.

69. Feng H, Shuda M, Chang Y, Moore PS. Clonal integration of a polyomavirus in human merkel cell carcinoma. *Science*. 2008;319(5866):1096–1100.

70. Newton R, Ziegler J, Ateenyi-Agaba C, et al. The epidemiology of conjunctival squamous cell carcinoma in Uganda. *Br J Cancer*. 2002;87(3):301–308.

71. Newton R, Ferlay J, Reeves G, Beral V, Parkin DM. Effect of ambient solar ultraviolet radiation on incidence of squamous-cell carcinoma of the eye. *Lancet*. 1996;347(9013):1450–1451.

72. Ateenyi-Agaba C. Conjunctival squamous-cell carcinoma associated with HIV infection in Kampala, Uganda. *Lancet*. 1995;345(8951):695–696.

73. Waddell KM, Lewallen S, Lucas SB, Atenyi-Agaba C, Herrington CS, Liomba G. Carcinoma of the conjunctiva and HIV infection in Uganda and Malawi. *Br J Ophthalmol*. 1996;80(6):503–508.

74. Ateenyi-Agaba C, Weiderpass E, Smet A, et al. Epidermodysplasia verruciformis human papillomavirus types and carcinoma of the conjunctiva: A pilot study. *Br J Cancer*. 2004;90(9):1777–1779.

75. Tornesello ML, Biryahwaho B, Downing R, et al. Human herpesvirus type 8 variants circulating in Europe, Africa and North America in classic, endemic and epidemic Kaposi's sarcoma lesions during pre-AIDS and AIDS era. *Virology*. 2010;398(2):280–289.

76. Yu JJ, Fu P, Pink JJ, et al. HPV infection and EGFR activation/alteration in HIV-infected East African patients with conjunctival carcinoma. *PLoS One*. 2010;5(5):e10477.

77. Babu K, Murthy KR, Krishnakumar S. Two successive ocular malignancies in the same eye of a HIV-positive patient: A case report. *Ocul Immunol Inflamm*. 2010;18(2):101–103.

78. Lanoy E, Rosenberg PS, Fily F, et al. HIV-associated Hodgkin lymphoma during the first months on combination antiretroviral therapy. *Blood*. 2011;118(1):44–49.

79. Pawlotsky JM, Belec L, Gresenguet G, et al. High prevalence of hepatitis B, C, and E markers in young sexually active adults from the central African republic. *J Med Virol*. 1995;46(3):269–272.

80. Sutcliffe S, Taha TE, Kumwenda NI, Taylor E, Liomba GN. HIV-1 prevalence and herpes simplex virus 2, hepatitis C virus, and hepatitis B virus infections among male workers at a sugar estate in Malawi. *J Acquir Immune Defic Syndr*. 2002;31(1):90–97.

81. Ocama P, Nambooze S, Opio CK, Shiels MS, Wabinga HR, Kirk GD. Trends in the incidence of primary liver cancer in central Uganda, 1960–1980 and 1991–2005. *Br J Cancer*. 2009;100(5):799–802.

82. Rong-Rong Y, Xi-En G, Shi-Cheng G, Yong-Xi Z. Interaction of hepatitis B and C viruses in patients infected with HIV. *J Acquir Immune Defic Syndr*. 2008;48(4):505–506.

83. Bonnet F, Burty C, Lewden C, et al. Changes in cancer mortality among HIV-infected patients: The mortalite 2005 survey. *Clin Infect Dis*. 2009;48(5):633–639.

84. Simard EP, Engels EA. Cancer as a cause of death among people with AIDS in the united states. *Clin Infect Dis*. 2010;51(8):957–962.

85. Casper C. The increasing burden of HIV-associated malignancies in resource-limited regions. *Annu Rev Med*. 2011;62:157–170.

86. Sitas F, Parkin DM, Chirenje M, Stein L, Abratt R, Wabinga H. Part II: Cancer in indigenous Africans—causes and control. *Lancet Oncol*. 2008;9(8):786–795.

87. Parkin DM. The global health burden of infection-associated cancers in the year 2002. *Int J Cancer*. 2006;118(12):3030–3044.

88. Mbulaiteye SM, Bhatia K, Adebamowo C, Sasco AJ. HIV and cancer in Africa: Mutual collaboration between HIV and cancer programs may provide timely research and public health data. *Infect Agent Cancer*. 2011;6(1):16.

CHAPTER 21

BREAST CANCER EARLY DETECTION AND CLINICAL GUIDELINES

DAVID B. THOMAS, RAUL MURILLO, KARDINAH, BENJAMIN O. ANDERSON

INTRODUCTION

Breast cancer mortality rates, which had been essentially unchanged in the United States for the six decades between the 1930s through the 1980s, have been dropping by nearly 2% each year since 1990.[1] Similar mortality reductions have been observed in other high resource countries such as Norway.[2] These improvements in breast cancer mortality can be attributed to early detection by screening combined with timely and effective treatment.[3] Randomized trials of screening mammography in the 1970s and 1980s demonstrated that early detection leads to down-staging of disease, improvement in breast cancer survival, and a reduction in mortality rates.[4] At the same time, randomized trials of systemic therapies for breast cancer showed that endocrine therapy for estrogen-receptor positive (ER+) cancers and cytotoxic chemotherapy for ER negative (ER–) cancers improve survival among lymph node negative, lymph node positive, and locally advanced breast cancers[5,6]. The relative contributions of screening and effective treatment to the reduction in breast cancer mortality are a source of controversy.[2]

In most low- and middle-resource countries (LMCs), breast cancer incidence rates are increasing more rapidly than in regions where incidence rates are already high. Despite the young age structure of most developing countries, 45% of the incident breast cancer cases and 54% of the breast cancer deaths in the world occur in LMCs.[7] The numbers of women who will develop breast cancer, and who will die from this disease, will increase by nearly 50% between the years 2002 and 2020, due solely to aging of current global populations. These increases will be greater among LMCs than in industrialized countries and are projected to reach a 55% increase in incidence and a 58% increase in mortality in fewer than 20 years.[7] These projected increases for LMCs are probably underestimates, because they do not take into account likely increases in age-specific breast cancer incidence and mortality rates, especially among recent birth cohorts and in urban women in LMCs that are at least partially attributable to changes in childbearing practices and the adoption of Western lifestyles.[8,9]

Low breast cancer survival rates in LMCs are largely attributable to late stage presentation and limited diagnostic and treatment capacity.[10] In India, between 50% and 70% of cases are initially diagnosed with disease that is locally advanced or metastatic.[11] By comparison, 38% of European and only 30% of American breast cancer cases were reported to be locally advanced at diagnosis between the years 1990 and 1992.[12] Therefore, efforts to promote early detection followed by appropriate treatment are essential components of population-based breast cancer control strategies. Three screening methods for the early detection of asymptomatic breast cancer have been promulgated: mammography, clinical breast examination (CBE), and breast self-examination (BSE).

BREAST CANCER SCREENING TOOLS

Definitions

Screening has been defined by the World Health Organization (WHO) as "the presumptive identification of unrecognized disease ... by the application of tests ... which can be applied rapidly ... [to] sort out apparently well persons who probably do not have a disease from those who probably do have the disease." *Secondary prevention* is the prevention of fatal outcome by presumptive early detection followed by definitive diagnosis and treatment. Thus, screening represents one component of secondary prevention, and can only be successful if adequate facilities for diagnosis and treatment are available.

Methodological Considerations

Since the ultimate goal of screening is to reduce deaths from the disease being screened, the strongest evidence for efficacy of screening is a reduction in mortality rates from the disease among screened persons. Randomized trials in which mortality rates from the disease of interest are compared in screened and unscreened persons provide the strongest evidence for efficacy. Observational studies conducted to estimate the disease-specific mortality rates in screened persons relative to those in unscreened persons can also provide useful evidence for or against efficacy if the studies are properly conducted so that bias is minimized.

Detection of disease at an earlier stage in screened persons than in unscreened persons is a necessary condition for there to be a reduction in mortality (Figure 21.1). Tumor size or stage of disease at diagnosis in screened and unscreened persons have thus been compared to assess efficacy of a screening modality. However, early detection may not necessarily alter the clinical disease course if the disease is still detected at an incurable stage (inadequate downstaging), or if tumors that are detected by screening would not progress to kill the person screened during her normal lifetime (overdiagnosis). Thus, downstaging by screening is a necessary but not a sufficient condition for a screening modality to be efficacious, and evidence for efficacy based solely on downstaging must be interpreted with some caution.

For a screening modality to be deemed efficacious, the disease-specific survival must be shown to be prolonged, i.e., the time from diagnosis to death must be a longer time period in screened persons than in unscreened persons. However, a longer survival time associated with screening can be artifactually increased and is not necessarily due to a true delay in the time of death. A longer time from diagnosis to death in screened than unscreened persons can also be observed if the disease is detected earlier in time in those persons screened than those not screened, even if the deaths occur at the same time in screened and unscreened persons, i.e., the longer survival time is due solely to increased lead time but does not actually reflect a shift in the course of disease.

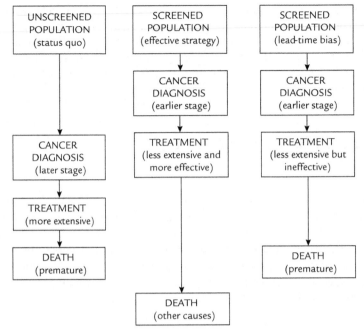

FIGURE 21.1 Comparison of effective screening strategy with ineffective screening strategy producing lead-time bias. Effective screening will provide cancer diagnoses at earlier stages where treatment is less extensive and/or costly and survival is improved. Ineffective screening strategies associated with lead time bias will lead to more cancer diagnoses and may involve less extensive therapies, but may not provide increased disease- specific survival. In screening populations, it can be inferred that some patients would not have died of their disease, meaning that they were by definition "overtreated." The magnitude of overtreatment represents cost to the system and unnecessary morbidity to the patient and therefore must be considered in a screening strategy.

It should also be recognized that the introduction of a screening strategy will initially diagnose more patients with disease, creating at least temporarily an increased disease incidence within the population. Once diagnosed, patients will require treatment, introducing a cost-burden to the healthcare system. This increased cost may be in part offset by lower treatment costs, if patients diagnosed with earlier stage disease in fact require less extensive therapy. The relative relationship between benefits and costs do need to be considered in the context of screening in an LMC where healthcare resources are significantly limited.

Mammographic Screening

The evidence for the efficacy of screening modalities for breast cancer has been summarized and evaluated by multiple organizations and independent investigators, including the International Agency for Research on Cancer (IARC)[13] and the US Preventive Services Task Force.[14] The evidence for the efficacy of screening mammography comes mainly from six trials in which women were randomized to either periodic mammographic screening alone, or no screening. By combining the results from these trials, the IARC working group estimated that periodic mammographic screening reduced mortality from breast cancer by about 25% in women 50–69 years old, and by about 19% in 40–49-year-old women. The results were consistent across studies in the older women but inconsistent for women in their 40s.

Younger premenopausal women tend to have more dense breasts on mammograms than older postmenopausal women, because as women age their mammary epithelial tissue is gradually replaced by fatty tissue. Therefore, the sensitivity of mammographic screening tends to be lower in younger than in older women. Benign lesions are also more common among younger women than older women, and more difficult to evaluate in their more dense breasts, so that there are more false positive screenings in younger women (lower specificity). Furthermore, the incidence of breast cancer increases with age in most populations, and therefore the proportion of women in a population who have breast cancer (the prevalence) is greater in older than younger women.

The predictive value of a positive screening test is the proportion of positive tests that ultimately lead to a diagnosis of the disease being screened. The lower the predictive value, the more additional diagnostic procedures must be performed to find one cancer. Its value increases with the specificity of the test, the prevalence of the disease, and to a smaller extent the sensitivity of the test. Therefore, the predictive value of a positive mammographic screening test increases with age, and is considerably lower in younger, premenopausal women.

There is considerable controversy as to whether women in their 40s should be screened for breast cancer with mammography. This controversy is based on the greater uncertainty as to its efficacy in these women, the smaller beneficial effect of mammography in reducing mortality from breast cancer if it is efficacious, and the greater cost of screening women in their 40s in terms of the numbers of women who must be screened, and the numbers of positive screenings that must be further evaluated to find one case of breast cancer. The limitations of screening in the 40s are aggravated, because breast cancers appear to progress more rapidly in premenopausal than postmenopausal women, more frequent mammograms (annual rather than every 2 years) are needed to optimize screening effectiveness.[15] It is thus less cost-effective to perform mammographic screening in women in their 40s than women age fifty and older, and in most situations, women in their 40s should receive lower priority for mammographic screening than older women.

In many LMCs, a relatively high proportion of women with breast cancers are in their 40s. This has led to the erroneous belief that breast cancer is more common in younger women in developing countries than in developed countries. The primary reason for the relatively high proportion of breast cancers in younger women in some developing countries is that there are few older women in the populations of these countries. This would not mean that rates of breast cancer were high in women in their 40s. The decision to screen or not to screen women in their 40s should be based in part on the prevalence of the disease in the women of this age in the population, and not on the proportion of cases that are in this age group.

The evidence for the efficacy of mammographic screening comes from trials that were conducted in high income countries with facilities to monitor mammograms for quality, and evaluate the performance of those who interpret mammograms. The efficacy of mammographic screening will obviously be reduced if mammograms are of inferior quality or if those who read mammograms are not adequately trained. Insuring that mammograms are of adequately high quality, and that those who read them are capable of doing so accurately, are particular challenges in LMCs.

Standard practice in developed countries is to perform two-view mammography, in which the breast is imaged in two planes (MLO, medial/lateral oblique; CC, craniocaudal), since this allows the radiologist to better distinguish true mammographic densities from overlapping shadows of normal dense tissues. However, in the randomized trials of mammographic screening, single view mammograms were found to be nearly as efficacious as 2-view mammograms. In LMCs with limited resources, consideration can be given to single view mammography if doing so can increase coverage in the population. Also, in women in the randomized trials between the ages of 50 and 69, screening every 33 months was as efficacious as screening every 18–24 months, although in women in their 40s, the reduction in mortality was inversely related to screening interval. When allocating limited resources for mammographic screening, it is generally better to screen women less frequently and reach a higher proportion of women in the population than to screen a smaller proportion of the population more frequently. The availability of film may also be an obstacle to screening in LMCs. Digital mammography may provide an alternative to analogue (film-based) mammography and would eliminate the concern about two-view versus one-view mammography, but this could only if the equipment and infrastructure costs of digital mammography can be reduced to an affordable level.

Because mammographic screening is expensive, consideration has been given to other methods of screening in LMCs that may be more cost effective such as clinical breast examination (CBE) and breast self-examination (BSE).

Clinical Breast Examination

No randomized trials to assess whether CBE alone reduces mortality from breast cancer have yet been completed. Evidence for the efficacy of CBE from observational studies is inconsistent. A case-control study in Japan showed a reduction in deaths from breast cancer in women who participated in a CBE screening program compared to women who did not participate;[16] and mortality rates from breast cancer decreased in the areas in which the screening program achieved a high level of coverage, but increased in areas in which the program was not promulgated.[17] Most studies based on the stage of disease at diagnosis have shown that breast cancers that were detected by CBE tended to be diagnosed at an earlier stage than breast cancers that were not detected by screening.[13] Also, an early trial, in which a combination of mammography and CBE was shown to reduce risk of dying from breast cancer, many of the tumors in the screened group were detected by CBE but not by mammography.[4] However, studies based on survival times have generally not revealed a longer survival from time of diagnosis in cases detected by CBE compared to cases not detected by screening;[13] and in randomized trials, a combination of mammography and CBE was not found to be more efficacious in reducing mortality from breast cancer than mammography alone.[13] The IARC working group and the US Preventive Services Task Force concluded that the evidence for the efficacy of CBE in reducing mortality from breast cancer is inadequate and insufficient, respectively.

Most of the evidence for the efficacy of CBE has come from studies in economically developed countries where women typically present with relatively small tumors. More information is needed from LMCs in which women with breast cancer more frequently present with large, advanced tumors. CBE has been advocated as a screening modality under such circumstances for several reasons: it has been hypothesized that CBE may be more efficacious in populations in which women tend to present with large tumors than in the populations in which most prior studies have been conducted; nonphysicians can be trained to perform CBE, thus making breast cancer screening less expensive and requiring less technical resources than mammography; and coverage of a higher proportion of a target population than with mammography should therefore also be feasible.

If CBE is initiated as a primary screening modality for breast cancer in LMCs, it should be done in such a way that its effectiveness can be evaluated. A randomized trial of CBE in the Philippines was unsuccessful because insufficient numbers women with positive findings on CBE received further diagnosis and treatment.[18] A randomized trial of CBE and visual inspection of the cervix by specially trained women with a 10th grade education is underway in Mumbai, India. Preliminary results show more breast cancers being detected at an early stage (stages 0, I, or II) in the screening group (62%) than in the control group (44%), but results based on breast cancer mortality rates are not yet available.[19] Feasibility and pilot studies of CBE, usually combined with the teaching of BSE, are also underway in Egypt, Indonesia, and other LMCs. All such efforts to evaluate the usefulness of CBE should include, in addition to assessments of its efficacy (sensitivity, down-staging, reduction in breast cancer mortality), a measure of its specificity. If large numbers of lesions are detected by CBE that are found not to be cancer on further evaluation, then this puts a heavy burden on local diagnostic facilities, which may be very limited in some LMCs. In addition, if large numbers of women must receive unnecessary breast biopsies in order to detect one case of breast cancer and to prevent one death, then this may not be either acceptable to the women who are targeted for screening or considered cost-effective by policy makers who decide how limited funds for health related activities are prioritized.

Some of the challenges facing CBE screening are the need to obtain good sensitivity and specificity, and the maintenance of standards. Since CBE accuracy depends on the level of skills among providers, the definition of a proper technique, the type of training, and the strategies for regular feedback are key. Standardized training using silicone models has shown increased detection of tumor lumps but also increased false positive results.[13] Regular evaluation and feedback of CBE performers has been implemented in several trials but no results of these interventions have been reported.

Breast Self-Examination (BSE)

BSE should be distinguished from programs to promote early treatment of *symptomatic* breast cancer. The aim of BSE is to detect *asymptomatic* breast conditions. BSE is the systematic search for an unapparent lump or other change in the breast suggestive of the presence of breast cancer. In formal BSE training, a woman receives instruction addressing four elements of the examination: visual inspection of the breasts in a mirror to look for asymmetry and dimpling; palpation in both the standing and lying positions with the arm above the head using a circular motion with the pads of the three middle fingers, with systematic coverage of the entire breast and axilla; squeezing the nipple to detect discharge; and regular practice on a monthly basis.

Most evidence as to the efficacy of BSE comes from two randomized trials that were conducted in Saint Petersburg, Russia,[20] and Shanghai, China.[21] In both studies, women were randomized to either an intervention group that received instruction in BSE and periodic reminders to practice the procedure, or to a control group that received no education regarding BSE or any formal breast cancer screening. Neither trial showed that mortality from breast cancer was reduced in women who received the BSE instruction. Both the IARC working group and the US Preventive Services Task Force concluded that the efficacy of BSE is unproven.

One possible reason for the negative results is that the woman may not have performed BSE well enough or frequently enough. Only 18% of the women in the St. Petersburg trial reported practicing BSE monthly. In the Shanghai trial, BSE practice was observed by medical workers every 4 to 5 month for the first 4 or 5 years of the study. There is some evidence that more frequent practice than this might be efficacious. The breast cancers in the women in Shanghai who attended all of the supervised sessions tended to be somewhat smaller than those in women who attended fewer than 70% of the sessions, and most of the observational studies summarized by the IARC working group (IARC) showed that breast cancers detected by BSE tended to be smaller than those not detected by screening. It is unlikely that BSE would be of values in LMCs unless means can be found to assure that women will practice it competently and frequently.

Another possible reason for the negative results of the two BSE trials is that they were conducted in situations in which women had easy access to medical care, such that women in the control groups tended to present with relatively small, localized tumors. Over 40% of the breast cancers diagnosed in the Shanghai control group were less than 2cm in diameter. This experience is in strong contrast to that in the Middle East, Africa and India where the median tumor size is commonly 4–6cm at presentation and the majority of women present with locally advanced or metastatic disease. It is unknown whether BSE might be efficacious in reducing mortality from breast cancer in populations in which women typically present with larger, more advanced tumors than what was observed in the randomized trials. It is therefore not unreasonable for BSE to still be advocated as a screening tool in LMCs, either as a primary screening modality, or in conjunction with CBE. No new trials of BSE alone have been undertaken, but BSE instruction has been included in some of the studies of CBE. This is reasonable, because a CBE offers an excellent opportunity to also provide BSE instruction.

It is unknown whether teaching women BSE in order to detect interval cancers that become detectable between periodic mammographic screenings would be beneficial, and the IARC working group recommended that randomized trials of BSE in women receiving mammographic screening be conducted to answer this question. In LMCs where mammographic screening as frequently as every two years is not feasible, it may be particularly useful to teach BSE in conjunction with mammographic screening, and this possibility should be investigated.

As with CBE, BSE should only be introduced as a screening tool in a manner in which its efficacy can be evaluated. Possible uses in LMCs that should receive particular consideration for trial and evaluation include use in conjunction with CBE, use to detect interval cancers in women who are screened with mammography less frequently than every two years, and use in countries in which women typically present with large, advanced breast cancers.

In both of the BSE trials, many more benign breast lesions were detected in the groups receiving BSE instruction than in the control groups. Since the trials did not show BSE to be of value in reducing mortality from breast cancer, teaching BSE clearly did more harm than good in these trials. Any evaluation of a BSE screening program should include a quantification of the benign lesions that must be evaluated, in addition to measures of its effectiveness.

Early Diagnosis and Treatment of Symptomatic Breast Cancer

Programs to promote early diagnosis and treatment of symptomatic breast cancer are not screening programs, because they are not designed to detect asymptomatic lesions. Their purpose is to encourage women who have symptoms suggestive of breast cancer to seek medical care. In some LMCs, women typically do not seek care until their breast cancers are very advanced, even if facilities for diagnosis and treatment of breast cancer are available, because of lack of knowledge about breast cancer, or because of social barriers to seeking evaluation for a breast problem. In such situations, screening would frequently either not be feasible, or could be viewed as unacceptable, and would hence not be the logical first step in addressing the breast cancer problem in the population. Instead, consideration should be given to programs to educate women about the symptoms of breast cancer and the importance of early diagnosis and treatment, to encourage them to be aware of their breast and any suspicious changes in them, and to empower them to overcome social barriers that prevent them from utilizing available diagnostic and treatment services.

As with screening programs, breast self-awareness programs should not be initiated unless adequate diagnostic and treatment facilities are available, and they should be established in such a way that they can be evaluated to determine the proportion of women in the target population who are reached by the program, and whether the program results in breast cancers being treated at an earlier stage than would be expected in the absence of the program.

PRIORITIZATION

The identification of a target group for screening in LMCs should be based on the burden of disease in the population, the potential benefit from screening, and available resources.[22] The only risk factor that is useful for establishing priorities for screening (in addition to sex) is age. In Western countries, the incidence rates of breast cancer increase sharply with age until the usual age at menopause, and then increase more slowly with age. In LMCs, the incidence rates in premenopausal women increase with age in a similar manner as in more developed countries but then either continue to increase less steeply with age than in Western countries, level off, or decrease with age.[23] This phenomenon is due to rates of breast cancer in developing countries increasing over time more rapidly in younger women than in older women (cohort effect).[24,25] As the women in the younger groups age, they will likely carry their increasing risks with them, and over time the age-specific incidence curves for LMCs will more closely approximate those observed in Western countries.[26]

Age-specific breast cancer incidence or mortality rates are useful in assessing which age groups should be targeted for screening. Ascertaining these rates and alternative means to assess the breast cancer problem in LMCs are discussed below in the section on guideline implementation. It is important to emphasize that incidence rates of breast cancer are lower in LMCs than in more developed countries at all ages. Since the efficacy and cost effectiveness of screening women under age 50 in developed countries are limited, screening such women in LMCs with even lower rates of disease is unlikely to be of much benefit. However, since the cohorts of younger women are experiencing the greatest increases in incidence, programs to begin to educate young women about breast cancer, and their likely future risks, should be considered in LMCs in which rates of breast cancer appear to be increasing.

In LMCs in which the incidence rates in women their 50s and older are beginning to show an increase with age, the frequency of the disease in the population may have approached a level at which screening will be cost effective and warrant sufficiently high priority for expenditure of health resources. It should also be noted that screening the elderly, perhaps women over 70, is of limited value because of their limited longevity, and their likelihood of dying of other causes even after a positive screening test.

When resources are limited, it is tempting to apply risk factor criteria in addition to age to reduce further the size of the target group. However, information on other risk factors is usually not readily available, and these factors do not distinguish sufficient numbers of women at high risk to warrant the effort and expense of preferentially screening women based on their presence.[27] Unlike some cancers with very strong risk factors, e.g., tobacco and lung cancer, breast cancer has multiple risk factors each of relatively small magnitude, markedly limiting their utility for identifying a clear high risk group where the majority of breast cancers occur[28]. For this reason, the two risk factors used for determining candidacy for breast cancer screening are limited to gender and age.

■ COVERAGE

Another concern of particular importance in LMCs is coverage of the target population. If a screening modality is efficacious in reducing mortality from breast cancer in those screened, but if only a small proportion of the women in the target population receive the service, then the impact of the screening program on breast cancer mortality in the population will be small. Consider the following simple formula:

Impact = Efficacy × Coverage

For example, if it is assumed that mammograms reduce mortality from breast cancer in those screened by 25%, and if 40% of the women in a target population are screened, then the screening program would be expected to reduce mortality in the target population by 10% $(0.25 \times 0.40 = 0.10)$. Mammographic screening programs in LMCs should be designed in such a way that the proportion of women in the target population who are screened can be assessed and maximized. Nonetheless, extending screening coverage necessarily requires access to proper tissue diagnosis and treatment for positively screened women, since a high coverage without follow-up is less cost-effective than a lower coverage with proper follow-up.

■ GUIDELINE DEVELOPMENT

Good research and timely publication of results are not sufficient to ensure the translation of scientific findings into general practice.[29,30] Translation of scientific discovery to clinical practice has been divided into two parts: clinical research to guidelines, and guidelines to practice.[31] The development of guidelines for breast cancer is discussed in this section, and their implementation is addressed in the next section.

In LMCs in which many women with breast cancer typically present with locally advanced or metastatic tumors, it can be reasonably assumed that down-staging of disease will be beneficial. Mortality from breast cancer will probably be reduced, and even if this effect is small, quality of life will be improved. Women will no longer present with large, sometimes infected, masses that are painful, offensive, socially ostracizing, and amenable only to palliative treatment. Breast preserving surgery will also be possible in more cases, further reducing morbidity and enhancing quality of life.

In high resource countries, evidence-based guidelines outlining optimal approaches to early detection, diagnosis, and treatment of breast cancer have been defined and disseminated.[27,32-35] These guidelines do not consider the deficits in infrastructure and resources in LMCs, making these guidelines of limited value in such countries.[36] Moreover, they do not consider implementation costs or provide guidance on how a suboptimal system can be improved incrementally toward an optimal system. Evidence-based, economically feasible and culturally appropriate guidelines that can be used in nations with limited health care resources to improve breast cancer outcomes have been developed by the Breast Health Global Initiative (BHGI). The BHGI held four Global Summits—in Seattle (2002), Bethesda (2005), Budapest (2007), and Chicago (2010)—focusing on health care disparities,[37] evidence-based resource allocation,[38] guideline implementation,[39] and optimization of resources,[40] in LMCs, respectively. Modeled after the approach of the National Comprehensive Cancer Network (NCCN),[41] the BHGI developed and applied an evidence-based consensus panel process now formally endorsed by the Institute of Medicine (IOM)[42] to create guidelines for early detection,[26] diagnosis,[43] treatment,[44] and health care delivery systems,[44] as related to breast cancer in countries with four different levels of available resources. This resource allocation system provides a general framework for strategy development and decision making, and should be consulted prior to the development of a breast cancer control program in an LMC. The same methodology has now been applied to the development of guidelines for management in Asia of hepatocellular carcinoma,[45] non–small cell lung carcinoma,[46] endometrial cancer,[47] head and neck cancer,[48] and HER-2/neu positive breast cancer.[49]

▧ GUIDELINE IMPLEMENTATION

Before a breast cancer control program is initiated in an LMC, careful assessment of the local situation must be made. This should consist of three parts: an assessment of the breast cancer problem in the population, an assessment of the existing infrastructure that will be utilized for the program, and an assessment of social and cultural barriers to women's participation in the program.

Assessing the breast cancer problem in a country

Larger numbers of women will have to be screened to prevent one death, and a higher proportion of positive screens will be false positives, if the disease is rare than if it is common. A realistic estimate of the numbers of women with the disease of interest in the population in which screening is proposed is therefore an essential part of the planning process.

Making an estimate of the frequency of breast cancer in LMCs can be a challenge, and in many situations less than ideal methods must be utilized. The ideal situation is one in which the numbers of women in the population to be screened (the target population) are known, and a population based cancer registry exists. If it can be assured that case finding for the registry is reasonably complete, and that coding of type of cancer is reasonably accurate, then incidence rates by age can be calculated. These rates can then be compared with rates in more developed countries, where breast cancer screening has been performed, and where it has been associated with a quantified reduction in the numbers of deaths due to breast cancer. With this information, the expected impact of the screening program can be estimated for specific age groups in the population. If the target population is well enumerated but does not have a population-based cancer registry, rates of cancer from comparable populations (if they exist) can be applied to the population of interest to estimate the numbers of breast cancer cases in that population, and the likely impact of screening. Cancer Incidence in Five Continents[50] is a good source of such rates.

Accurate mortality rates can also serve as good measures of the breast cancer problem. In fact, since the ultimate purpose of screening is to reduce mortality from breast cancer, breast cancer mortality rates provide a direct measure the problem for which the screening program is to be established. However, mortality rates can be misleading if the population size is not accurately enumerated, if many deaths are unreported, or if certification of cause of death is not accurately recorded.

In the absence of adequate information on the population to be screened, reviews of deaths certificates can be useful. The numbers of deaths certified as due to breast cancer during specific years can be obtain, and this can provide a rough estimate of the numbers of breast cancer deaths in the population per year. In addition, the proportion of all deaths due to breast cancer can be calculated. Such proportional mortality ratios can provide a rough estimate of the magnitude of the breast cancer problem in relation to other causes of death in the population. If breast cancer is a small problem relative to other preventable causes of death, then a screening program may not be warranted, but if breast cancer deaths constitute a relatively high proportion of preventable deaths, then this information can be used to justify the development of breast cancer screening activities, and can provide an indication that such activities would have a meaningful impact on the numbers of deaths in the population. Such analyses should, of course be age specific, so that the relative impact of a screening program in various age groups can be estimated.

A review of hospital records can also be useful in assessing the magnitude of the breast cancer problem. If a single hospital serves all cancer patients in a defined population, then a review of the hospital records for a specific number of years can provide an estimate of the numbers of cases of breast cancer to be expected annually. A record review can also provide an indication of the importance of breast cancer relative to other cancers in the population, and relative to other reasons for hospitalization. If admissions for breast cancer constitute a reasonably high proportion of all preventable causes of admission, or a high proportion of all admissions for cancer, then a screening program may be justifiable, but if breast cancer is a rare cause of hospitalization, then it may not warrant high priority consideration for screening.

It must be emphasize that none of the above means of assessing the breast cancer problem in a population will be satisfactory in populations in which social or financial barriers to diagnosis and treatment of breast cancer prevent large numbers of women with breast cancer from seeking care. If such a situation is suspected, then special efforts will have to be made to overcome these barriers as a first step in assessing and addressing the breast cancer problem.

In addition to assessing the magnitude of the breast cancer problem, it is important to also determine the stage at which breast cancers are typically diagnosed. This information can be obtained either from population based cancer registries, or from registries in individual hospitals. In the absence of cancer registries, the records in clinics, hospitals, and pathology laboratories can be reviewed. If a high proportion of breast cancers are diagnosed at an advanced stage, then a screening program, or an educational program to encourage earlier diagnosis of symptomatic breast cancers, has the potential to exert a large impact on morbidity and mortality due to breast cancer. Conversely, if a high proportion of breast cancers is already being diagnosed at an early stage, then screening programs based on BSE, and probably also on CBE, are unlikely to have a large impact on either mortality or morbidity.

Assessing the Screening Infrastructure

Mammography is the only screening method of proven efficacy, and it will serve as an example for assessing infrastructure. In LMCs, as elsewhere, for a mammographic screening program to result in meaningful down-staging of breast cancers in the population, 6 elements will need to be adequately functioning: (1) a means to recruit a sufficiently high proportion of women in the target population to have a meaningful impact on the breast cancer problem in the population, (2) facilities to ensure that the mammograms are of high quality, (3) sufficient number of radiologists who can properly interpret the mammograms in a timely manner, (4) means to recontact women with suspicious findings and ensure that they come to a facility for further evaluation in a timely fashion, (5) adequate diagnostic facilities and trained pathologists to provide timely and accurate tissue diagnoses, and (6) sufficient facilities and personnel to provide timely and appropriate treatment. Regardless of the screening modality used (BSE, CBE, or screening mammography), gaps in this system at any level must be identified and addressed before a program of early detection is established.

Assessing Social and Cultural Barriers

Women in LMCs may be unaware of breast cancer or may have major misconceptions about its nature or curability, or have fatalistic attitudes toward diseases in general.[26] Under such circumstances, programs to enhance public awareness of breast cancer, and to teach that breast cancer outcomes are improved through early detection, are critical to improving participation in early detection programs, regardless of the methods for early detection that are utilized.

Cultural barriers to participation must also be identified, and strategies developed to overcome them. These barriers may include both women's attitudes and those of their husband's. In some cultures, women must obtain their husband's permission to seek medical services. Under such circumstances, efforts to empower women and educate men may be needed for a program to succeed. Cultural and social barriers are highly specific to different countries, religions, and ethnic groups, and cannot be comprehensively reviewed here. However, an example of the assessment of such barriers is provided to illustrate how they may be addressed. In a survey in the Palestinian Authority,[51] it was found that women were more likely to undergo screening mammography if they were (1) less religious, (2) described having fewer personal barriers to examinations, and (3) indicated a lower degree of cancer fatalism. Women who consented to CBE had a higher perceived effectiveness of CBE and described lower levels of cancer fatalism. Muslim women were half as likely as Christian women to participate in CBE screening. Women were more likely to perform breast self-examination (BSE) if they were more highly educated, resided in cities, were Christian, were less religious, and had a first-degree relative with breast cancer. These results suggest one approach to improved participation in breast cancer screening might be to recruit religious leaders as spokespersons for early detection messages. Having special screening clinics staffed by women physicians and nurses sensitive to the needs of conservative Muslim women who must remain covered in public might also be beneficial.

As shown in Figure 21.2, women who are correctly diagnosed and properly treated for early stage breast cancer can become survivors of the disease, and organize breast cancer survivor groups, like Reach for Recovery. Such groups can play a vital role in educating the public about the value of early detection, and in providing newly diagnosed women

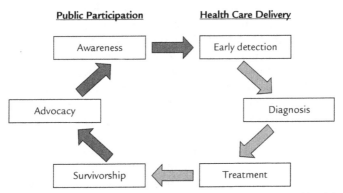

FIGURE 21.2 Synergistic relationship between public participation and health care delivery in down-staging breast cancer and improving cancer outcomes (used with permission).

with practical and emotional support.[52] Survivor groups also can organize into political advocacy groups that have real and positive impact on healthcare policy or national cancer research agendas.[53,54]

▪ EXAMPLES OF FIELD STUDIES

The evidence for the efficacy of mammography, clinical breast examination, and breast self-examination that has been summarized above is based largely on studies in developed countries, and the results may not be directly applicable to LMCs. A basic principle that should therefore be followed in implementing a breast cancer early detection program in a LMC is that the program should be designed in advance in such a way that it can be evaluated.[55] Methods that have been employed for program evaluation include both observational studies and randomized trials. Two types of observational studies are comparisons of screening modalities and assessing temporal trends in stage of disease. Randomized trials may be clinic or population based. Examples of each of these methods of evaluation follow.

Comparison of modalities. In an ongoing program in Jakarta, Indonesia, midwives are trained to perform CBE. Volunteers recruit women to come to clinics for the screening. The screened women are then independently screened by mammography without knowledge of the results of the CBE screening. Women with a positive screening by any method are clinically evaluated by a physician and receive further diagnostic procedures if indicated; and those found to have breast cancer are treated. In order to determine the efficacy of CBEs performed by the midwives, the breast cancer detection rates by CBE alone, by mammography alone, and by both methods will be compared. The false positive rates for CBE alone, mammography alone, and by both methods will be similarly compared, as will the size and stage of tumors detected by each method alone and by both methods. If the results for CBE are similar to those for mammography, this will provide evidence that CBE performed by midwives will likely be efficacious as a screening modality in urban Jakarta. This method of evaluation is only of value if the mammographic screening is competently conducted, and methods to ensure that it is must be incorporated into such a program.

Temporal trends in stage of disease. Almost all diagnosed cancers are treated in a single referral hospital in the State of Sarawak, Malaysia (population approximately 2 million). Therefore, by reviewing the medical records of all women with breast cancer at that hospital before and after an early detection initiative, it was possible to assess the impact of the program on breast cancer in the population.[56] The intervention consisted of: training community nurses who worked in rural clinics to perform CBE and teach BSE; circulating pamphlets and posting posters to motivate women to go to their nearest clinic at the earliest signs of a breast problem; instructing community nurses to hold health education talks and discussion groups on early diagnosis during monthly visits to villages, to teach BSE, and to perform CBE; and strengthening the system for referring women with signs and symptoms of breast cancer to district hospitals for diagnosis. The proportion of breast cancers that were diagnosed at late stage (stages III or IV) was 77% in 1993, before the program, and 37% in 1998, after the program was initiated. Since these statistics are for nearly all women in the population who were treated for breast cancer, regardless of whether they participated in the program or not, they reflect the impact of the program on the breast cancer problem in the population, and suggest that the program had a positive impact.

Population based randomized trial. In a study of CBE, and visual inspection of the cervix after acetic acid application (VIA), by lay women in Mumbai, India,[19] 20 slums were randomly allocated to a screening or a control group (10 slums in each group), and the 35 to 64 year old women in each slum were considered eligible for the trial. Over 75, 000 women were identified for inclusion into each arm of the study. Women with a 10th grade education were trained to perform CBE and VIA, and women in the screening arm of the trial were invited for screening by these specially trained workers. Women in the control arm received no screening. Four rounds of screening at 2 year intervals were performed on women in the screening arm, and women in both arms are being monitored for breast and cervical cancer incidence and mortality for an additional 8 years. Preliminary results after 3 rounds of screening have been reported. More breast cancers have been detected in the screening arm than in the control arm, and the proportion of cancers detected at an early stage is higher in the screened than control arm. These results suggest that CBE performed by specially trained lay women may be efficacious in reducing mortality from breast cancer in the slums of India, and clearly indicate that continuation of the trail is warranted in order to provide direct evidence for a reduction in breast cancer mortality by CBE. The analyses of the data from this trial include all women and all breast cancers in the screening group, whether or not the women were actually screened. This is analogous to an intent-to-treat analysis in a clinical trial. The results will indicate the efficacy of the screening modality as it was actually implemented in the target population (i.e. its impact).

Clinic based randomized trial. The National Cancer Institute of Colombia (*Instituto Nacional de Cancerología / INC*) adapted the BHGI guidelines for middle income countries[57] to develop a pilot breast cancer screening program in Bogota. The *INC* guidelines recommend screening with annual clinical breast examination (CBE) and biennial mammography for women aged 50 to 69. Based on these guidelines, the *INC* designed a pilot study aimed at evaluating opportunistic screening as a programmatic approach to improve early detection in the country.[58, 59] Opportunistic screening is defined as the systematic offer of CBE and mammography for all women aged 50 to 69 who visit health centers on their own (regardless of motivation). It implies that screening is clinic-based and no outreach strategies or follow-up are carried out for women outside the health centers. The primary objectives of the study are to evaluate the effect of opportunistic screening on population coverage, to determine the impact of opportunistic screening on clinical stage at diagnosis, and to identify basic requirements for implementing opportunistic screening within the Colombian health system. A randomized cluster trial was implemented, in which health centers were the units of randomization. Women attending the health centers on a regular basis were assigned to the opportunistic screening arm of the trial, or to the nonintervention (control) branch according to the random allocation of their clinic. Since the Colombian health system is insurance-oriented, randomization was stratified by health insurance company in order to control for the effect of administrative factors on access to screening and diagnosis.

Before recruiting women for screening, the general practitioners in the intervention clinics attended a two day training course on breast cancer epidemiology, breast cancer screening, benign and malignant clinical presentation of breast diseases, and cancer diagnosis based on screening results. The training course includes lectures, discussions, review of clinical cases, and CBE clinical experience in health centers. The nurses attend a one day training course with similar content but without clinical practice. Radiologists and their technicians were given a standard one day course on quality of mammographic screening and the essentials of the BIRADS system.

The screening consists of recruitment in the clinics (and follow up) by health care assistants (auxiliary nurses, backed up by registered nurses), CBE performed by general practitioners (GPs), and mammography by radiologists and radiology technicians. Mammography quality control comprises examination and adjustment of mammography machines before starting screening, quality control of mammography films, and evaluation of mammography reading according to international standards. CBE quality control is done by breast surgeons who periodically visit health centers to evaluate GP's practice of CBE; agreement between breast surgeons and GP's CBE results is monitored. In the control group, women who would be eligible for screening if they had been in the intervention group are given general information about breast cancer but are not offered screening.

After the enrollment of approximately 12,000 women (about 6000 per branch), 88.9% and 99.8% in the opportunistic screening branch who were offered screening had a mammogram and a CBE, respectively, compared to 11.7% and 5% of the control women. Preliminary results show a three-fold greater rate of detection in the screened group than in the control group (15 and 5 cases, respectively), and a higher proportion of cases at an early stage at diagnosis (13/15=86.6% vs. 3/5=60%). Furthermore, the enrollment rate (2.9 patients per center per day) does not over-burden the GPs or other clinic staff. When the trial is completed, it will be possible to compare the stage of disease at diagnosis in the women who are screened vs. the women given information on breast cancer in the control group. This is an analysis analogous to an on protocol analysis in a clinical trial. It will also be possible to compare the stage at diagnosis in all of the breast cancers that occur in the populations served by the clinics in which this trial is conducted. This is analogous to an analysis on intent to treat in a clinical trial, and will provide a measure of the impact of the screening program in the population of women served by the clinics that participated in the trial.

■ SUMMARY

In response to an increasing burden of breast cancer in LMICs, due to an increase in incidence rates and the growth and aging of their populations, programs are being advocated, initiated or expanded to provide early detection, diagnostic, and treatment services. Early detection efforts should only be initiated if adequate diagnostic and treatment facilities are available. In countries in which women with breast cancer typically present with advanced tumors, programs to promote earlier treatment of symptomatic disease may be the most appropriate initial activities. Mammography, clinical breast examination (CBE), and breast self-examination (BSE) are methods available for screening for inapparent disease. Only mammography has been shown in randomized trials to reduce mortality from breast cancer, but its use in some LMICs is precluded by lack of resources. Evidence for the efficacy of CBE is insufficient, and two randomized trials have not shown teaching BSE to reduce deaths from breasts cancer, but studies of these two methods have been conducted largely in populations in which women typically present with small tumors. They may be more efficacious in LMICs in which women more often present with larger, more advanced tumors. Evidence-based guidelines for the provision of screening, diagnostic and treatment services commensurate with varying levels of available resources have been developed, and their use should be promulgated. All programs for the early detection of breast cancer should be conducted in such a manner that they can be evaluated to determine whether down-staging of disease at diagnosis has been achieved, and to assess the level of coverage in the population.

■ REFERENCES

1. Jemal A, Siegel R, Ward E, Hao Y, Xu J, Thun MJ. Cancer statistics, 2009. *CA Cancer J Clin.* 2009; 59(4):225–249.
2. Kalager M, Zelen M, Langmark F, Adami HO. Effect of screening mammography on breast-cancer mortality in Norway. *N Engl J Med.* 2010;363(13):1203–1210.

3. Weir HK, Thun MJ, Hankey BF, et al. Annual report to the nation on the status of cancer, 1975–2000, featuring the uses of surveillance data for cancer prevention and control. *J Natl Cancer Inst.* 2003; 95(17):1276–1299.

4. Chu KC, Smart CR, Tarone RE. Analysis of breast cancer mortality and stage distribution by age for the health insurance plan clinical trial. *J Natl Cancer Inst.* 1988;80(14):1125–1132.

5. Perloff M, Lesnick GJ, Korzun A, et al. Combination chemotherapy with mastectomy or radiotherapy for stage III breast carcinoma: A cancer and leukemia group B study. *J Clin Oncol.* 1988;6(2):261–269.

6. Clarke M. Meta-analyses of adjuvant therapies for women with early breast cancer: The early breast cancer trialists' collaborative group overview. *Ann Oncol.* 2006;17 Suppl 10:x59–x62.

7. Ferlay J, Bray F, Pisani P, Parkin DM. GLOBOCAN 2002: Cancer incidence, mortality and prevalence worldwide. IARC CancerBase no. 5. version 2.0. 2004.

8. Parkin DM, Fernandez LM. Use of statistics to assess the global burden of breast cancer. *Breast J.* 2006;12 Suppl 1:S70–S80.

9. Porter P. "Westernizing" women's risks? Breast cancer in lower-income countries. *N Engl J Med.* 2008;358(3):213–216.

10. Hisham AN, Yip CH. Spectrum of breast cancer in Malaysian women: Overview. *World J Surg.* 2003;27(8):921–923.

11. Chopra R. The Indian scene. *J Clin Oncol.* 2001;19(18 Suppl):106S–111S.

12. Sant M, Allemani C, Berrino F, et al. Breast carcinoma survival in Europe and the United States. *Cancer.* 2004;100(4):715–722.

13. Screening for breast cancer. In: Boyle P, Levin B, eds. *World cancer report. 2008.* Lyon: IARC Press; 2008:296–301.

14. US Preventive Services Task Force. Screening for breast cancer: U.S. preventive services task force recommendation statement. *Ann Intern Med.* 2009;151(10):716–726, W-236.

15. Tabar L, Fagerberg G, Chen HH, et al. Efficacy of breast cancer screening by age. New results from the Swedish two-county trial. *Cancer.* 1995;75(10):2507–2517.

16. Kanemura S, Tsuji I, Ohuchi N, et al. A case control study on the effectiveness of breast cancer screening by clinical breast examination in Japan. *Jpn J Cancer Res.* 1999;90(6):607–613.

17. Kuroishi T, Hirose K, Suzuki T, Tominaga S. Effectiveness of mass screening for breast cancer in Japan. *Breast Cancer.* 2000;7(1):1–8.

18. Pisani P, Parkin DM, Ngelangel C, et al. Outcome of screening by clinical examination of the breast in a trial in the Philippines. *Int J Cancer.* 2006;118(1):149–154.

19. Mittra I, Mishra GA, Singh S, et al. A cluster randomized, controlled trial of breast and cervix cancer screening in Mumbai, India: Methodology and interim results after three rounds of screening. *Int J Cancer.* 2010;126(4):976–984.

20. Semiglazov VF, Moiseyenko VM, Manikhas AG, et al. Role of breast self-examination in early detection of breast cancer: Russia/WHO prospective randomized trial in St. Petersburg. *Cancer Strategy.* 1999;1:145–151.

21. Thomas DB, Gao DL, Ray RM, et al. Randomized trial of breast self-examination in Shanghai: Final results. *J Natl Cancer Inst.* 2002;94(19):1445–1457.

22. Humphrey LL, Helfand M, Chan BK, Woolf SH. Breast cancer screening: A summary of the evidence for the U.S. preventive services task force. *Ann Intern Med.* 2002;137(5 Part 1):347–360.

23. Freedman LS, National Cancer Institute (U.S.), Middle East Cancer Consortium. Cancer incidence in four member countries (Cyprus, Egypt, Israel, and Jordan) of the Middle East cancer consortium (MECC) compared with US SEER. . 2006:1 online resource (http://seer.cancer.gov/publications/mecc/mecc_monograph.pdf).

24. Wong IO, Cowling BJ, Schooling CM, Leung GM. Age-period-cohort projections of breast cancer incidence in a rapidly transitioning Chinese population. *Int J Cancer.* 2007;121(7):1556–1563.

25. Chia KS, Reilly M, Tan CS, et al. Profound changes in breast cancer incidence may reflect changes into a westernized lifestyle: A comparative population-based study in Singapore and Sweden. *Int J Cancer.* 2005;113(2):302–306.

26. Yip C, Smith RA, Anderson BO, et al. Guideline implementation for breast healthcare in low—and middle—income countries. *Cancer.* 2008;113(S8):2244.

27. Smith RA. Risk-based screening for breast cancer. is there a practical strategy? *Seminars in Breast Disease.* 1999;2:280–291.

28. McTiernan A, Porter P, Potter JD. Breast cancer prevention in countries with diverse resources. *Cancer.* 2008;113(8 Suppl):2325–2330.

29. National Academy Press (U.S.), Institute of Medicine (U.S.). *Crossing the quality chasm a new health system for the 21st century.* Washington, D.C.: National Academy Press; 2001.

30. IOM committee calls for complete revamping of health care system to achieve better quality. *Qual Lett Healthc Lead.* 2001;13(3):14–15.

31. Rubenstein LV, Pugh J. Strategies for promoting organizational and practice change by advancing implementation research. *J Gen Intern Med.* 2006;21 Suppl 2:S58–S64.

32. Carlson RW, Allred DC, Anderson BO, et al. Breast cancer. Clinical practice guidelines in oncology. *J Natl Compr Canc Netw.* 2009;7(2):122–192.

33. Morrow M, Strom EA, Bassett LW, et al. Standard for breast conservation therapy in the management of invasive breast carcinoma. *CA Cancer J Clin.* 2002;52(5):277–300.

34. Smith RA. Breast cancer screening among women younger than age 50: A current assessment of the issues. *CA Cancer J Clin.* 2000;50(5):312–336.

35. Abrams JS. Adjuvant therapy for breast cancer—results from the USA consensus conference. *Breast Cancer.* 2001;8(4):298–304.

36. World Health Organization (WHO). Executive summary of the national cancer control programmes: Policies and managerial guidelines. Geneva: WHO2002.

37. Anderson BO, Braun S, Carlson RW, et al. Overview of breast health care guidelines for countries with limited resources. *Breast J.* 2003;9 Suppl 2:S42–S50.

38. Anderson BO, Shyyan R, Eniu A, et al. Breast cancer in limited-resource countries: An overview of the breast health global initiative 2005 guidelines. *Breast J.* 2006;12 Suppl 1:S3–S15.

39. Anderson BO, Yip CH, Smith RA, et al. Guideline implementation for breast healthcare in low-income and middle-income countries: Overview of the breast health global initiative global summit 2007. *Cancer.* 2008;113(8 Suppl):2221–2243.

40. Anderson BO, Cazap E, El Saghir NS, et al. Optimisation of breast cancer management in low-resource and middle-resource countries: Executive summary of the breast health global initiative consensus, 2010. *Lancet Oncol.* 2011;12(4):387–398.

41. Winn RJ, Botnick WZ. The NCCN guideline program: A conceptual framework. *Oncology (Williston Park).* 1997;11(11A):25–32.

42. Summary. In: Institute of Medicine (U.S.)., Sloan FA, Gelband H, eds. *Cancer control opportunities in low- and middle-income countries.* Washington, DC: National Academies Press; 2007:1–16.

43. Shyyan R, Sener SF, Anderson BO, et al. Guideline implementation for breast healthcare in low- and middle-income countries: Diagnosis resource allocation. *Cancer.* 2008;113(8 Suppl):2257–2268.

44. Eniu A, Carlson RW, El Saghir NS, et al. Guideline implementation for breast healthcare in low- and middle-income countries: Treatment resource allocation. *Cancer.* 2008;113(8 Suppl):2269–2281.

45. Poon D, Anderson BO, Chen LT, et al. Management of hepatocellular carcinoma in Asia: Consensus statement from the Asian oncology summit 2009. *Lancet Oncol.* 2009;10(11):1111–1118.

46. Soo RA, Anderson BO, Cho BC, et al. First-line systemic treatment of advanced stage non-small-cell lung cancer in Asia: Consensus statement from the Asian oncology summit 2009. *Lancet Oncol.* 2009;10(11):1102–1110.

47. Tangjitgamol S, Anderson BO, See HT, et al. Management of endometrial cancer in Asia: Consensus statement from the Asian oncology summit 2009. *Lancet Oncol.* 2009;10(11):1119–1127.

48. Wee JT, Anderson BO, Corry J, et al. Management of the neck after chemoradiotherapy for head and neck cancers in Asia: Consensus statement from the Asian oncology summit 2009. *Lancet Oncol.* 2009;10(11):1086–1092.

49. Wong NS, Anderson BO, Khoo KS, et al. Management of HER2-positive breast cancer in Asia: Consensus statement from the Asian oncology summit 2009. *The lancet oncology*. 2009;10(11):1077.

50. Curado MP, International Agency for Research on Cancer. International Association of Cancer Registries. *Cancer incidence in five continents, volume IX.* Lyon :Geneva: International Agency for Research on Cancer; Distributed by WHO Press, World Health Organization; 2008:lx, 837 p.

51. Azaiza F, Cohen M, Awad M, Daoud F. Factors associated with low screening for breast cancer in the Palestinian authority: Relations of availability, environmental barriers, and cancer-related fatalism. *Cancer*. 2010;116(19):4646–4655.

52. Ashbury FD, Cameron C, Mercer SL, Fitch M, Nielsen E. One-on-one peer support and quality of life for breast cancer patients. *Patient Educ Couns*. 1998;35(2):89–100.

53. Visco F. The national breast cancer coalition: Setting the standard for advocate collaboration in clinical trials. *Cancer Treat Res*. 2007;132:143–156.

54. Schmidt C. Komen/ASCO program aims to swell ranks of minority oncologists. *J Natl Cancer Inst*. 2009;101(4):224.

55. McCannon CJ, Berwick DM, Massoud MR. The science of large-scale change in global health. *JAMA*. 2007;298(16):1937–1939.

56. Devi BC, Tang TS, Corbex M. Reducing by half the percentage of late-stage presentation for breast and cervix cancer over 4 years: A pilot study of clinical downstaging in Sarawak, Malaysia. *Ann Oncol*. 2007;18(7):1172–1176.

57. Instituto Nacional de Cancerología (INC). Recomendaciones para la tamización y la detección temprana del cáncer de mama en Colombia. Bogotá: INC. 2006.

58. Murillo R, Diaz S, Sanchez O, et al. Pilot implementation of breast cancer early detection programs in Colombia. *Breast Care (Basel)*. 2008;3(1):29–32.

59. Harford JB, Otero IV, Anderson BO, et al. Problem solving for breast health care delivery in low and middle resource countries (LMCs): Consensus statement from the breast health global initiative. *Breast*. 2011;20 Suppl 2:S20–S29.

5

Future Directions and Recommendations

CHAPTER 22

EMERGING OPPORTUNITIES AND CHALLENGES

AMR S. SOLIMAN, DAVID SCHOTTENFELD, PAOLO BOFFETTA

In 2008, in a global population of 6.8 billion, the WHO estimated that there were 12.7 million incident cancer cases and 7.6 million cancer deaths. Of approximately a total of 59 million global deaths in 2008, 31% were attributed to cardiovascular diseases, and 12–13% to cancers in all sites. Approximately, 64% of cancer deaths and 56% of cancer cases were registered in low-and middle-income countries (LMICs) that comprised at least 80% of the world's population. By 2020, the projected global cancer mortality will exceed 10 million cancer deaths.[1,2] The burden of cancer in LMICs is projected to increase because of increasing urbanization and expansion of the population at risk, in conjunction with increasing prevalence of major risk factors, such as use of various forms of tobacco and alcohol consumption, obesity and/or micro-and macronutrient deficiencies that are accompanied by lipid and immune dysfunction, exposures to oncogenic infectious agents, and to occupational and environmental chemical and physical carcinogenic agents.[3]

When compared with industrialized countries, LMICs experienced a higher proportion of uterine cervical, stomach, liver, oral cavity and pharyngeal, esophageal, and HIV-associated cancers. Lung cancer and breast cancer were leading causes of mortality in both LMICs and industrialized countries. More than half of global breast cancer deaths were registered in LMICs. While incidence rates in men and women for all cancers combined in economically developed countries were nearly twice the rates in economically developing countries, after allowing for differences in age distribution, cancer mortality rates in developed countries were only 21% higher in men, and 2% higher in women. The proportion of incident cancers diagnosed in LMICs that were attributed to infectious agents was estimated to vary from 20% to 30%, in contrast to that of ≤5% to 10% in the USA and developed countries.[4,5] Of the 12.7 million new cancer cases that were diagnosed worldwide in 2008, about 2 million were attributable to infectious agents, of which 1.6 million (80%) were diagnosed in LMICs.[6]

BURDEN OF CANCER IN DEVELOPING COUNTRIES

LMICs are constrained by limited budgetary resources and the availability of trained health professionals for planning and implementing comprehensive cancer control programs.[7]

Cancer control interventions are designed to alleviate the burden of cancer mortality, incidence, and disability in a population. Ideally the control of the global burden of cancer will be achieved by integrating (1) population-based primary preventive practices (e.g., controlling tobacco and alcohol consumption, obesity, physical inactivity, and the prevalence of persistent and transmissible cancer-causing infectious agents), (2) facilitating access to effective cancer screening examinations (e.g., HPV and cervical cancer, breast and colorectal cancer), (3) increasing the availability of cost-effective programs in cancer curative therapy, palliation, and rehabilitation and their administration by trained health professionals, and (4) active governmental regulation of hazardous levels of occupational and environmental carcinogenic chemicals and ionizing radiation. Governmental regulatory actions may also facilitate the implementation of preventive interventions that serve to constrain adverse lifestyle behavioral practices, such as tobacco smoking.

Cancer surveillance may be defined as the systematic and continuous collection, analysis, and interpretation of cancer incidence data in a defined population or geographic region. Cancer registration that is either population- or hospital-based in LMICs, although generally recognized as vital for cancer control programs, has been, in general, assigned a low priority in resource allocation. Global cancer incidence data have been published since 1962 at regular intervals by the International Union Contra Cancer (UICC), and subsequently by the WHO International Agency for Research on Cancer (IARC). The ninth volume of *Cancer Incidence in Five Continents* provided comparable data from 225 registries in 60 countries covering the period, 1998–2002. The statistics for 2008 were based on GLOBOCAN 2008 provided by IARC.[8] Country-specific incidence and mortality rates were age-standardized (per 100,000 person-years) using the World Standard Population. Cancer-specific cumulative risks of developing or dying from cancer before the age of 75 years were calculated and expressed as a percentage. For example, age-standardized cancer mortality, all causes, in the LMICs for men was 119.3, and for women, 85.4 per 100,000; cumulative risks of developing cancer from birth to age 74 were 12.7% in men and 9.0% in women.

Cancers of the lung, stomach, breast, liver, head and neck, esophagus, large intestine, and lymphopoietic and hematopoietic neoplasms accounted for nearly four-fifths of all cancers in the LMICs. Thus, cancer control measures directed to these cancer sites will have maximum impact on the cancer burden in these countries. The high burden of stomach, liver, and uterine cervix cancers was related to the lack of basic preventive health care and screening services, and the lack of a well-developed public health infrastructure for the control of cancer-causing infectious agents. The high burden of squamous-cell esophageal cancer was likely due to dietary deficiencies, use of tobacco, and the consumption of traditional beverages at extremely high temperatures. The incidence rates of lung, breast and large intestine cancers were increasing due to increasing "westernization" of lifestyles, longer life expectancy, and globalization of markets for tobacco. These cancers will present a heavy future burden unless prompt control measures are implemented. Cancer control measures and research priorities that will target these cancer sites are listed in Table 1.With the exception of the lymphohematopoietic neoplasms, all cancers with high incidence in low- and medium-income countries are amenable to primary and secondary preventive interventions.

A section of the monograph is devoted to curriculum and training requirements in cancer epidemiology and preventive oncology for graduate students who wish to pursue etiologic research studies and program evaluation research in developing countries. The emphasis is on reviewing illustrative projects that demonstrate methodologic principles, multidisciplinary perspectives, and instructive examples of collaborative field studies. The setting and context for didactic instruction and training mentoring may be based at

TABLE 1 Summary of cancer prevention and early detection interventions that target major cancer sites in low- and middle-income countries

CANCER SITE	CANCER CONTROL INTERVENTIONS		RESEARCH PRIORITY
	PREVENTION	EARLY DETECTION	
Head and neck	+++ Tobacco control; reduced alcohol consumption; increased consumption of vegetables and fruits	+++ Awareness, early clinical diagnosis; screening by visual inspection	Implementation and evaluation of tobacco/alcohol control measures and population-based visual screening for oral cancer Evaluation of clinical down-staging Formulation of locally feasible, cost-effective management protocols and evaluating their adherence and effectiveness
Esophagus	+++ Tobacco control; reduced alcohol use; healthy diet	+	Evaluation of the effectiveness of tobacco/alcohol control measures and promotion of healthy eating practices. Evaluation of chemoprevention
Stomach	+++ Prevention and eradication of *H. pylori* infection; healthy diet; tobacco control; improved living conditions	+ Early clinical diagnosis	Evaluation of the efficacy and cost-effectiveness of screening individuals for infection with *H. pylori* and then eradicating *H. pylori* with antibiotic therapy Vaccination to prevent *H. pylori* infection
Large bowel	++ Control of overweight/obesity, promotion of healthy diet and physical activity	+++ Awareness; early clinical diagnosis; screening by fecal occult blood test; endoscopy	Evaluation of efficacy and cost-effectiveness of colorectal cancer screening Evaluation of clinical down-staging Formulation of locally feasible, cost-effective management protocols and evaluating their adherence and effectiveness
Liver	+++ Hepatitis B (HBV) vaccination in infancy Prevention of exposure to liver flukes Reduced fungal contamination of stored grains Blood supply and injection safety measures to prevent exposure to hepatitis C virus (HCV) Reduced alcohol use Tobacco control	+	Evaluation of long-term protection from HBV vaccination; need for booster doses Evaluation of methods to cure chronic HBV and HCV infection

(continued)

TABLE 1 (Continued)

CANCER SITE	CANCER CONTROL INTERVENTIONS		RESEARCH PRIORITY
	PREVENTION	EARLY DETECTION	
Lung	+++ Tobacco control Dietary improvements Regulation of automobile exhaust and industrial combustion products Ventilation and improved low-technology heating and cooking Workplace regulation and controls	+	Implementation and evaluation of primary prevention measures
Breast	+ Control of obesity; promotion of physical activity; reduced alcohol use	+++ Breast awareness; early clinical diagnosis	Evaluation of chemoprevention Evaluation of breast awareness and physical examination Evaluation of clinical down-staging Formulation of locally feasible, cost-effective management protocols and evaluating their adherence and effectiveness
Uterine cervix	+++ HPV vaccination; tobacco control	+++ Awareness; early clinical diagnosis; screening with cytology, visual inspection with acetic acid (VIA) or HPV testing	Implementation and evaluation of HPV vaccination and alternative methods of screening. Integration of HPV vaccine and screening programs Effectiveness of screening with fast HPV testing followed by VIA triage and treatment in preventing cervical cancer Evaluation of clinical down-staging Formulation of locally feasible, cost-effective management protocols and evaluating their adherence and effectiveness
Lymphohematopoietic neoplasms	+ Workplace regulation and controls; improved medical practices; tobacco control	++	Evaluation affordable forms of chemotherapy regimes in low-resource settings Formulation of locally feasible, cost-effective management protocols and evaluating their adherence and effectiveness

schools of public health, schools of medicine, comprehensive or designated cancer centers, or government-sponsored research institutions. These may function independently or collaboratively.

HIV/AIDS

By 2007, the Joint United Nations Program on HIV/AIDS (UNAIDS) estimated the global prevalence of HIV-1 infection to be 33 million. HIV prevalence proportions ranged from less than 0.5% in most developed countries to an upper limit of 25% to 30% in Central and Southern Africa. UNAIDS estimation of national HIV incidence relied on indirect estimates based on trends in serial prevalence surveys from antenatal clinics and population subgroups. The estimates reflected assumptions about the stability of survival rates and migration patterns.[9,10] In 2007, UNAIDS assumed that the median survival in the infected population increased from 9 years to 11 years, which resulted in a reduction in the estimated global incidence from 4.1 million in 2006 to 2.5 million in 2007. UNAIDS estimated that 2.5 million deaths in LMICs were averted since 1995 since the introduction of anti-retroviral therapy. Refinements in future estimates will depend on the enhanced specificity and availability of immunoassays for diagnosing new infections.

Higher risks were evident in migratory and malnourished populations. HIV-1 infection may be transmitted by anal or vaginal intercourse, transfusion of infected blood or sharing of infected injection equipment among intravenous drug users, and transmission from HIV-infected mother to infant. Before the introduction of highly active anti-retroviral therapy (HAART), a number of cancers were identified as AIDS-defining cancers (ADCs). These included Kaposi sarcoma; non-Hodgkin lymphoma, most commonly of B-cell phenotype, that included entities classified as primary central nervous system lymphoma, large-cell immunoblastic lymphoma, and Burkitt lymphoma; and cancer of the uterine cervix. During the period following the introduction of HAART, the relative risks of ADCs changed substantially. In addition, cancers that were not designated as ADCs were reported in patients with HIV. The non-ADCs included Hodgkin lymphoma, anogenital cancers, keratinocytic (non-melanoma) skin cancer, squamous cell carcinoma of the conjunctiva, and hepatocellular carcinoma.[11,12] HIV. infection is indirectly carcinogenic as a result of severe lymphocyte depletion and impaired immune function. The pattern of neoplastic sequellae results from increased expression of oncogenic viruses, namely Kaposi sarcoma herpes virus, Epstein-Barr virus, human papillomaviruses, hepatitis B and C viruses, or interactions with environmental agents such as ultraviolet radiation and tobacco.

CANCER IN AFRICA

Cancer mortality and incidence patterns varied substantially in Africa when analyzed by anatomic site, pathology, demographic characteristics, and the prevalence of causal agents. For example, for the year 2000, in West Africa, the age-standardized cancer incidence rate per 100,000 in men was 81.2, and in women, 94.1. Liver cancer was the predominant cancer in men, and cancer of the uterine cervix in women. In contrast to West Africa, the age-standardized cancer incidence in Southern Africa was 2.7 times higher in men, and 1.6 times higher in women. In addition to liver and uterine cervix cancers, the residents in Southern Africa exhibited higher rates of lung and esophageal cancers, and HIV infection.

Africa is a heterogeneous and genetically diverse continent with an estimated population of 965 million. About 41% of the population is under the age of 15 years. The major causes of death include infant and maternal mortality, and the communicable diseases.

Thus the provision of services for cancer prevention and cancer treatment has received a lower priority by governmental agencies. According to the WHO, the 2008 cancer burden in Africa was estimated to be 681,000 incident cases, and 512,000 deaths. The projected increase by the year 2030 would be 1.6 million cases and 1.2 million deaths per year.[13] The most common cancers in men were Kaposi sarcoma, non-Hodgkin lymphoma, cancers of the liver, esophagus, prostate, and urinary bladder. In women, the most common cancers were uterine cervix, breast, Kaposi sarcoma, liver, and non-Hodgkin lymphoma.[14]

■ CANCER IN INDIA AND CHINA

Asian Indians (AIs) represented one-sixth of the world`s population, exceeding one billion, in addition to 20 million living outside of India. More than 70% of AIs lived in rural areas that tended to be under-enumerated by population cancer registries. However, cancer incidence patterns among Indian males have underscored the relative significance, when compared with European and North American white males, of cancers of the oral cavity and pharynx, esophagus, stomach, lung and larynx. Among Indian females, the most prominent cancers were of the uterine cervix, breast, oral cavity and pharynx, esophagus, and stomach.[15] The Singapore Cancer Registry has described for Indian and Pakistani males, elevated risks for cancers of the stomach, oral cavity and pharynx, esophagus, and lung. Among females, cancers of the uterine cervix, breast, and oral cavity and pharynx ranked among the most common. The prominence of upper digestive tract cancers in AIs may be attributed to the common use of multiple tobacco products. Such products included chewing tobacco, the common practice of chewing betel quid, with or without tobacco, and smoking bidi cigarette tobacco. Bidis are hand-rolled cigarettes, where the tobacco, often fruit flavored, is wrapped in temburni leaf.

Between 2010 and 2030, annual incident cancer cases are estimated to increase in the LMICs from 7.5 to 12.9 million. Approximately 1.9 million of the additional cancer cases will be registered in China, 0.7 million in India, 1.6 million in the rest of Asia, 0.6 million in Africa, and 0.7 million in Latin America and the Caribbean.[16] The highest incidence rates for stomach cancer were in Eastern Asia, South America and Eastern Europe. Stomach cancer incidence rates have been decreasing in most parts of the world, in part due to reductions in prevalence of chronic cytopathogenic Helicobacter pylori infection, and the increasing availability of fresh fruits and vegetables, improving hygienic conditions and their association with decreasing fecal-oral transmission of the bacteria, and decreased reliance on salted, processed, and preserved foods.

Hepatocellular carcinoma (HCC) in men was the fifth most frequently diagnosed cancer worldwide, and the second most common cause of cancer mortality. In women, HCC was the seventh most commonly diagnosed cancer worldwide, and the sixth leading cause of cancer mortality. In 2008, an estimated 696,000 HCC deaths occurred worldwide, with 50% of deaths estimated to have occurred in China. The highest rates were registered in East and Southeast Asia, and in sub-Saharan and Western Africa. The elevated HCC rates largely reflected the prevalence of chronic hepatitis B virus (HBV) infection, where over 8% of the population was chronically infected. Chronic HBV infection accounted for about 60% of liver cancer incidence in developing countries, compared with chronic infection with hepatitis C virus (HCV), which accounted for about 33%[1]. The magnitude of the relative risk of HCC due to chronic HBV infection was correlated with HBV viral load and pathologic indicators of cirrhosis, and amplified by co-infections with HCV, HIV, and Delta hepatitis virus, or interactive with exposures to ethanol, tobacco, and obesity.[17]

FUTURE CHALLENGES IN CANCER CONTROL

Future cancer trends in the LMICs will reflect global shifts in population distributions of lifestyle practices, such as tobacco exposure (i.e., smoking, environmental and smokeless forms of tobacco), alcohol consumption, excess body weight and physical inactivity, malnutrition and the control of cancer-causing infectious agents and of sources of environmental chemical pollution Assessment of global trends assumes an increasing commitment to developing more complete and accurate cancer surveillance registries that are maintained by trained health professionals with the collaboration and support of medical and public health organizations. The sophistication of a committed public health infrastructure will enable the implementation of effective interventions in cancer treatment and palliation, cancer screening (e.g., breast, uterine cervical, colorectal and oral cavity cancers), immunization (i.e., HPV vaccine against types 16 and 18 viruses and cervical cancer, HBV and hepatocellular carcinoma), and treatment of Helicobacter pylori for stomach cancer, and treatment and prevention of transmission of HIV.

Epidemiologic methods applied in populations offer the basic tools for estimating the current and future burden of disease, and for assessing the effectiveness of cancer prevention and control measures. Investing in the training of epidemiologists, establishing the requisite infrastructure in Ministries of Health, in conjunction with regional health authorities and major medical centers, and participating in inter-regional and international surveillance and research programs, comprise the essential components of an integrated and cost-effective program. In the context of other chronic disease control programs, there are the opportunities in sharing resources, research methodologies and skilled personnel that unify concerns with the consequences of tobacco, alcohol, obesity, physical inactivity, imprudent dietary practices, and the exposures to toxic environmental physical, chemical, and biologic agents.

REFERENCES

1. Jemal A, Bray F, Center MM, Ferlay J, Ward E, Forman D. Global cancer statistics. *CA Cancer J Clin.* 2011;61(2):69–90.
2. Jemal A, Center MM, DeSantis C, Ward EM. Global patterns of cancer incidence and mortality rates and trends. *Cancer Epidemiol Biomarkers Prev.* 2010;19(8):1893–1907.
3. Vineis P, Xun W. The emerging epidemic of environmental cancers in developing countries. *Ann Oncol.* 2009;20(2):205–212.
4. Parkin DM. The global health burden of infection-associated cancers in the year 2002. *Int J Cancer.* 2006;118(12):3030–3044.
5. Kanavos P. The rising burden of cancer in the developing world. *Ann Oncol.* 2006;17 Suppl 8: viii15–viii23.
6. de Martel C, Ferlay J, Franceschi S, et al. Global burden of cancers attributable to infections in 2008: A review and synthetic analysis. *Lancet Oncol.* 2012;13(6):607–615.
7. Valsecchi MG, Steliarova-Foucher E. Cancer registration in developing countries: Luxury or necessity? *Lancet Oncol.* 2008;9(2):159–167.
8. Ferlay J, Shin HR, Bray F, Forman D, Mathers C, Parkin DM. GLOBOCAN 2008 v1.2, cancer incidence and mortality worldwide: IARC CancerBase no. 10 [internet]. Lyon, France: International Agency for Research on Cancer2010. Available from: http://globocan.iarc.fr, accessed 07/02/2012.
9. Brookmeyer R. Measuring the HIV/AIDS epidemic: Approaches and challenges. *Epidemiol Rev.* 2010;32(1):26–37.
10. Walker N, Grassly NC, Garnett GP, Stanecki KA, Ghys PD. Estimating the global burden of HIV/AIDS: What do we really know about the HIV pandemic? *Lancet.* 2004;363(9427):2180–2185.
11. Casper C. The increasing burden of HIV-associated malignancies in resource-limited regions. *Annu Rev Med.* 2011;62:157–170.

12. Grulich AE, van Leeuwen MT, Falster MO, Vajdic CM. Incidence of cancers in people with HIV/AIDS compared with immunosuppressed transplant recipients: A meta-analysis. *Lancet.* 2007;370(9581): 59–67.

13. Lingwood RJ, Boyle P, Milburn A, et al. The challenge of cancer control in Africa. *Nat Rev Cancer.* 2008; 8(5):398–403.

14. Parkin DM, Sitas F, Chirenje M, Stein L, Abratt R, Wabinga H. Part I: Cancer in indigenous Africans— burden, distribution, and trends. *Lancet Oncol.* 2008;9(7):683–692.

15. Rastogi T, Devesa S, Mangtani P, et al. Cancer incidence rates among South Asians in four geographic regions: India, Singapore, UK and US. *Int J Epidemiol.* 2008;37(1):147–160.

16. Yang JD, Roberts LR. Hepatocellular carcinoma: A global view. *Nat Rev Gastroenterol Hepatol.* 2010;7(8):448–458.

17. El-Serag HB. Hepatocellular carcinoma. *N Engl J Med.* 2011;365(12):1118–1127.

INDEX

CPSIA information can be obtained
at www.ICGtesting.com
Printed in the USA
BVOW07s0019150816
458826BV00001B/2/P

9 780199 733507